New Directions
in Affective Disorders

Bernard Lerer   Samuel Gershon
Editors

New Directions
in Affective Disorders

With 51 Figures

Springer-Verlag
New York Berlin Heidelberg
London Paris Tokyo Hong Kong

BERNARD LERER, M.D.
Director of Research
Jerusalem Mental Health
  Center-Ezrath Nashim;
Associate Professor
Department of Psychiatry
Hebrew University
Jerusalem 91001
Israel

SAMUEL GERSHON, M.D.
Vice President for Research in the
  Medical and Health Care Division;
Associate Vice President for Research in
  the Health Sciences
University of Pittsburgh;
Professor of Psychiatry
Associate Research Director for
  Neurosciences
Department of Psychiatry
University of Pittsburgh School of
  Medicine
Pittsburgh, PA 15213
USA

Library of Congress Cataloging in Publication Data
New directions in affective disorders.
    ''This volume originated from the International
Conference on New Directions in Affective Disorders
held in Jerusalem in April 1987''—Intro.
    Includes index.
    1. Affective disorders—Congresses. I. Lerer,
Bernard. II. Gershon, Samuel. III. International
Conference on New Directions in Affective Disorders
(1987 : Jerusalem) [DNLM: 1. Affective Disorders—
congresses. WM 207 N532 1987]
RC537.N488 1989   616.85'27   88-35580

Printed on acid-free paper

Typeset by David E. Seham Associates Inc., Metuchen, New Jersey.
Printed and bound by R.R. Donnelley & Sons, Harrisonburg, Virginia.
Printed in the United States of America.

9 8 7 6 5 4 3 2 1

ISBN 0-387-96769-9 Springer-Verlag New York Berlin Heidelberg
ISBN 3-540-96769-9 Springer-Verlag Berlin Heidelberg New York

Introduction

This book is presented as a 1989 update on the task set by Robert Burton in his "Anatomy of Melancholy," published in 1621. Burton's treatise addressed questions regarding depression which are still highly relevant today: ". . . What is it, with all the kinds, causes, symptoms, prognostickes and several cures of it. . . ." These remain the core issues in affective disorders notwithstanding the remarkable progress that has been made in addressing them. *New Directions in Affective Disorders* sets out to provide an overview of what has been achieved with particular emphasis on developing trends and novel initiatives in both fundamental research and treatment. The overriding objective of the book is to integrate significant contributions from basic and clinical science into a comprehensive format which will be of value to both clinicians and researchers.

Intensive interest in affective illness is an inevitable consequence of the frequency with which these disorders occur. Depression is the most common psychiatric condition, affecting as many as 50% of people in Western countries at some time in their lives. National Institute of Mental Health Statistics estimate that 15% of adults between 18 and 74 years of age may be suffering from serious depressive disorders in any given year. Depression is a serious condition with a high mortality. A suicide rate of approximately 20,000 deaths per year as a result of this illness is almost certainly a conservative estimate. When morbidity as a result of manic and hypomanic states as well as of related conditions with a significant affective component is added, the magnitude of the public health problem posed by affective illness is strikingly apparent.

In 1621, Burton posed the question: ". . . How far the power of spirits and devils doth extend, and whether they can cause this, or any other disease, is a serious question and worthy to be considered. . . ." Etiology and pathogenesis are a central focus of the first two sections of this volume, which encompass the results of animal and human studies relevant to these issues. Neurotransmitter hypotheses have been a cornerstone of theorizing regarding the underlying causes of affective illness and this emphasis is reflected in the contributions to these sections. A move away from unitary transmitter hypotheses towards the interrelated involvement of different systems is inevitably acknowledged and the role of receptor and post-receptor mediated signal amplification processes is emphasized.

It is intriguing that in spite of their enormous clinical impact, the basic mechanisms underlying the therapeutic efficacy of antidepressant and mood stabilizing drugs are not definitively known. Contributions in the first two sections address this question and also consider the extent to which therapeutic mechanisms might be of relevance to our understanding of the underlying causes of the syndromes in which they are effective. Animal models of affective disorder are a classical component of research of this type. Recently developed paradigms are presented from the standpoint of pathogenesis and also emphasize a move away from retroactive modelling based on the actions of drugs shown to be clinically efficacious towards more novel approaches to clinical predictability.

Contributions on the neurobiology of affective disorder focus on the most productive strategies currently applied in biologically oriented clinical investigation. The recent genetic findings that have galvanized this area of research are comprehensively presented and the further application of molecular genetic techniques to the elucidation of single major loci responsible for the transmission of affective illness is considered. The search for biological markers characteristic of affective illness has harnessed a variety of technologically sophisticated methods, the results of which are presented in this section. Studies presented involve the use of peripheral blood cell markers, cerebrospinal fluid metabolites and the electroencephalogram. Chronobiological approaches are also discussed as well as the contribution of psychoneuroendocrinological strategies to our understanding of pathophysiology and the mechanism of drug action.

The "symptoms and prognostickes" of affective disorders referred to by Burton are addressed in the first clinical section of this volume, which focuses on populations specifically at risk. Affective disorders in childhood and adolescence, in the elderly, and in relation to reproductive cyclicity in women are the topics of separate sections. Factors specific to these populations demand that affective illness by approached within the context in which it is encountered and that treatments be appropriately tailored. In the case of children, the interrelationship between depression in parents and their offspring is a striking example. In elderly populations co-existing depression and cognitive impairment is a central issue as well as the association between depression, somatic illness, and excess mortality in late life.

Suicide is a highly significant risk in all populations affected by depression. The section dealing with this topic considers epidemiologic and genetic factors as well as specific aspects of suicidal behavior in children and adolescents. The role of neurotransmitter abnormalities in the pathogenesis in suicidal behavior is then addressed by studies of monoamine metabolites in suicidal individuals and postmortem neurochemical studies in the brains of completed suicides.

This book recognizes that the boundaries of affective disorder are not clearly defined and takes a broad position on this question. A number of syndromes are related to affective illness to a varying degree, have a significant affective component, or respond to antidepressant or mood stabilizing treatments. The nature of their relationship to affective illness is an important direction for future research. Contributions dealing with Anxiety Disorders, Posttraumatic Stress Disorder, Eating Disorders, and Schizoaffective Disorder are presented in the section dealing with specific and related affective syndromes.

The final section of this volume deals with new directions in treatment. It opens with a consideration of the interrelationship between classification and phomacotherapy. The revolutionary impact of antidepressant agents and lithium on the clinical management of affective illness has highlighted the clinical problem posed by the significant minority of individuals who do not respond to these conventional treatments. The use of anticonvulsant agents in the treatment of lithium-resistant bipolar patients represents a major advance and is therefore highlighted. A further section deals with treatment strategies for the management of resistant depression, recognizing the clinical difficulties posed by this group of patients. A section dealing with important aspects of the use of antidepressants in clinical practice is also included, focusing on the role of placebo response in depression, monitoring of plasma levels of antidepressants, and the potentially serious adverse effects of these agents. A section on the use of GABA-mimetic agents follows and encompasses the theoretical background to this approach as well as the outcome of clinical trials. Electroconvulsive therapy is also discussed in this section. The contributions stress the increasingly rigorous approach to technical issues such as electrode placement, stimulus intensity, and wave form that now characterizes ECT practice as well as novel suggestions regarding pharmacological potentiation of ECT seizures. Contributions on the use of psychotherapy in the treatment of depression conclude this section.

This book originated from the International Conference on New Directions in Affective Disorders held in Jerusalem in April 1987 but is not limited to material presented at that meeting. The editors express their thanks to the multiple contributors for their painstaking efforts. We recognize that many fundamental questions posed by Burton in 1621 regarding the anatomy of melancholia remain unanswered. We trust that the material presented in this volume will serve to stimulate further progress by pinpointing emergent trends while consolidating the close interaction between basic and clinical investigation that has characterized the major advances already achieved.

Jerusalem, Israel   Bernard Lerer
Pittsburgh, Pennsylvania, USA   Samuel Gershon

Contents

I PATHOGENESIS OF AFFECTIVE DISORDERS AND BASIC MECHANISMS OF DRUG ACTION

I.A. ANIMAL MODELS AND ANTIDEPRESSANT PREDICTABILITY

II NEUROBIOLOGY OF AFFECTIVE DISORDERS

II.A. NEW GENETIC FINDINGS

III AFFECTIVE DISORDERS IN POPULATIONS AT RISK

III.A. AFFECTIVE DISORDERS AND SUICIDE

III.B. AFFECTIVE DISORDERS DURING CHILDHOOD AND ADOLESCENCE

V NEW DIRECTIONS IN TREATMENT

V.A. CLASSIFICATION AND PHARMACOTHERAPY

V.B. ANTICONVULSANTS IN AFFECTIVE DISORDER

Contributors

LUIGI F. AGNATI, M.D., Professor of Human Physiology, University of Modena, Modena, Italy

HANS ÅGREN, M.D., PH.D., Associate Professor, Department of Psychiatry, University Hospital, Uppsala, Sweden

C. ALBANO, M.D., Associate Professor, Department of Neurology, University of Genoa-Medical School, Genoa, Italy

JOSEF B. ALDENHOFF, M.D., Senior Lecturer, Department of Psychiatry, Johannes Gutenberg University, Mainz, Federal Republic of Germany

CLEONA R. ALLEN, B.A., Research Associate, Department of Psychiatry, University of Miami School of Medicine, Miami, Florida, USA

PETER ALLERUP, CAND. STAT., Assistant Professor, Department of Statistics, Danish Institute for Educational Research, Copenhagen, Denmark

ENRIQUE ALVAREZ, M.D., Psychiatrist, Department of Psychiatry, Hospital de Sant Pau (Medical School), Barcelona, Spain

CHARLES ANELLO, SC.D., Deputy Director, Office of Epidemiology and Biostatistics, Center for Drug Evaluation and Research, Food and Drug Administration, Department of Health and Human Services, Rockville, Maryland, USA

MARC ANSSEAU, M.D., PH.D., Assistant Hospital Specialist, Psychiatric Unit, University of Liège, Centre Hospitalier Universitaire, Domaine Universitaire du Sart Tilman, Liège, Belgium

ALAN APTER, M.D., Senior Lecturer in Psychiatry, University of Tel Aviv, Sackler School of Medicine, Tel Aviv, Israel; Geha Psychiatric Hospital, Petah Tikva, Israel

GREGORY ASNIS, M.D., Associate Professor of Psychiatry, Department of Psychiatry, Albert Einstein College of Medicine; Director, Outpatient Clinic, Montefiore Medical Center, Bronx, New York, USA

EYTAN BACHAR, PH.D., Senior Psychologist, Jerusalem Mental Health Center-Ezrath Nashim, Jerusalem, Israel

JAMES C. BALLENGER, M.D., Chairman and Professor, Department of Psychiatry and Behavioral Sciences, Medical University of South Carolina, Charleston, South Carolina, USA

T.A. BAN, M.D., Professor of Psychiatry, Department of Psychiatry, Vanderbilt University, Nashville, Tennessee, USA

WILLIAM A. BARKER, M.B., B.S., M.R.C.P., M.R.C.PSYCH., Consultant Psychiatrist, St. Mary's Hospital, Stannington, Morpeth, Northumberland, United Kingdom

MIRON BARON, M.D., Associate Professor, Department of Psychiatry, Columbia University College of Physicians and Surgeons; Director, Division of Psychogenetics, Department of Medical Genetics, New York State Psychiatric Institute, New York, New York, USA

FAOUZIA BAROUCHE, M.D., Department of Psychiatry, New York University School of Medicine, New York, New York, USA

GIUSEPPE BARTHOLINI, M.D., Professor and President Synthélabo Recherche (L.E.R.S.), Paris, France

PER BECH, M.D., Associate Professor, Department of Psychiatry, Frederiksborg General Hospital, Hillerød, Denmark

WOLFGANG BELLAIRE, M.D., Head Physician, University Hospital, Psychiatric Hospital, Hamburg, Federal Republic of Germany

R.H. BELMAKER, M.D., Hoffer-Vickar Professor of Psychiatry, Ben Gurion University School of Medicine, Beersheva, Israel

M. STROLIN BENEDETTI, PH.D., Department of Metabolism and Pharmacokinetics, Research and Development, Farmitalia Carlo Erba, Milan, Italy

JONATHAN BENJAMIN, M.D., Instructor, Department of Psychiatry, School of Medicine, Ben Gurion University, Beersheva, Israel

EDNA BEN-TZVI, B.A., Clinical Psychologist (Trainee), Ministry of Health, Jaffa, Israel

M. BERGER, M.D., Central Institute of Mental Health, Mannheim, Federal Republic of Germany

BIRGIT BERING, PH.D., Psychopharmacological Laboratory, Central Institute of Mental Health, Mannheim, Federal Republic of Germany

LEIF BERTILSSON, PH.D., Associate Professor, Department of Clinical Pharmacology, Huddinge University Hospital, Huddinge, Sweden

AVRAHAM BLEICH, M.D., Lieutenant Colonel, Director, Israel Defense Forces Central Psychiatric Clinic, Tel Hashomer, Israel

JEAN-PHILIPPE BOULENGER, M.D., Research Fellow, I.N.S.E.R.M., Caen, France

FRANCESCA BRAMBILLA, M.D., Professor, Director of the Psychoendocrine Center, Pini Psychiatric Hospital, Milan, Italy

PETER BRAUN, M.D., Eitanim Psychiatric Hospital, D.N. Shimshon, Israel

PETER BRÄUNIG, M.D., Nervenklinik, Psychiatry, University of Bonn, Bonn, Federal Republic of Germany

DIRK E. BREMER, M.D., Research Fellow, Department of Psychiatry, Max-Planck-Institute of Psychiatry, Munich, Federal Republic of Germany

PAUL K. BRIDGES, M.D., PH.D., F.R.C.PSYCH., Physician in Psychological Medicine and Senior Lecturer, Guy's Hospital and the United Medical and Dental Schools of Guy's and St. Thomas's Hospitals, University of London, London, United Kingdom

IAN F. BROCKINGTON, M.D., Professor of Psychiatry, University of Birmingham, Birmingham, United Kingdom

MARIEKE BROEKMAN, M.D., Resident, Bloemendaal Psychiatric Center, The Hague, The Netherlands

KIM BRØSEN, M.D., Assistant Professor of Clinical Pharmacology, Department of Clinical Pharmacology, Odense University, Odense, Denmark

GREGORY M. BROWN, M.D., PH.D., F.R.C.P.C., Professor, Departments of Biomedical Sciences and Psychiatry, McMaster University, Hamilton, Ontario, Canada

RICHARD P. BROWN, M.D., Assistant Professor of Psychiatry, Columbia University College of Physicians and Surgeons, New York, New York, USA

WALTER A. BROWN, M.D., Professor of Psychiatry and Human Behavior, Brown University, Providence, Rhode Island, USA

NICOLETTA BRUNELLO, PH.D., Assistant Professor, Center of Neuropharmacology, University of Milan, Milan, Italy

WILLY P. BURKARD, PH.D., Department of PF/CNS, F. Hoffman-La Roche & Co., Ltd., Basel, Switzerland

GRAHAM D. BURROWS, M.D., CH.B., B.SC., D.P.M., F.R.C.PSYCH., Department of Psychiatry, University of Melbourne, Parkville, Victoria, Australia

JACQUELINE BUTLER, B.SC., PH.D., Postdoctoral Research Fellow, Department of Pharmacology, University College, Galway, Republic of Ireland

AVRAHAM CALEV, PH.D., Principal Research Psychologist, Jerusalem Mental Health Center-Ezrath Nashim, Jerusalem, Israel

MAGDA CAMPBELL, M.D., Professor of Psychiatry; Director, Division of Child and Adolescent Psychiatry, Department of Psychiatry, New York University Medical Center, New York, New York, USA

MIGUEL CASAS, M.D., Head of the Psychopharmacology Section, Department of Psychiatry, Hospital de Sant Pau (Medical School), Barcelona, Spain

MARCO CATALANO, M.D., Assistant, University Psychiatry Clinic III, Institute of Biomedical Sciences, San Paolo University, Milan, Italy

S.M. CHANNABASAVANNA, M.D., Department of Psychiatry, National Institute of Mental Health and Neurosciences, Bangalore, India

BRUCE G. CHARLTON, M.B.B.S., Wellcome Clinical Research Fellow, MRC Neuroendocrinology Unit, Newcastle General Hospital, Newcastle upon Tyne, United Kingdom

DENNIS S. CHARNEY, M.D., Associate Professor, Department of Psychiatry, Yale University School of Medicine, New Haven, Connecticut, USA

STUART A. CHECKLEY, B.M., M.R.C.P., M.R.C.PSYCH., Consultant Psychiatry, Maudsley Hospital, London, United Kingdom

SHARON C. CHEETHAM, B.SC., M.SC., Department of Pharmacology and Clinical Pharmacology, St. George's Hospital Medical School, London, United Kingdom

LARS CLEMMESEN, M.D., Senior Resident, Department of Psychiatry, Frederiksborg General Hospital, Hillerød, Denmark

EMIL F. COCCARO, M.D., Medical Director of Specialty Clinic Programs, Psychiatry Service, Bronx Veterans Administration Medical Center, Bronx, New York, USA

C. EDWARD COFFEY, M.D., Assistant Professor, Departments of Psychiatry and Medicine (Neurology), Duke University Medical Center, Durham, North Carolina, USA

BRIAN L. COOK, D.O., Assistant Professor, Department of Psychiatry, University of Iowa, Iowa City, Iowa, USA

JOHN C. COOKSON, B.M., PH.D., M.R.C.P., F.R.C.PSYCH., Consultant Psychiatrist, The London Hospital (St. Clement's), London, United Kingdom

BRYAN CORRIDAN, M.A., M.B., B.CHIR., Senior House Officer, Department of Psychiatry, Charing Cross Hospital, London, United Kingdom

R. COUPEZ-LOPINOT, M.D., Head, Department of Clinical Research, Laboratoires d'Etudes et de Recherches Synthélabo (L.E.R.S.), Brussels, Belgium

M. RUFUS CROMPTON, M.D., PH.D., D.M.J., F.R.C.PATH., Department of Forensic Medicine, St. George's Hospital Medical School, London, United Kingdom

JACQUELINE A. CROSS, B.SC., Department of Pharmacology and Clinical Pharmacology, St. George's Hospital Medical School, London, United Kingdom

JOSEPH T. CUMMINS, PH.D., Veterans Administration Medical Center, Sepulveda, California, USA

GERALD CURZON, PH.D., D.SC., Professor of Neurochemistry, Institute of Neurology, London, United Kingdom

CAROLE Z. CZUDEK, B.SC., Department of Pathology, University of Nottingham Medical School, Queens Medical Center, Nottingham, United Kingdom

MOSÉ DA PRADA, M.D., Professor of Pharmacology, University of Milan, Milan, Italy

HAIM DASBERG, M.D., Director, Jerusalem Mental Health Center-Ezrath Nashim; Associate Professor, Department of Psychiatry, Hebrew University, Jerusalem, Israel

JOHN M. DAVIS, M.D., Professor, Department of Psychiatry, College of Medicine, University of Illinois at Chicago; Director of Research, Illinois State Psychiatric Institute, Chicago, Illinois, USA

KENNETH L. DAVIS, M.D., Chairman, Department of Psychiatry; Professor of Psychiatry and Pharmacology, Mt. Sinai School of Medicine, New York, New York, USA

WILLIAM REES DAVIS, PH.D., Research Scientist, Department of Psychiatry, New York State Psychiatric Institute, New York, New York, USA

PAOLA DELLA MAGGIORA, M.D., Medical Fellow, University Psychiatric Clinic III, Institute of Biomedical Sciences, San Paolo Hospital, Milan, Italy

KLAUS DEMISCH, M.D., Professor and Head, Psychiatric Hospital, Hanau City Hospital, Hanau, Federal Republic of Germany

DAVID DE WIED, M.D., PH.D., Professor of Pharmacology, Rudolf Magnus Institute for Pharmacology, Medical Faculty, University of Utrecht, Utrecht, The Netherlands

JUUL E. DE WILDE, M.D., Medical Director, St. Camillus Neuropsychiatric Hospital, Ghent-St. Denys-Westrem, Belgium

STEVEN C. DILSAVER, M.D., Assistant Professor of Psychiatry, Department of Psychiatry, University of Michigan, School of Medicine, Ann Arbor, Michigan, USA

G. DIRLICH, PH.D., Staff Scientist, Department of Biostatistics, Max Planck Institute of Psychiatry, Munich, Federal Republic of Germany

REGINA DITTRICH, PH.D., Department of Psychiatry, University of Vienna, Vienna, Austria

MATTHIAS DOSE, M.D., Senior Research Associate, Department of Adult Psychiatry, Max Planck Institute of Psychiatry, Munich, Federal Republic of Germany

PHILIPPE DOSTERT, PH.D., Research and Development, Farmitalia Carlo Erba, Milan, Italy

HEINZ DREXLER, M.D., Anesthesiologist, Jerusalem Mental Health Center-Ezrath Nashim, Jerusalem, Israel

HENRI DUFOUR, M.D., Professor of Clinical Psychiatry, Hôpital de la Timone, Marseilles, France

MICHEL DUGAS, M.D., Professor, Service de Psychopathologie de l'Enfant et de L'Adolescent, Faculté de Médecine Lariboisière-Saint Louis, Hôpital Robert Debré, Paris, France

PILAR DURO, M.D., Psychiatrist, Department of Psychiatry, Hospital de Sant Pau (Medical School), Barcelona, Spain

DONALD ECCLESTON, M.B., PH.D., D.SC., F.R.C.PSYCH., Professor of Psychiatry, Department of Psychiatry, University of Newcastle upon Tyne, The Royal Victoria Infirmary, Newcastle upon Tyne, United Kingdom

JAMES E. EDWARDSON, PH.D., Director, MRC Neuroendocrinology Unit, Newcastle General Hospital, Newcastle upon Tyne, United Kingdom

JANICE A. EGELAND, PH.D., Professor, Department of Psychiatry, University of Miami School of Medicine, Miami, Florida, USA

JANE L. EISEN, M.D., Assistant Professor, Department of Psychiatry and Human Behavior, Butler Hospital, Providence, Rhode Island, USA

HINDERK M. EMRICH, M.D., Professor and Head, Department of Adult Psychiatry, Max Planck Institute for Psychiatry, Munich, Federal Republic of Germany

L. ERLENMEYER-KIMLING, PH.D., Professor, Departments of Psychiatry, and of Genetics and Development, Columbia University, New York, New York, USA

JEAN-LUC EVRARD, M.D., Chief, Department of Psychiatry, Day Hospital, Santa Theresa Hospital, Montignies Sur Sambre, Belgium

IRL EXTEIN, M.D., Medical Director, Fair Oaks Hospital at Boca/Delray, Delray Beach, Florida, USA

CAROL J. FAIRCHILD, M.S., Clinical Research Associate, Bristol-Myers Company, Wallingford, Connecticut, USA

FRANCOIS FERRERO, M.D., University Institutions of Psychiatry, Geneva, Switzerland

IAN NICOL FERRIER, B.SC. (HONS), M.R.C.P., M.R.C.PSYCH., M.D.(HONS), MRC Clinical Scientist, Honorary Consultant Psychiatrist, MRC Neuroendocrinology Unit, Newcastle General Hospital, Newcastle upon Tyne, United Kingdom

RONALD R. FIEVE, M.D., Professor of Clinical Psychiatry, New York State Psychiatric Institute, New York, New York, USA

JOHN P.M. FINBERG, PH.D., Associate Professor, Department of Pharmacology, Rappaport Institute of Medical Research and Faculty of Medicine, Technion, Haifa, Israel

NAOMI FINEBERG, M.A., M.B., Lecturer, St. Mary's Hospital Medical School, London, United Kingdom

ALISON S. FLEMING, PH.D., Professor, Department of Psychology, Erindale College, University of Toronto, Mississauga, Ontario, Canada

CHRISTOPHER J. FOWLER, M.A., PH.D., Research Scientist, Research and Development Laboratories, Astra Lakemedel AB, Sodertalje, Sweden

HENRIETTE FRANCES, PH.D., Research Fellow, I.N.S.E.R.M. U-302; Department of Pharmacology, Faculty of Medicine, Pitié-Salpêtrière, Paris, France

ELLEN FRANK, PH.D., Associate Professor of Psychiatry and Psychology, Department of Psychiatry, University of Pittsburgh School of Medicine, Western Psychiatric Institute and Clinic, Pittsburgh, Pennsylvania, USA

RICHARD FRIEDMAN, M.D., Attending Physician, Payne Whitney Clinic, New York, New York, USA

KJEN G. FUXE, M.D., Professor, Department of Histology and Neurobiology, Karolinska Institute, Stockholm, Sweden

ROBERTO GALIMBERTI, PH.D., Research Assistant, Center of Neuropharmacology, University of Milan, Milan, Italy

JESÚS A. GARCÍA-SEVILLA, M.D., Professor, Department of Pharmacology and Therapeutics, Medical School, University of the Basque Country, Leioa, Biscay, Spain

MARTINE GARREAU, M.D., Psychiatrist, Clinical Research, Laboratoires d'Etudes et de Recherches Synthélabo (L.E.R.S.), Paris, France

MARIANGELA GASPERINI, M.D., Assistant, Department of Clinical Psychiatry, Milan University School of Medicine, San Paolo Hospital, Milan, Italy

ARNE GEISLER, M.D., Associate Professor, Department of Pharmacology, University of Copenhagen, Copenhagen, Denmark

BARBARA GELLER, M.D., Professor of Psychiatry, University of South Carolina, Columbia, South Carolina, USA

ANASTASIOS GEORGOTAS, M.D., Professor of Psychiatry and Director, Depression Studies Program, New York University School of Medicine; Director of Biological Psychiatry-Psychopharmacology, New York University-Bellevue Medical Center, New York, New York, USA

DANIELA S. GERHARD, PH.D., Assistant Professor, Department of Genetics, Washington University School of Medicine, St. Louis, Missouri, USA

ELLIOT S. GERSHON, M.D., Chief, Clinical Neurogenetics Branch, Division of Intramural Research, National Institute of Mental Health, Bethesda, Maryland, USA

SAMUEL GERSHON, M.D., Vice President for Research in the Medical and Health Care Division; Associate Vice President for Research in the Health Sciences, University of Pittsburgh; Professor of Psychiatry, Associate Research Director for Neurosciences, Department of Psychiatry, University of Pittsburgh School of Medicine, Pittsburgh, Pennsylvania, USA

DAVID GILL, M.B., CH.B., F.R.C.PSYCH., D.P.M., D.T.M & H., D. OBST., R.C.O.G., Consultant Psychiatrist, Mapperley Hospital, Nottingham Mental Illness Service; Clinical Teacher, Nottingham University Medical School, Nottingham, United Kingdom

J. CHRISTIAN GILLIN, M.D., Professor of Psychiatry; Director, UCSD Mental Health Clinical Research Center; Director, UCSD Fellowship in Clinical Psychopharmacology and Psychology, Department of Psychiatry, University of California, San Diego; San Diego Veterans Administration Medical Center, La Jolla, California, USA

ANNETTE GJERRIS, M.D., Research Associate, Department of Psychiatry, Rigshospitalet, Copenhagen, Denmark

MARK S. GOLD, M.D., Director of Research, Fair Oaks Hospital, Summit, New Jersey and Delray/Beach, Florida, USA

LYNN R. GOLDIN, PH.D., Senior Staff Fellow, Clinical Neurogenetics Branch, National Institute of Mental Health, Bethesda, Maryland, USA

SHAHKROKH GOLSHAN, PH.D., Chief Statistician, Department of Psychiatry, University of California, San Diego, La Jolla, California, USA

NUNO GONÇALVES, M.D., Head of General Psychiatry I, Psychiatric Hospital, Giessen, Federal Republic of Germany

PAUL J. GOODNICK, M.D., Department of Psychiatry, University of Miami, Miami, Florida; Director, Affective Disorders Program, Fair Oaks Hospital, Boca-Delray, Florida, USA

LARS F. GRAM, M.D., Professor, Department of Clinical Pharmacology, Odense University, Odense C, Denmark

DAVID GREENBERG, M.D., Director, Outpatient Clinic, Jerusalem Mental Health Center; Lecturer, Department of Psychiatry, Hebrew University, Jerusalem, Israel

STEVEN GREENWALD, M.A., Health Science Specialist, Bronx Veterans Administration Medical Center, Bronx, New York, USA

WALDEMAR GREIL, M.D., Psychiatric Hospital, University of Munich, Munich, Federal Republic of Germany

ORNA GRUCHOVER, M.A., Department of Psychology, Bar-Ilan University, Ramat-Gan, Israel

WILLY E. HAEFELY, M.D., Professor of Pharmacology, Department of PF/CNS, F. Hoffmann-La Roche & Co., Ltd., Basel, Switzerland

ANGELOS HALARIS, M.D., PH.D., Professor of Psychiatry and Pharmacology; Vice Chairman and Director, Department of Psychiatry, Case Western Reserve University, Cleveland Metropolitan General Hospital, Cleveland, Ohio, USA

URIEL HALBREICH, M.D., Professor of Psychiatry; Director, Biobehavioral Research, Department of Psychiatry, State University of New York at Buffalo, Buffalo, New York, USA

DARAKSHAR J. HALEEM, M.SC., Department of Neurochemistry, Institute of Neurology, London, United Kingdom

JAMES P. HALPER, M.D., Assistant Professor of Psychiatry, Cornell University Medical College, New York, New York, USA

M. HARIHARAN, PH.D., Scientific Director, Clinical Laboratory, Department of Psychiatry, Mental Health Research Institute, University of Michigan, Ann Arbor, Michigan, USA

SHAVI HAR-ZAHAV, M.A., Department of Psychology, Bar-Ilan University, Ramat-Gan, Israel

REINHOLD HATZINGER, PH.D., Department of Psychiatry, University of Vienna, Vienna, Austria

GEORGE R. HENINGER, M.D., Professor, Department of Psychiatry, Yale University School of Medicine, New Haven, Connecticut, USA

P.H. HERMANNS, M.D., Assistant, Clinical Research Department, Laboratoires d'Etudes et de Recherches Synthélabo (L.E.R.S.), Brussels, Belgium

PETER HERRIDGE, M.D., Director, Neuropsychiatric Evaluation, Fair Oaks Hospital, Summit, New Jersey, and Delray Beach, Florida, USA

ROBERT M.A. HIRSCHFELD, M.D., Chief, Affective and Anxiety Disorders Research Branch, Division of Clinical Research, National Institute of Mental Health, Rockville, Maryland, USA

P. HOFF, M.D., Department of Psychiatry, University of Munich, Munich, Federal Republic of Germany

FLORIAN HOLSBOER, M.D., PH.D., Professor and Chairman, Department of Psychiatry, University of Freiburg, Freiburg, Federal Republic of Germany

EDITH HOLSBOER-TRACHSLER, M.D., Department of Psychiatry, University of Basel, Basel, Switzerland

ULRICH E. HONEGGER, PH.D., Chief Assistant, Department of Pharmacology, University of Bern, Bern Switzerland

ROGER W. HORTON, PH.D., Department of Pharmacology and Clinical Pharmacology, St. George's Hospital Medical School, London, United Kingdom

ABRAM M. HOSTETTER, M.D., Clinical Professor, Department of Psychiatry, University of Miami School of Medicine, Miami, Florida, USA

DAVID E. HOUSMAN, PH.D., Professor, Department of Biology, Massachusetts Institute of Technology, Cambridge, Massachusetts, USA

DOROTHEA HUBER, M.D., Psychiatric Hospital, University of Munich, Munich, Federal Republic of Germany

CARROLL W. HUGHES, PH.D., Investigator, Psychiatric Research Institute, St. Francis Regional Medical Center; Research Associate Professor, Department of Psychiatry, University of Kansas School of Medicine; Wichita, Kansas, USA

DAVID S. JANOWSKY, M.D., Professor and Chair, Department of Psychiatry, University of North Carolina, Chapel Hill, North Carolina, USA

G. SEBASTIAAN JANSEN, PH.D., Biochemist, Head of Laboratory, Bloemendaal Psychiatric Center, The Hague, The Netherlands

ANN MARI JANSSON, M.D., Department of Histology and Neurobiology, Karolinska Institute, Stockholm, Sweden

MAREK JAREMA, M.D., PH.D., Associate Professor of Psychiatry, University of Szczecin, School of Medicine, Department of Psychiatry, Szczecin, Poland

DONALD A.W. JOHNSON, M.D., M.SC., F.R.C.PSYCH., D.P.M., Consultant Psychiatrist, University Hospital of South Manchester, Manchester, United Kingdom

ANTHONY G. JOLLEY, M.B., B.S., M.R.C.PSYCH., Lecturer in Psychiatry, Department of Psychiatry, Charing Cross Hospital, London, United Kingdom

LEWIS L. JUDD, M.D., Director, National Institute of Mental Health, Rockville, Maryland, USA

H.P. KAPFHAMMER, M.D., Department of Psychiatry, University of Munich, Munich, Federal Republic of Germany

ALLAN S. KAPLAN, M.D., F.R.C.P.C., Assistant Professor; Department of Psychiatry, University of Toronto; Director, Eating Disorder Center; Post-Graduate Education Coordinator, Staff Psychiatrist, Toronto General Hospital, Toronto, Ontario, Canada

ZEV KAPLAN, M.D., Instructor, Department of Psychiatry, Ben Gurion University, School of Medicine, Beersheva, Israel

CORNELIUS L.E. KATONA, M.B., M.R.C.PSYCH., Department of Psychiatry, The Middlesex Hospital Medical School, London, United Kingdom

JACK L. KATZ, M.D., Professor of Clinical Psychiatry, Cornell University Medical College, New York Hospital-Cornell Medical Center, Westchester Division, White Plains, New York, USA

SIDNEY H. KENNEDY, M.B., B.CH., M.R.C.PSYCH., F.R.C.P.(C)., Associate Professor, Department of Psychiatry, University of Toronto; Head of Nutrition and Affective Disorder Service, Toronto General Hospital, Toronto, Ontario, Canada

GUY A. KENNETT, PH.D., Research Scientist, Department of Neurochemistry, Institute of Neurology, London, United Kingdom

T. ALAN KERR, M.D., F.R.C.PSYCH., Consultant Psychiatrist, St. Nicholas Hospital, Gosforth, Newcastle upon Tyne, United Kingdom

ROLF KETTLER, PH.D., Department of PF/CNS, F. Hoffmann-La Roche & Co., Ltd., Basel, Switzerland

SUMANT KHANNA, D.P.M., M.D., Lecturer, Department of Psychiatry, National Institute of Mental Health and Neurosciences, Bangalore, India

JUDITH R. KIDD, B.A., Associate in Research, Department of Human Genetics, Yale University School of Medicine, New Haven, Connecticut, USA

KENNETH K. KIDD, PH.D., Professor, Department of Human Genetics, Yale University School of Medicine, New Haven, Connecticut, USA

SETH KINDLER, M.D., Senior Resident, Jerusalem Medical Health Center-Ezrath Nashim, Jerusalem, Israel

ISAO KITAYAMA, M.D., Department of Psychiatry, Mie University School of Medicine, Mie-Ken, Japan

EHUD M. KLEIN, M.D., Clinical Instructor, Techion School of Medicine, Haifa, Israel

GRETA KOINIG, M.D., Department of Psychiatry, University of Vienna, Vienna, Austria

PER KRAGH-SØRENSEN, M.D., Associate Professor, Institute of Psychiatry, Odense University, Odense, Denmark

JÜRGEN-CHRISTIAN KRIEG, M.D., Assistant Head, Psychiatric Department, Max-Planck-Institute of Psychiatry, Munich, Federal Republic of Germany

HOWARD KRIEGER, M.D., Toronto General Hospital, Toronto, Ontario, Canada

HANS-LUDWIG KRÜBER, M.D., Head Physician in Clinic, Ruprecht-Karls-University, Psychiatric Hospital, Heidelberg, Federal Republic of Germany

DAVID J. KUPFER, M.D., Professor and Chairman, Department of Psychiatry, University of Pittsburgh School of Medicine, Western Psychiatric Institute and Clinic, Pittsburgh, Pennsylvania, USA

MALCOLM T. LAMBERT, M.B., CH.B., M.R.C.PSYCH., Lecturer/Honorary Senior Registrar, Academic Department of Psychiatry, St. Mary's Hospital Medical School, London, United Kingdom

GERHARD LANGER, M.D., Associate Professor of Psychiatry, Department of Psychiatry, University of Vienna, Vienna, Austria

SALOMON Z. LANGER, M.D., Director, Department of Biology, Laboratoires d'Etudes et de Synthélabo Recherches (L.E.R.S.), Paris, France

YVES LECRUBIER, M.D., Department of Pharmacology, Faculty of Medicine, Pitié-Salpêtrière, Paris, France

HEINZ E. LEHMANN, M.D., Professor Emeritus, Department of Psychiatry, McGill University, Montreal, Québec, Canada

BRIAN E. LEONARD, PH.D., D.SC., Professor of Pharmacology, Department of Pharmacology, University College, Galway, Republic of Ireland

BERNARD LERER, M.D., Director of Research, Jerusalem Mental Health Center-Ezrath Nashim; Associate Professor, Department of Psychiatry, Hebrew University, Jerusalem, Israel

JAMES E.B. LINDESAY, M.A., M.R.C.PSYCH., Lecturer in Psychogeriatrics, United Medical Schools of Guys and St. Thomas Hospitals, Guys Hospital, London, United Kingdom

KENNETH GEORGE LLOYD, PH.D., Vice Director, Biology Department, Synthélabo Recherches (L.E.R.S.), Paris, France

CARLO LOEB, M.D., Professor of Neurology and Chairman, Department of Neurology, Medical School, University of Genoa, Genoa, Italy

ADELIO LUCCA, M.D., Medical Fellow, University Psychiatric Clinic III, Institute of Biomedical Sciences, San Paolo Hospital, Milan, Italy

WOLFGANG LUDWIG, PH.D., Psychiatric Hospital, University of Munich, Munich, Federal Republic of Germany

FABIO MACCIARDI, M.D., Assistant in Clinical Psychiatry, Milan University School of Medicine, Milan, Italy

KAY P. MAGUIRE, B.SC., M.SC., PH.D., Professional Officer, Department of Psychiatry, University of Melbourne, Victoria, Australia

MARIO MAJ, M.D., PH.D., Professor of Mental Hygiene, First Medical School, University of Naples, Naples, Italy

J. JOHN MANN, M.D., Professor of Psychiatry, Cornell University Medical College, New York, New York, USA

ELIZABETH G. MARSHALL, PH.D., Lecturer, Department of Psychiatry, University of Newcastle upon Tyne, Newcastle upon Tyne, United Kingdom

JUAN MASANA, M.D., Head, Neurophysiology Section, Department of Psychiatry, Clinical Hospital (Medical School), Barcelona, Spain

ROY J. MATHEW, M.D., Professor, Department of Psychiatry; Associate Professor, Department of Radiology, Duke University Medical Center, Durham, North Carolina, USA

LOU ANN MCADAMS, PH.D., Biostatistician, Population Research Center, Research and Education Institute, Harbor-UCLA Medical Center, Torrance, California, USA

P. ANNE MCBRIDE, M.D., Assistant Professor of Psychiatry, Cornell University Medical College, New York, New York, USA

ROBERT E. MCCUE, M.D., Research Assistant Professor of Psychiatry, New York University School of Medicine, New York, New York, USA

IAIN M. MCINTYRE, B.SC., M.SC., PH.D., Research Fellow, Department of Psychiatry, University of Melbourne, Austin Hospital, Heidelberg, Victoria, Australia

TODD MCINTYRE, PH.D., Staff Fellow, Laboratory of Neuroscience, National Institute of Diabetes, Digestive and Kidney Diseases (N.I.D.D.K.), National Institutes of Health, Bethesda, Maryland, USA

IAN G. MCKEITH, M.B.B.S., M.R.C.PSYCH, Consultant Psychiatrist and Honorary Lecturer, Department of Psychiatry, University of Newcastle upon Tyne, Newcastle upon Tyne, United Kingdom

JULIEN MENDLEWICZ, M.D., PH.D., Professor and Chairman, Department of Psychiatry, University Clinics of Brussels, Erasme Hospital, Free University of Brussels, Brussels, Belgium

CLAUDINE J.H.M. MERTENS, M.D., Medical Director, Psychiatry Center, Sleidinge, Belgium

NORMAN A. MILGRAM, PH.D., Professor, Department of Psychology, Tel-Aviv University, Ramat-Aviv, Israel

EDITH MITRANY, M.D., Psychosomatic Service Chief, Child and Adolescent Psychosomatic Unit, The Chaim Sheba Medical Center, Tel Hashomer, Israel; Tel-Aviv University, Sackler School of Medicine, Tel-Aviv, Israel

HANS W. MOISES, M.D., Central Institute of Mental Health, Psychiatric Clinic, Mannheim, Federal Republic of Germany

J. DROGO MONTAGU, M.R.C.S., L.R.C.P., Late Assistant Clinician, Department of Neurophysiology, Charing Cross Hospital, London, United Kingdom

DEIDRE B. MONTGOMERY, B.A., Research Psychologist, St. Mary's Hospital Medical School, London, United Kingdom

STUART A. MONTGOMERY, M.D., Reader, Department of Psychiatry, St. Mary's Hospital Medical School, London, United Kingdom

ARNE MØRK, CAND. SCIENT., Department of Pharmacology, University of Copenhagen, Copenhagen, Denmark

PAOLO LUCIO MORSELLI, M.D., Director of Clinical Research Department, Laboratoire d'Etudes et de Recherches Synthélabo (L.E.R.S.), Paris, France

JAN MOS, PH.D., Head, Behavioral Pharmacology, Department of Pharmacology, Duphar B.V., Weesp, The Netherlands

C.R. MUKUNDAN, PH.D., Department of Clinical Psychology, National Institute of Mental Health and Neurosciences, Bangalore, India

WALTER E. MÜLLER, PH.D., Head, Psychopharmacological Laboratory, Central Institute of Mental Health; Professor of Pharmacology and Toxicology, Faculty of Clinical Medicine at Mannheim, University of Heidelberg, Mannheim, Federal Republic of Germany

ELAINE MURPHY, M.D., F.R.C.PSYCH., Professor of Psychogeriatrics, United Medical Schools of Guys and St. Thomas Hospitals, Guys Hospital, London, United Kingdom

BRUNO MUSCH, M.D., Vice-Director, Laboratoires d'Etudes et de Recherches Synthélabo (L.E.R.S.), Paris, France

NARMADA NAGACHANDRAN, M.D., Postdoctoral Fellow, New York University School of Medicine, New York, New York, USA

R. SWAMI NATHAN, M.D., Associate Professor of Psychiatry, Department of Psychiatry; Medical Director of Clinical Research Unit, Western Psychiatric Institute and Clinic, University of Pittsburgh School of Medicine, Pittsburgh, Pennsylvania, USA

J. CRAIG NELSON, M.D., Associate Professor of Psychiatry, Yale University School of Medicine, New Haven, Connecticut, USA

CHARLES B. NEMEROFF, M.D., PH.D., Associate Professor, Departments of Psychiatry and Pharmacology, Duke University Medical Center, Durham, North Carolina, USA

MICHAEL E. NEWMAN, PH.D., Senior Biochemist, Jerusalem Mental Health Center-Ezrath Nashim, Jerusalem, Israel

NIELS PETER NIELSEN, M.D., Consultant Psychiatrist, Unita Socio Sanitario Locale 11, Como, Italy

WILLEM A. NOLEN, M.D., PH.D., Head, Department of Biological Psychiatry, Bloemendaal Psychiatric Center, The Hague, The Netherlands

CONNY NORDIN, M.D., Department of Psychiatry, Huddinge University Hospital, Huddinge, Sweden

TREVOR R. NORMAN, B.SC.(HONS), PH.D., Research Fellow, Department of Psychiatry, University of Melbourne, Austin Hospital, Heidelberg, Victoria, Australia

ANNE-MARIE O'CARROLL, B.A., PH.D., Research Scientist, Department of Biochemistry, Trinity College, Dublin, Republic of Ireland

WILLIAM T. O'CONNOR, B.SC., PH.D., Postdoctoral Fellow, Pharmacology Department, Karolinska Institute, Stockholm, Sweden

SVEN OVE ÖGREN, M.D., Associate Professor of Neurobiology, Department of Histology, Karolinska Institute, Stockholm, Sweden

TERUO OKUMA, M.D., D.M.S., Director, National Center Hospital for Mental, Nervous and Muscular Disorders, National Center of Neurology and Psychiatry, Tokyo, Japan

BEREND OLIVIER, PH.D., Head, CNS Pharmacology, Duphar B.V., Weesp, The Netherlands

BERNADETTE O'NEILL, B.SC., PH.D., Pharmacology Department, University College, Galway, Republic of Ireland

GERALD OPPENHEIM, M.B., B.S., F.R.A.N.Z.C.P, Director, Alzheimer's Disease Treatment and Study Program, Department of Psychiatry, Shaare Zedek Medical Center, Jerusalem, Israel

ISRAEL ORBACH, PH.D., Associate Professor, Department of Psychology, Bar-Ilan University, Ramat-Gan, Israel

SCOTT P. ORR, PH.D., Research Psychologist, Veterans Administration Medical Center, Manchester, New Hampshire; Adjunct Research Associate, Dartmouth Medical School, Hanover, New Hampshire, USA

ANGELA ORSINI, M.D., Assistant in Clinical Psychiatry, Milan University School of Medicine, Milan, Italy

HELEN ORVASCHEL, PH.D., Associate Professor and Director of Child Psychology, Division of Child Psychiatry, Medical College of Pennsylvania, Eastern Pennsylvania Psychiatric Institute, Philadelphia, Pennsylvania, USA

DAVID H. OVERSTREET, PH.D., Associate Professor, School of Biological Sciences, The Flinders University of South Australia, Bedford Park, South Australia, Australia

MICHAEL J. OWENS, B.S., Doctoral Candidate, Department of Pharmacology, Duke University Medical Center, Durham, North Carolina, USA

ANDREW J. PAKSTIS, PH.D., Associate Research Scientist, Department of Human Genetics, Yale University School of Medicine, New Haven, Connecticut, USA

GHANSHYAM N. PANDEY, PH.D., Professor, Department of Psychiatry, College of Medicine, University of Illinois at Chicago; Director, Biological Research, Illinois State Psychiatric Institute, Chicago, Illinois, USA

STEPHEN J. PARKER, B.SC., Department of Pharmacology and Clinical Pharmacology, St. George's Hospital Medical School, London, United Kingdom

DAVID L. PAULS, PH.D., Assistant Professor, Child Study Center, Yale University School of Medicine, New Haven, Connecticut, USA

ROBERT H. PERRY, M.R.C.P., M.R.C.PATH., Consultant Neuropathologist and Honorary Lecturer, Department of Neuropathology, Newcastle General Hospital, Newcastle upon Tyne, United Kingdom

ERIC D. PESELOW, M.D., Assistant Professor, Department of Psychiatry, New York University School of Medicine, New York, New York, USA

ANN PETERS, M.S., Research Specialist, Department of Psychiatry, Cornell University Medical College, New York, New York, USA

BERTALAN PETHO, M.D., M.PSYCHOL., Professor of Psychiatry, Semmelweis Medical University, Budapest, Hungary

THEODORE A. PETTI, M.D., M.P.H., Associate Professor of Child Psychiatry, Department of Psychiatry, University of Pittsburgh School of Medicine, Pittsburgh, Pennsylvania, USA

CYNTHIA R. PFEFFER, M.D., Associate Professor of Clinical Psychiatry, Cornell University Medical College; Chief, Child Psychiatry, Inpatient Unit, White Plains, New York, USA

PHILIPPE PICHAT, PHAR.D., Laboratoire Delagrange, Chilly Mazarin, France

M. CRISTINA PINET, M.D., Department of Psychiatry, Hospital de Sant Pau (Medical School), Barcelona, Spain

K.M. PIRKE, PH.D., Department of Clinical Chemistry, Max Planck Institute for Psychiatry, Munich, Federal Republic of Germany

ROGER K. PITMAN, M.D., Clinical Investigator, Veterans Administration Medical Center, Manchester, New Hampshire; Adjunct Assistant Professor of Clinical Psychiatry, Dartmouth Medical School, Hanover, New Hampshire, USA

ROGER D. PORSOLT, PH.D., Scientific Director, I.T.E.M.-Labo, Kremlin-Bicêtre, France

ROBERT M. POST, M.D., Chief, Biological Psychiatry Branch, National Institute of Mental Health, Bethesda, Maryland, USA

ASHOKA JAHNAVI PRASAD, M.D., Consultant Psychiatrist, Claybury Hospital, London, United Kingdom

SHELDON H. PRESKORN, M.D., Director, Psychiatric Research Institute, St. Francis Reginal Medical Center; Professor and Vice-Chairman, Department of Psychiatry, University of Kansas School of Medicine-Wichita; Chief, Psychiatry Service, Veterans Administration Medical Center-Wichita, Wichita, Kansas, USA

PAOLO PRIORE, M.D., Director, L.E.R.S. Clinical Unit, Milan, Italy

MARCELLA PROVENZA, M.D., Assistant in Clinical Psychiatry, Milan University School of Medicine, Milan, Italy

FRANK W. PUTNAM, JR., M.D., Chief, Unit on Dissociative Disorders, Laboratory of Developmental Psychology, National Institute of Mental Health, Bethesda, Maryland, USA

GIORGIO RACAGNI, PH.D., Professor of Pharmacology, Center of Neuropharmacology, Milan, Italy

OLE J. RAFAELSEN, M.D., Professor and Head, Department of Psychiatry and Psychochemistry, University of Copenhagen, Rigshospitalet, Copenhagen, Denmark

WILLIAM A. RAFULS, M.D., Assistant Director, Neuropsychiatric Evaluation Unit, Fair Oaks Hospital at Boca/Delray, Delray Beach, Florida, USA

ANKE RAM, M.D., Resident in Psychiatry, Geha Psychiatric Hospital, Petah Tikva, Israel

MARIE LUISE RAO, PH.D., Universitätsnervenklinik, Psychiatrie, Venusburg, Federal Republic of Germany

CONSTANTIN RAPTIS, R.C., M.D., Research Fellow, Department of Psychiatry, Max-Planck-Institute of Psychiatry, Munich, Federal Republic of Germany

STEVEN A. RASMUSSEN, M.D., Assistant Professor, Department of Psychiatry and Human Behavior, Butler Hospital, Providence, Rhode Island, USA

MOSHE REHAVI, PH.D., Senior Lecturer, Department of Physiology and Pharmacology, Sackler Faculty of Medicine, Tel-Aviv University, Tel-Aviv, Israel

NIELS REISBY, M.D., Professor in General Psychiatry, University of Århus, Risskov, Denmark

GAVIN P. REYNOLDS, PH.D., Department of Pathology, University of Nottingham Medical School, Queen's Medical Center, Nottingham, United Kingdom

J. STEVEN RICHARDSON, B.A.(HONS), M.A., PH.D., Professor, Departments of Pharmacology and Psychiatry, College of Medicine, University of Saskatchewan, Saskatoon, Saskatchewan, Canada

S. CRAIG RISCH, M.D., Professor of Psychiatry, Director of Clinical Research, Department of Psychiatry, Emory University School of Medicine, Atlanta, Georgia, USA

MARCO RIVA, PH.D., Research Assistant, Center of Neuropharmacology, University of Milan, Milan, Italy

ASHLEY A. ROBIN, M.D., F.R.C.PSYCH., D.P.M., Honorary Consulting Psychiatrist, Charing Cross Hospital, London, United Kingdom

CLIVE ROBINS, PH.D., Associate Professor of Psychology, Duke University Medical Center, Durham, North Carolina, USA

JOSE RODRIGUEZ-ESPINOSA, M.D., Endocrinologist, Head, Section of Neuroendocrinology, Hospital de Sant Pau (Medical School), Barcelona, Spain

GREGORY ROITMAN, M.D., Instructor, Department of Psychiatry, Ben Gurion University School of Medicine, Beersheva, Israel

SIR MARTIN ROTH, M.D., SC.D.(HON), F.R.C.P., F.R.C.PSYCH., Fellow of Trinity College; Professor Emeritus of Psychiatry, University of Cambridge, Cambridge, United Kingdom

ALESSANDRA C. ROVESCALLI, PH.D., Research Assistant, Center of Neuropharmacology, University of Milan, Milan, Italy

ALEC ROY, M.B., Visiting Associate, National Institutes of Health, Bethesda, Maryland, USA

KAREN RUBENSTEIN, M.ED., M.A., Psychologist, Bronx Veterans Administration Medical Center, Bronx, New York, USA

DIANE N. RUBLE, PH.D., Professor, Department of Psychology, New York University, New York, New York, USA

A. JOHN RUSH, M.D., Betty Jo Hay Professor, Department of Psychiatry and Affective Disorders, University of Texas, Health Science Center, Dallas, Texas, USA

JEAN CLAUDE SAMUELIAN, M.D., Department of Psychiatry, La Timone Hospital, Marseilles, France

ELAINE SANDERS-BUSH, PH.D., Professor of Pharmacology, Tennessee Neuropsychiatric Institute, Nashville, Tennessee, USA

DAVID J. SANGER, B.SC., PH.D., Assistant Group Leader, CNS Pharmacology, Laboratories d'Etudes et de Recherches Synthélabo (L.E.R.S.), Bagneux, France

BERNARD SCATTON, PH.D., Section Head, Biology Department, Laboratoires d'Etudes et de Synthélabo Recherche (L.E.R.S.), Paris, France

CLAUDIA SCHMAUSS, M.D., Department of Psychopharmacology, Max Planck Institute for Psychiatry, Munich, Federal Republic of Germany

MAX SCHMAUSS, M.D., Head Physician, Psychiatric Hospital, University of Munich, Munich, Federal Republic of Germany

STEPHAN SCHMIDT, M.D., Psychiatric Hospital, University of Munich, Munich, Federal Republic of Germany

HANS SCHOEMAKER, PH.D., Project Leader, Department of Biology, Laboratoires d'Etudes et de Synthélabo Recherches (L.E.R.S.), Paris, France

GEORG SCHOENBECK, M.D., Department of Psychiatry, University of Vienna, Vienna, Austria

GABRIELLA SCIUTO, M.D., Fellow, Institute of Clinical Psychiatry, University of Milan School of Medicine, Milan, Italy

BRUCE A. SCOGGINS, MAGRSC., PH.D., Senior Principal Research Fellow (NH-MRC), Howard Florey Institute of Experimental Physiology and Medicine, Parkville, Australia

JANINE L. SCOTT, M.B., B.S., M.R.C.PSYCH., Lecturer in Psychiatry, Department of Psychiatry, University of Newcastle upon Tyne, Royal Victoria Infirmary, Newcastle upon Tyne, United Kingdom

C. SERRATI, M.D., Assistant, Department of Neurology, University of Genoa Medical School, Genoa, Italy

BARUCH SHAPIRA, M.D., Director, Affective Disorder Program, Jerusalem Mental Health Center-Ezrath Nashim; Lecturer, Department of Psychiatry, Hebrew University, Jerusalem, Israel

RICHARD SHINDLEDECKER, M.A., Biostatistician, Department of Psychiatry, Cornell University Westchester Division, White Plains, New York, USA

SASHI SHUKLA, M.D., Assistant Professor, Department of Psychiatry and Behavioral Sciences, State University of New York at Stony Brook, Stony Brook, New York, USA

LARRY J. SIEVER, M.D., Director, Out-Patient Psychiatry Clinic, Bronx Veterans Administration Medical Center, Bronx, New York; Associate Professor of Psychiatry, Mount Sinai School of Medicine, New York, New York, USA

STUART SILVERMAN, M.D., Fellow, Child Psychiatry, Columbia University College of Physicians of Surgeons, New York, New York, USA

TREVOR SILVERSTONE, D.M., F.R.C.P., F.R.C.PSYCH., Professor of Clinical Psychopharmacology, Academic Unit of Human Psychopharmacology, Medical College of St. Bartholomew's Hospital, London, United Kingdom

PIERRE SIMON, PH.D., Department of Pharmacology, Faculty of Medicine, Pitié-Salpêtrière, Paris, France

PHIL SKOLNICK, PH.D., Chief, Laboratory of Neuroscience, National Institute of Diabetes, Digestive and Kidney Diseases (N.I.D.D.K.), National Institutes of Health, Bethesda, Maryland, USA

ENRICO SMERALDI, M.D., Professor and Director, University Psychiatric Clinic III, Institute of Biomedical Sciences, San Paolo Hospital, Milan, Italy

ZAHAVA SOLOMON, PH.D., Head, Research Branch, Department of Mental Health, Medical Corps, Israel Defense Forces, Israel

STEPHEN M. STAHL, M.D., PH.D., Professor of Psychiatry, UCSD; Chief, Psychiatry Service, V.A. Medical Center, San Diego, California, USA

MICHAEL STANLEY, PH.D., Associate Professor, Departments of Psychiatry and Pharmacology, Columbia University College of Physicians and Surgeons; Department of Neurochemistry, New York State Psychiatric Institute, New York, New York, USA

AXEL STEIGER, M.D., Department of Psychiatry, University of Freiburg, Freiburg, Federal Republic of Germany

MEIR STEINER, M.D., PH.D., F.R.C.P.(C), Professor of Psychiatry and Neurosciences, Faculty of Health Sciences, McMaster University; Head, Clinical Studies Program, McMaster Psychiatric Unit, St. Joseph's Hospital, Hamilton, Ontario, Canada

KLAUS-DIETER STOLL, PH.D., Sponsor for Neuropsychopharmacology, Clinical Research, Ciby-Geigy GmbH, Frankfurt, Federal Republic of Germany

JAMES P. SULLIVAN, B.A., Research Scientist, Department of Biochemistry, Trinity College, Dublin, Republic of Ireland

FRIDOLIN SULSER, M.D., Professor of Pharmacology and Psychiatry, Tennessee Neuropsychiatric Institute, Nashville, Tennessee, USA

JAMES N. SUSSEX, M.D., Professor, Department of Psychiatry, University of Miami School of Medicine, Miami, Florida, USA

JOHN A. SWEENEY, PH.D., Assistant Professor of Psychology in Psychiatry, Cornell University Medical College, New York, New York, USA

JOHN F. TALLMAN, PH.D., Associate Professor, Department of Psychiatry, Ribicoff Research Facility, Yale University School of Medicine, New Haven, Connecticut, USA

JOHN TEASDALE, PH.D., Senior Scientist, Medical Research Council Applied Psychology Unit, Cambridge, United Kingdom

ANTONIO TEJERO, PH.D., Psychologist, Department of Psychiatry, Hospital de Sant Pau (Medical School), Barcelona, Spain

PHILIPPE THERMOZ, M.D., Department of Psychiatry, Hôpital de la Timone, Marseilles, France

KEITH F. TIPTON, M.A., PH.D., Professor, Department of Biochemistry, Trinity College, Dublin, Republic of Ireland

JOSE TOMAS-VILALTELLA, M.D., Head, Child Psychiatry Department, Hospital del Valle de Hebron (School of Medicine), Barcelona, Spain

M. TOSCANO, M.D., Medical Director, Neuropsychiatric Institute Fond'Roy, Brussels, Belgium

RAMON TRULLAS, PH.D., Fogarty International Fellow, Laboratory of Neuroscience, National Institute of Diabetes, Digestive and Kidney Diseases (N.I.D.D.K.), National Institutes of Health, Bethesda, Maryland, USA

SAM TYANO, M.D., Professor of Psychiatry, University of Tel Aviv, Sackler School of Medicine, Tel Aviv, Israel; Geha Psychiatric Hospital, Petah Tikva, Israel

CLAUDI UDINA, M.D., Department of Psychiatry, Hospital de Sant Pau (Medical School), Barcelona, Spain

THOMAS W. UHDE, M.D., Chief, Unit on Anxiety and Affective Disorders; Unit Chief, 3-West Clinical Research Unit, Biological Psychiatry Branch, National Institute of Mental Health, Bethesda, Maryland, USA

DIETRICH VAN CALKER, M.D., Psychiatric Hospital, University of Munich, Munich, Federal Republic of Germany

BESSEL A. VAN DER KOLK, M.D., Director, MMHC Trauma Center, Harvard Medical School, Boston, Massachusetts, USA

HERMAN M. VAN PRAAG, M.D., PH.D., Silverman Professor and Chairman, Department of Psychiatry, Albert Einstein College of Medicine; Psychiatrist-in-Chief, Department of Psychiatry, Montefiore Medical Center, Bronx, New York, USA

JAN M. VAN REE, PH.D., Rudolf Magnus Institute for Pharmacology, Medical Faculty, University of Utrecht, Utrecht, The Netherlands

PER VESTERGAARD, M.D., Head, Department A, University of Aarhus; Department of Psychiatry, Psychiatric Hospital, Risskov, Denmark

FRIEDRICH VOGEL, M.D., Director, Institute of Human Genetics and Anthropology, University of Heidelberg, Heidelberg, Federal Republic of Germany

ULRICH VON BARDELEBEN, M.D., Department of Psychiatry, University of Freiburg, Freiburg, Federal Republic of Germany

GABRIEL VON EULER, M.D., Department of Histology and Neurobiology, Karolinska Institute, Stockholm, Sweden

DETLEV VON ZERSSEN, M.D., Head, Psychiatric Evaluation Research Unit, Max-Planck-Institute of Psychiatry; Associate Professor, Ludwig-Maximillians-University, Munich, Federal Republic of Germany

MATTHIAS M. WEBER, M.D., Research Fellow, Clinical Department, Max-Planck-Institute for Psychiatry, Munich, Federal Republic of Germany

RICHARD D. WEINER, M.D., PH.D., Associate Professor, Department of Psychiatry, Duke University Medical Center, Durham, North Carolina, USA

SUSAN R.B. WEISS, PH.D., Biological Psychiatry Branch, National Institute of Mental Health, Bethesda, Maryland, USA

ABRAHAM WEIZMAN, M.D., Lecturer, Geha Hospital and Sackler Faculty of Medicine, Tel-Aviv University, Tel-Aviv, Israel

RONIT WEIZMAN, M.D., Lecturer, Hasharon Hospital and Sackler Faculty of Medicine, Tel-Aviv University, Tel-Aviv, Israel

ELIZABETH WELLER, M.D., Professor and Chief, Division of Child Psychiatry, Department of Psychiatry, Ohio State University, Columbus, Ohio, USA

RONALD WELLER, M.D., Professor and Director of Residency Training, Department of Psychiatry, Ohio State University, Columbus, Ohio, USA

CAROL A. WHITFORD, PH.D., Research Fellow, MRC Neuroendocrinology Unit, Newcastle General Hospital, Newcastle upon Tyne, United Kingdom

DANIEL WIDLÖCHER, PH.D., Department of Pharmacology, Faculty of Medicine, Pitié Salpêtrière, Paris, France

KLAUS WIEDEMANN, M.D., Department of Psychiatry, University of Freiburg, Freiburg, Federal Republic of Germany

JEAN WILMOTTE, M.D., Head, Psychiatric Department, Vincent Van Gogh Hospital, Marchienne-Au-Pont, Belgium; Neuropsychiatrist and Assistant·Lecturer, Department of Psychiatry, Free University of Brussels, Brussels, Belgium

PHILIP J. WILNER, M.D., Instructor in Psychiatry, Cornell University Medical College, New York, New York, USA

WILLIAM H. WILSON, PH.D., Associate Professor, Department of Psychiatry, Duke University Medical Center, Durham, North Carolina, USA

RONALD M. WINCHEL, M.D., Research Psychiatrist, Departments of Psychiatry and Pharmacology, Columbia University College of Physicians and Surgeons; Department of Neurochemistry, New York State Psychiatric Institute, New York, New York, USA

ADAM WOLKIN, M.D., Assistant Professor, Department of Psychiatry, New York University School of Medicine, New York, New York, USA

P.Y. WONG, M.D., Director, Radioassay Laboratory, Toronto General Hospital, Toronto, Ontario, Canada

SCOTT W. WOODS, M.D., Assistant Professor, Department of Psychiatry, Yale University School of Medicine, New Haven, Connecticut, USA

MOUSSA B.H. YOUDIM, M.SC., PH.D., Professor and Chairman, Department of Pharmacology, Faculty of Medicine-Technion, Haifa, Israel

BRANIMIR ZIVKOVIC, PH.D., Vice Director, Biology Department, Laboratoires d'Etudes et de Synthélabo Recherche (L.E.R.S.), Paris, France

JUERGEN ZULLEY, PH.D., Psychologist, Max-Planck-Institute for Psychiatry, Munich, Federal Republic of Germany

I PATHOGENESIS OF AFFECTIVE DISORDERS AND BASIC MECHANISMS OF DRUG ACTION

I.A. ANIMAL MODELS AND ANTIDEPRESSANT PREDICTABILITY

1. Neurochemical and Behavioral Effects of Stress: A Rat Model of Depression

G. Curzon, D.J. Haleem, and G.A. Kennett

We have established a model for depression that has behavioral and neurochemical analogies to the human illness and also responds to antidepressant drugs. The model is based on effects of 2 h of restraint stress in the rat: (a) increased plasma corticosterone; (b) decreased locomotion and increased defecation on placement 24 h later in an open field; and (c) anorexia. Figure 1.1 shows typical results and that daily restraint leads to adaptation; behavior becomes normal.[1]

Similar stress-induced changes have been widely used as models of depression because of their similarities with clinical findings[2] and the putative link between life event stress and depression.[3] Therefore failure to adapt provides a rational model.[4] The anorexia is not merely due to stress-induced gastric ulceration,[5] and is of interest as anorexia nervosa may be a nontypical form of depression.[6]

As there is evidence that 5-hydroxytryptamine (serotonin, 5-HT) has a role in depression,[7,8] it is relevant that some components of the 5-HT behavioral syndrome induced by the 5-HT agonist 5-MeODMT are increased 24 h after repeated stress, particularly forepaw treading and tremor.[1]

These results lead one to ask if the increased responsiveness to 5-HT mediates adaptation and how corticosterone is involved in adaptation, especially as glucocorticoids are reported to both influence 5-HT function[9,10] and cause affective changes clinically.[11] Investigation revealed that although plasma corticosterone rises during stress and has acute adaptive and anxiolytic effects, repeated corticosterone injection is maladaptive, causing deficits in open field activity and body weight, as well as a decreased postsynaptic response to 5-MeODMT.[12] Conversely, the corticosterone synthesis inhibitor metyrapone accelerates behavioral adaptation to repeated stress and augments the increased response to the 5-HT agonist.[13]

These findings lead to a model in which high glucocorticoid response to stress and low 5-HT functional activity oppose adaptation and therefore predispose to depression. This model is plausible in view of (a) the high corticoid levels during depression[14] and (b) the evidence for a 5-HT abnormality in the illness.

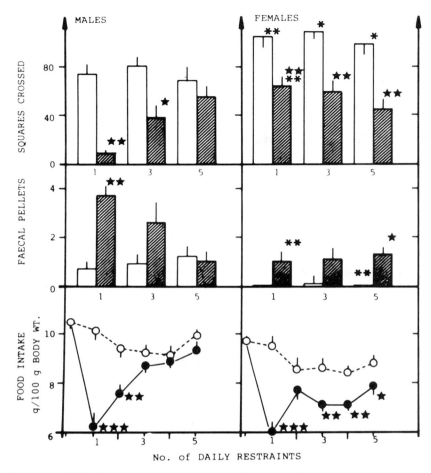

FIGURE 1.1. Behavior during first exposure in a 5-min open field test of male and female controls (open columns) and rats restrained daily (2 h/day) for 1, 3, or 5 days 24 h after the last restraint (hatched columns). Daily food intakes of controls (open circles) and rats restrained daily for up to 5 days (closed circles) are also shown. Number of daily restraints are shown on the y-axis. All points are means ± SEM; n = 10 per group. Differences from respective controls: ★$p < 0.05$; ★★$p < 0.01$; ★★★$p < 0.001$. Differences from male group: *$p < 0.05$; **$p < 0.01$ by two-tailed Mann-Whitney U-test after appropriate analysis of variance. (Results from Kennett et al.[17])

Effects of Stress on Male and Female Rats

All the above work was on male rats. As stress increases corticosterone more in female animals[15] and as depression is more common in women,[16] we compared the effects of stress on male and female rats.[17] Figure 1.1 shows that the open field behavior of female rats was less affected by a single stress than that of the male rats, though food intake was comparably decreased. However, in striking contrast to the male rats, these effects were still present or were even greater after repeated stress. Also, on repeated stress the female rats did not develop the increased response to 5-MeODMT shown by the male rats.

The model thus conforms to the sex difference in incidence seen with the human illness, the higher corticosterone responses of the female animals and their failure to increase 5-HT functional activity on repeated stress being associated with defective behavioral adaptation. Extrapolation to humans implies that the higher incidence of depression in women may involve not only social factors but also maladaptation to stress or to altered internal milieu.

We have now confirmed the higher corticosterone response of female rats to stress and have shown that it may cause their defective adaptation to repeated stress. Thus when the response was decreased to the male level with metyrapone, the behavioral effects of stress were altered to the male pattern. Thus open field activity 24 h after a single stress was impaired but returned to normal after repeated stress. Similarly, the response to 5-MeODMT was increased and food intake became normal after repeated stress.

Effects of Drugs

An obvious requirement of any depression model is that it should respond appropriately to antidepressants. We have found this situation to be the case as chronic pretreatment with two antidepressant 5-HT reuptake inhibitors, desipramine and sertraline, significantly normalized open field locomotion (but not anorexia) after a single stress.[18] The effects of 5-HT$_{1A}$ agonists were also studied because the responses to 5-MeODMT that were increased in association with adaptation largely involve 5-HT$_{1A}$ receptors.[19] It was found that single doses of the 5-HT$_{1A}$ agonists 8-OH-DPAT, buspirone, and ipsapirone (TVXQ 7821) given 2 h after release from restraint significantly normalized open field activity measured on the next day[18] and somewhat opposed the anorexia.[20] However, the two 5-HT reuptake inhibitors and the benzodiazepine anxiolytics chlordiazepoxide and diazepam were inactive when given using the above dose schedule.

The remarkably rapid effects of 5-HT$_{1A}$ agonists on behavioral deficits following stress suggests that some of these drugs could be effective antidepressants. Their attenuation of the effects of stress may involve rapid desensitization of presynaptic 5-HT$_{1A}$ receptors. This hypothesis can be studied using acute hyperphagia, which depends on activation of these receptors.[21] Thus a single large dose of an agonist appears to desensitize them because a second injection 24 h later is markedly less hyperphagic.[22] Desensitization would probably prevent feedback inhibition of 5-HT release, thereby increasing postsynaptic 5-HT function.

Our results as a whole reveal a depression model with psychodynamic, biochemical, and therapeutic analogies to numerous findings on the human illness. Thus, (a) The model (i.e., failure to adapt to repeated stress) is associated with elevated corticosterone levels and female sex. (b) Adaptation is associated with increased response to the 5-HT agonist 5-MeODMT. (c) Both this response and adaptation are enhanced by the corticosterone synthesis inhibitor metyrapone and by chronic treatment with antidepressants. Results also suggest that 5-HT$_{1A}$ agonists may not only be anxiolytic but may also have antidepressant effects probably mediated by different mechanisms and perhaps activated by different dose schedules.

References

1. Kennett GA, Dickinson S, Curzon G. Enhancement of some 5-HT dependent behavioural responses following repeated immobilisation in rats. Brain Res 1985;330:253–263.
2. Willner P. The validity of animal models of depression. Psychopharmacology 1984;83:1–16.
3. Brown T, Bifulco A, Harris OT. Life events, vulnerability and onset of depression: some refinements. Br J Psychiatry 1987;150:30–42.
4. Katz RJ, Roth KA, Carroll BJ. Acute and chronic stress effects on open field activity in the rat: implications for a model of depression. Neurosci Biobehav Rev 1981;5:247–251.
5. Donohoe T, Kennett GA, Curzon G. Immobilisation stress-induced anorexia is not due to gastric ulceration. Life Sci 1987;40:467–472.
6. Brambilla F, Cavagnini F, Invitti C, et al. Neuroendocrine and pseudopathological measures in anorexia nervosa: resemblance to primary affective disorders. Psychiatr Res 1985;16:165–176.
7. Curzon G, Kantamaneni BD, Van Boxel P, et al. Substances related to 5-hydroxytryptamine in plasma and in lumbar and ventricular fluids of psychiatric patients. Acta Psychiatr Scand [Suppl 280] 1980;3–19.
8. Van Praag HM. Neurotransmitters and CNS disease: depression. Lancet 1982;1:1259—1264.
9. Buckett WR, Luscombe GP. Chronic hydrocortisone induces central serotonergic supersensitivity without affecting a behavioural paradigm for depression. Brt J Pharmacol 1984;81:132P.
10. Nausieda PA, Carvey PM, Weiner WJ. Modification of central serotonergic and dopaminergic behaviours in the course of chronic corticosteroid administration. Eur J Pharmacol 1982;78:335–343.
11. Carpenter WT, Gruen PH. Cortisol's effects on human mental functioning. J Clin Psychopharmacol 1982;2:91–101.
12. Dickinson SC, Kennett GA, Curzon G. Reduced 5-hydroxytryptamine dependent behaviour in rats following chronic corticosterone treatment. Brain Res 1985;345:10–18.
13. Kennett GA, Dickinson SL, Curzon G. Central serotonergic responses and behavioural adaptation to repeated immobilisation: the effect of the corticosterone synthesis inhibitor metyrapone. Eur J Pharmacol 1985;119:143–152.
14. Carroll BJ. The dexamethasone suppression test for melancholia. Brt J Psychiatry 1982;140:292–304.
15. Kant GT, Lennox RH, Bunnell BN, et al. Comparison of stress receptors in male and female rats: pituitary cyclic AMP and plasma prolactin, growth hormone and corticosterone. Psychoneuroendocrinology 1983;8:421–428.
16. Weissman MM, Klerman GL. Sex differences and the epidemiology of depression. Arch Gen Psychiatry 1977;34:98–111.
17. Kennett GA, Chaouloff F, Marcou M, et al. Female rats are more vulnerable than males in an animal model of depression: the possible role of serotonin. Brain Res 1986;382:416–421.
18. Kennett GA, Dourish CT, Curzon G. Antidepressant-like action of 5-HT$_{1A}$ agonists and conventional antidepressants in an animal model of depression. Eur J Pharmacol 1987;134:265–274.
19. Tricklebank MD, Forler C, Fozard JR. Subtypes of the 5-HT receptor mediating the behavioural response to 5-methoxy-N,N-dimethyltryptamine in the rat. Eur J Pharmacol 1985;117:15–24.
20. Dourish CT, Kennett GA, Curzon G. The 5-HT$_{1A}$ agonists 8-OH-DPAT, buspirone and ipsapirone attenuate stress-induced anorexia in rats. J Brt Assoc Psychopharmacol 1987;1:23–30.
21. Hutson PH, Dourish CT, Curzon G. Neurochemical and behavioural evidence for mediation of the hyperphagic action of 8-OH-DPAT by 5-HT cell body autoreceptors. Eur J Pharmacol 1986;129:347–352.
22. Kennett GA, Marcou M, Dourish CT, et al. Single administration of 5-HT$_{1A}$ agonists decreases presynaptic, but not postsynaptic receptor-mediated responses. Eur J Pharmacol 1987;138:53–60.

2. Study of Olfactory Bulbectomized Rats: Revelations About Major Depressive Disorder

J. STEVEN RICHARDSON

The idea of using rats to learn about human psychiatric conditions such as major depressive disorder raises many questions and poses several conceptual difficulties. However, on the neuroanatomical and neurochemical levels, the rat brain and the human brain are roughly congruent, and all available evidence indicates that antidepressant drugs act on brain tissue from both species in similar ways. The main problem appears to be that whereas most interaction with major depressive disorder patients is on the verbal level the investigator must interact with the rat in a nonverbal manner.

Traditionally, the study of depression has involved introspection by the depressed person and verbal communication of the depressed person's feelings and thoughts to the therapist or researcher. Although the mood state and cognitive processes of the depressed person are strikingly abnormal, major depressive disorder is considerably more than just unusual feelings and thoughts. Indeed, the verbalization of depressed mood and negative cognitions by a person does not differentiate between the pathological state of a person needing treatment and the accurate account of an individual with an unpleasant existence. Nor are verbal reports alone helpful in predicting if the depressed person will benefit from antidepressant drug therapy. A successful therapeutic response to drugs is generally seen in patients with the behavioral and neurovegetative symptoms of depression. Depressed people with the characteristic sleep disturbance and a loss of interest in food, sex, hobbies, and other usual daily activities have a much better chance of responding to drug therapy than do those with only the mood and cognitive symptoms. This situation suggests that a careful analysis of the depressed patient's nonverbal behavior is at least as important as the patient's introspective reports for identifying and understanding major depressive disorder.

At the present time it appears that the patient with major depressive disorder has some neurochemical abnormality that disrupts the normal activity of the limbic system and produces a syndrome with abnormal behavioral, hormonal, cognitive, and emotional components reflecting this abnormal limbic activity. The hypothesis that major depressive disorder involves a dysregulation of the homeostatic control of neural activity in limbic and related structures[1,2] is supported by an ever growing body of neurochemical and neuroendocrinological data. Numerous mechanisms are involved in maintaining brain neural activity within homeostatic limits. Nerve impulse traffic is regulated by a complex interplay of excitatory and inhibitory neurotransmitters, numerous neuromodulators, a variety of autoreceptors that control the release of the neurotransmitters, and numerous membrane functions such as ion channel regulation, second messenger transduction, and the up- and down-regulation of the receptors for neurotransmitters, neuromodulators, and neurally active hormones. Because an abnormality in any one of these parameters could disrupt the normal function of a given part of the brain, it is not surprising that a single neurochemical cause of major depressive disorder has not been discovered. Theoretically, limbic dysregulation would be produced by disruptions in any one, or more, of these numerous neurochemical factors. Perhaps a detailed analysis of the behavioral differences and similarities between major depressive disorder patients would provide clues for establishing subgroups of depressed patients sharing a single specific neurochemical abnormality, which would in turn provide homogeneous patient populations and a more rational basis for the search for specific neurochemical causes and specific genetic markers. However, regardless of the specific neurochemical defect, the chronic administration of antidepressant drugs appears to return the overall neural activity in the limbic system to the homeostatic range, thereby restoring normal behavior and emotional expression. Because the major depressive disorder patient is characterized by specific behavior patterns and a specific drug response, the analysis of comparable behaviors and drug responses in animals is appropriate and sufficient for providing information relevant to the major depressive disorder patient.

Nevertheless, major depressive disorder is predominantly an emotional one, and analysis of the mechanisms of emotional function is crucial to the understanding of this syndrome. The structures of the limbic system, generally considered to be involved with the creation and expression of emotion, have evolved to a fairly sophisticated level in the rat and seem to be comparable to the same structures in the human. Moreover, it is commonly observed that similar brain structures have analogous functions in different species. Consequently, it is to be expected that the limbic systems of rats and humans should share common functions. By introspection, emotions can be classified as pleasant or unpleasant. On a behavioral level, pleasant emotions are positive reinforcers and increase the frequency of behavior that leads to the pleasant emotional state. On the other hand, unpleasant emotions are negative reinforcers and reduce the frequency of preceding behavior. Thus, the quality of an emotion can be deduced from observable behavior patterns as well as from the verbal report of introspection. In evolutionary terms, emotional states can also be characterized on the basis of survival value. The attainment of a pleasant emotional state and the avoidance of a negative emotional state increase the probability of survival of the organism. Consequently, normal emotional activity increases survival-oriented behavior and reduces behavior that jeopardizes survival. In pathological emotional states such as mania, rage, or depression, the individual has lost contact with reality and acts as though normal reinforcement contingencies are meaningless. Indeed, the depressed person appears to be unable to respond to any form of reinforcement, cannot form or retrieve pleasant memories, and cannot interpret incoming sensory data in terms of survival value. Perhaps not surprisingly, much behavior in these pathological states seems to be with total disregard of survival. However, this line of reasoning suggests a rather unusual conclusion. If emotional mechanisms evolved by increasing the probability of survival of the organism by creating and directing memory storage and learning, rein-forcing survival oriented behavior, and attaching survival value to incoming sensory data, is the converse also true? Does behavior lacking survival value also lack emotion? Perhaps new insight could be gained by considering major depressive disorder as a condition lacking emotion rather than a condition of extreme emotion. Perhaps in major depressive disorder the neural substrates of emotion are disrupted and the individual is forced to exist without the benefit of emotional reactivity rather than the traditional view of the depressed person as being driven by excessive emotion. Antidepressant drug therapy restores normal neural activity in the emotion pathways, restores normal emotional function, and restores survival-oriented be-havior. Although the validity and usefulness of this novel conceptual framework for viewing major depressive disorder can be established only by future research, at the present time the evidence is consistent with the major depressive disorder patient having some dysregulation of the limbic system and related brain areas that results in pathological behaviors that are normalized specifically by the chronic administration of antidepressant drugs.

Removing the olfactory bulbs in the rat causes a dysregulation of neural activity in the limbic system[3,4] and produces abnormal behaviors that are normalized spe-cifically by the chronic administration of antidepressant drugs.[5-7] This remarkable pharmacological similarity between patients with major depressive disorder and rats with olfactory bulbectomy does not necessarily mean that there is neuro-chemical and neuroanatomical congruence or that the drugs are working on similar substrates in these two conditions. However, it does suggest that the bulbectomized rat might be a fertile model in which to evaluate hypotheses concerning major depressive disorder. To be testable in bulbectomized rats, these hypotheses cannot involve verbalization or introspection but, rather, must be based on observable behavior patterns. In addition to providing hypotheses to test in bulbectomized rats, the analysis of the nonverbal behavior of major depressive disorder patients might provide clues that could be used to improve the accuracy of diagnosis, the predictability of drug selection, and the homogeneity of subgroups of major de-pressive disorder patients for neurochemical and genetic analyses. At the very least, the bulbectomized rat could contribute to the study of major depressive disorder by requiring a fresh approach to depressed patients that would have ben-efits in other areas of depression research. Although it is unlikely that the neural dysfunction in the bulbectomized rat is exactly the same as in the major depressive disorder patient, there are compelling pharmacological parallels, and there may be some neurochemical similarities as well. The olfactory bulbectomized rat ap-pears to be a sensitive and specific, but time-consuming and labor-intensive, screening system for the preclinical evaluation of new compounds for potential antidepressant properties. As reported so far in the literature, the olfactory bul-bectomized rat has made only two errors in identifying drugs with antidepressant properties in humans. The monoamine oxidase inhibitor tranylcypromine screens as a false negative, and the antispasmodic γ-aminobutyric acid (GABA) agonist baclofen screens as a false positive.[8] The neurochemical analysis of specific brain regions in bulbectomized rats could provide hypotheses that can be tested in major depressive disorder patients by neuroendocrine challenge tests or in postmortem studies. Although there is no evidence of brain lesions or selective brain cell death in major depressive disorder patients, as reviewed elsewhere,[9] a high percentage of stroke patients, particularly those with cell loss in the anterior cortex, develop a syndrome that is nearly identical to major depressive disorder in terms of presenting symptoms and specific response to chronic antidepressant drug treatment. Thus there are numerous interesting parallels between olfactory bulbectomized rats, stroke patients, and patients with major depressive disorder.

In summary, the study of the olfactory bulbectomized rat can contribute to the study of major depressive disorder by identifying potential antidepressant drugs; providing behavioral, neurochemical, and neuroanatomical hypotheses for evaluation in major depressive disorder patients; and encouraging a more detailed and rigorous analysis of the behavioral profiles of depressed people.

References

1. Richardson JS. Neurochemical psychiatry as a source of hypotheses concerning the role of homeostatic mechanisms in brain function. Int J Neurosci 1984;24:197–202.
2. Siever LJ, Davis KL. Overview: toward a dysregulation hypothesis of depression. Am J Psychiatry 1985;142:1017–1031.
3. Cain DP. The role of the olfactory bulb in limbic mechanisms. Psychol Bull 1974;81:654–671.
4. Jesberger JA, Richardson JS. Brain output dysregulation induced by olfactory bulbectomy: an approximation in the rat of major depressive disorder in humans? Int J Neurosci 1988;38:241–265.
5. Cairncross KD, Cox B, Forster C, et al. Olfactory projection systems, drugs and behavior: a review. Psychoneuroendocrinology 1979;4:253–272.
6. Leonard BE, Tuite M. Anatomical, physiological and behavioral aspects of olfactory bulbectomy in the rat. Int Rev Neurobiol 1981;22:251–286.
7. Jesberger JA, Richardson JS. Effects of antidepressant drugs on the behavior of olfactory bulbectomized and sham-operated rats. Behav Neurosci 1986;100:256–274.
8. Leonard BE. The olfactory bulbectomized rat as a model of depression. Pol J Pharmacol Pharm 1984;36:561–569.
9. Richardson JS, Jesberger JA. Models for the experimental analysis of depression. Acta Psychiatr Belg 1986;86:733–747.

3. Bilaterally Olfactory Bulbectomized Rat Model of Depression

B.E. LEONARD, J. BUTLER, B. O'NEILL, AND W.T. O'CONNOR

In the rat the integrity of the olfactory system is necessary for the normal functioning of the limbic system; disruption of the olfactory system results in behavioral abnormalities that are unrelated to a deficit in olfaction.[1] There is evidence that lesions of the olfactory bulbs result in degeneration of limbic and nonlimbic regions that receive afferent projections from the bulbs. Such changes could be responsible for the specific behavioral effects as a consequence of the changes in the response of the animal to external and internal stimuli. Changes in social behaviors (e.g., increased aggression, territorial activity, and increased irritability), sexual behavior (e.g., maternal and mating behaviors), and such nonsocial behaviors as exploratory activity and passive avoidance learning have been reported to occur in rats following bulbectomy. These behavioral deficits have been reviewed by Leonard and Tuite.[2] Of the nonsocial behaviors that are disrupted following bulbectomy, active avoidance performance is largely facilitated, whereas passive avoidance shows behavioral deficits.[3,4] Anosmia, caused by the irrigation of the olfactory mucosa with zinc sulfate solution, does not cause any of the behavioral deficits reported to occur following bilateral bulbectomy.[5]

When the multitude of behavioral changes that occur following bulbectomy are considered, it is tempting to speculate that they bear similarities with the major symptoms found in the depressed patient. Thus disturbances of the sleep pattern, particularly the rapid eye movement (REM) phase, and food intake are frequently associated with the symptoms of endogenous depression; changes in these parameters have also been reported in the bulbectomized rat.[6,7] Anhedonia is also a common feature of the depressed patient. Cain[1] has suggested that the disruptive effects of bulbectomy on behavior are at least partially attributable to a lesion of arousal system II of Routtenberg,[8] which has been associated with incentive and reward. Thus it may be concluded that at least some of the principal behavioral changes appear to be common to both the bulbectomized rat and the depressed patient.

In addition to such similarities, it is also apparent that the functional activity of biogenic amine neurotransmitters in the limbic regions of the brain (e.g., amygdaloid cortex) is abnormal following bulbectomy. Thus Jancsár and Leonard[9] showed that the turnover of norepinephrine and serotonin in this region of the rat brain was significantly reduced following bulbectomy and the density of β-adrenoceptors was increased. Despite the controversy regarding the relevance of changes in norepinephrine, serotonin, and their metabolites in body fluids of depressed patients to the etiology of the illness,[10] it is nevertheless widely assumed that depression is associated with a defect in the functional activity of these amines. It may therefore be concluded that the bulbectomized rat resembles the depressed patient in terms of the behavioral and biochemical changes that result from unknown pathological/genetic causes or from surgical lesions.

Perhaps the most convincing evidence for the view that the bulbectomized rat has behavioral features in common with the depressed patient arises from the effects of chronic drug treatment. Cairncross and co-workers[11] clearly demonstrated that many of the behavioral deficits shown by the bulbectomized rat could be largely counteracted by the chronic administration of therapeutically effective antidepressants but not by psychotropic drugs that lack such clinical activity. From the initial studies of Cairncross and other investigators,[2,11] it appears that antidepressant drugs normalize deficits in passive avoidance behavior irrespective of the presumed mode of action of the antidepressant on central neurotransmission. We have extended such studies to show that antidepressants affecting the noradrenergic, serotonergic, dopaminergic, γ-aminobutyric acid (GABA)ergic,[12] and other (? peptidergic) systems can be detected using the bulbectomy model of depression. In addition, the time of onset of the behavioral response to antidepressant treatment approximately coincides with that found in humans. Thus the ability of the novel tetracyclic antidepressant mianserin to attentuate the hyperactivity of the bulbectomized rat in the "open field" apparatus requires that the drug be administered for approximately 7 days, an optimal response to treatment becoming apparent only after 14 days of administration. Furthermore, the activity of the individual isomers of antidepressants that exist in enantiomeric forms may be evaluated using the bulbectomized rat model.[13,14]

The effects of different classes of antidepressants and other drugs with effects on various neurotransmitter systems in the central nervous system (CNS) are summarized in Table 3.1. It is of interest that monoamine oxidase inhibitors, lofepramine, fluvoxamine, and rolipram do not appear to be active in the bulbectomized model. Earley (unpublished data) has shown that REM sleep deprivation is associated with an attenuation of hyperactivity in the "open field" (i.e., an antidepressant effect).

In addition to the behavioral and physiological changes and effects of antidepressants that appear to be similar in both the depressed patient and the bulbectomized rat, studies have indicated that changes in serotonin transport into the platelet and the phagocytic activity of neutrophils are similar in the depressed patient and the rodent model of depression. Studies undertaken here[15,16] and elsewhere[17] have shown that the uptake of [3H]serotonin into platelets from depressed patients is decreased. However, following effective treatment with any class of antidepressant (i.e., drugs that may or may not affect the transport of serotonin) or with electroconvulsive therapy (ECT), the [3H]serotonin transport returns to control values. Patients failing to respond to therapy persist in showing the defect in serotonin uptake. Studies have shown that platelets from the bulbectomized rat show defects in serotonin transport similar to those seen in the depressed patient.[18] Following chronic treatment with either sertraline, a specific serotonin uptake inhibitor, or desipramine, which is presumed to show selectivity

TABLE 3.1. Effects of various antidepressants and other centrally acting drugs on the behavior of bulbectomized rats in the "open field" apparatus.

Drug	Activity	Drug	Activity
Antidepressants		Novel or putative antidepressants	
Desipramine	+	Progabide	+
Imipramine	+	Sulpiride	+
Lofepramine[a]	−	ε-Flupenthixol	+
Nomifensine	+	Alprazolam	+
Mianserin		Adinazolam	+
Isomers (±)	+	Salbutamol	+
Isomers (+)	+	Fluvoxamine	−
Isomers (−)	−	Sertraline	+
Mianserin metabolites		Other compounds	
Desmethylmianserin	−	γ-Vinyl GABA	+
8-Hydroxymianserin	−	Baclofen	+
Mepirzepine (Org. 3770)	−	Diazepam	−
Isomers (±)	+	Reserpine	−
Isomers (+)	+	Clonidine	−
Isomers (−)	−	Yohimbine	+
		Methysergide	+
		Phenobarbitone	−
		Atropine	−

[a]High doses of lofepramine (30 mg/kg i.p.) are active. At this dose it seems probable that the activity is due to the major metabolite, desipramine, rather than the parent compound.
+ = active, − = inactive.

for the norepinephrine transport site, the uptake of [^{3}H]serotonin was normalized. This change paralleled the attenuation of the hypermotility of the bulbectomized rat when placed in the "open field."

In addition to the changes in platelet function, which are corrected by antidepressant treatment, O'Neill et al.[19] have shown that bulbectomy is associated with suppression of neutrophil phagocytosis, which returns to control values following chronic desipramine treatment. Previous studies have shown that neutrophil function was subnormal in depressed patients but returned to normal following effective treatment with mianserin.[20] It therefore appears that abnormalities in some immune functions, in addition to neurotransmitter activities, are similar in depressed patients and the bulbectomized rat.

It may be concluded that the olfactory bulbectomized rat resembles the depressed patient: (a) in response to antidepressant treatment; (b) in behavioral and physiological changes; (c) in terms of defects in central and peripheral neurotransmitter function; and (d) in some immunological functions. It therefore appears that the bulbectomized rat is a relevant animal model for depression in addition to being a useful model for the detection of antidepressants.

Acknowledgments. The authors thank the MRCI for financial support. We also thank Pfizer, U.K., Merck, U.K., and Organon International B.V., Holland, for supplying many of the drugs used in these studies and for financial assistance toward the cost of these projects.

References

1. Cain DP. The role of the olfactory bulb in limbic mechanisms. Psychol Bull 1974;81:654–671.
2. Leonard BE, Tuite M. Anatomical, physiological and behavioural aspects of olfactory bulbectomy in the rat. Int Rev Neurobiol 1981;22:251–286.
3. Marks HE, Remley NR, Seago, JD, et al. Effects of bilateral lesions of the olfactory bulb of rats as measures of learning and motivation. Physiol Behav 1971;7:1–6.
4. Sieck MH, Gordon BL. Selective olfactory bulb lesions, reactivity changes and avoidance learning in rats. Physiol Behav 1973;9:545–552.
5. Sieck MH. Selective olfactory lesions in rats and changes in appetite and aversive behaviour. Physiol Behav 1973;10:705–710.
6. La Rue DG, Le Magneu J. The olfactory control of meal patterns in rats. Physiol Behav 1972;9:817–821.
7. Sakurada, J, Shima K, Jadano I, et al. Sleep wakefulness rhythms in olfactory bulb lesioned rats. Jpn J Pharmacol 1976;26:605–610.
8. Routtenberg A. The two-arousal hypothesis: reticular formation and limbic system. Psychol Rev 1968;75:51–80.
9. Jancsár SM, Leonard BE. Changes in neurotransmitter metabolism following olfactory bulbectomy in the rat. Prog Neuropsychopharmacol Biol Psychiatry 1984;263–269.
10. Leonard BE. Neurotransmitter receptors, endocrine responses, and the biological substrates of depression: review. Hum Psychopharmacol 1986;3–21.
11. Cairncross KD, Cox B, Forster C, et al. Olfactory projection systems, drugs and behaviour: a review. Psychoneuroendocrinology 1979;4:253–272.
12. Lloyd KG, Morselli, PL Depoortere H, et al. The potential use of GABA agonists in psychiatric disorders: evidence from studies with progabide in animal models and clinical trials. Pharmacol Biochem Behav 1985;18:957–966.
13. Jancsár S, Leonard BE. The effect of the racemates of mianserin and its enantiomers on the behavioural hyperactivity of the olfactory bulbectomized rat. Neuropharmacology 1985;23:1065–1070.
14. O'Connor WT, Leonard BE. Effect of chronic administration of the 6-aza analogue of mianserin (Org. 3770) and its enantiomers on behaviour and changes in noradrenaline metabolism of olfactory bulbectomized rats in the ''open field'' apparatus. Neuropharmacology 1986;25:267–270.
15. Healy D, Carney PA, O'Halloran A, et al. Peripheral adrenoceptors and serotonin receptors in depression: changes associated with response to treatment with trazodone or amitriptyline. J Affective Disord 1985;9:285–296.
16. Butler J, Leonard BE. Post-partum depression and the effects of nomifensine treatment. Int Clin Psychopharmacol 1986;1:244–252.
17. Coppen A, Wood KM. Platelet 5-hydroxytryptamine uptake in depressive illness. Acta Psychiatr Scand [Suppl 280] 1980;21–28.
18. Butler J, Leonard BE. The effects of a novel serotonin uptake inhibitor on the behaviour and the serotonergic system of the olfactory bulbectomized rat model of depression. In: Proceedings of the British Association of Psychopharmacology, Cambridge, August 1986.
19. O'Neill B, O'Connor WT, Leonard BE. Is there an abnormality in neutrophil phagocytosis in depression? IRCS Med Sci 1986;802–803.
20. O'Neill B, Leonard BE, O'Connor WT. Depressed neutrophil phagocytosis in the rat following olfactory bulbectomy reversed by chronic desipramine treatment. IRCS Med Sci 1987;15:267–268.

4. Behavioral Despair: Past and Future

ROGER D. PORSOLT

"Behavioral despair" is the term that has been applied to the recognizable immobile posture observed in rats or mice forced to swim in a restricted space from which there is no escape.[1] The phenomenon was first observed during experiments with a water maze. Rats placed at one end of a water maze generally found the exit within less than a minute. Some rats, however, after swimming around for a few minutes did not find the exit and remained immobile in the water, making only those movements necessary to keep their heads above water. Intuitively it seemed that for these rats the situation was insoluble and that they had simply given up hope ("behavioral despair"). The behavior was conceptually similar to the "learned helplessness" that can be induced in some animals exposed to inescapable aversive stimulation, and parallels could also be drawn with the "protest–despair" reactions described in young primates separated from their mothers or their peers. In any case, it was predicted that the characteristic behavior would be reduced by anti-depressant treatments.

Pharmacology of Behavioral Despair

During the time since the model was first described the test procedure and variants of it have been subjected to testing in many laboratories. The general conclusion from these studies is that most known clinically active antidepressant treatments, particularly after repeated treatment, reduce the duration of immobility in rats or mice forced to swim for a few minutes.[1-4] The list of active compounds includes many so-called atypical compounds (mianserin, iprindole, rolipram, idazoxan), which are not readily detected using classical pharmacological tests. The findings with these compounds are important, as they suggest that this behavioral model may be capable of detecting antidepressants acting by mechanisms other than those of traditional agents. An important false negative is constituted by the 5-hydroxytryptamine (serotonin, 5-HT) uptake inhibitors, which although clinically active show little or no activity in the behavioral despair test, particularly in the rat. The test has often been criticized for the presence of false positives, including several psychostimulants, anticholinergics, and antihistamines. False positives represent a less serious limitation as they can usually be eliminated using additional tests; furthermore, the absence of clinical efficacy of some potential false positives (e.g., anticholinergics) cannot be regarded as proven. Other compounds such as neuroleptics and anxiolytics are not active or even enhance immobility, with the exception of some atypical compounds (e.g., *t*-chlorprothixene, clozapine, sulpiride, carpipramine) whose clinical profiles are also mixed. Further validation is provided by the findings that nonpharmacological antidepressant treatments such as electroshock and rapid eye movement (REM) sleep deprivation also reduce immobility and the fact that repeated (in contrast to single) drug administrations are more effective in reducing immobility, an effect unrelated to brain concentrations of the drug.[5]

Other pharmacological studies[1-3] indicate that behavioral despair is mediated primarily by central catecholamine systems; increasing central catecholamine activity decreases immobility, whereas immobility is enhanced by agents that decrease central catecholamine transmission. Conflicting or opposite findings have been reported after manipulation of central serotonin. A role for central γ-aminobutyric acid (GABA) is also suggested by the findings that immobility is enhanced by agents that facilitate GABAergic transmission and decreased by GABAergic blockers at least in subconvulsive doses.[6] These pharmacological findings are corroborated by direct neurochemical investigations[7] and by studies where specific brain regions rich in either catecholamines or indoleamines are subjected to stimulation or lesion. For example, electrical stimulation of the locus ceruleus mimicked the effect of desipramine,[8] whereas catecholaminergic but not serotonergic lesions of the amygdala abolished desipramine effects.[9]

New Directions

Available pharmacological evidence suggests that the behavioral despair test is a useful model for detecting antidepressant effects of novel compounds. A variant of the test where escape-directed activity is measured automatically by wheel-turning has been proposed for eliminating false positives such as psychostimulants and anticholinergics.[10] More interestingly, another procedure, where immobility is induced by suspending rodents by the tail,[11] avoids the marked hypothermia caused by forced swimming and furthermore is sensitive to a wide range of antidepressants, including serotonin uptake inhibitors, which represented an important false negative for the traditional behavior despair test (Fig. 4.1). The tail suspension test, which is automated, offers promise therefore of a rapid, sensitive procedure for evaluating novel compounds.

The model could also be further exploited for investigating regionally specific neurochemical changes accompanying induced immobility and antidepressant treatment. One study[12] has indicated that combined forced swimming and antidepressant treatment is more effective in inducing β down-regulation in rat forebrain but not striatum than either treatment alone, suggesting the value of studying these phenomena in an animal model of induced psychopathology.

Another direction that has not been exploited is the possibility of selectively breeding animals that show a greater propensity for developing immobility. Important strain differences have been shown to exist in both the swimming model[13] and the tail suspension procedure (unpublished data), with some strains showing greater reactivity to certain categories of drugs. Demonstration of a genetic factor

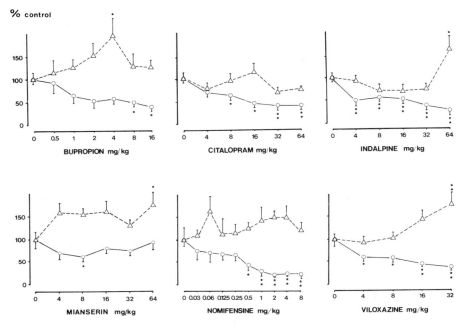

FIGURE 4.1. Effects of six atypical antidepressants on the duration of immobility (o–o) and the power of movements (△---△) in the automated tail suspension test.[11] Compounds were administered intraperitoneally 30 min before a 6-min test. Mean differences from control were evaluated using the Dunnett test (*$p < 0.05$; **$p < 0.01$). Note the significant immobility reducing effects of citalopram and indalpine, specific inhibitors of serotonin uptake. [Reprinted with permission from ref. 11, Copyright 1987, Pergamon Press plc.]

would provide an important argument against the criticism that behavioral despair is a model only of reactive depression.

In general, however, it should be clear that any one rodent model must represent a gross oversimplification of the complexities of human depressive illness. The usefulness of such a model must therefore crucially depend on its capacity to provide new insights into the neurobiology of affective disorder or to detect new drugs for use in therapeutics.

References

1. Porsolt RD. Behavioral despair. In Enna SJ, Malick JB, Richelson E (eds): Antidepressants: Neurochemical, Behavioral and Clinical Perspectives. New York: Raven Press, 1981;121–139.
2. Porsolt RD. Animal models of affective disorders. In Dewhurst WG, Baker GB (eds): Pharmacotherapy of Affective Disorders: Theory and Practice. New York: Croom Helm, 1985;108–150.
3. Kulkarni SK, Parale MP. Despair behaviour: a tool in experimental psychopharmacology: a review. Methods Find. Exp. Clin. Pharmacol 1986;8:741–744.
4. Willner P. The validity of animal models of depression. Psychopharmacology 1984;83:1–16.

5. Poncelet M, Gaudel G, Danti S, et al. Acute versus repeated administration of desipramine in rats and mice: relationships between brain concentrations and reduction of immobility in the swimming test. Psychopharmacology 1986;90:139–141.
6. Nagatani T, Sugihara T, Kodaira R. The effect of diazepam and of agents which change GABAergic functions on immobility in mice. Eur J Pharmacol 1984;97:271–276.
7. Weiss JM, Simson PG. Depression in an animal model: focus on the locus ceruleus. In Porter R, Bock G, Clark S (eds): Antidepressants and Receptor Function. Ciba Foundation Symposium 123. Chichester: Wiley, 1986;191–209.
8. Plaznik A, Danysz W, Kostowski W. Mesolimbic noradrenaline but not dopamine is responsible for organization of rat behavior in the forced swim test and an anti-immobilizing effect of desipramine. Pol J Pharmacol Pharm, 1985;37:347–357.
9. Araki H, Kawashima K, Uchiyama Y, et al. Involvement of amygdaloid catecholaminergic mechanism in suppressive effects of desipramine and imipramine on duration of immobility in rats forced to swim. Eur J Pharmacol 1985;113:313–318.
10. Nomura S, Shimizu J, Kinjo M, et al. A new behavioral test for antidepressant drugs. Eur J Pharmacol 1982;83:171–175.
11. Stéru L, Chermat R, Thierry B, et al. The automated tail suspension test: a computerized device which differentiates psychotropic drugs. Prog Neuropsychopharmacol Biol Psychiatry 1987;11:659–671.
12. Duncan GE, Paul I, Harden TK, et al. Rapid down regulation of beta adrenergic receptors by combining antidepressant drugs with forced swim: a model of antidepressant-induced neural adaptation. J Pharmacol Exp Ther 1985;234:402–408.
13. Porsolt RD, Bertin A, Jalfre M. Behavioural despair in rats and mice: strain differences and the effects of imipramine. Eur J Pharmacol 1978;51:291–294.

5. Genetically Nervous and Normal Pointer Dogs: Relation Between Hearing and Behavioral Abnormalities

EHUD KLEIN AND THOMAS W. UHDE

Genetically nervous pointer dogs have been characterized in earlier works as an animal model for pathological anxiety.[1-3] Individual differences in fearfulness were initially used to create two lines of pointer dogs.[4,5] These lines have been maintained now for more than 20 years with continuous selection for the most fearful dogs in the nervous line and for the least fearful dogs in the normal line. Each line originated from a single male–female pair of each type. The behavioral traits of both fearfulness and normality have bred essentially true since the first generation.[2] The nervous dogs begin to demonstrate from the age of 3–9 months a highly characteristic and reproducible pattern of fear-related behaviors to certain exogenous stimuli.[6] In the absence of such stimuli, these dogs do not appear to be markedly different from the normal dogs: they move freely, play with other dogs, breed as well as the normal dogs, and adequately rear their pups or foster pups from the normal line.[1] In contrast to these normal behaviors, exposure to humans, a sudden blast of a loud noise, and certain other stimuli elicit a dramatic expression of fear-related behaviors such as excessive timidity, hyperstartle, reduced exploratory activity, marked avoidance of the human observer, catatonic freezing cardiovascular changes, urination, and defecation.[1,2] The normal dogs behave differently under those conditions as evidenced by friendly play with humans. They are active and inquisitive and comply without protest to experimental tasks,[1,3] and despite such tasks they continue to approach man in a friendly fashion.[1,3] The phenotypic expression of the nervous behavior in these dogs is not prevented by cross-rearing or by extra home-rearing, which produces only temporary changes compared to kennel rearing.[7] Studies done in our group with these dogs included the evaluation of a hearing deficit and its relation to the abnormal behavior.

Evaluation of Deafness and Abnormal Behaviors

In the course of our work with these dogs, the existence of a hearing deficit was suspected. Obviously such a deficit could contribute to or largely determine this abnormal behavior. We thus decided to evaluate the hearing status of both nervous and normal dogs using the brainstem auditory evoked response (BAER) technique that has been applied to dogs[8] and further assess the relation between a possible hearing deficit and the abnormal behavior.

Twenty-seven anxious (10 male, 17 female) and 16 control (8 male, 8 female) dogs were selected from our colony for hearing assessment. The same dogs were later rated blindly using three rating scales: (a) The dog morbidity scale described by Murphree and Dykman.[9] (b) A rating scale developed in our laboratory that covers a wide range of behaviors in these dogs under stressful (e.g., presence of a human) and nonstressful conditions. Behaviors that were rated included exploration, tail wagging, immobilization, tremor, urination, and defecation. (c) A global subjective rating of the dogs' degree of abnormality in each condition.

Results of Hearing and Behavioral Testing

Of 16 normal dogs tested, all showed normal responses bilaterally. Figure 5.1A shows a characteristic BAER recording from a hearing dog. In contrast, the testing in the "nervous" dogs revealed that 20 of 27 dogs had no brainstem evoked response in either ear. The remaining seven dogs had normal responses. Figure 5.1B shows a characteristic BAER recording from a deaf dog where no response was obtained. Examination of the pedigree revealed that one female and six of her nine progeny in one litter accounted for all of the hearing "nervous" dogs.

The analysis of the behavioral ratings revealed a highly significant difference

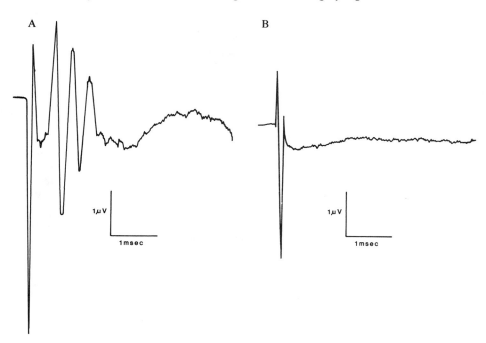

FIGURE 5.1. Characteristic brainstem auditory evoked responses.
A. Recording from a hearing dog.
B. Recording from a deaf dog.

TABLE 5.1. Results of the behavioral ratings in normal, deaf nervous, and nondeaf nervous dogs obtained with three rating scales.

Rating	Mean scores			ANOVA		Post HOC tests ($p \leqslant$)		
	Control dogs	Deaf nervous dogs	Nondeaf nervous dogs	F DF 2/28	$p \leqslant$	Control dogs vs. deaf nervous dogs	Control dogs vs. nondeaf nervous dogs	Deaf vs. nondeaf nervous dogs
Dog morbidity scale								
Weighted activity	2.0±0.9	3.8±1.0	4.6±0.5	13.23	0.0001	0.0003	0.0001	0.09
Weighted nervousness	3.2±1.8	4.3±1.1	4.0±0.6	1.92	NS	NS	NS	NS
Morbidity score	6.7±2.4	11.9±9.4	13.1±1.2	16.30	0.0001	0.0001	0.0001	0.22
Dog rating scale								
Dog alone	1.7±3.0	−1.4±2.4	−2.6±2.6	4.62	0.018	0.018	0.007	0.34
Human sitting	6.0±6.2	−3.1±1.6	−3.6±2.9	20.84	0.0001	0.0001	0.0001	0.96
Human calling	3.3±6.0	−3.5±1.6	−3.7±0.9	16.24	0.0001	0.0001	0.0001	0.96
Human approaching	1.7±6.5	−3.8±1.6	−3.6±2.3	7.42	0.003	0.0008	0.0006	0.79
Total	12.7±20.1	−11.8±5.7	−13.4±8.1	15.23	0.0001	0.0001	0.0001	0.82
Global rating								
Dog alone	2.7±1.4	6.7±1.7	7.7±0.9	20.84	0.0001	0.0001	0.0001	0.15
Human sitting	3.8±2.1	7.7±1.2	8.1±0.7	22.0	0.0001	0.0001	0.0001	0.55
Human calling	4.3±2.3	8.1±0.9	8.3±0.5	23.43	0.0001	0.0001	0.0001	0.83
Human approaching	5.2±2.5	8.2±0.8	8.4±0.5	15.3	0.0001	0.0001	0.0001	0.79
Total	16.0±8.1	30.7±4.3	32.6±2.5	24.38	0.0001	0.0001	0.0001	0.46

between nervous and normal dogs on almost all behavioral ratings and no differences between deaf and nondeaf dogs within the nervous group. Table 5.1 summarizes the results obtained from the analysis of all components of the rating scales.

Relation Between Hearing Deficit and Behavioral Abnormality

The BAER results provide evidence that 20 of 27 (74%) "nervous" dogs and none of the normal dogs had a bilateral hearing loss. Interestingly, earlier work had found loud noise (100-dB horn blast) to provoke the characteristic fear-related behaviors in the nervous dogs.[6] The possibility of a very high hearing threshold, above the intensity we employed in the BAER tests, thus cannot be ruled out. It is also possible that deafness appeared sometime later in the breeding of the colony after these earlier studies had already been completed.

The available data are insufficient to draw any firm conclusions about the mode of inheritance of the deafness trait; it can only be assumed that because there is male-to-male transmission of the deafness, the trait is not X-linked but could be autosomal dominant or recessive.

The results of the behavioral ratings, on the other hand, show that regardless of the hearing status there is a robust difference between nervous and normal dogs, as has been shown repeatedly in earlier studies,[2] whereas deaf and nondeaf nervous dogs do not differ significantly on any of the ratings. These results thus support a conclusion that hearing status does not affect the behavioral outcome in these dogs and that these traits are not causatively related, although genetic linkage between the behavioral abnormality and the deafness might be expected.

These findings underscore an issue that is well known to those working with genetic animal models, i.e., that breeding of animals for a particular genetic trait (e.g., nervousness) is often associated with the emergence of other less desirable traits (e.g., deafness). Such traits, when they emerge, need to be evaluated as to their causal relation and genetic linkage to the trait of interest.

References

1. Reese WG. Familial vulnerability for experimental neurosis. Pavlov J Biol Sci 1978;13:169–173.
2. Lucas LA, DeLuca DC, Newton JEO, et al. The nervous pointer dog in genetic research strategies for psychobiology and psychiatry. In Gershon ES, et al (eds): Animal Models for Human Psychopathology. Pacific Grove: Boxwood Press, 1981.
3. Angel C, DeLuca DC, Newton JEO, et al. Assessment of pointer dog behavior, drug effects and neurochemical correlates. Pavlov J Biol Sci 1982;17:84–88.
4. Murphree OD, Peters J, Dykman R. Behavioral comparisons of nervous, stable and crossbred pointers at ages 2, 3, 6, 9 and 12 months. Cond Reflex 1969;4:20–23.
5. Brown CJ, Murphree OD, Newton JEO. The effect of inbreeding on human aversion in pointer dogs. J Hered 1978;69:362–365.
6. Murphree OD, Angel C, DeLuca DC, et al. Nervous dogs: a partial model for psychiatric research. Lab Anims 1974;3:16–19.
7. Murphree OD, Angel C, DeLuca DC, et al. Longitudinal studies of genetically nervous dogs. Biol Psychiatry 1977;12:573–576.
8. Morgan JL, Coulter DB, Marshall AE, et al. Effects of neomycin on waveform of auditory-evoked brain stem potentials in dogs. Am J Vet Res 1980;41:1077–1081.
9. Murphree OD, Dykman RA. Litter patterns in the offsprings of nervous and stable dogs. I. Behavioral tests. J Nerv Ment Dis 1965;141:321–332.

6. Agonist-Induced Down-Regulation of β_1-Adrenergic Receptors: Possible Biochemical Rationale for Novel Antidepressants

S.M. STAHL

Changes in the linkage between the serotonergic and noradrenergic neuronal systems at the level of the norepinephrine (NE) receptor coupled adenylate cyclase is currently the favored hypothesis to explain the mechanism of action of antidepressant drugs. In particular, the down-regulation of β-adrenoceptors (βARs), which is associated with a subsensitivity of the receptor-coupled adenylate cyclase, has been postulated as a marker of antidepressant efficacy as the time course for this action corresponds closely with the onset of clinical therapeutic effects. It has also been proposed that centrally acting βAR agonists, which interact directly with the receptor, could down-regulate βARs in the brain more quickly than classical antidepressants and would therefore cause rapid-onset antidepressant effects in patients.

In order to explore this hypothesis, investigators have attempted to demonstrate rapid-onset down-regulation of central nervous system β-receptors by βAR agonists and a rapid-onset antidepressant effect in patients. In fact, long-term exposure to βAR agonists does lead to an attenuation of tissue responsiveness to β-adrenergic stimulation due to decreased receptor density and/or to diminished adenylate cyclase activity.[1] In particular, clenbuterol and salbutamol are claimed to possess fast-acting antidepressant properties.

In our laboratory we have been interested not only in the time course of βAR regulation but also in determining which, if either, of the βAR subtypes is preferentially down-regulated by classical antidepressants and by potential fast-acting "βAR agonists type antidepressants."

In this study in rats, the effects of chronic dosing with the βAR agonists clenbuterol and prenalterol were compared with those of the tricyclic desipramine. The drugs or vehicle were administered subcutaneously to male Sprague-Dawley rats at a rate of 20 mg/kg/day using osmotic Alzet pumps. The pumps were removed after 8 days, and the rats were killed 24 h later. The total βAR population was determined, in cerebral cortex, by saturation analysis on crude synaptosomal membrane preparations. The chosen radioligand was $(-)[^{125}I]$pindolol (20–800pm) and $(-)$isoprenaline (200 μM) was used to define nonspecific binding. The addition of the highly selective β_1-adrenoceptor antagonist CGP 20712A (100 nM) to the assay medium converted the heterogeneous populations of βAR populations to essentially homogeneous β_2-adrenoceptor populations. They were then available for measurement with $(-)[^{125}I]$pindolol. The remaining β_1-adrenoceptor population was then estimated by subtraction.

Using these techniques we have been able to confirm that desipramine is a selective down-regulator of β_1-adrenoceptors, by 40% in cerebral cortex (Fig. 6.1; Table 6.1). This finding was previously suggested by Minneman et al.,[2] who employed the β_1-adrenoceptor selective agonist zinterol in displacement-type binding studies; by Dooley et al.,[1] who used various tissue types; and by Kitada et al.,[3] who conducted behavioral studies. Hence any potential fast-acting "βAR agonist

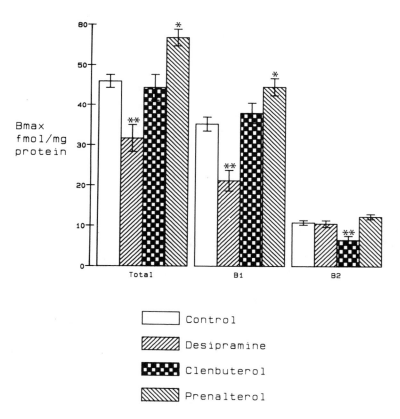

FIGURE 6.1. Effects of 8 days of treatment with vehicle ($n = 9$), desipramine ($n = 7$), clenbuterol ($n = 7$), or prenalterol ($n = 6$) on the maximal binding capacity of $(-)-[^{125}I]$pindolol to total β_1-adrenoceptors, and β_2-adrenoceptors in rat cerebral cortex. Each column represents the mean value, and the vertical lines show SEMs. Significantly different from control: **$p < 0.01$; *$p \le 0.05$.

TABLE 6.1. Effects of treatments on the maximal binding capacities and the dissociation constants for $(-)-[^{-125}I]$pindolol binding to rat cerebral cortex.

Treatment	Control (n = 9)	Desipramine 20 mg/kg/day (n = 7)	Clenbuterol 20 mg/kg/ day (n = 7)	Prenalterol 20 mg/kg/ day (n = 6)
Total				
Bmax (fmol/mg)	45.9 ± 1.6	31.6 ± 3.3[a]	44.3 ± 3.2	56.8 ± 2.1[b]
Kd (pM)	250 ± 14.7	210 ± 12.3	372 ± 14.7[a]	267 ± 18.3
β_1				
Bmax (fmol/mg)	35.1 ± 1.7	21.1 ± 2.5[a]	37.8 ± 2.6	43.5 ± 2.1[b]
Kd (pM)	—	—	—	—
β_2				
Bmax (fmol/mg)	10.7 ± 0.6	10.5 ± 0.8	6.5 ± 1.0 [a]	12.3 ± 0.7
Kd (pM)	118 ± 9.5	124 ± 8.7	266 ± 33.4[a]	116 ± 9.7

Results are given as the means ± SEM.
[a]$p \leq 0.01$.
[b]$p < 0.05$.

type antidepressant'' would have to mimic this action if it is a primary antidepressant action of desipramine.

The βAR agonists clenbuterol and prenalterol were chosen for comparison with desipramine in this study because of their known ability to penetrate the blood–brain barrier. In addition, clenbuterol has been reported to possess antidepressant-like properties in clinical evaluations.

In this study, however, neither compound was shown to mimic the action of desipramine. It was found that the centrally nonselective agonist clenbuterol selectively down-regulated β_2-adrenoceptors by 40% in cerebral cortex. Conversely, the β_1 selective agonist prenalterol was shown to cause an up-regulation of β_1-adrenoceptors in cerebral cortex, by 123% (Fig. 6.1; Table 6.1).

The partial agonist prenalterol was shown to act on the receptor for which it is selective, and the up-regulation is possibly due to the antagonistic properties of the partial agonist. In fact, a similar up-regulation of β_1-adrenoceptors has been demonstrated by receptor blockade with the antagonist propranolol.[4]

The findings with clenbuterol, however, are not so readily explained. This agonist is known to display a lack of selectivity for β_1:β_2 adrenoceptors in radioligand binding studies with brain tissue. Therefore why is the preferential down-regulation of β_2-adrenoceptors seen? Similar findings have been reported by Frazer et al.,[5] who failed to find any evidence that clenbuterol acts at β_1-adrenoceptors in cerebral cortex or cerebellum from autoradiographic studies and after investigating the reduced adenylate cyclase responsiveness to $(-)$isoprenaline and clenbuterol.[5]

One possible explanation is that β_2-adrenoceptors are more tightly coupled to the adenosine 3',5'-cyclic phosphate (cAMP) secondary messenger system, which would preferentially increase their rate of internalization when acted on by such a nonselective agonist. A second possibility is that endogenous norepinephrine is tightly bound to βARs in the central nervous system, as has been demonstrated to be the case in the heart.[6] As norepinephrine has a higher affinity for β_1-adrenoceptors, the latter are more likely to be masked from the action of clenbuterol.

Conclusion

The centrally active βAR agonists clenbuterol and prenalterol do not mimic the actions of desipramine on βARs and thus would not be predicted to be rapid-acting desipramine-like antidepressants. The possibility remains that a centrally active β_1 selective full agonist could still produce down-regulation of brain β_1-adrenoceptors in a time course faster than that of desipramine. If such a compound could be produced, it would be an intriguing possibility for an effective rapid-onset antidepressant.

References

1. Dooley DJ, Hauser KL, Bittiger H. Differential decrease of the central beta-adrenergic receptor in the rat after subchronic infusion of desipramine and clenbuterol. Neurochem Int 1983;5:333–338.
2. Minneman KP, Hegstrand LR, Molinoff PB. Simultaneous determination of beta-$_1$ and beta-$_2$-adrenergic receptors in tissue containing both receptor subtypes. Mol Pharmacol 1979;16:34–46.
3. Kitada Y, Miyauchi T, Kosasa T, et al. The significance of beta-adrenoceptor downregulation in the desipramine action in the forced swimming test. Naunyn Schmiedebergs Arch Pharmacol 1986;333:31–35.
4. Wolfe BB, Minneman KP, Molinoff PB. Selective increases in the density of cerebellar beta$_1$-adrenergic receptors. Brain Res 1982;234:474–479.
5. Frazer A, Ordway G, O'Donnell J, et al. Effect of repeated administration of clenbuterol on the regulation of beta-adrenoceptors in the central nervous system of the rat. In: Antidepressants and Receptor Function. Ciba Foundation Symposium 123. Chichester: Wiley, 1986;170–190.
6. Nerme V, Severne Y, Abrabamsson T, et al. Endogenous noradrenaline masks beta-adrenergic receptors in rat heart membranes via tight agonist binding. Biochem Pharmacol 1985;34:2917–2922.

7. Behavioral Pharmacology and Clinical Antidepressant Effects of β-Adrenergic Agonists

H. FRANCES, P. SIMON, Y. LECRUBIER, AND
D. WIDLÖCHER

In rodents the psychopharmacological profile of β-adrenergic stimulants is similar to that of classical antidepressants on a battery of tests used for screening antidepressant drugs[1] (Table 7.1). One exception is the behavioral despair test, on which none of the β-adrenergic stimulants act. Two behavioral effects are shared by β-adrenergic stimulants and not by tricyclic antidepressants: decreased interest for food in mice starved for 24 h and decrease in spontaneous motor activity in rats and mice.

Because imipramine inhibits the reuptake of catecholamines, its mechanism of action may involve an indirect stimulation of β-adrenergic receptors. To test this hypothesis, we tried to antagonize imipramine and salbutamol effects with the β-blocking drug propranolol. Regarding each of the four tests—antagonism of the hypothermia induced by reserpine, oxotremorine, or a high dose of apomorphine, and potentiation of yohimbine-induced toxicity—it is possible to reduce significantly the effect of imipramine and of salbutamol with propranolol.[2] Regarding the learned helplessness test, propranolol dose-dependently impairs the effect of imipramine. Therefore participation of the β-adrenergic system in these tests appears highly probable. However, several questions remain unresolved. The first is that propranolol is primarily a β-blocking drug but secondarily a 5-hydroxytryptamine (5-HT_1) blocking drug, and we do not know which property is involved in these tests. The second question is that on the reserpine test the effect of imipramine is significantly but not completely suppressed by either propranolol or betaxolol, a specific $β_1$-blocking drug. There is a ceiling, and increasing the doses from 0.25 up to 16 mg/kg does not increase the antagonism. As a consequence, we have to keep in mind that a component other than the β-adrenergic one is part of the imipramine action in the reserpine test.

Because it has been shown that chronic antidepressant treatment reduces the number of β-adrenergic receptors or the effect of their stimulation, we wondered if chronic treatment with the β-adrenergic stimulant clenbuterol would make its behavioral effects disappear. Clenbuterol was administered to mice intraperitoneally at a dose of 0.25 mg/kg (9 a.m. and 6 p.m.) during 12 days. Under these conditions the administration of a clenbuterol test dose may increase or decrease. The increase is called *facilitation* and the decrease *tachyphylaxis*.

Table 7.1. Comparison of clenbuterol and imipramine in psychopharmacological tests.

Tests	Acute clenbuterol	"Chronic" + acute clenbuterol	Imipramine
Antagonism of reserpine hypothermia (2.5 mg/kg)	+	+ +	+
Antagonism of apomorphine hypothermia (16 mg/kg)	+	+	+
Antagonism of oxotremorine hypothermia (0.5 mg/kg)	+	+ +	+
Potentiation of yohimbine-induced toxicity (25 mg/kg)	+	+ +	+
Reversal of learned helplessness	0	+	+
Behavioral despair test	0	0	+
Decrease in spontaneous motor activity	+	0	0
Decreased interest for food in starved mice	+	0	0

The facilitation is observed for the tests on which imipramine and β-stimulants are active. On the contrary, the tachyphylaxis appears for the tests that are specific to β-stimulants, not shared by tricyclic antidepressants. Another difference between these two effects is in their delay of onset. The tachyphylaxis is obtained with a small number (three to five) of administrations (2–3 days). The facilitation becomes higher as the number of treatments increases; and the full effect is obtained after 20 administrations.

To investigate if one or both effects could be explained by a modification of drug metabolism, we measured the plasma levels of clenbuterol under conditions that simultaneously induced tachyphylaxis and facilitation. Thirty minutes after an acute administration of 0.5 mg/kg, the plasma level of clenbuterol was 125 ng/ml in clenbuterol-treated mice and 140 ng/ml in control mice: The metabolism of clenbuterol is unchanged.

The number and affinity of β-adrenoceptors have been measured in rats and mice after chronic clenbuterol treatment by R. Raisman and R. Cash at the Pitié-Salêtrière in Paris. We observed a decrease of 70% in the rat cerebellum and 29% in the cerebral cortex; as the β_2-adrenoceptors are predominant in the cerebellum and represent only 30% in the cerebral cortex, these results seem to indicate that only the β_2-adrenoceptors are reduced by clenbuterol. In the cerebral cortex of mice receiving clenbuterol according to the protocol that induces tachyphylaxis and facilitation, the number of β_1-adrenoceptors is unchanged, and the number of β_2-adrenoceptors is decreased by 17%. The affinity is unchanged.

In addition to a reduction in the response of the β_2-adrenoceptors, chronic clenbuterol treatment induces hypersensitivity in the response of the β_1-adrenoceptors. Using the specific β_1- and β_2-blocking drugs betaxolol and ICI 118 551, we showed (Fig. 7.1) that in control mice clenbuterol antagonism of reserpine hypothermia is more sensitive to the β_1-blocking drug, whereas in chronically treated mice the clenbuterol effect is more sensitive to the β_2-blocking drug. Because β_2-adreno-ceptors are down-regulated after chronic treatment, less ICI 118 551 is required to block the remaining receptors. Inversely, more betaxolol is required to block the β_1-adrenoceptors. Therefore the hypersensitivity of the response may be mediated through β_1-adrenoceptors. Taken together, these results suggest that, on one hand, tachyphylaxis could be explained through a down-regulation of β_2-adrenoceptors. On the other hand, facilitation could involve an increase in the re-

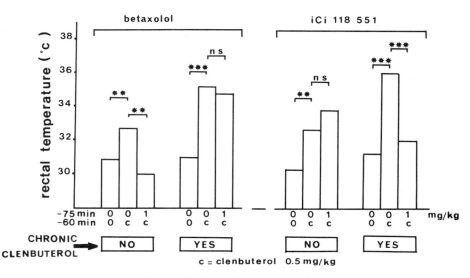

FIGURE 7.1. Reserpine hypothermia.

sponse of β_1-adrenoceptors but cannot be explained by an increase in their number or affinity.

Because the serotonergic system is involved in the depressive states, we investigated its modifications after repeated clenbuterol treatments. This work was carried out by G. Fillion at the Pasteur Institute. Under the conditions inducing facilitation, the number of 5-HT$_1$ receptors increased progressively with the number of repeated clenbuterol administrations.[3]

After a lesion of the 5-HT system induced by 5,7-DHT, clenbuterol still antagonized reserpine-induced hypothermia, but no facilitation occurred after chronic treatment.[4] Therefore the serotonergic system must be intact for the facilitation to occur.

These pharmacological data led our group to start clinical studies with salbutamol and clenbuterol. A clinical pilot study[5] was followed by an open study of 50 patients. A first controlled study comparing salbutamol (6 mg/day) to clomipramine (150 mg/day), both given by intravenous infusion, was performed on depressed inpatients (ten per group).[6] Both treatments effectively alleviated the overall symptomatology, as measured by the Hamilton rating scale (HRS), but the onset of action of salbutamol was more rapid.

A second controlled study comparing salbutamol to clomipramine was undertaken[7] that included a larger number ($n = 126$) of patients. To be included patients had to: (a) be considered as appropriate for classical antidepressant treatments; and (b) meet Feighner's criteria.

Allocation to treatment was made using a random number table. There were two treatments:

1. Clomipramine 150 mg daily by intravenous infusion. This dosage, commonly used in France, was reached within 3 days according to tolerance.
2. Salbutamol in two daily infusions, each given over 2–3 h according to tolerance. Dosage was progressively increased by 0.5-mg steps from 1.5 mg to 3.0 mg in each infusion (i.e., up to 6 mg/day).

The raters were two psychiatrists blind to treatment and not in charge of the patients. Ratings were made before daily treatment administration at day 0 and on days 8 and 28 of treatment between 9 and 10 a.m. The number of responders was studied in each group according to the following criteria: global score of the HRS less than 10 after treatment and improvement more than 10 on the same scale. No difference between treatments appeared in any scale at day 8 due to a partial improvement of most patients treated with clomipramine, whereas in the salbutamol group most patients were either greatly improved or unchanged at this time. The responders group appeared to be the bipolar group and probably part of the unipolar groups.

A third controlled study comparing clenbuterol and clomipramine was performed in 60 depressed inpatients.[7] The two drugs were given by the oral route during 4 weeks. No difference appeared at day 8 for the global population, but some patients appeared to be rapid responders to clenbuterol, especially some bipolar patients. Clenbuterol (merely B_2) appeared to present a better tolerance than salbutamol $(B_1 + B_2)$ but a weaker efficacy, suggesting that the antidepressant effect observed in a subgroup of depressed (endogenous ?) patients is more linked to a B_1- than to a B_2-stimulating property.

Conclusion

These results show that, in animals, β-adrenergic stimulants have a profile similar to that of antidepressants. Their activity is increased after repeated treatments despite a down-regulation of β_2-adrenoceptors. This increased effect is linked to the hypersensitivity of the response of β_1-adrenoceptors and requires the integrity of the serotonergic system; it occurs concomitantly with an up-regulation of 5-HT_1 receptors. In patients, β-stimulants are effective antidepressants acting rapidly, but only in bipolar and some unipolar patients. Globally they are equally or less effective than clomipramine. They are difficult to use because of cardiac tolerance at effective dosage. The antidepressant effect does not seem to be linked to down-regulation of the β_1-adrenoceptors but merely to an increase in their reactivity.

References

1. Frances H, Poncelet M, Danti S, et al. Psychopharmacological profile of clenbuterol. Drug Dev Res 1983;3:349–356.
2. Souto M, Frances H, Lecrubier Y, et al. Antagonism by d-l-propranolol of imipramine effects in animals. Eur J Pharmacol 1979;60:105–108.
3. Frances H, Bulach C, Simon P, et al. Chronic beta-adrenergic stimulation increases in mice the sensitivity to methysergide and the number of cerebral high affinity serotonin binding sites (5-HT-1). J Neural Transm 1986;67:215–224.
4. Frances H, Raisman R, Simon P, et al. Lesions of the serotonergic system impair the facilitation of but not the tolerance to the effects of chronic clenbuterol administration. Psychopharmacology 1987;91:496–499.
5. Lecrubier Y, Jouvent R, Puech AJ, et al. Effect antidépresseur d'un stimulant bêta-adrénergique. Nouv Presse Med 1977;6:2786.
6. Lecrubier Y, Puech AJ, Jouvent R, et al. A beta-adrenergic stimulant (salbutamol) versus clomipramine in depression: a controlled study. Br J Psychiatry 1980;136:354–358.
7. Simon P, Lecrubier Y, Jouvent R, et al. Beta-receptor stimulation in the treatment of depression. In Usdin E, et al (eds): Frontiers in Biochemical and Pharmacological Research in Depression. New York: Raven Press, 1984.

I.B. MONOAMINES AND NEUROPEPTIDES

8. Beyond Nosology in Biological Psychiatry: Prolegomena of a Functional Psychopathology

HERMAN M. VAN PRAAG

Serotonin and Depression

Disturbances in central serotonin (5-hydroxytryptamine, 5-HT) have been reported to occur in a variety of psychiatric disorders, e.g., depression, certain anxiety states, schizophrenia, and alcoholism. The situation has been called chaotic, with 5-HT disorders classified as being nonspecific and 5-HT having been qualified, ironically, as a "neurotransmitter of all seasons."[1] I disagree with these viewpoints and clarify my point of view by summarizing some old data and then focusing on some recent findings of my own group.

Serotonin disturbances in the brain were first reported in depression.[2] They were inferred to exist based on the finding of lowered basal and postprobenecid concentrations of 5-hydroxyindoleacetic acid (5-HIAA) in cerebrospinal fluid (CSF) in a subgroup of patients suffering from major depression, melancholic type. Initially, depressed patients with and without demonstrable disturbances in central 5-HT seemed psychopathologically indistinguishable. Interpreting the available data at that time, we introduced in 1971 the concept of biochemical heterogeneity of (endogenous) depression.[3] Some forms, we postulated, are linked to disturbances in 5-HT functions, whereas others are not or are but to a much lesser extent. The same syndrome, we postulated, could be the ultimate outcome of various pathophysiological processes.

Subsequent studies of our group, however, made the postulate of a separate 5-HT depression untenable. They indicated that increasing 5-HT availability *alone* is not a sufficient antidepressant measure.[4] This finding argues against a predominantly 5-HT-related type of depression.

First, we demonstrated in a double-blind, placebo-controlled comparative study that 5-hydroxytryptophan (5-HTP) is an active antidepressant, whereas tryptophan is not. Next, we showed that both 5-HT precursors increase central 5-HT metabolism to an equal extent but differ in their effect on catecholamine (CA) metabolism: 5-HTP augments it, tryptophan does not.

In some patients, moreover, the therapeutic effect of 5-HTP wears off during the second month of treatment. This phenomenon is paralleled by normalization of CA metabolism, whereas 5-HT metabolism remains increased. Addition of tyrosine restores the therapeutic effect and the enhancement of CA metabolism.

Combining tryptophan with tyrosine, finally, raises the therapeutic effect of tryptophan above the significance level. These data argure against the existence of a separate 5-HT depression and suggest that combined augmentation of 5-HT and CA availability provide the best conditions for antidepressant activity.

Another hypothesis regarding the presence of 5-HT disturbances in only a subgroup of depression is their relatedness to a particular psychopathological dimension that might occur in depression but might be absent as well. This hypothesis seems plausible in the light of recent observations, the relevant dimensions being disregulation of aggression, anxiety, and (possibly) mood.

5-HT and Aggression

In 1976 Asberg et al.[5] reported that depression with and without 5-HT disturbances are distinguishable in that suicide attempters accumulate in the 5-HT-disturbed group. This finding was confirmed by many, though not all, investigators.[6] Low CSF 5-HIAA appeared not to be restricted to depressed suicide attempters but was also found in those who were not depressed and not psychotic as well as in the suicide attempters who were not depressed but were psychotic.

Low CSF 5-HIAA not only relates to inwardly directed aggression but was also found in individuals in whom disturbed aggression regulation manifested in outwardly directed aggression (murders, violent offences, severe personality disorders).

Therefore it appears that 5-HT disturbances are related to disregulation of aggression, irrespective of the direction the aggression takes. In one study we found additional evidence in favor of the hypothesis. We compared 25 patients with major depression and low 5-HIAA with 25 patients who had the same syndrome and normal 5-HIAA in terms of suicide frequency and interpersonal hostility. The low 5-HIAA group exceeded the normal 5-HIAA group in both suicide frequency and frequency of signs of outwardly directed aggression.

In summary, 5-HT disorders (suggestive of decreased central 5-HT metabolism), originally linked to (a subgroup of) depression, seem to be related to a particular psychopathological dimension—disturbed aggression regulation—irrespective of the direction the aggression takes and irrespective of diagnosis.

5-HT and Anxiety

A second psychopathological dimension seems to be 5-HTergically regulated: anxiety. The subject only recently became an issue of systematic study, but the preliminary data seem intriguing.[7] The biological psychiatry group in Utrecht reported the apparent therapeutic effect of clomipramine and 5-HTP in panic disorder using a double-blind, placebo-controlled design. Both drugs are strong 5-HT agonists but not selective ones. The involvement of the 5-HT component, however, became plausible when it was demonstrated that the selective 5-HT uptake inhibitors zimelidine and fluvoxamine had the same antipanic and antianxiety effects in panic disorder patients. The effectiveness of selective 5-HT reuptake inhibitors in panic disorder patients was confirmed by several authors using fluoxetine and trazodome.

Clomipramine has been reported to be effective in obsessive compulsive disorder, which in the present classification is also considered to be an anxiety disorder.

When treating panic disorder patients with indirect 5-HT agonists, an interesting observation was made, i.e., that in the initial phases of treatment anxiety *increased* in approximately 40% of patients, only to subside gradually over the course of 2–3 weeks. These phenomena were explained by postulating *hypersensitivity* of postsynaptic 5-HT receptors in panic disorder. Increasing 5-HT availability would under those circumstances first lead to additional stimulation of an already hyperactive system and hence to clinical deterioration. Down-regulation of the receptor system would eventually lead to amelioration of the anxiety disorder. *Evidence confirmatory to this hypothesis* has been found.

1. Panic disorder patients were challenged with the selective 5-HT$_1$ agonist *m*-chlorophenylpiperazine (MCPP). Panic disorder patients showed a substantial increase in anxiety during the test compared to placebo-treated patients. In normals and in patients with major depression, no significant behavioral response occurred. Depression and hostility scores also increased, albeit to a lesser degree. The same was true for the score for physical complaints.

2. The cortisol response to MCPP was augmented in panic disorder patients compared to placebo-treated patients, normal controls, and patients with major depression.

3. Another piece of confirmatory evidence can be found in the development of two new drugs efficacious in generalized anxiety disorder (but not yet well studied in panic disorder) buspirone and ritanserin. The latter is a selective 5-HT$_2$ antagonist; the former has high affinity for 5-HT$_{1A}$ receptors and probably decreases 5-HT activity—additional evidence that decreasing 5-HT function induces anxiolytic effects.

4. If 5-HT receptor hypersensitivity exists, we would expect 5-HT metabolism and 5-HIAA production to be reduced. However, no CSF 5-HIAA studies have been conducted in panic disorder. We analyzed our own 5-HIAA data for depression as to correlations with anxiety scores on the Hamilton Depression Scale. No such correlation was found, but the six patients with the highest anxiety scores clustered in the group with the lowest 5-HIAA concentration.

In conclusion, preliminary evidence suggests that 5-HT disturbances are related to the psychopathological dimension of anxiety, at least in the groups of anxiety disorders we presently distinguish.

5-HT and Mood

Serotonin disturbances do not specifically relate to depression as a disease entity. Is there linkage with depressed mood (as a symptom)? This is a moot point. Some data, however, make it seem likely. The important data are as follows:

1. Low CSF 5-HIAA is found in depressives without suicidal histories and without undue outward aggression.
2. Lowest CSF 5-HIAA levels were found in depressed suicide attempters.[8]
3. Low CSF 5-HIAA was found in parkinsonian patients with depressed mood.[9]
4. Manipulating 5-HT induces mood changes. 5-HTP has been reported to induce euphoria in normals; lowering of tryptophan content of diet was mood-lowering.

For a more definitive answer, individuals should be studied with lowered mood but without depression, such as might occur after bereavement.

Conclusions

Serotonin disturbances in psychiatric disorders lack nosological specificity; they are, in other words, not linked to particular psychiatric disorders. Rather, they seem to be correlated to particular psychopathological dimensions, specifically to dysregulated aggression, increased anxiety, and possibly lowering of mood.

If one particular brain system is involved in the regulation of several behavioral dimensions, one would expect those dimensions to be highly intercorrelated; to the extent that data are available, they are indeed correlated. Anxiety and depression are mutually linked. Panic disorder and obsessive compulsive disorder, for example, are frequently accompanied by major depression; and in depressed patients panic attacks and generalized anxiety are common. Depression and aggression are also linked. Depression, for example, is the common precursor of suicide. In depression, outwardly directed aggression is accentuated. Suicide rates are increased in individuals with histories of violent behavior and in homicidal criminals.

The interrelation between anxiety and aggression has been less well studied. It seems clear, however, that strong aggressive impulses can either induce or suppress fear and apprehension. Induction of fear by aggressive impulses is seen in certain phobias (e.g., fear of knives) and obsessions (e.g., fear of killing one's children). Suppression of fear by aggressive impulses occurs in certain forms of antisocial personality disorder.

The dimensional 5-HT hypothesis is compatible with the cerebral distribution of 5-HT. Ascending projections of the raphe nuclei are directed to different discrete areas of the brain, such as septum, amygdala, hypothalamus, and hippocampus. Different projection areas could conceivably be involved in the regulation of different psychological functions.

The 5-HT data look chaotic only if one's major concern is discovery of markers of *disease entities,* and this area has indeed been the major concern of biological psychiatric research so far. The 5-HT data, however, appear interpretable if we were to look for meaningful correlations between biological and psychological dysfunctions, realizing that psychological dysfunctions, which are generally nosologically nonspecific, do occur across diagnoses.

We have advocated this approach for a long time—not as an alternative for, but as a complement to, the nosological approach. The term we coined for it was *functional psychopathology.*[10-12] The approach calls for dissection of a given psychopathological syndrome into its component parts, i.e. the psychological dysfunctions, and then a search for possible relations between the psychological and biological dysfunctions.

Serotonin research in psychiatry illustrates the appropriateness and viability of this approach. It is for this reason that 5-HT, rather than being a "neurotransmitter of all seasons," seems to be a neurotransmitter heralding a new season of biological research in psychiatry.[13]

References

1. Van Kammen DP. 5-HT, a neurotransmitter for all seasons? Biol Psychiatry 1987;22: 1–3.
2. Van Praag HM. Neurotransmitters and CNS disease: depression, Lancet 1982;2:1259–1264.

3. Van Praag HM, Korf J. Endogenous depressions with and without disturbances in the 5-hydroxytryptamine metabolism: a biochemical classification? Psychopharmacology 1971;19:148–152.
4. Van Praag HM, Lemus C. Monoamine precursors in the treatment of psychiatric disorders. In Wurtman JJ, Wurtman RJ (eds): Nutrition and the Brain. New York: Raven Press, 1986.
5. Asberg M, Traskman L, Thoren P. 5-HIAA in the cerebrospinal fluid: a biochemical suicide predictor? Arch Gen Psychiatry 1976;33:1193–1197.
6. Van Praag HM. Biological suicide research: outcome and limitations. Biol Psychiatry 1986;21:1305–1323.
7. Kahn RS, van Praag HM, Wetzler S, et al. Serotonin and anxiety revisited. Biol Psychiatry 1988;23:189–208.
8. Traskman L, Asberg M, Bertillson L, et al. Monoamine metabolites in CSF and suicidal behavior. Arch Gen Psychiatry 1981;38:631–636.
9. Mayeux R, Stern Y, Cote L, et al. Altered serotonin metabolism in depressed patients with Parkinson's disease. Neurology 1984;34:642–646.
10. Van Praag HM, Leijnse B. Neubewertung des sydroms: Skizze einer funktionellen pathologie. Psychiatr Neurol Neurochir 1965;68:50–66.
11. Van Praag HM, Korf J, Lakke JPWF, et al. Dopamine metabolism in depression, psychoses and Parkinson's disease: the problem of the specificity of biological variables in behaviour disorders. Psychol Med 1975;5:138–146.
12. Van Praag HM, Kahn R, Asnis GM, et al. Therapeutic indications for serotonin-potentiating compounds: a hypothesis. Biol Psychiatry 1987;22:205–212.
13. Van Praag HM, Kahn R, Asnis GM, et al. Densologization of biological psychiatry or the specificity of 5-HT disturbances in psychiatric disorders. J Affective Disord 1987;13:1–8.

9. Serotonergic Aspects of Agonistic Behavior

BEREND OLIVIER AND JAN MOS

For a number of decades serotonin (5-hydroxytryptamine, 5-HT) has been implicated in the control of aggressive behavior. Early work on 5-HT and aggression indicated that general 5-HT activation decreased aggression, whereas overall inactivation of 5-HT by various means enhanced it.[1]

However, the anatomical distribution and localization of cell groups and pathways of 5-HT in the central nervous system and their differential projections[2] are strong arguments against a simple general inhibitory role of 5-HT in any aggression paradigm. Moreover, the differentiations in 5-HT receptor (sub)types[2] and their distinct functional roles delineate the possibility that the same applies with regard to different kinds of agonistic behavior. The present contribution therefore focuses on the role the various types of serotonergic receptor may play in agonistic behavior.

Apart from a general modulatory role, it may well be possible that a more specific role of 5-HT in aggression is dependent on the type of paradigm used. Therefore we used not only several aggression paradigms reflecting diverse aspects of agonistic behavior, including offensive and defensive paradigms, but also a paradigm of predatory aggression. Moreover, different species and genders have been used. By applying psychoactive drugs with several serotonergic mechanisms of action in those various agonistic behavior paradigms, we hoped to be able to give a uniform description of the mode of action of 5-HT in agonistic behavior and to delineate whether 5-HT is involved in a uniform way in aggression or that its role differs depending on the paradigm used.

Isolation-Induced Aggression and Intermale Aggression in Mice

When a male mouse is isolated for some time and then confronted with a male intruder, fighting may occur, including threat, chasing, and biting.[3] The behavior of aggressive isolated male mice has been considered as offensive, and effects of drugs can be studied using ethological methodology.[4] Several behavioral elements are used to describe the behavior and changes therein. A simple first approach is determination of an ED_{50} for lowering the number of aggressive interactions[4] (IIA mouse). This approach is shown in Table 9.1, where arrows depict the main effects on aggressive behavior. A substantial number of drugs inhibit aggression, but from this paradigm it is unclear which behavioral inhibitory mechanisms are involved. This area was further investigated by extensive ethological observations. By subdividing the behavior into several categories (i.e., exploration, social interest, aggression, defense, avoidance, and inactivity[4]) one can get a general view of the main effects of the drugs (Table 9.1). Such an analysis[4] shows that several drugs exert a nonspecific antiaggressive action because the decreasing effects on aggression are accompanied by simultaneous decreasing effects in, for example, social interest and exploratory activities and/or increases in inactivity indicative of a nonspecific reduction in aggression, e.g., by sedation, muscle relaxation, or motor disturbances.[4,5] Serenics [eltoprazine (DU 28853), fluprazine], TFMPP, and RU24969 exert a behavioral specific profile: reduction in aggression without concomitant reduction in exploration, social interest (even enhanced), and inactivity.

Resident-Intruder Aggression in Rats

Introduction of a strange male rat into the territory of another male rat (resident) evokes a rich repertoire of natural agonistic activities, which can be used in an ethopharmacological approach.[3,4] This analysis shows that a number of drugs exert nonspecific antiaggressive actions caused by sedation (5-Me-O-DMT, quipazine, buspirone, and fenfluramine), which is evident in increases in inactivity concomitant with decreases in social interest and exploration. Detailed ethological analysis[5] reveals the specific nature of the antiaggressive action of serenics (eltoprazine, fluprazine) also in this model; the animals show no decrease in social interest, a slight increase in exploration, and no increase in inactivity.

Brain-Stimulation-Induced Aggression in Rats

Electrical stimulation of certain areas in the hypothalamus may evoke aggressive responses; however, using the same electrodes, locomotion, teeth-chattering, and switch-off behavior can be induced as well.[6] Measurement of drug effects on these parameters gives direct clues to the specificity of the behavioral effects on aggression. By estimating threshold current intensities of the different behaviors, it is possible to determine whether drugs exert specific antiaggressive effects (only enhancing aggression and teeth-chattering thresholds) or affect other behaviors as well (locomotion thresholds primarily).[7]

Serenics have a specific profile in this electrical stimulation of the brain (EBS) paradigm. They enhance current thresholds for aggression without affecting thresholds for locomotion or switch-off behavior. 8-OH-DPAT has no effect in this paradigm up to doses that completely incapacitate animals. Quipazine and fluvoxamine have a nonspecific antiaggressive influence indicated by a concomitant enhancement of locomotion thresholds.

Maternal Aggression in Rats

Lactating female rats attack intruders with short attack latencies and a high intensity form of attack.[4] The lactation period between 3 and 12 days postpartum is a relatively stable period to measure aggression, using the female rats as their own

TABLE 9.1. Effects of several serotonergic drugs with different mechanisms of action in various animal paradigms in rats and mice.

Drug	IIA mouse	IMA mouse	RI rat	EBS rat	MA rat	MK rat	FID mouse	DB rat	Putative serotonergic mechanism of action
TFMPP	↓	φ	φ	φ	φ	φ	φ	–	1B Agonist (partial)
Eltoprazine	↓	φ	φ	φ	φ	φ	φ	–	1A/1B Agonist (partial)
Fluprazine	↓	φ	φ	φ	φ	φ	nt	–	Weak 1A/1B/2 agonist
RU24969	↓	φ	nt	nt	↓	φ	nt	nt	1A/1B Agonist
5-Me-O-DMT	–	↓	↓	↓	nt	↓	↓	nt	1A Agonist
Quipazine	↓	nt	↓	↓	↓	↓	–	nt	Weak 1/2 agonist
8-OH-DPAT	–	↓	nt	–	↓	–	nt	nt	1A Agonist
Buspirone	–	nt	↓	nt	↓	↓	nt	nt	1A Agonist
Ipsapirone	↓	nt	nt	↓	↓	–	nt	nt	1A Agonist
Fluvoxamine	–	φ	↓	–	–	↓	nt	nt	Reuptake blocker
Methysergide	–	nt	nt	nt	–	–	nt	nt	1/2 Antagonist
Ritanserine	–	nt	nt	nt	↓	–	nt	nt	2 Antagonist
Fenfluramine	↓	nt	nt	nt	–	↓	nt	nt	Release

φ = specific decrease. ↓ = nonspecific decrease. – = no effect. nt = not tested.
IIA = isolation-induced aggression. IMA = intermale aggression. RI = resident-intruder. EBS = electrical stimulation of the brain.
MA = maternal aggression. MK = mouse killing. FID = foot-shock-induced defense. DB = defensive behavior. [Reprinted from ref. 4, with permission.]

controls. The behavior performed by lactating female rats against intruders differs in morphology and causation from that in male rat aggression paradigms. Therefore drug effects were evaluated after extensive ethological analysis of the behavioral "makeup" of this paradigm.[4] Table 9.1 indicates that this paradigm also clearly differentiates between different drugs: Sedation (increased inactivity, disruption of pup care) or inattentiveness to the pups occurred in a number of cases (e.g., with quipazine, 8-OH-DPAT, ipsapirone, fenfluramine), whereas serenics exerted specific behavioral effects.

Mouse Killing by Rats

Although mouse killing reflects aspects of aggression other than intraspecific agonistic behavior (predation), it is of value in determining psychoactive properties of drugs. By measuring concomitantly other behavioral effects, e.g., sedation, a subjective rating of the specificity of a drug's inhibitory effect is obtained.[4] A number of drugs (8-OH-DPAT, ipsapirone, methysergide, ritanserine) do not inhibit mouse killing (unless very high doses are used, which completely debilitate animals), whereas all other drugs do, although not always in a specific way (quipazine, buspirone, fluvoxamine).

Defensive Behavior

When animals are attacked, they normally defend themselves adequately or, if necessary, flee. This aspect of agonistic behavior is of importance for species survival, and antiaggressive drugs should preferably not interfere with adequate defense/flight capacities of animals. Two paradigms to test defense/flight effects of drugs have been used: (a) foot-shock-induced defense in which pairs of mice are shocked via their paws and consequently perform defensive behaviors; and (b) a more natural intruder paradigm.[7]

Although only a limited number of drugs has been tested, the available data suggest that serenics do not adversely affect defensive capabilities of animals. The decrease observed in foot-shock-induced fighting after TFMPP and fluprazine presumably can be ascribed to the analgesic properties of these drugs, which is absent with eltoprazine.

Conclusions

The available evidence points to a specific modulatory role of the $5-HT_{1B}$ receptor site in aggression. Agonists mainly affecting the $5-HT_{1B}$ receptors (TFMPP) or mixed $5-HT_{1A/1B}$ agonists (eltoprazine, fluprazine, RU24969) exert specific antiaggressive effects in several aggression paradigms, whereas drugs with other serotonergic mechanisms of action have either no or nonspecific antiaggressive effects.

Although it is too early to exclude the involvement of other 5-HT sites in aggression, the $5-HT_{1B}$ receptor site seems an attractive candidate that may be used to modulate agonistic behavior in a specific manner. The development of a new class of drugs, serenics, which have high affinity for the $5-HT_{1B}$ receptor, awaits further investigation in other species, including humans, to validate the specific $5-HT_{1B}$ role in aggression.

The available evidence suggests that the differential role of the various 5-HT receptor mechanisms holds for most if not all aggression paradigms used. This finding, in turn, may point to a general role of the 5-HT_{1B} subsystem in the central nervous system in aggression.

References

1. Valzelli L. Psychopharmacology of aggression: an overview. Int Pharmacopsychiatry 1981;16:39–48.
2. Peroutka SJ, Heuring RE, Mauk MD, et al. Serotonin receptor subtypes: biochemical, physiological, behavioural, and clinical implications. Psychopharmacol Bull 1986;22:813–817.
3. Miczek KA. The psychopharmacology of aggression. In Iversen LL, Iversen SD, Snyder SH (eds): Handbook of Psychopharmacology, Vol 19: Behavioral Pharmacology. New York: Plenum Press, 1987;183–328.
4. Olivier B, Mos J, Schipper J, et al. Serotonergic modulation of agonistic behaviour. In Olivier B, Mos J, Brain PF (eds): Ethopharmacology of Agonistic Behaviour in Humans and Animals. Dordrecht: Martinus Nijhoff, 1987;162–186.
5. Olivier B, Van Aken H, Jaarsma I, et al. Behavioural effects of psychoactive drugs on agonistic behaviour of male territorial rats (resident-intruder paradigm). In Miczek KA, Kruk MR, Olivier B (eds): Ethopharmacological Aggression Research. New York: Alan R Liss, 1984;137–156.
6. Kruk MR, Van der Poel AM, Lammers JHCM, et al. Ethopharmacology of hypothalamic aggression in the rat. In Olivier B, Mos J, Brain PF (eds): Ethopharmacology of Agonistic Behaviour in Humans and Animals. Dordrecht: Martinus Nijhoff, 1987;33–45.
7. Olivier B, Mos J. Serenics and aggression. Stress Med 1986;2:197–209.

10. Noradrenergic and Serotonergic Dysfunction in the Affective Disorders

LARRY J. SIEVER, EMIL F. COCCARO, RICHARD FRIEDMAN, KAREN RUBINSTEIN, AND KENNETH L. DAVIS

The catecholaminergic system[1] and the indoleaminergic system[2] have been postulated to be abnormal in the affective disorders. Considerable support exists for at least some disturbance in these systems in a substantial proportion of affective disorder patients. The exact character of these abnormalities remains to be determined. However, abnormalities in noradrenergic metabolites in body fluids[3] as well as abnormalities in adrenergic receptor responsiveness[4] have been found in depressed patients. Decreased concentrations of the serotonin metabolite 5-hydroxyindoleacetic acid (5-HIAA)[5] and prolactin responses to serotonergic challenges[6,7] have also been demonstrated in patients with major depressive disorder.

It has not yet been established which of the abnormalities are state-dependent and which are state-independent (trait). However, indices of monoaminergic presynaptic output such as noradrenergic metabolite concentrations[8] and serotonergic metabolite concentrations[9] tend to normalize with recovery. Decreased adrenergic receptor responsiveness, as reflected in the blunted growth hormone (GH) response to clonidine, however, appears to persist in the remitted state in preliminary studies,[4] and serotonergic receptor responsiveness has not been evaluated in acute and remitted patients.

Thus we have initiated systematic investigations of serotonergic and noradrenergic activity in depressed patients and their relation to state. In the noradrenergic system the absolute concentrations and circadian/ultradian rhythms of norepinephrine and its metabolite 3-methoxyhydroxyphenylglycol (MHPG) were evaluated in both acute and remitted depressed patients, including a subset of patients in both states.

Several preliminary studies, however, have suggested that the GH response to clonidine is reduced in depressed patients in both the acute and the remitted state.[10,11] Preliminary data from our laboratory are shown in Table 10.1. As the prevalence of blunted GH responses between acute and remitted patients is similar and, in general, the response in specific patients does not seem to change between states, the blunted GH response to clonidine has characteristics of a trait marker for depression and may be related to the vulnerability to depression.[11,12] Whether the blunted GH response to clonidine represents a direct or indirect reflection of

TABLE 10.1. Growth hormone response to clonidine.

Group	No.	Age	Average baseline (ng/ml)	Average GH response (ng/ml)	Peak GH response (ng/ml)	Blunters No. %	Nonblunters No. %
Acute depressed	21	55.9 ± 86	1.1 ± 0.7	4.0 ± 6.3	6.0 ± 9.7	15 71.4[a]	6 28.6
Remitted depressed	16	52.7 ± 9.6	1.0 ± 0.5	3.7 ± 4.4	7.4 ± 11.1	11 68.7[a]	5 31.3
Normal control	11	52.4 ± 13.7	1.0 ± 0.6	6.5 ± 7.8	9.9 ± 11.8	4 36.4	7 63.6
Normal controls (< 70 years)	9	48.0 ± 10.9	1.0 ± 0.6	7.3 ± 8.4	11.2 ± 12.7	2 22.2	7 77.8

All patients have a baseline of < 3 ng/ml. Those with a peak response of < 5 ng/ml are blunters.
Combined depressed group significantly increased from all normal controls (Fisher's Exact Test, $p < 0.05$).
[a]Each significantly increased in prevalence compared with normal controls < 70 years (Fisher's Exact Test, $p < 0.05$).

the underlying genetic predisposition to depression or it is a residual marker of depressive episodes is unknown. It could conceivably represent an interaction of the two possibilities, e.g., a genetically determined defect in receptor plasticity predisposing to persistent α_2-adrenergic receptor down-regulation in the face of excessive release of norepinephrine during repeated depressive or other stressful episodes. Studies of family members of depressed patients and "high risk" volunteers using the clonidine challenge, as well as strategies to evaluate receptor plasticity in depressed patients and controls are required to explore these possibilities.

Although presynaptic activity of the serotonergic system may change between the acute and remitted state, there are few data available regarding changes in this system using measures that include serotonergic receptor responsiveness. The prolactin response to fenfluramine is a measure that apparently depends on both presynaptic serotonergic integrity and postsynaptic serotonergic receptor responsiveness resulting in an index of "net" serotonergic activity.[6] The prolactin response to fenfluramine is blunted in approximately half of depressed patients, and this proportion does not seem to be different in medication-free remitted patients.[10] Patients studied across two states show modest increases from the acute to the remitted states but are correlated between the two states. In addition, those patients blunted in their prolactin responsiveness in the acute state remain blunted in the remitted state. The results of the fenfluramine study cannot distinguish between presynaptic and postsynaptic changes accompanying remission. However, as presynaptic serotonergic activity may increase with remission, this study might be consistent with persistently reduced serotonergic receptor responsiveness. This possibility requires exploration with the use of direct serotonergic receptor agonists in patients across states.

The identification of state-independent correlates of depression is important in the understanding of pathophysiological and genetic mechanisms in depression and their interaction with environmental events. The suggestions of persistent receptor defects in depression point to further exploration of receptor regulation in depression.

References

1. Schildkraut JJ: The catecholamine hypothesis of affective disorders: a review of supporting evidence. Am J Psychiatry 1965;122:509–522.
2. Murphy DL, Campbell LC, Costa JL. The brain serotonergic system in the affective disorders. Prog Neuropsychopharmacol 1978;2:1–31.
3. Koslow JJ, Maas JW, Bowden CL, et al. CSF and urinary biogenic amines and metabolites in depression and mania. Arch Gen Psychiatry 1983;40:999–1010.
4. Siever LJ, Uhde TW: New studies and perspectives on the noradrenaline receptor system in depression: effects of the alpha-adrenergic agonist clonidine. Biol Psychiatry 1984;190:131–156.
5. Van Praag HM. Neurotransmitters and CNS disease. Lancet 1982;2:1259–1264.
6. Siever LJ, Murphy DL, Slater S, et al. Plasma prolactin changes following fenfluramine in depressed patients compared to controls: an evaluation of central serotonergic responsivity in depression. Life Sci 1984;34:1029–1039.
7. Heninger GR, Charney DS, Sternberg DE: Serotonergic function in depression. Arch Gen Psychiatry 1984;41:398–402.
8. Pickar D, Sweeney DR, Maas JW, et al: Primary affective disorder, clinical state change and MHPG excretion: a longitudinal study. Arch Gen Psychiatry 1978;35:1378–1381.
9. Asberg M, Thoren P, Traskman L, et al: "Serotonin depression"—a biochemical subgroup within the affective disorders? Science 1976;191:478–480.

10. Siever LJ, Coccaro EF, Benjamin E, et al. Adrenergic and serotonergic receptor responsiveness in depression. In: Depression, Antidepressants and Receptor Sensitivity. CIBA Foundation Symposium 123 Chichester UK: John Wiley & Sons, Ltd. 1986;148–169.
11. Hoehe M, Valido G, Matussek N. Growth hormone response to clonidine in endogenous depressive patients: evidence for a trait marker in depression. In Shagass C, et al (eds): Proceedings of the World Congress of Biologic Psychiatry. New York: Elsevier, 1986.
12. Siever LJ, Davis KL. Overview: towards a dysregulation hypothesis of depression. Am J Psychiatry 1985;142:1017–1031.

11. Neuropeptides and Affective Disorders

JAN M. VAN REE AND DAVID DE WIED

Pituitary hormones regulate the endocrine organs, are involved in many home-ostatic mechanisms in the body, and have direct effects on processes in the central nervous system. The latter was initially demonstrated by animal behavioral experiments[1] and confirmed by neurochemical and electrophysiological studies in animals.[2] Fragments of pituitary hormones may have similar effects on behavior as the parent hormones, but interestingly they hardly elicit the classical endocrine actions of the parent hormones. The central effects of pituitary hormones and their fragments indicate that they belong to the category of neuropeptides, which are peptide molecules that affect nerve function and/or are present in nerve tissue. Research during the last decade has disclosed that many peptide molecules, including the pituitary hormones, are present in the central nervous system, and that they are presumably located in neuronal pathways. They are synthesized in large proteins, and several are formed in the same molecule. A cascade of processes evolve in peptidergic neurons to express the genetic information into biologically active neuropeptides. These processes control the quantities of neuropeptides synthesized as well as the nature of their biological activity through size, form, and derivation of the endproduct. In this way sets of neuropeptides with different, opposite, and more selective properties are formed from the same precursor.

The symptomatology of affective disorders is heterogeneous. Prominent are mood changes and disturbances in appetite, sleep, libido, energy, and circadian rhythms. Some of these functions are controlled by brain centers located in the hypothalamus and lower brainstem, and they are innervated by particular peptidergic neurons. Neuroendocrine dysfunctions have been demonstrated in patients with affective disorders, such as diminished suppression of cortisol after dexamethasone administration[3] and a blunted thyroid-stimulating hormone (TSH) response to thyrotropin-releasing hormone (TRH).[4] Cognitive dysfunctions may accompany the mood disturbances in affective disorders. Interestingly, neuropeptides related to adrenocorticotropic hormone (ACTH) and vasopressin have been implicated in cognitive processes; and the opioid peptide β-endorphin, which like ACTH is derived from proopiomelanocortin, may be involved in mood changes. These findings and suggestions may indicate a relation between affective disorders and neuropeptides, especially those related to pituitary hormones and the hypothalamic peptides controlling the release of these hormones.

Animal Studies

Three strategies can be followed in animal experiments to search for potential antidepressant entities, i.e., physiological, pharmacological, and pathological approaches. These strategies may also contribute to the unraveling of possible relations between endogenous substances, including neuropeptides, and affective disorders.

The *physiological approach* determines physiological processes in the brain that are disturbed in affective disorders. These processes may be related to one or a set of symptoms characteristic for the disease. Knowledge about the substances involved in the regulation and control of these processes may lead to prediction of entities with antidepressant action. Information about brain processes disrupted in affective disorders, however, is limited. The symptomatology of affective disorders is rather heterogeneous, and key symptoms can hardly be designated. One characteristic feature is mood changes. It has been suggested that intracranial self-stimulation behavior in animals, investigating the brain systems that mediate reward, may bear some relation with mood in humans. This behavior procedure also fulfills other validating criteria for an animal model related to depression, including that under certain conditions subchronic treatment with antidepressants facilitates reward.[5]

Research so far has mainly been concentrated on the *pharmacological approach,* which determines the actions in animals of drugs known to be effective in treating affective disorders. However, little information about the relation between such actions and the therapeutic effect of the antidepressants is available. Not all antidepressant treatments, including the second generation of antidepressants and electroconvulsive shock, share the same effects in these models. Furthermore, most of these models deal with acute effects of antidepressants, whereas their therapeutic action is visible after chronic administration only. Thus until now the pharmacological approach—including, for example, yohimbine, dopa, or amphetamine potentiation, reserpine reversal, olfactory bulbectomy, and kindling—has not yielded new classes of antidepressants. One interesting lead has, however, been explored during the last decade, suggesting that chronic treatment with antidepressants may desensitize hypersensitive adrenoceptors.[6]

The *patho (physio) logical approach,* which tries to mimic the pathology of affective disorders in animals, is hampered by the fact that the pathological process underlying affective disorders is unknown. Most animal studies in this respect have concentrated on phenomena related to stress. They include the responses of infant monkeys to maternal separation, reversal of the light-dark cycle in rats, the exposure of rodents to chronic unpredictable stress, the performance deficit in learning tasks after exposure to uncontrolled stress (learned helplessness), and the enhanced immobility after a previous experience of an unsuccessful escape attempt (behavioral despair). In most of these models an activation phase is followed by an inhibition phase. Interestingly, in three of these models the inhibitory phase has been shown to be associated with a decrease in positively reinforced behavior, which characterizes the intracranial self-stimulation model.[5] (Sub)chronic treatment with antidepressant alleviates the induced behavioral changes in these models, but the specificity of some of these tests for antidepressants has been questioned. It has been proposed that in depressed patients α_2- and β-adrenoceptors are supersensitive. However, a valid animal model mimicking this pathology is not available.

Neuropeptides have not been studied extensively in the above-mentioned models. Increased sensitivity to brain stimulation reward is induced by oxytocin and its C-terminal tripeptide prolyl-leucyl-glycinamide (PLG), α-endorphin, and some ACTH neuropeptides, including the ACTH-(4-9) analog Org 2766[7]. The opioid peptides may be physiologically involved in brain stimulation reward, as opioid antagonists decrease sensitivity to this reward especially during and after chronic treatment.[8] Peptides related to ACTH and vasopressin have been implicated in certain cognitive processes that are disturbed in a number of depressed patients. In a learned immobility test TRH was found to mimic the action of antidepressants.[9] Readjustment of a normal circadian cycle after disruption of the light-dark cycle is facilitated by some antidepressants and by the peptides desglycinamide-(Arg[8])-vasopressin and the ACTH-(4-9) analog Org 2766.[10,11] In some other tests similar actions of neuropeptides and antidepressants have been found. Short-term (7 days) social isolation of rats increases social activities in a dyadic encounter test, and this increase is prevented by treatment with some antidepressants and the neuropeptides PLG, TRH, and the ACTH-(4-9) analog Org 2766.[12,13] The behavioral changes induced by injection of melatonin into the nucleus accumbens are antagonized by local pretreatment with some antidepressants, serotonin, and α- and γ-type endorphins, including the peptide β-endorphin-(10-16).[14,15] These findings warrant research leading to a more detailed profile of some of these peptides using animal behavioral tests in current use to detect potential antidepressants.

Human Studies

Human research with respect to neuropeptides and affective disorders concerns the measurement of peptide levels in body fluids of patients and in postmortem brains, peptide challenge tests, and treatment of patients with peptides (for references see refs. 16,17).

Peptide Levels

Plasma cortisol levels are elevated in a number of patients suffering from affective disorders. This finding may be due to increased ACTH secretion. The reports on plasma ACTH levels, however, are not uniform. β-Lipotropin and β-endorphin have been reported to be increased in plasma of certain depressed patients. A number of peptides have been determined in cerebrospinal fluid (CSF) of depressed patients. Increased levels have been reported for corticotropin-releasing hormone (CRH), thyrotropin-releasing hormone (TRH), and substance P and decreased levels for somatostatin (growth hormone release-inhibiting hormone), vasopressin, cholecystokinin, and vasoactive intestinal peptide. The levels of β-endorphin, bombesin, calcitonin, and delta sleep-inducing peptide were found to be unaltered. Most of this information is based on single reports, however, and therefore more studies are needed before definite conclusions can be drawn. This need also holds true for manic patients, in whom calcitonin and vasopressin levels in CSF may be decreased and increased, respectively.

Challenge Tests

Peptides have been administered to patients suffering from affective disorders, and the endocrine responses on this challenge have been determined. Most studies have concentrated on the pituitary-adrenal and pituitary-thyroid axis. The ACTH and cortisol responses to CRH infusion were reduced in depressed patients, whereas administration of ACTH produced a normal or increased cortisol response. In some depressed patients the cortisol response to vasopressin was decreased. Thus the pituitary may be subsensitive to the factors normally stimulating ACTH release. It is not clear if this subsensitivity is secondary to the hypercortisolemia observed in a number of depressed patients. The TSH response to TRH administration is diminished in about 30% of the depressed patients, whereas an exaggerated TSH response to TRH may be present in a limited number of these patients. The release of follicle-stimulating hormone and luteinizing hormone on challenge with luteinizing hormone-releasing hormone seems to be normal in depressed patients.

Treatment with Peptides

Some neuropeptides have been studied as a possible therapeutic agent in depression. Most studies to data have used the tripeptide TRH. The peptide appeared to be ineffective in most of the double-blind studies using oral administration. However, after intravenous administration, a short-lasting antidepressant effect was observed in about half of the studies, which include more than 500 patients. The C-terminal fragment of oxytocin, the tripeptide PLG, was reported to exert an antidepressant effect in three of four studies. Interestingly, in these studies the peptide was given orally. The antidepressant effect of PLG occurred rather rapidly and was long-lasting. An analog of vasopressin, 1-desamino-8-D-arginine-vasopressin, given intranasally to a limited number of depressed patients improved cognition, and in some an antidepressant effect was observed as well. A number of depressed patients has been treated with β-endorphin. A positive effect of β-endorphin was found in only one of three double-blind studies. Conversely, the opioid antagonist naloxone may worsen the conditions of depressed patients, although there are some reports of a beneficial effect of naloxone in manic patients. The nonopiate fragment of β-endorphin, Des-Tyr[1]-γ-endorphin, which possesses an antipsychotic effect in a number of schizophrenic patients,[18] has been reported to induce an antidepressant effect in some depressed patients.[19]

Conclusions

More research on affective disorders and neuropeptides is needed, especially related to pituitary hormones, because (a) certain pituitary functions are disturbed in a category of depressed patients; (b) affective disorders are accompanied by changes in the CSF levels of certain neuropeptides; (c) treatment with some neuropeptides, particularly PLG and TRH, may alleviate symptomatology in some depressed patients; (4) neuropeptides affect brain functions in animals that may be disturbed in human affective disorders; (5) some neuropeptides mimic the action of antidepressants in animals; (6) certain neuropeptides may be effective in animal models of affective disorders. Detailed animal and human research in this respect may eventually disclose neuropeptides with therapeutic action in affective disorders.

References

1. De Wied D. Effects of peptide hormones on behavior. In Ganong WF, Martini L (eds): Frontiers in Neuroendocrinology. New York: Oxford University Press, 1969;97–140.
2. De Wied D, Jolles J. Neuropeptides derived from pro-opiocortin: behavioral, physiological and neurochemical effects. Physiol Rev 1982;62:976–1059.
3. Carroll BJ. Dexamethasone suppression test: a review of contemporary confusion. J Clin Psychiatry 1985;46:13–24.
4. Loosen PT, Prange AJ Jr. Serum thyrotropin response to thyrotropin-releasing hormone in psychiatric patients: a review. Am J Psychiatry 1982;139:405–416.
5. Willner P. The validity of animal models of depression. Psychopharmacology 1984;83:1–16.
6. Leonard BE. Pharmacological properties of some "second generation" antidepressant drugs. Neuropharmacology 1980;19:1175–1183.
7. Van Ree JM, De Wied D. Behavioral effects of endorphins: modulation of opiate reward by neuropeptides related to pro-opiocortin and neurohypophyseal hormones. In Smith JE, Lane JD (eds): The Neurobiology of Opiate Reward Processes. Amsterdam: Elsevier, 1983;109–145.
8. Van Wolfswinkel L, Seifert WF, Van Ree JM. Long-term changes in self-stimulation threshold by repeated morphine and naloxone treatment. Life Sci 1985;37:169–176.
9. Ogawa N, Mizuno S, Mori A, et al. Potential antidepressive effects of thyrotropin releasing hormone (TRH) and its analogues. Peptides 1984;5:743–746.
10. Baltzer V, Weiskrantz L. Antidepressant agents and reversal of diurnal activity cycles in the rat. Biol Psychiatry 1973;10:199–209.
11. Fekete M, Van Ree JM, De Wied D. The ACTH-(4-9) analog ORG 2766 and des-glycinamide⁹-(Arg;8)-vasopressin reverse the retrograde amnesia induced by disrupting circadian rhythms in rats. Peptides 1986;7:563–568.
12. Niesink RJM, Van Ree JM. Antidepressant drugs normalize the increased social behavior of pairs of male rats induced by short term isolation. Neuropharmacology 1982;21:1343–1348.
13. Niesink RJM, Van Ree JM. Neuropeptides and social behavior of rats tested in dyadic encounters. Neuropeptides 1984;4:483–496.
14. Gaffori O, Van Ree JM. Serotonin and antidepressant drugs antagonize melatonin-induced behavioural changes after injection into the nucleus accumbens of rats. Neuropharmacology 1985;24:237–244.
15. Gaffori O, Van Ree JM. β-Endorphin-(10-16) antagonizes behavioral responses elicited by melatonin following injection into the nucleus accumbens of rats. Life Sci 1985;37:357–364.
16. Prange AJ Jr. Garbutt JC, Loosen PT, et al. The role of peptides in affective disorders: a review. Prog Brain Res 1987;572:235–247.
17. Prange AJ Jr, Loosen PT. Peptides in depression. In Usdin E, Asberg M, Bertilsson L, et al. (eds): Frontiers in Biochemical and Pharmacological Research in Depression. New York: Raven Press, 1984;127–145.
18. Van Ree JM, Verhoeven WMA, Claas FHJ, et al. Antipsychotic action of γ-type endorphins: animal and human studies. Prog Brain Res 1986;65:221–235.
19. Chazot G, Claustrat B, Brun J, et al. Rapid antidepressant activity of Des Tyr gamma endorphin: correlation with urinary melatonin. Biol Psychiatry 1985;20:1026–1030.

12. Antemortem and Postmortem Measures of Central Nervous System Serotonergic Function: Methodological Issues

MICHAEL STANLEY AND RONALD M. WINCHEL

Recent years have seen the emergence of great interest in the function of the serotonergic neurotransmitter system. Research in this area, however, is complicated by the relative inaccessibility of central measures (i.e., cerebrospinal fluid and brain tissue). Compounding this difficulty is the sensitivity of the serotonergic system to a number of variables. We review here a variety of factors that may influence measures of serotonergic activity and briefly discuss the evidence for their impact on these measures.

Evidence for the validity of cerebrospinal fluid (CSF) measures as reflective of CSF function is derived from the work of Stanley and colleagues[25], who measured 5-hydroxyindoleacetic acid (5-HIAA) and Homovanillic acid (HVA) in both CSF and frontal cortex simultaneously obtained at autopsy. A significant positive correlation was found between these two measures, demonstrating that CSF concentrations of 5-HIAA and HVA do accurately reflect changes in this region of the brain. These data validate the use of CSF analysis for evaluating central serotonergic and dopaminergic activity in living patients. It is interesting to note, however, that CSF HVA concentrations did not correlate with HVA measured in the caudate ($r = -0.09$; $N = 35$; n.s.).

Age

Evaluation of the effect of the subject's age on CSF levels of 5-HIAA yield inconsistent findings. Gottfries et al.[1] reported a significant positive correlation between age and CSF levels of 5-HIAA for 100 individuals ranging in age from 18 to 81 years. Traskman-Bendz[2] reported a weak positive correlation between age and 5-HIAA concentration. Bowers and Gerbode,[3] however, noted a much more complex relation between age and 5-HIAA levels. They found CSF concentrations of 5-HIAA to be much lower in the 35–55 years age group than in individuals who were either younger than 35 or older than 55.

Wode-Helgodt and Sedvall[4] and our group have found no correlation between age and 5-HIAA level. Post and co-workers[5] were also unable to find an age effect.

The latter studies, which find no evidence for an age effect, are consistent with some postmortem work that has also found no age effect for both 5-HIAA and serotonin (5-hydroxytryptamine, 5-HT) levels in the human frontal cortex.[6] These inconsistencies may be in part attributed to different proportions of individuals in the age groups. If an age effect were indeed present within certain age ranges, the different age distributions in the various samples may have obscured the effect. Reevaluation of this issue within more restricted age groups may settle the question.

Postmortem studies have addressed the age effect issue as well. Stanley and co-workers[7] examined the impact of age on 5-HT and 5-HIAA levels and [³H]imipramine binding in the human frontal cortex. Although no effect was seen on levels of 5-HT and 5-HIAA, age does appear to be positively correlated with [³H]imipramine binding. Severson et al.[8] studied [³H]imipramine binding in post-mortem samples and found that, although age did not appear to affect 5-HT and 5-HIAA levels, a strong positive correlation between age and imipramine binding was observed.

Gender

The influence of gender has also been investigated by several researchers; and as with the effect of age, there are inconsistencies in the findings. Whereas Traskman-Bendz reported differences in the mean values of CSF 5-HIAA concentration for male and female subjects[2] three other laboratories have not observed such differences.[1,3,9,]

Circadian Variation

Nicoletti and colleagues[10] studied circadian variations in CSF 5-HIAA with the use of a ventricular drain. Starting at 0600 hours and sampling fluid every 6 h, they observed a progressive increase in 5-HIAA up to 2400 hours with a return to starting levels again at 0600 hours.

Seasonal Influence

Traskman-Bendz[2] reported a nonsignificant trend in seasonal changes of 5-HIAA. They studied 155 controls and depressed patients and found the highest values during July and August. Losonczy et al.[11] found a significant seasonal variation in 5-HIAA levels in 24 schizophrenic patients. In their studies, however, they found the lowest 5-HIAA values at the same time of the year that Asberg's group[29] found the highest values. In our studies[12] we have not found a significant seasonal variation for CSF 5-HIAA. In contrast with Asberg's[29] data, we observed the highest monthly values in February and the lowest in January.

Variations Within Individual Patients

Multiple samplings of CSF obtained from the same subjects at different times appear to yield consistent values of 5-HIAA concentration. Post and Goodwin[13] observed a significant positive correlation between 5-HIAA values obtained from depressed patients on two occasions. Traskman-Bendz and co-workers[14] have reported the same findings for normal controls as well as depressed patients.

In our study[15] three lumbar punctures (LPs) were done on each patient at 1-week intervals. Values obtained at week 1 were highly correlated with values obtained at weeks 2 and 3. These findings suggest that, independent of drug effects, a single CSF 5-HIAA measurement in a patient is likely to be a representative one. It should be noted that in the foregoing experiment we took no particular dietary precautions when performing these measurements (other than an overnight fast), which suggests a relative lack of dietary influence on this measure. An intentionally enhanced diet of tryptophan-rich foods or extreme variations in nutritional states may still affect CSF 5-HIAA values,[16] but the random dietary variations in the sample studied did not significantly influence outcome.

Body Height

Height has been shown to have an impact on 5-HIAA levels. Several investigators have reported weak but significant inverse correlations between body height and 5-HIAA levels[2] (unpublished data).

This difference has been attributed to the presence of a concentration gradient of 5-HIAA in the CSF. 5-HIAA concentration in the ventricular fluid is higher than in the lumbar sac. An additional consideration related to this gradient is the site or lumbar interspace used to obtain the sample. Nordin et al.[17] have shown that by simply shifting the site of the LP in the same individual different 5-HIAA values can be obtained.

Activity

Some data indicate that it is possible to produce alterations in the level of 5-HIAA by changing the activity level of the patient prior to CSF sampling. Post et al.[18] asked patients to simulate mania for 4 h prior to an LP. (Among other behaviors, the patients ran through the corridors and turned cartwheels.) The results demonstrated a rise in 5-HIAA levels. Banki[19] also reported an activity-related rise in CSF 5-HIAA in depressed patients but not in controls. However, Kirstein et al.[20] reported lower levels of 5-HIAA as a function of increased motor activity. Although these studies differ in their results, CSF 5-HIAA concentrations do appear to change with motor activity. It therefore seems prudent to restrict activity in some uniform way prior to LP. (It is our practice to keep patients at bed rest for 8 h prior to the LP.)

Position

It has been suggested that changes such as those related to activity may result from mixing of the concentration gradient. To evaluate this possibility we performed LPs with patients in the lateral recumbent and sitting positions. We did not find any apparent difference.[21]

Drug Exposure

Drugs clearly affect 5-HIAA levels. Consistent findings demonstrate that medications that act as precursors or inhibitors of 5-HT synthesis, respectively, increase or decrease CSF 5-HIAA levels.[22] Similarly, drugs that alter the neuronal firing rate or receptor responsivity, such as tricyclic antidepressants, have been shown to alter 5-HIAA levels. In an attempt to evaluate how long a drug-free interval may be needed to avoid this medication effect, Traskman et al.[23] studied patients after washout periods ranging from 2 to 60 days (mean 15.7 days). No correlations were observed between the drug-free interval and CSF 5-HIAA. Similar results have been reported in a study of a large number of patients ($n = 120$) with a history of receiving a wide range of psychoactive compounds for various treatment intervals.[24]

Postmortem Studies

Except for the age-related effects noted by Stanley et al.[7] and Severson et al.[8] all of the investigational work described above was carried out with living patients. Although postmortem research allows for the direct study of central measures of serontonergic function, such work also creates several other confounding variables.

Postmortem Interval

The postmortem interval (PMI) represents the amount of time between death and the time the brain tissue is removed and frozen. Stanley et al.[25] assessed the impact of the PMI on 5-HT and 5-HIAA levels. The PMI range was 6–45 h. There was a significant positive correlation between the PMI and 5-HT levels in the frontal cortex. They did not find evidence for a significant effect of PMI on levels of 5-HIAA. Severson's group[8] also found evidence for a PMI effect on 5-HT, but they found an affect in the opposite direction, i.e., a decrease in 5-HT with increasing PMI. This difference between the two studies may be explained by the different postmortem interval ranges they studied. In the study conducted by Stanley and colleagues the average PMI was approximately 15 h. In Severson's sample the average was 36 h (in some cases more than 72 h). It may be that there is an initial rise in 5-HT levels after death with a subsequent fall. Severson's group, however, also found no significant effect of the PMI on 5-HIAA. Consistent with the absence of the PMI effect on 5-HIAA is previously published data that have shown that amines are more sensitive to the PMI than are their acidic metabolites.[26]

Regional Specificity in Dissection

In an attempt to evaluate the possible regional differences in 5-HT and 5-HIAA levels in the cortex, McIntyre and Stanley[27] dissected homogeneous samples corresponding to frontal, temporal, and occipital cortex. In this study the frontal cortex showed significantly higher concentrations of 5-HT and 5-HIAA compared with that in the temporal or occipital region. In a second experiment, three progressive (rostral to caudal) 1-mm slices of the frontal cortex were examined for regional concentration differences in 5-HT and 5-HIAA levels. A significant variation was noted with a rostral to caudal increase in 5-HIAA levels; that for 5-HT was consistent. Therefore significant differences exist among the general areas of the cortex (i.e., frontal, occipital, and temporal) as well as within each area.

Mode of Death

The mode of death can have an significant impact on serotonergic measures. Patients who die secondary to massive doses of certain drugs (e.g., tricyclic antidepressants, cocaine) may have an alteration in central nervous system 5-HIAA as a direct result of the drug.[28]

We (unpublished data) compared several modes of death in a sample in which we measured 5-HT and 5-HIAA levels in frontal cortex specimens. Our comparisons included death by hanging versus gunshot, hanging and overdose versus gunshot, cardiovascular versus gunshot, and gunshot to the head versus gunshot to the body. Among all of these comparisons we found no significant differences. Nevertheless, it is difficult to draw a general conclusion from these data, and we suggest that postmortem studies of serotonergic activity include descriptions of modes of death. Case-control grouping of patients by the nature of the death should be used because of this unknown variable.

Acknowledgment. Supported in part by U.P.H.S. Grants MH42242 and MH41847 and by the Scottish Rite Schizophrenia Research Program and the Lowenstein Foundation.

References

1. Gottfries CG, Gottfries I, Johansson B, et al. Acid monoamine metabolites in human CSF and their relation to age and sex. Neuropharmacology 1971;10:665–672.
2. Traskman-Bendz L. Depression and suicidal behavior. M.D., Ph.D. thesis, Karolinska Institute, Stockholm, 1980.
3. Bowers MB, Gerbode F. Relationship of monoamine metabolites in human CSF to age. Nature 1968;219:1256–1257.
4. Wode-Helgodt B, Sedvall G. Correlations between height of subject and concentrations of monoamine metabolites in CSF from psychotic men and women. Commun Psychopharmacol. 1978;2:177–183
5. Post RM, Ballenger JC, Goodwin FK. CSF studies of neurotransmitter function in manic and depressive illness. In Wood JH (ed): Neurobiology of CSF. New York: Plenum Press, 1980;690.
6. Stanley M, Mann JJ, Cohen L. Role of the serotonergic system in the post-mortem analysis of suicide. Psychopharmacol Bull 1986;22:735–40.
7. Stanley M. Presynaptic measures of serotonin in suicide. Paper delivered at the convention of the American College of Neuropsychopharmacology, Maui, 1985.
8. Severson JA, Marwsson JO, Osterburg HH. Elevated density of [³H]imipramine binding in aged human brain. J Neurochem 1985;45:1382–1389.
9. Sedvall G, Gyro B, Gullberg B, et al. Relationships in healthy volunteers between concentrations of monoamine metabolites a CSF and family history of psychiatric morbidity. Br J Psychiatry 1980;136:366–374.
10. Nicoletti F, Raffaele R, Falsaperla A, et al. Circadian variation in 5-HIAA levels in human CSF. Eur Neurol 1984;20:834–838.
11. Losonsczy MF, Mohs RC, Davis KL. Seasonal variation in human lumbar CSF neurotransmitter metabolite concentrations. Psychiatr Res 1984;12:79–87.
12. Stanley M. Relationship of platelet imipramine binding to CNS serotonergic functioning in man: autopsy and CSF correlations. Paper delivered at the convention of the American College of Neuropsychopharmacology, Puerto Rico, 1984.
13. Post RM, Goodwin FK. Studies of CSF amine metabolites in depressed patients. In Mendels J (ed): Biological Aspects of Depression. New York: Spectrum, 1975;47–67.
14. Traskman-Bendz L, Asberg M, Bertilsson L, et al. CSF monoamine metabolites in depressed patients during illness and after recovery. Acta Psychiatr Scand 1984;69:333–342.
15. Stanley M. CSF measures: basic and clinical correlates. Address at the Convention of the American Psychiatric Association, Chicago, 1987.
16. Kaye WH, Ebert MH, Raleigh M, et al. Abnormalities in CNS monoamine metabolism in anorexia nervosa. Arch Gen Psychiatry 1984;41:350–355.

17. Nordin C, Siwers B, Bertilsson L. Site of lumbar puncture influences level of monoamine metabolites (letter to the editor). Arch Gen Psychiatry 1982;39:1445.
18. Post RM, Kotin J, Goodwin FK, et al. Psychomotor activity and CSF amine metabolites in affective illness. Am J Psychiatry 1973;130:67–72.
19. Banki CM. Correlation between CSF amine metabolites and psychomotor activity in affective disorders. J Neurochem 1977;28:255–257.
20. Kirstein L, Bowers MB Jr, Heninger G. CSF amine metabolites, clinical symptoms and body movement in psychiatric patients. Biol Psychiatry 1976;2:241–234.
21. Gateless D, Stanley M, Traskman-Bendz L, et al. The influence of the lying and sitting positions on the gradients of 5-HIAA and HVA in lumbar CSF. Biol Psychiatry 1984;19:1585–1589.
22. Post RM, Goodwin FK. Effects of amitriptyline and imipramine on amine metabolites in the CSF of depressed patients. Arch Gen Psychiatry 1974;30:234–239.
23. Traskman L, Asberg M, Bertilsson L, et al. Monoamine metabolites in CSF and suicidal behavior. Arch Gen Psychiatry 1981;38:63.
24. Koslow SH, Maas JW, Davis JM, et al. Tricyclic antidepressant washout effects of CSF and urinary monoamines and metabolites (letter to the editor). Arch Gen Psychiatry 1986;43:1012–1013.
25. Stanley M, Traskman-Bendz L, Dorovini-Zis K. Correlations between aminergic metabolites simultaneously obtained from samples of CSF and brain. Life Sci. 1985;37:1279–1286.
26. Wilk S, Stanley M. Dopamine metabolites in human brain. Psychopharmacology 1978;57:77.
27. McIntyre IM, Stanley M. Post morterm anmd regional changes in serotonin, 5-HIAA and tryptophan in the brain. J Neurochem 1984;42:1589–92.
28. Petrouka S, Snyder SH. Long-term antidepressant treatment lowers spiroperidol labeled serotonin receptor binding. Science 1980;210:88–90.
29. Asberg M, Bertilsson L, Rydin E, et al. Monoamine metabolites in cerebrospinal fluid in relation to depressive illness, suicidal behavior and personality. In Angrist B, Burrows G, Lader M, et al. (eds): Recent Advances in Neuropsychopharmacology. New York: Pergamon Press, 1981;257–271.

13. Postmortem Investigation of Serotonergic and Peptidergic Hypotheses of Affective Illness

I.N. Ferrier, I.G. McKeith, B.G. Charlton, C.A. Whitford, E. Marshall, R.H. Perry, D. Eccleston, and J.A. Edwardson

Some pharmacological[1,2] and neuroendocrinological[3] data support the notion that in depression there is an increase in postsynaptic serotonin (5-hydroxytryptamine, 5-HT) receptor function consequent to a diminished presynaptic availability of 5-HT. Each of these lines of evidence has been criticized, and all are indirect. An alternative approach has been to examine parameters of serotonergic function in postmortem tissue. Studies to date have largely involved suicide cases. Conflicting results on 5-hydroxyindoleacetic acid (5-HIAA) levels and 5-HT receptors have been reported.[4] Mann et al.[5] reported a significant increase in the number of 5-HT sites in drug-free suicides compared with matched controls, but this was not replicated in another study.[6] Such discrepancies may arise from the use of data from suicide patients, a heterogeneous group for whom clinical documentation is often lacking and of whom fewer than half may have a history of affective disorder.[4]

Corticotropin-releasing factor (CRF) has an extensive distribution in human brain. Hyperactivity of the hypothalamo-pituitary-adrenal axis is a common observation in patients with major depression, and hypersecretion of hypothalamic CRF is at least partly responsible. Patients with major depression have a significantly higher cerebrospinal fluid (CSF) level of CRF than controls.[7] CRF has a number of behavioral effects in animals that are similar to those seen in depressed patients, and so a generalized central nervous system (CNS) hypersecretion of CRF hypothesis of depression has been formulated. Somatostatin (SRIF) has an extensive CNS distribution in human brain, and reduced CSF concentrations of SRIF have been reported in major depression.[8] In the present study we have measured these peptides and 5-HT receptors in tissue from well documented depressed patients.

Materials and Methods

Full methodological details are given elsewhere.[4,9] Diagnoses were made by DSM-III criteria,[10] and cases were excluded if there was a history of drug or alcohol abuse, severe physical disease, prolonged anoxia before death, or clinical or neuropathological evidence of organic brain disease. Eight patients were assigned a

DSM-III diagnosis of major depressive disorder, one bipolar disorder, and seven dysthymic disorder. A similar percentage (60%) of both the major depressive disorder and dysthymic disorder patients were on antidepressants before death, but the remainder were drug-free for at least 4 weeks. Six aged-matched drug-free controls were studied. Delay between death and postmortem examination was similar for the three groups.

Tissue was taken from frontal pole gray matter (Brodmann area 10). Membranes were prepared by standard methods, the details of which are described elsewhere.[9] Tissue for radioimmunoassay (RIA) was extracted using 0.1 M hydrochloric acid in 0.005 M ascorbic acid.

[3H] Serotonin was used to estimate 5-HT$_1$ binding and [3H]ketanserin to estimate 5-HT$_2$ binding, both at a radioligand concentration of 2.0 nM. Membrane suspensions were then pooled equally for each patient within diagnostic groups, and saturation curves were obtained using six concentrations (0.25–4.00 nM) of [3H]ketanserin and [3H]5-HT. Scatchard analysis gave values for Bmax and Kd. CRF RIA was performed according to the protocol of Linton and Lowry.[11] SRIF RIA was performed using the technique and reagents supplied by Amersham International, UK, with standard SRIF 14 from CRB, UK. The antiserum cross-reacts with SRIF 14, 25, and 28.

Results

Results are shown in Table 13.1 (mean ± SEM). 5-HT$_1$ and 5-HT$_2$ bindings were both higher in major affective disorder cases (51% and 37% increase over control values, respectively). The differences just failed to reach a 1 in 20 level of significance. The dysthymic group values were similar to those of the controls. Bmax values for 5-HT$_1$ binding showed only a modest increase (13%) over control values for major affective disorder, whereas the increase in 5-HT$_2$ binding (33%) was similar to that seen for the single concentration experiment. CRF levels were identical in the three groups. SRIF levels were lower in the major depressive group (with a subgroup below the lowest control value), but the difference failed to reach significance ($0.1 > p > 0.05$). No significant correlation between any of

TABLE 13.1. 5HT binding sites and peptides in frontal cortex of depressed patients and controls.

Group	Major depressive disorder	Dysthymic disorder	Control
5HT$_1$ specific binding using 2 nM ^{3}H–5-HT (fmol/mg protein)	47 ± 15	34 ± 7	31 ± 7
5 HT$_1$ Bmax (fmol/mg protein)	94.7	78.4	83.8
5-HT$_1$ Kd (nm)	2.8	2.61	3.91
5-HT$_2$ specific binding using 2nM ^{3}H-ketanserin (fmol/mg protein)	103 ± 19	68 ± 12	75 ± 14
5 HT$_2$ Bmax (fmol/mg protein)	131.7	91.8	98.8
5-HT$_2$ Kd (nm)	0.77	0.71	0.49
CRF (pg/mg protein)	338 ± 72 (7)	354 ± 100 (3)	361 ± 241
SRIF (fmol/mg tissue)	39.7 ± 4.3 (7)	45.3 ± 8.5 (3)	46.7 ± 5.3

The numbers of patients are as in the text unless stated in parentheses.

the measured values was found, and no significant relations between clinical variables (e.g., presence or absence of melancholia, psychosis, drug treatment) were established.

Discussion

The results of the single concentration assays demonstrate a tendency toward increased 5-HT$_1$ and 5-HT$_2$ receptor binding in the frontal cortex of elderly patients known to have suffered from major affective disorder compared to age-matched dysthymic disorder patients and normal controls. Care was taken to exclude any patient with degenerative brain disease. Aging has been shown to be associated with decreases in 5-HT receptors,[12] but the influence of such an effect on our results should be minimized by age matching. The strategy of using an inpatient depressed group for such a study offers advantages of diagnostic accuracy over the use of suicide cases. For 5-HT$_2$ binding to membranes from patients with major affective disorder, the increase in single concentration values is reflected by a similar increase in Bmax using pooled material. For 5-HT$_1$ binding the large increase in binding observed in the single concentration experiments is not reflected by a similarly large increase in Bmax, illustrating the difficulty of extrapolating from single point estimations in this type of study. There are several factors that may account for the apparently conflicting results[5,6] on 5-HT receptors in postmortem brain from suicide patients. There is a large variation in normal values probably due to sampling effects, as there are large variations in 5-HT receptor density in different parts and layers of the same area of cortex.[13]

Despite these methodological considerations, these results are similar, in terms of both relative and absolute values, to the findings from suicide brains obtained by Mann et al.[5] An increase in 5-HT$_2$ binding sites in frontal cortex in major affective disorder is compatible with both a hypothesis of an abnormality in the ascending 5-HT system from the dorsal raphe nucleus and the observed effects of antidepressants on 5-HT binding.[14]

No change in CRF or SRIF immunoreactivity was found, although there was a trend for lower levels of SRIF that requires further study. These results therefore do not provide support for the notion that the altered levels of CRF[7] and SRIF[8] in CSF from major depressives reflects a similar change in brain. However, concentrations of peptides measured by RIA do not give a measure of the functional activity and/or turnover of that peptide. Our results indicate that there is no gross change in these peptide levels in depressed brain. Changes in peptides have been shown to be markers for neuropathological change in a number of neuropsychiatric conditions, and therefore our results are evidence that cells containing these peptides are not damaged in depression, as seems to be the case with Alzheimer's disease. Further studies of these peptides and their receptors are under way in an enlarged series of brains.

References

1. Asberg M, Bertilsson L, Martenson B, et al. CSF monoamine metabolites in melancholia. Acta Psychiatr Scand 1984;69:201–219.
2. Van Praag HM. Management of depression with serotonin precursors. Biol Psychiatry 1981;16:290–310.

3. Meltzer HY, Umberkoman-Witta B, Robertson A, et al. Effect of 5-hydroxytryptophan on serum cortisol levels in major affective disorders. Arch Gen Psychiatry 1984;41:366–374.
4. Ferrier IN, McKeith IG, Cross AJ, et al. Post-mortem neurochemical studies in depression. Ann NY Acad Sci 1986;47:128–142.
5. Mann JJ, Stanley M, McBride PA, et al. Increased serotonin and β-adrenergic receptor binding in the frontal cortices of suicide victims. Arch Gen Psychiatry 1986;43:954–959.
6. Owen FJ, Chambers DR, Cooper SJ, et al. Serotonergic mechanisms in brains of suicide victims. Brain Res 1986;362:185–188.
7. Nemeroff CB, Widerlov E, Bissette G, et al. Elevated concentrations of CSF corticotropin-releasing factor-like immunoreactivity in depressed patients. Science 1984; 226:1342–1344.
8. Bissette G, Widerlov E, Walleus H, et al. Alterations in cerebrospinal fluid concentrations of somatostatin-like immunoreactivity in neuropsychiatric disorders. Arch Gen Psychiatry 1986;43:1148–1151.
9. McKeith IG, Marshall E, Ferrier IN, et al. 5HT receptor binding in post-mortem brain from patients with affective disorder. J Affective Disord 1987;13:67–74.
10. American Psychiatric Association. DSM III, Diagnostic and Statistical Manual of Mental Disorders. 3rd ed. Washington, DC: APA, 1980.
11. Linton E, Lowry PJ. Comparison of a specific two-site immunoradiometric assay with radioimmunoassay for rat/human CRF-41. Regul Peptides 1986;14:69–84.
12. Marcusson JO, Morgan DG, Winblad B, et al. Serotonin-2 binding sites in human frontal cortex and hippocampus: selective loss of S-2A sites with age. Brain Res 1984;311:51–56.
13. Bigeon A, Kargman S, Snyder L, et al. Characterisation and localisation of serotonin receptors in human brain post-mortem. Brain Res 1986;353:91–98.
14. Peroutka SJ, Snyder SH. Long term antidepressant treatment decreased spiperidol labelled serotonin receptor binding. Science 1980;210:88–90.

I.C. CHOLINERGIC MECHANISMS

14. Genetic Animal Model of Depression with Cholinergic Supersensitivity

DAVID H. OVERSTREET

There has been renewed interest in cholinergic mechanisms underlying affective disorders because of the increased sensitivity of affective disorder patients to cholinergic agonists[1] and cholinergically mediated rapid eye movement (REM) sleep abnormalities in depressed patients.[2] The Flinders Sensitive Line (FSL) and Flinders Resistant Line (FRL) of rats were selectively bred to differ in their sensitivity to the anticholinesterase compound diisopropyl fluorophosphate (DFP).[3,4] Later the FSL rats were found to be more sensitive to muscarinic agonists, and it became apparent that they may be an animal model of depression that focuses on cholinergic supersensitivity.[5] The present chapter reviews the evidence that supports the FSL rats as an animal model of depression.

Genetics

An earlier study found evidence for DFP sensitivity to be genetically regulated differently in the sexes: Sensitivity to DFP was related to one or more recessive genes in male rats, but additive genetic variance was involved in the female rats.[6] A more recent study has examined responses to muscarinic agonists in the FSL and FRL rats and genetic crosses. Biometrical genetic analyses of the data indicated that all of the differences among the groups could be explained by additive and dominance genetic variance (Overstreet et al., in preparation). Thus the increased muscarinic sensitivity of FSL rats has a clear genetic basis.

Behavioral Differences

Because the cholinergic system is involved in many behavioral and physiological processes, the genetically influenced cholinergic supersensitivity in the FSL may result in some behavioral or physiological changes. Indeed, a number of baseline differences between the FSL and FRL rats have been observed, including decreased body weight and locomotor activity, changes that are well documented to occur in humans who become depressed.[4,5] One report, however, has indicated that euthymic patients with a history of affective disorders also showed reduced activity compared to control subjects.[7]

The FSL and FRL rats also exhibit differences on avoidance tasks. The FSL rats perform poorly on an active avoidance task.[8] In contrast, they have a significantly better memory on a passive avoidance task.[5] These differences in avoidance behavior between the FSL and FRL rats could be accountable by differences in shock-induced suppression in activity.[9] The FSL rats were much more inactive in an open field after exposure to foot shock.[5,10] This difference was not the consequence of differences in shock sensitivity because the FSL and FRL rats exhibited comparable shock sensitivities.[10] The FSL rats also exhibited longer periods of immobility in the forced swim test.[5,10] Thus the FSL rats are more sensitive to mild stressors and may therefore resemble depressed humans, who may also be more sensitive to stressors.[11]

A final parallel between human depressives and the FSL rats is in REM sleep. It is well known that human depressives have a more rapid onset of REM sleep and increased REM density. We have completed sleep studies in eight FSL rats and six FRL rats. These studies indicated that FSL rats had an increased amount of REM sleep and tended to go into REM sleep from the drowsy state more frequently than the FRL rats.[12]

In summary, the FSL rats exhibit a number of behavioral and physiological characteristics that resemble those seen in human depressives, as indicated in Table 14.1.

Cholinergic Differences

Several studies have confirmed the increased sensitivity of the FSL rats to muscarinic agonists using a range of behavioral and physiological indices.[5,13] These findings, which are summarized in Table 14.1, are similar to the findings for depressed humans, who also exhibit increased behavioral and hormonal sensitivity to muscarinic agonists.[1]

The data on muscarinic receptor (mAChR) binding in humans is not straightforward. The promising early report of increased mAChR binding on fibroblasts from human depressives and their ill relatives has not been confirmed. Similarly, there has been one positive report of increased mAChR binding in the brain of suicides but two negative reports.[14] This lack of uniformity may be a consequence of the brain region selected for the binding studies—the cortex. We have found that the increased mAChR binding in the FSL rats occurs in the hippocampus and striatum but not in the cortex. Instead, in this region we have observed an increase in acetylcholine synthesis.[15] There is a need to look at mAChR binding in other human brain regions.

TABLE 14.1. Parallels between FSL rats and depressed humans.

Phenomenology	Cholinergic System
Reduced activity	Increased behavioral sensitivity to muscarinic agonists
Reduced body weight	Increased hormonal sensitivity to muscarinic agonists
Reduced REM latency	Increased muscarinic receptor density
Increased REM density	
Increased sensitivity to stress	

Neurotransmitter Interactions

The cholinergic system interacts with other neurotransmitter systems to regulate many functions. Because FSL rats have a genetically influenced muscarinic su-persensitivity, secondary changes in other neurotransmitter systems may have occurred. Our approach to this question has been to employ receptor agonists and to study operant responding for water reward, general activity, and core body temperature. To date, every agonist studied has induced hypothermia that was significantly greater in FSL rats; agonists included apomorphine, a dopamine ag-onist; m-chlorophenylpiperazine, a serotonin agonist; diazepam, a benzodiazepine agonist; and muscimol, a GABA agonist.[16,17] The FSL rats also tended to be more sensitive to the depressive effects of m-chlorophenylpiperazine, diazepam, and muscimol but less sensitive to the stereotypy-inducing effects of apomorphine. Studies suggest that the increased benzodiazepine-γ-amino-butyric acid (GABA) sensitivity in the FSL rats may be related to increased binding sites.[17] Data on serotonin and dopamine binding sites have not been collected as yet. Thus there are changes in the sensitivity of drugs acting on other neurotransmitter systems in the FSL rats.

Conclusions

The FSL rats resemble depressed humans in many respects (Table 14.1). We submit that they are a genetic animal model of depression with cholinergic supersensitivity.

References

1. Risch SC, Kalin NH, Janowsky DS. cholinergic challenge in affective illness: behavioral and neuroendocrine correlates. J Clin Psychopharmacol 1981;1:186–192.
2. Sitaram N, Nurnberger JI, Gershon E, et al. Faster cholinergic regulation of mood and REM sleep: a potential model and marker for vulnerability to depression. Am J Psychiatry 1982;139:571–576.
3. Overstreet DH, Russell RW, Helps SC, et al. Selective breeding for sensitivity to the anticholinesterase, DFP. Psychopharmacology 1979;65:15–20.
4. Russell RW, Overstreet DH, Messenger M, et al. Selective breeding for sensitivity to DFP: generalisation of effects beyond criterion variables. Pharmacol Biochem Behav 1982;17:885–891.
5. Overstreet DH. Selective breeding for increased cholinergic function: development of a new animal model of depression. Biol Psychiatry 1986;21:49–58.
6. Overstreet DH, Russell RW. Selective breeding for differences in cholinergic function: sex differences in the genetic regulation of sensitivity to the anticholinesterase, DFP. Behav Neurol Biol 1984;40:227–238.
7. Wolff EA, Putnam FW, Post RM. Motor activity and affective illness: the relationship of amplitude and temporal distribution to changes in affective state. Arch Gen Psychiatry 1985;42:288–294.
8. Overstreet DH, Measday M. Impaired active avoidance performance in rats with cho-linergic supersensitivity: its reversal with chronic imipramine. Presented at the 4th In-ternational Congress of Biological Psychiatry, Philadelphia, 1985.
9. McAllister TW. Cognitive functioning in the affective disorders. Comp Psychiatry 1981;22:572–586.
10. Overstreet DH, Janowsky DS, Gillin JC, et al. Stress-induced immobility in rats with cholinergic supersensitivity. Biol Psychiatry 1986;21:657–664.
11. Anisman HS, Zacharko RM. Depression: the predisposing influence of stress. Behav Brain Sci 1982;5:89–137.

12. Shiromani PJ, Overstreet DH, Levy D, et al. Increased REM sleep in rats selectively bred for cholinergic hyperactivity. Neuropsychopharmacology 1988;1:127–133.
13. Overstreet DH, Booth RA, Dana R, et al. Enhanced elevation of corticosterone following arecoline administration to rats selectively bred for increased cholinergic function. Psychopharmacology 1986;88:129–130.
14. Dilsaver SC. cholinergic hypothesis of depression. Brain Res Rev 1986;11:285–316.
15. Overstreet DH, Russell RW, Crocker AD, et al. Selective breeding for differences in cholinergic function: pre- and post-synaptic mechanisms involved in sensitivity to the anticholinesterase, DFP. Brain Res 1984;294:327–332.
16. Wallis E, Overstreet DH, Crocker AD. Selective breeding for increased cholinergic function: psychopharmacological evidence for altered serotonergic sensitivity. Pharmacol Biochem Behav (in press).
17. Pepe S, Crocker AD, Overstreet DH. Altered GABA-benzodiazepine sensitivity in an animal model of depression with cholinergic supersensitivity. Presented at the Conference on New Directions in Affective Disorders, Jerusalem, 1987.

15. Impact of the Cholinergic System on the Hypothalamic-Pituitary-Adrenocortical Axis and on REM Sleep

J-C. KRIEG AND M. BERGER

The activation of the hypothalamic-pituitary-adrenocortical (HPA) axis and the regulation of rapid eye movement (REM) sleep are believed to be mediated by cholinergic neurons. The finding that depressed patients display an increased responsiveness of the HPA axis or of REM sleep to a cholinergic stimulus has been interpreted as a sign of a supersensitivity of cholinergic neurons.[1,2] However, as the application of cholinomimetics such as physostigmine or arecoline is frequently accompanied by unpleasant side effects, the question was posed whether in those experiments the HPA axis was directly activated by the cholinergic agonists or more indirectly via a stress stimulus.[3,4] In addition, considerable doubts about a depression-related supersensitivity of cholinergic neurons activating the cortisol system were expressed by Berger and co-workers,[5] who demonstrated that after dexamethasone suppression the HPA axis of depressed patients was no more sensitive to a physostigmine challenge than was that of healthy subjects.

A suitable drug for studying the effect of a cholinergic stimulus on the HPA axis and on REM sleep and for elucidating a possible supersensitivity of cholinergic neurons in depression is the centrally acting muscarinic agonist RS 86. It has an alleged preference for M1 receptors, lacks nicotinic properties, has a half-life of 6–8 hrs, and produces only minor peripheral side effects in the dose range used.

HPA Axis

At approximately weekly intervals and in a random design, 12 healthy volunteers aged 18–43 years received placebo or 1.5 or 3.0 mg RS 86 at 5:00 p.m. For cortisol analysis blood samples were drawn at half-hour intervals between 4:00 p.m. and 8:00 p.m. Figure 15.1 shows the mean plasma cortisol profile of the 12 volunteers prior to and after the intake of placebo and RS 86. All three profiles display a decline, which apparently reflects the circadian secretion pattern of cortisol. No statistically significant increase in plasma cortisol levels could be observed after the 5:00 p.m. intake of RS 86.

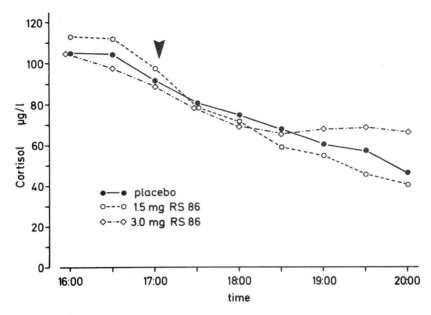

FIGURE 15.1. Mean plasma cortisol profiles of 12 healthy subjects prior to and after the intake of placebo or 1.5 or 3.0 mg RS 86 at 5 p.m.

REM Sleep

Eighteen healthy volunteers aged 21–65 years as well as seven patients aged 21–50 years with a major depressive disorder took part in the study. Seven of the healthy subjects served as an age- and sex-matched control group for the depressed patients. After a night of adaptation, all subjects received placebo and 1.5 mg RS 86, respectively, at 10:00 p.m. the two following nights. Sleep was recorded using standard procedures (electroencephlography, electrooculography, electromyography). Blood samples for cortisol analysis were obtained at 11:15 p.m.

The volunteers displayed a significant RS 86-induced shortening of REM latency as well as an increase in REM sleep. However, no significant difference was observed in the plasma cortisol levels between the placebo and the RS 86 experiment. In the depressed patients, the RS 86-induced effect on REM sleep was even more pronounced than in the matched control subjects. Again, there was no significant difference in the mean plasma cortisol concentration between the placebo and RS 86 situation (Table 15.1).

Discussion

The findings reported here may indicate a depression-related supersensitivity of muscarinic neurons regulating REM sleep. The results, however, fail to demonstrate that the HPA axis is activated by the muscarinic agonist RS 86 or is supersensitive to an RS 86 challenge in depression.

There are two possible explanations for the absence of an activating effect of RS 86 on the cortisol system. First, Cortisol secretion is mediated by muscarinic

TABLE 15.1. REM sleep and cortisol response to the muscarinic agonist RS 86 in depressed patients and healthy subjects.

	Depressives ($n = 8$)			Controls ($n = 8$)		
Parameter	Placebo	RS 86	Wilcoxon test (two-tailed)	Placebo	RS 86	Wilcoxon test (two-tailed)
REM latency (min)	68.4 ± 34.3	14.2 ± 18.9	$p < 0.05$	65.9 ± 12.6	39.2 ± 26.2	$p < 0.08$
REM sleep (%SPT)	21.6 ± 4.3	29.5 ± 4.6	$p < 0.05$	19.2 ± 3.4	23.4 ± 6.8	NS
Cortisol (μg/l)	25 ± 14	21 ± 21	NS	57 ± 70	50 ± 55	NS

Means ± SD given
%SPT = sleep period time. NS = not significant.

receptors different from those on which RS 86 acts. According to respective studies, the idea of nicotinic receptors activating the HPA axis also must be considered.[6] On the other hand, nothing is known about a disturbed functioning of nicotinic receptors in depression. The second explanation, which we favor, is that cholinergic neurons do not directly activate the HPA axis in humans at all. Like weight loss, inner turmoil, or drug withdrawal, the noxious side effects of physostigmine or arecoline activate the HPA axis in a nonspecific way, resulting in hypercortisolemia. Thus hypercortisolism or dexamethasone nonsuppression frequently observed in depression can be explained as a consequence of stressful emotional arousal and is not due to a supersensitivity of cholinergic neurons alleged to activate the HPA axis.

References

1. Carroll BJ, Greden JF, Haskett R, et al. Neurotransmitter studies of neuroendocrine pathology in depression. Acta Psychiatr Scand [Suppl 280] 1980;183–199.
2. Sitaram N, Nurnberger JJ, Gershon ES, et al. Cholinergic regulation of mood and REM sleep: potential model and marker of vulnerability to affective disorder. Am J Psychiatry 1982;139:571–576.
3. Doerr P, Berger M. Physostigmine-induced escape from dexamethasone suppression in normal adults. Biol Psychiatry 1983;18:261–268.
4. Lewis DA, Sherman BM, Kathol RG. Analysis of the specificity of physostigmine stimulation of adrenocorticotropin in man. J Clin Endocrinol Metab 1984;58:570–573.
5. Berger M, Doerr P, Zerssen von D. Physostigmine's influence on DST results. Am J Psychiatry 1984;141:469–470.
6. Wilkins JN, Carlson HE, van Vunakis H, et al. Nicotine from cigarette smoking increases circulating levels of cortisol, growth hormone, and prolactin in male chronic smokers. Psychopharmacology 1982;70:305–308.

16. Relation Between m-Cholinoceptor Density on Human Blood Cells and Psychological Predisposition Factors for Depression

WALTER E. MÜLLER, BIRGIT BERING, AND HANS W. MOISES

A variety of experimental evidence indicate that disturbances of cholinergic neurotransmission are involved in the etiology of affective disorders, with some evidence for sensitivity changes at the level of the central muscarinic cholinergic receptors.[1-3] However, direct experimental evidence for this hypothesis is still missing, as a suitable model to study m-cholinoceptor sensitivity in man and especially in psychiatric patients is not available. Accordingly, we have started to investigate the use of human blood cells as easily accessible tissues to study the properties of m-cholinoceptors in man.[4,5]

Muscarinic cholinergic receptor binding to human erythrocyte membranes and to intact circulating human lymphocytes was determined using tritiated quinuclidinyl benzilate (^{3}H-QNB) or tritiated N-methylscopolamine (^{3}H-NMS) as radioligands. The experimental details have been reported elsewhere.[4,5] β-Adrenergic receptor binding to intact circulating human lymphocytes was determined using tritiated dihydroalprenolol (^{3}H-DHA) as radioligand.

Using the radioligands indicated above, low levels of specific binding could be demonstrated in both of the human tissues, with average densities of about 80 fmol/mg protein for the erythrocyte membranes and about 15 fmol/10^6 lymphocytes.[4,5] Specific binding in both tissues could be inhibited by a variety of cholinergic agonists and antagonists in a fashion typical for muscarinic cholinergic receptor binding (Table 16.1), e.g., with Hill coefficients close to 1.0 for antagonists but significantly smaller than 1.0 for agonists and with a pronounced stereospecificity for the enantiomers of QNB with a much higher inhibition constant for the pharmacologically active (R) enantiomer. However, in most cases muscarinic antagonists showed a considerable lower affinity in both human tissues than in parallel experiments using rat heart and rat brain membranes (Table 16.1). The same observation was made for the dissociation constants of the radioligands, where again a lower affinity was found in both human tissues than in the two rat tissues when investigated in parallel experiments. The drug pirenzepine, a rather specific antagonist of the M_1 m-cholinoceptor subclass, exhibited a relatively high affinity

TABLE 16.1. Inhibition constants of several cholinergic agonists and antagonists for muscarinic cholinergic receptor binding to various human and rat tissues.

	Human tissues				Rat tissues			
	Erythrocyte membranes		Intact lymphocytes		Brain		Heart membranes	
Drug	K_i	n_H	K_i	n_H	K_i	n_H	K_i	n_H
Atropine	21	1.04	10	0.93	1	1.04	1	0.97
Scopolamine	0.4	0.86	8	0.88	3	0.96	7	1.10
(R,S) QNB	2	0.91	10	0.89	1	0.99	0.4	0.98
(R) QNB	1		9		0.5		0.3	
(S) QNB	25		142		17		20	
Pirenzepine	169	0.68	1,440	0.84	178	0.68	2,100	0.89
Oxotremorine	580	0.57	3,320	0.67	187	0.63	264	0.61
Carbachol	1,150	0.49	5,500	0.51	39,000	0.70	1,400	0.52

K_i = inhibition constants. n_H = apparent Hill coefficients. For further details, see refs 4,5. [Reprinted by permission of the publisher from ref. 5, Copyright 1987 by Elsevier Science Publishing Co., Inc., and from ref. 4, with permission.]

for the m-cholinoceptors on human erythrocyte membranes and a rather low affinity for the m-cholinoceptors on human lymphocytes; these findings are similar to those for rat brain (a predominantly M_1 tissue) and rat heart (an M_2 tissue), providing evidence for a predominance of M_1 receptors on human erythrocytes and a predominance of M_2 receptors on human lymphocytes. This assumption could be supported by experiments using the stable GTP analogue GppNHp, which reduced agonist affinity but increased antagonist affinity for m-cholinoceptor binding to human lymphocytes, an effect that seems to be a specific response of the M_2 subclass only.[5] Similar experiments on human erythrocyte membranes did not show any effect of GppNHp.[4] The individual densities of both m-cholinoceptors varied in healthy volunteers over more than one order of magnitude but seemed to be a stable individual characteristic when assayed repeatedly over several weeks.[4,5]

In an attempt to investigate if different densities might represent predisposition factors for affective disorders we studied m-cholinoceptor density correlates with some personality traits known to predispose for depression.[6] In order to avoid biases resulting from disease and drug effects, the study was carried out on 16 healthy drug-free male volunteers (age 27 ± 4 years). For evaluation of personality traits, the Premorbid Personality Inventory (PP-I),[7] Freiburger Personality Inventory (FPI),[8] and Minnesota Multiphasic Personality Inventory (MMPI)[9] were used. The results are given in Table 16.2. Interestingly, significant correlations were found only for personality factors that have already been suggested as predisposing to depression; e.g., erythrocyte receptors correlated with reactive aggressiveness (dominance) on the FPI and extraversion on the PP-I as well as highly significantly negatively with depression on the MMPI. Lymphocyte receptors correlated with the orderliness scale on the PP-I, a psychometric measure of Tellenbach's melancholic type, and negatively with spontaneous aggressiveness. Furthermore, β-adrenoceptor density on the lymphocytes correlated negatively with spontaneous aggressiveness and extraversion on the FPI. A detailed discussion of these data is given elsewhere.[6]

In conclusion, our data give some preliminary evidence that premorbid personality traits of depressives might be related to the individual densities of m-cholinoceptors and/or β-adrenoceptors in such a way that increased as well as

TABLE 16.2. Spearmen's correlation coefficients[a] between receptor and personality measures ($n = 16$).

Personality scales	Bmax muscarinic receptors on erythrocytes (M1)	Bmax muscarinic receptors on lymphocytes (M2)	Bmax β-adrenergic receptors on lymphocytes
MMPI—depression	−71[c]	5	9
MMPI—Hypomania (k)[b]	18	11	−19
MMPI—paranoia	−25	−16	−11
MMPI—schizophrenia (k)	−24	24	24
FPI—depression	− 5	10	− 2
FPI—extraversion	25	−30	−38
FPI—neuroticism	− 8	22	2
FPI—spontaneous aggressiveness	3	−39	−51[d]
FPI—reactive aggressiveness dominance	48[d]	8	−15
PPI—orderliness	11	36	9
PPI—extraversion	46[d]	−19	−32
PPI—neuroticism	−17	28	32
PPI—frustration intolerance	9	23	4
PPI—schizoidea	−15	−31	−20
PPI—motivation	10	6	5
PPI—Social conformity	− 5	6	−13

[Reprinted from ref. 6, with permission.]
[a] Decimal points omitted.
[b] k = K-corrected.
[c] $p < .001$ (two-tailed).
[d] $p < 0.05$ (two-tailed).

decreased densities of these receptors might predispose an individual to the development of depression. Moreover, the findings are compatible with the postulated relation between personality and neurobiological predisposition factors of depressive disorders. Thus *m*-cholinoceptor as well as β-adrenoceptor densities could be part of a presumably genetically determined vulnerability to depression. However, because all of our volunteers were not depressive, these factors are not specific for depression and are probably neither a sufficient nor a necessary cause of this disorder. Additional biological or psychological factors seem to be required for the development of clinical depression.

Acknowledgment. Supported by a grant of the Deutsche Forschungsgemeinschaft.

References

1. Janowski DS, El-Yousef ML, Davis JM, et al. A cholinergic-adrenergic hypothesis of mania and depression. Lancet 1972;2:632–635.
2. Sitaram N, Nurnberger JI Jr, Gershon ES, et al. Cholinergic regulation of mood and REM sleep: potential model and marker of vulnerability to affective disorders. Am J Psychiatry 1982;139:571–576.
3. Snyder S. Cholinergic mechanisms in affective disorders. N Engl J Med 1984;311:254.
4. Bering B, Müller WE. Stereospecific ³H-QNB binding to human erythrocyte membranes associated with muscarinic cholinergic receptors. J Neural Transm 1987;68:97–111.

5. Bering B, Moises HW, Müller WE. Muscarinic cholinergic receptors on intact human lymphocytes: properties and subclass characterization. Biol Psychiatry 1987;22:1451–1458.
6. Moises HW, Bering B, Müller WE. Relationships between psychological and biological predisposition factors for depression. Eur Arch Psychiatry Neurol Sci (in press).
7. Dietzfelbinger T. Quantifizierende Erfassung biographischer Aspekte und prämorbider Persönlichkeitsdimensionen bei Neurosen und endogenen Psychosen. MD thesis, Technical University, Munich, 1985.
8. Fahrenberg J, Selg H, Hampel R. Das Freiburger Persönlichkeitsinventar FPI. 3. Auflage. Göttingen: Hogrefe, 1978.
9. Hathaway SR, McKinley JC. Minnesota Multiphasic Personality Inventory. New York: Psychological Corporation, 1942–1967.

17. Differential Effects of Physostigmine in Alcoholics, Alcoholics with Affective Disorder, and Normal Individuals

DAVID S. JANOWSKY AND S. CRAIG RISCH

Depression and anxiety are common among alcoholic populations, but interrelations with actual drinking behaviors are not particularly clear. Winokur et al.[1] have suggested that there may be at least three types of alcoholism, one occurring independently of other psychiatric illnesses and the others as part of either sociopathy or unipolar affective disorder. It also appears that excessive drinking occurs during bipolar affective episodes, and an association may exist between unipolar affective disorder and excessive drinking. Thus primary affective disorder patients do appear to increase drinking during periods of mania and perhaps depression.[2] It appears that alcoholic women with an affective disorder represent a separate population from alcoholic women without an affective disorder, having distinct demographic and prognostic patterns and family histories.[3,4]

The differentiation of patients with primary alcoholism from those with primary affective disorder and secondary alcoholism is complicated by the fact that alcoholics, when they drink, can develop a pharmacologically induced depressive syndrome. It may appear to be a major depressive disorder but is more often defined as sadness and feelings of depression. This depressive syndrome may occur when an alcoholic is drinking or during detoxification; in most alcoholics it disappears or dramatically decreases after up to 3 weeks of detoxification, regardless of whether antidepressants have been given.[5]

Therefore to distinguish whether a patient with alcoholism (a) is depressed due to the alcohol or (b) has a primary affective disorder and secondary alcoholism may require (a) observation of the patient for affective symptoms during prolonged "dry" intervals; (b) an obvious history of affective disorder antedating the alcoholism; (c) persistence of depressive symptoms long after detoxification has occurred; or (d) an apparent history that the depression occurs at times other than in the midst of chronic drinking and is noted independently.

The relevance of distinguishing between alcoholics with associated primary affective disorder and those in whom depression is secondary to alcohol consumption is important for several reasons. First, affective disorder alcoholic women have a better prognosis on short-term follow-up than nonaffective disorder alcoholic women. Second, in subjects who have continuing depression after a bout of alcoholism, the alcoholic relapse rate is higher. Third, although there is hard evidence that primary alcoholics and patients with primary affective disorders (and secondary alcoholism) respond differently to antidepressants and lithium with respect to their alcoholism, differentiation of these two subclasses during antidepressant trials may help ensure the uncovering of a successful treatment response. Furthermore, because primary affective disorder, with or without alcoholism is treatable and can be persistent and dangerous without treatment, antidepressant treatment is indicated in such patients.[3,4]

In a variety of studies we have observed that the centrally acting cholinesterase inhibitor/cholinomimetic agent physostigmine causes increases in negative affect and emesis, as well as plasma prolactin, cortisol, β-endorphin, and ACTH levels.[6,7] Furthermore, as described below, we have also noted that our alcoholic psychiatric controls were especially unreactive to physostigmine compared to affective disorder patients and patients with a combination of alcoholism and major affective disorder. Therefore it is possible that a cholinomimetic challenge may be a useful technique to discriminate between primary alcoholics with and without depression and secondary alcoholics whose alcoholism is associated with a major affective disorder.

TABLE 17.1. Significant differential effects of physostigmine (0.022 mg/kg i.v.) on various groups.

Parameter	Ratings		
	Primary alcoholics ($n = 15$)	Alcoholics + affective disorder ($n = 25$)	Normal controls ($n = 42$)
Beigel-Murphy Mania Scale			
Grandiosity	-0.1 ± 0.5	-1.6 ± 0.3	-2.8 ± 0.2*,a,b
Total	-1.0 ± 1.2	-1.8 ± 0.6	-3.7 ± 0.5***,a
BPRS: excitement	0.1 ± 0.2	0.6 ± 0.2	-0.1 ± 0.1**,b
Activation-Inhibition Scale			
Rater inhibition	8.6 ± 3.0	18.5 ± 3.0	16.6 ± 1.6****,c
Rater activation	-6.6 ± 0.6	-3.6 ± 0.6	-3.6 ± 0.3****,a
Rater dysophoria	0.8 ± 0.5	2.1 ± 0.5	1.1 ± 0.2*****
POMS			
Anxiety	1.8 ± 1.3	8.5 ± 2.1	7.8 ± 1.1***,a,c
Depression	-2.7 ± 1.8	4.0 ± 2.8	6.9 ± 1.5***,a
Hostility	-2.4 ± 2.5	3.5 ± 2.0	2.9 ± 1.1*****
Vigor	-4.1 ± 1.2	-6.0 ± 1.4	-9.7 ± 1.0**,a
Confusion	1.2 ± 0.6	5.9 ± 1.4	6.3 ± 0.7**,a,c
Elation	-1.1 ± 0.8	-3.4 ± 1.1	-4.9 ± 0.7**,a
Friendliness	-2.8 ± 0.7	-5.3 ± 1.6	-7.9 ± 0.9***,a
Cardiovascular parameters			
Systolic BP (mm Hg)	3.1 ± 1.9	9.4 ± 2.1	14.4 ± 2.0**,a
Diastolic BP (mm Hg)	3.3 ± 1.7	7.2 ± 1.3	10.2 ± 1.5**,a
Pulse (beats/min)	10.0 ± 3.5	14.2 ± 2.9	22.3 ± 2.6****,a
Gastrointestinal emesis	0.6 ± 0.2	1.5 ± 0.2	1.2 ± 0.2****,c

Overall significant differences among the three diagnostic groups: $*p < 0.001$; $**p < 0.01$; $***p < 0.025$; $****p < 0.05$; $*****p < 0.1$.
Significant specific comparisons between the three diagnostic groups: [a]Significance between normals and alcoholics. [b]Significance between alcoholics + affective disorder and normals. [c]Significance between alcoholics and alcoholics + affective disorder.

In the study described below, our experimental group consisted of 84 people who had remained off psychotropic medications for at least 1 week. Subgroups were as follows:

1. Patients with alcoholism and major affective disorder ($n = 25$)
2. Patients with primary alcoholism ($n = 15$)
3. Normal volunteers ($n = 42$)

All alcoholics had been detoxified for at least 2 weeks, and all subjects were diagnosed using Schedule of Affective Disorders and Schizophrenia-Research Diagnostic Criteria (SADS-RDC).

The experimental protocol, which has been described in detail elsewhere, is as follows: Physostigmine (0.022 mg/kg i.v.) was given crossed over 2 days or more later or before with placebo, using a double-blind counterbalanced order design. Behavioral and cardiovascular changes before (15 min) and after (10 min) were compared across groups on the active drug day using ANOVA techniques.[7]

As illustrated in Table 17.1, primary alcoholics showed a blunted response to physostigmine compared to either affective disorder patients with alcoholism or normals. This blunted response was noted with respect to the behavioral and cardiovascular effects of physostigmine.

If this finding is accurate, it may be of theoretical and practical importance, as it may be useful for differentiating primary and secondary alcoholics, and it may give insights into the pathophysiology of alcoholism.

However, it should be noted that our study consisted of relatively small subgroups of subjects. Furthermore, our data do not rule out the possibility that the results given are due to the differential metabolism of physostigmine in alcoholic patients.

References

1. Winokur G, Rimmer J, Reich T. Alcoholism. IV. Is there more than one type of alcoholism? Br J Psychiatry 1971;118:525–531.
2. Morrison JR. Bipolar affective disorder and alcoholism. Am J Psychiatry 1974;131:1130–1134.
3. Schuckit MA. Alcoholism and affective disorder: diagnostic confusion. In Goodwin DW, Erickson CK (eds): Alcoholism and Affective Disorders: Clinical, Genetic and Biochemical Studies. New York: Spectrum, 1979.
4. Schuckit MA. Alcoholism and other psychiatric disorders. Hosp Community Psychiatry 1983;34:1022–1027.
5. Weissman MM, Myers JK. Clinical depression in TC alcoholism. Am J Psychiatry 1980;137:372–373.
6. Janowsky DS, El-Yousef MK, Davis JM, et al. Parasympathetic suppression of manic symptoms by physostigmine. Arch Gen Psychiatry 1973;28:542–547.
7. Risch SC, Kalin NH, Janowsky DS. Cholinergic challenges in affective illness, behavioral and neuroendocrine correlates. J Clin Psychopharmacol 1981;1:185–192.

I.D. BASIC MECHANISMS OF ANTIDEPRESSANTS AND ANXIOLYTICS

18. Serotonin/Norepinephrine/Steroid Receptor Link in Brain and the Mode of Action of Antidepressants: Update and New Perspectives

FRIDOLIN SULSER AND ELAINE SANDERS-BUSH

New developments on the dual requirements of noradrenergic and serotonergic neuronal systems in the antidepressant-induced deamplification of the norepinephrine signal

The implications of the desensitization of the norepinephrine (NE) receptor coupled adenylate cyclase system as a mechanism common to most if not all clinically effective antidepressant treatments have been reviewed.[1] More selective serotonin (5-hydroxytryptamine, 5-HT) uptake inhibitors, e.g., fluvoxamine, sertraline, and fluoxetine, can now be added to the long list of antidepressant treatments causing down-regulation of β-adrenoceptors. Moreover, prolonged treatment with the atypical antidepressant rolipram attenuates the NE-sensitive adenylate cyclase system linked to down-regulation of β-adrenoceptors.[2] This effect of rolipram seems to be mediated via stereospecific and isozyme-specific inhibition of cyclic AMP–phosphodiesterase. Rolipram thus is the first antidepressant drug to cause desensitization of the NE receptor-coupled adenylate cyclase system by a mechanism distal to the receptor.

Studies on mechanisms of regulation of the NE β-adrenoceptor-coupled adenylate cyclase system in brain and its in vivo alteration by antidepressants have revealed two basic requirements: (a) The synaptic availability of NE and an unhindered occupancy of the receptor by NE are necessary for down-regulation. (b) A co-requirement of 5-HT is suggested by the finding that selective lesions of serotonergic neurons with 5,7-dihydroxytryptamine (5,7-DHT) prevent the down-regulation of β-adrenoceptors after chronic administration of desipramine (DMI), monoamine oxidase (MAO) inhibitors, and electroconvulsive therapy (ECT). However, despite the failure to down-regulate after 5,7-DHT lesions, the neurohormonal responsiveness to NE is reduced following DMI to essentially the same degree in tissue preparations from normal rats and those from rats with selective lesions of serotonergic neurons. Nonlinear regression analysis of competition binding curves revealed that the reduction in the density of β-adrenoceptors following DMI is confined to the β-adrenoceptor population displaying high agonist affinity. Moreover, nonlinear regression analysis of agonist competition curves obtained with cortical tissue from 5,7-DHT-lesioned animals showed that the high agonist affinity fraction of β-adrenoceptors is reduced by DMI to the same level as in cortical membrane preparations of normal animals. Because it is the high agonist affinity state of the β-adrenoceptor formed in the presence of the agonist NE that determines stimulation of adenylate cyclase, the results can satisfactorily explain the apparent discrepancy between β-adrenoceptor number and agonist-induced stimulation of the adenylate cyclase system. Although the basic phenomena of regulation of receptor number and function of the β-adrenoceptor-coupled adenylate cyclase system in brain are now fairly well established—with NE regulating the population of β-adrenoceptors in the high-affinity conformation (down-regulated by antidepressants) and 5-HT regulating those receptors in the low agonist affinity conformation—the molecular basis of the substantial and exclusive loss by DMI of β-adrenoceptors in the high agonist affinity conformation and of the shift in the ratio of high to low agonist affinity β-adrenoceptors following 5,7-DHT remains to be elucidated.

Biochemical Effector Systems Coupled to 5-HT Receptors

Radioligand binding studies have led to the classification of central 5-HT receptors into four subtypes: 5-HT_{1a}, 5-HT_{1b}, 5-HT_{1c}, and 5-HT_2. Advances have been made in understanding the molecular events linked to activation of these receptors. Effector systems, physiological roles, and regulation of central 5-HT receptors have been reviewed by Conn and Sanders-Bush.[3] Briefly, central 5-HT receptors have been reported to be both positively and negatively coupled to adenylate cyclase. The negatively coupled receptor, which has been characterized in rat and guinea pig hippocampus and in primary cultures of striatal and cortical neurons, is similar to the 5-HT_{1a} binding site. 5-HT_{1a}-like receptors also apparently mediate stimulation of adenylate cyclase in rat hippocampus. The possibility that the same receptor is both positively and negatively linked to adenylate cyclase is unprecedented and is difficult to understand in functional terms. These responses are measured under artificial conditions, and the important issue is whether one or the other or both mediate the physiological action of 5-HT. This question awaits further investigations.

Other cell surface receptors are linked to the membrane-associated enzyme phospholipase C, leading to the hydrolysis of membrane inositol lipids. The most common substrate is phosphatidylinositol-4,5-bisphosphate, whose two hydrolytic products, inositol-1,4,5-triphosphate (IP3) and diacylglycerol, serve as second messengers. Both of these messengers regulate cellular functions via protein kinase activation and protein phosphorylation. With regard to central 5-HT receptors, evidence suggests that the phospholipase C/phosphoinositide hydrolysis pathway is positively coupled to the 5-HT_2 receptor in cerebral cortex and to the 5-HT_{1c} receptor, which is highly localized in the choroid plexus. The demonstration that central 5-HT_2 and 5-HT_{1c} receptors are linked to phospholipase C permitted investigation of the regulation of signal transfer across the membrane at these sites. Chronic administration of the tricyclic antidepressant imipramine and the atypical antidepressant mianserin induces desensitization of 5-HT-stimulated phosphoinositide hydrolysis in conjunction with a down-regulation of the 5-HT_2 site. However, the 5-HT_2 receptor does not develop functional supersensitivity after 5,7-DHT lesions, suggesting that changes in this receptor system do not play a role in the β-adrenoceptor changes after this neurotoxin. On the other hand, the 5-

HT_{1c} site develops functional supersensitivity after 5,7-DHT lesions, leaving open the possibility that this receptor may be involved in the 5-HT/NE receptor link.

Biochemical Mechanisms of Desensitization

Although multiple mechanisms are involved in regulating the responsiveness of β-andrenoceptor-coupled adenylate cyclase systems, protein kinase-mediated phosphorylation seems to be the common final pathway.[4] A novel cyclic AMP-independent kinase has been discovered that preferentially phosphorylates the agonist-occupied β-adrenoceptor. This kinase exists in various tissues including brain and may explain the intimate linkage of agonist receptor activation and desensitization.

Studies from our laboratory have demonstrated that glucocorticoids are also involved in the regulation of the sensitivity of the β-adrenoceptor-coupled adenylate cyclase system in brain.[5] Adrenalectomy specifically enhances the formation of cyclic AMP by NE but not by isoproterenol. Moreover, the density of β-adrenoceptors remains unchanged under conditions of supersensitivity to NE, and the sensitivity is normalized by the administration of corticosterone to adrenalectomized animals. Glucocorticoids seem to affect the β-adrenoceptor-mediated cyclic AMP formation via the α-adrenergic component of NE receptors. The findings that protein kinase C activation by phorbol esters enhances the cyclic AMP response to isoproterenol are compatible with this view.[6] This regulatory role by glucocorticoids has gained significance as glucocorticoid receptors have been demonstrated immunocytochemically in the nuclei of NE, 5-HT, and epinephrine cell bodies.[7] Because glucocorticoids are known to influence the regulation of gene expression, it is tempting to speculate that glucocorticoids affect the diffusely projecting stress-responsive monoamine systems in brain via changes in transcription of pivotal proteins of the transmembrane signaling cascade.

Another potentially important clue to regulation of β-adrenoceptor-mediated signal transfer derives from studies with human fibroblasts. Chronic but not short-term exposure of fibroblasts to DMI leads to a dose-dependent accumulation of membrane phospholipids, particularly phosphatidylinositol and to a dose-dependent decrease in the number of β-adrenoceptors. Enna and Karbon[6] have reviewed the evidence for the biological significance of the relation between phospholipid metabolism and neurotransmitter receptor-mediated cyclic AMP formation and the implications for regulation of receptor sensitivity in brain.

Some Perspectives

Two events should enhance our understanding of the linked aminergic receptor-mediated transmembrane signaling on a molecular level: the cloning of the genes for β-adrenoceptors and the elucidation of oncogene expression. The avian $β_1$-adrenoceptor is an integral membrane glycoprotein that is arranged in seven membrane-spanning sequences with a long cytoplasmic hydroxyl-reach carboxyl terminus[8] that offers numerous potential sites for protein kinase-mediated regulatory phosphorylation. The mammalian $β_2$-adrenoceptor appears also to contain seven membrane-spanning domains that appear to be a feature of membrane receptors coupled to signal-transducing guanine nucleotide regulatory proteins. Using in situ hybridization to metaphase chromosomes, the gene for the $β_2$-adrenoceptor has been assigned to bands q31–q32 of the human chromosome 5.[9] These developments make possible genetic and immunological investigations of the receptor's regulatory functions, which in turn should provide new approaches to the development of more selective agents for the pharmacotherapy of affective disorders.

Oncogenes have been linked to the phosphatidylinositol (PI) transducing system, and evidence indicates that the *ras* gene encodes an N protein for the PI system, and activation of the PI system results in increased expression of the *fos* and *myc* oncogenes.[10] Whereas the receptors for neurohormones provide a means of communication between molecules on the outside of the cell with those in the cytoplasm, oncogene products may provide communication between molecules in the cytoplasm and the nucleus of the cell. Though speculative at this time, the experimental pursuit of such ideas promises a new understanding of the serotonin/norepinephrine/steroid receptor link in brain and the mode of action of antidepressants at a molecular level.

Acknowledgement. Studies from our laboratories have been supported by USPHS grants MH-29228 and MH-26463 and by the Tennessee Department of Mental Health and Mental Retardation.

References

1. Sulser F, Sanders-Bush E. The serotonin-norepinephrine link hypothesis of affective disorders: receptor–receptor interactions in brain. In Ehrlich Y, Lenox R (eds): Molecular Basis in Neuronal Responsiveness. New York: Plenum Press, 1987;489–502.
2. Schultz JE, Schmidt BH. Rolipram, a stereospecific inhibitor of calmodulin-indephosphodiesterase, causes beta-adrenoceptor subsensitivity in rat cerebral cortex. Naunyn Schmiedebergs Arch Pharmacol 1986;333:23–30.
3. Conn PJ, Sanders-Bush E. Central serotonin receptors: effector systems, physiological roles and regulation. Psychopharmacology 1987;92:267–277.
4. Sibley DR, Lefkowitz RJ. Adenylate cyclase coupled beta-adrenergic receptors—biochemical mechanisms of desensitization. Clin Neuropharmacol 1986;9:3–5.
5. Mobley PL, Manier DH, Sulser F. Norepinephrine-sensitive adenylate cyclase system in rat brain: role of adrenal corticosteroids. J Pharmacol Exp Ther 1983;226:71–77.
6. Enna SJ, Karbon EW. Receptor regulation: evidence for a relationship between phospholipid metabolism and neurotransmitter receptor-mediated cAMP formation in brain. Trends Pharmacol Sci 1987;8:21–24.
7. Harfstrand A, Fuxe K, Cintra A, et al. Demonstration of glucocorticoid receptor immunoreactivity in monoamine neurons of the rat brain. Proc Natl Acad Sci USA 1986;83:9779–9783.
8. Yarden Y, Rodriquiz H, Wong, SKF, et al. The avian beta-adrenergic receptors: primary structure and membrane topology. Proc Natl Acad Sci USA 1986;83:6795–6799.
9. Kobilka BK, Dixon RAF, Frielle TH, et al. cDNA for the human beta$_2$ adrenergic receptors: a protein with multiple membrane-spanning domains and encoded by a gene whose chromosomal location is shared with that of the receptor for platelet-derived growth factor. Proc Natl Acad Sci USA 1987;84:46–50.
10. Marx TL. Polyphosphoinositide research update. Science 1987;235:974–976.

19. Presynaptic Sites of Antidepressant Action: Monoamine Transport Systems and Release-Modulating Autoreceptors

SALOMON Z. LANGER AND HANS SCHOEMAKER

Most antidepressant drugs known to date increase the synaptic efficacy of mono-aminergic neurotransmission, in particular that of serotonergic and/or noradrenergic neurotransmission, by inhibiting metabolism, i.e., monoamine oxidase (MAO) inhibitors, or neuronal reuptake. Additionally, drug antagonism of presynaptic serotonergic or α_2-adrenergic autoreceptors, through which serotonin and nor-epinephrine exert an autoinhibitory effect on their release from the nerve terminal, may be expected to increase the synaptic efficacy of these neurotransmitters. The mechanism of clinical efficacy of antidepressant drugs is complex and may involve neuronal adaptation to their acute effects. Thus there is considerable interest in the identification and characterization of the primary site of action of antidepressant drugs. This chapter reviews the identification and characterization of the primary mechanism of action of antidepressant drugs by means of radioligand binding studies using [3H]-labeled antidepressants, particularly for those antidepressants for which the neuronal monoaminergic transporter is a primary target of pharmacological action. In addition, putative novel mechanisms of action for anti-depressant drugs having preferential activity as antagonists of the presynaptic serotonergic or noradrenergic α_2-autoreceptors are also discussed.

Radioligand binding studies have identified high affinity recognition sites for [3H]-labeled antidepressants associated with the monoamine transporter system. Thus [3H]imipramine labels, with high affinity, a site associated with the serotonin transporter in brain and platelets.[1] High affinity [3H]imipramine binding in the brain is heterogeneously distributed, closely following the regional density of serotonergic innervation; in subcellular fractionation studies it is recovered largely from the nerve terminal fraction. High affinity [3H]imipramine binding sites may further be demonstrated on the cell body of serotonergic neurons and during axonal transport.[2]

The pharmacological profile of [3H]imipramine binding is closely correlated with that of inhibition of serotonin transport into serotonergic nerve terminals or platelets. Nevertheless, significant discrepancies exist between the ability of some individual drugs, mainly tricyclic antidepressants, to inhibit [3H]imipramine binding and [3H]serotonin uptake, and between the affinity of serotonin transporter sub-strates for [3H]imipramine binding and transport itself. The high affinity of tricyclic antidepressants such as imipramine for [³H]imipramine binding in platelets determined at 0°C (K_d 0.79 nM) compared to its inhibition of platelet [³H]serotonin uptake at 37°C (IC_{50} 30 nM) appears to be related to thermodynamic considerations.[3] The affinity of tricyclic antidepressants for the serotonin transporter is temperature-dependent and is progressively lower at higher incubation temperatures. Radioligand binding to the serotonin transporter at 37°C may be studied using [³H]paroxetine, a novel, nontricyclic, high affinity (K_d 0.2 nM) marker of the serotonin transporter, even at 37°C. Drug K_i values for inhibition of [³H]imipramine and [³H]paroxetine binding to human platelet membranes are highly significantly correlated. However, the temperature sensitivity of tricyclic but not of nontricyclic serotonin uptake inhibitors for the transporter is reflected in a significantly better correlation of drug K_i values between inhibition of [³H]serotonin transport and [³H]paroxetine binding, both carried out at 37°C, than between inhibition of transport at 37°C and [³H]imipramine binding at 0°C.[3] The temperature dependence of the affinity of [³H]imipramine for the serotonin transporter also explains its selectivity as a radioligand at 0°C. Thus although imipramine is a nonselective inhibitor of serotonin and norepinephrine uptake, its affinity for the noradrenergic transporter is independent of the incubation temperature,[4] whereas its affinity for the serotonergic transporter is higher at 0°C than at 37°C. Moreover, the affinity of imipramine for the serotonergic transporter at 0°C is higher than its affinity for H_1-histaminergic, α_1-adrenergic, and serotonin (5-hydroxytryptamine, 5-HT) 5-HT_2 receptors.[5]

[³H]Imipramine binding has been studied extensively in affective disorders and has been proposed as a biological marker in depression.[6] Indeed most (23 studies) of the 36 studies published to date report a significant decrease in the Bmax of platelet [³H]imipramine binding in depression (Table 19.1), although an increase was reported in one study. The remaining 12 studies (for review, see ref. 1) failed to demonstrate a significant difference in platelet [³H]imipramine binding between untreated depressed patients and the control population. Data indicate that following antidepressant therapy platelet [³H]imipramine binding in the depressed patient is normalized but only well after clinical improvement.[7] These data support the hypothesis that platelet [³H]imipramine binding is a state-dependent biological marker in depression, which recovers to control levels only when remission is well consolidated. At least two studies reported that the B_{max} of [³H]imipramine binding in the postmortem brain is similarly decreased in suicides and depressives.[8,9] Although a decrease in platelet [³H]imipramine binding is largely specific to depression (Table 19.1), similar findings have been reported in patients with enuresis, Cushing's disease, anorexia nervosa, and obsessive-compulsive disorders (for review see ref. 1).

High affinity binding sites for ³H-labeled antidepressants have also been identified in association with the neuronal transporter for norepinephrine, dopamine, and most recently epinephrine.[10] The binding of [³H]desipramine to the transporter for epinephrine was demonstrated in the frog heart and, in contrast to [³H]desipramine binding to the noradrenergic transporter, is inhibited with high affinity by imipramine and the atypical antidepressants mianserin and iprindol (Table 19.2). The hypothesis[10] that the affinity of some antidepressants for the epinephrine transporter, in particular imipramine, mianserin, and iprindol, contributes to their clinical effects remains to be evaluated but may constitute a novel and so far unrecognized mechanism of antidepressant activity.

TABLE 19.1. Specificity of the variation in platelet [^{3}H]imipramine binding density as a biological marker in depression.

Disease	[^{3}H]Imipramine binding
Depression	↓ (23/36)
Panic disorders	− (5/6)
Schizophrenia	− (3/3)
Autism	− (2/2)
Alzheimer's disease	− (1/1)
Parkinson's disease	− (1/1)
Essential hypertension	− (1/1)
Cirrhosis	− (1/1)
Obsessive-compulsive disorders	− (1/2)
Anorexia nervosa	↓ (1/1)
Enuresis	↓ (2/2)
Postpartum depressive mood	− (1/1)
Cushing's disease	↓ (1/1)

Shown is a compilation of the variation of platelet [^{3}H]imipramine B_{max} values as measured in different diseases. ↓ = significant decrease. − = no significant variation. In parentheses are the number of studies that arrived at this conclusion/number of studies reported. For references, see Langer and Schoemaker.[1]

Novel mechanisms for antidepressant activity that remain to be fully explored also include an antagonism toward presynaptic autoreceptors on noradrenergic and serotonergic nerve terminals. These presynaptic autoreceptors function as a negative feedback mechanism that modulates neurotransmitter release.[11] Antagonists of such presynaptic autoreceptors, by blocking this feedback mechanism, increase the release and synaptic concentration of norepinephrine and serotonin, and hence may possess antidepressant properties. Presynaptic autoreceptors on the noradrenergic nerve terminal are of the α_2-adrenoceptor subtype,[11] whereas those on the serotonergic nerve terminal belong to the 5-HT$_{1B}$ receptor subtype.[12]

TABLE 19.2. Comparative affinity of desipramine and other antidepressants for the neuronal epinephrine and norepinephrine transporter as determined by radioligand binding studies.

Drug	Neuronal transporter for	
	Epinephrine	Norepinephrine
[^{3}H]Desipramine	$K_d = 1.94 \pm 0.39$ nM	$K_d = 1.5 \pm 0.4$ nM
	$B_{max} = 816 \pm 66$ fmol/mg protein	$B_{max} = 63 \pm 11$ fmol/mg protein
Other drugs IC$_{50}$ (μM)		
Desipramine	0.004	0.006
Nisoxetine	0.010	0.007
(+) Oxaprotiline	0.050	0.020
Imipramine	0.005	0.220
Mianserin	0.043	0.950
Iprindol	0.20	10.7

[^{3}H]Desipramine binding to the epinephrine transporter was determined in the frog heart, whereas [^{3}H]desipramine binding to the norepinephrine transporter was measured in the rat heart, except for mianserin, which was measured in the rat cortex.
Data were taken from refs. 10,13,14.

Conclusion

Several receptor-mediated mechanisms of antidepressant action may be identified as their primary site of interaction within monoaminergic neurotransmission. A better understanding of these sites of action may be expected to contribute to the elucidation of their mechanism of clinical efficacy.

References

1. Langer SZ, Schoemaker H. Effects of antidepressants on monoamine transporters. Prog Neuropsychopharmacol Biol Psychiatry 1988;12:193–196.
2. Dawson TM, Gehlert DR, Snowhill EW, et al. Quantitative autoradiographic evidence for axonal transport of imipramine receptors in the central nervous system of the rat. Neurosci Lett 1985;55:261–266.
3. Segonzac A, Schoemaker H, Langer, SZ. Temperature-dependence of drug interaction with the platelet 5HT transporter: a clue to the imipramine selectivity paradox. J Neurochem 1986;48:331–339.
4. Javitch JA, Blaustein RO, Snyder SH. [^{3}H]Mazindol binding associated with neuronal dopamine and norepinephrine uptakes sites. Mol Pharmacol 1984;26:35–44.
5. Laduron PM. Criteria for receptor sites in binding studies. Biochem Pharmacol 1984;33:833–839.
6. Langer SZ, Zarifian E, Briley MS, et al. High-affinity ^{3}H-imipramine binding: a new biological marker in depression. Pharmacopsychiatry 1982;15:3–10.
7. Langer SZ, Sechter D, Loo H, et al. Electroconvulsive shock therapy and maximum binding of platelet ^{3}H-imipramine binding in depression. Arch Gen Psychiatry 1986;53:949–952.
8. Stanley M, Virgilio S, Gershon S. Tritiated imipramine binding sites are decreased in the frontal cortex of suicides. Science 1982;216:1337–1339.
9. Perry EK, Marshall EF, Blessed G, et al. Decreased imipramine binding in the brain of patients with depressive illness. Br J Psychiatry 1983;142:188–192.
10. Pimoule C, Schoemaker H, Langer SZ. [^{3}H]Desipramine labels with high affinity the neuronal transporter for adrenaline in the frog heart. Eur J Pharmacol 1987;137:277–280.
11. Langer SZ. Presynaptic regulation of the release of catecholamines. Pharmacol Rev 1981;32:337–362.
12. Engel G, Göthert M, Schlicker E, et al. Identity of inhibitory presynaptic 5-hydroxytryptamine (5-HT) autoreceptors in the rat brain cortex with 5-HT$_{1B}$ binding sites. Naunyn Schmiedebergs Arch Pharmacol 1986;332:1–7.
13. Raisman R, Sette M, Pimoule C, et al. High-affinity [^{3}H]-despiramine binding in the peripheral and central nervous system: a specific site associated with the neuronal uptake of noradrenaline. Eur J Pharmacol 1982;78:345–351.
14. Lee CM, Javitch JA, Snyder SH. Characterization of [^{3}H]-desipramine binding associated with neuronal norepinephrine uptake sites in rat brain membranes. J Neurochem 1982;2:1515–1525.

20. Light–Dark-Related Changes in the Serotonin Uptake Molecular Complex in Rat Brain: Involvement in Antidepressant Action

GIORGIO RACAGNI, ALESSANDRA C. ROVESCALLI,
ROBERTO GALIMBERTI, MARCO RIVA, AND
NICOLETTA BRUNELLO

Clinical studies have clearly indicated that acute episodes and relapses of major depressive illness are characterized by a rhythmic cycle during the year, their incidence being highest during the spring and autumn.[1] In addition, circadian modifications in the mood of depressed patients and in the efficacy of antidepressive therapies have been observed[2–4] together with disruption or desynchronization of hormonal circadian patterns.[5] Based on the above observations, it has been postulated that in those depressed patients susceptible to seasonal bouts of the illness, a circadian and/or seasonal desynchronization occurs and may be corrected by antidepressant drugs[1,6] or light therapy.[4]

The discovery in the brain and thrombocytes of specific recognition sites for tritiated imipramine ([³H]IMI)[7] distinct from but functionally coupled to the high affinity serotonin (5-hydroxytryptamine, 5-HT) transporter[8–10] has led to several biochemical studies in which human platelets from normal and depressed subjects were employed as a model of brain serotonergic synapsis.[11] As concerns seasonal rhythms, these studies have revealed that rhythmic changes in the kinetic properties of platelet [³H]IMI binding and 5-HT uptake are present in either control volunteers or depressed patients.[12–14] Although these papers reported controversial data on the precise moment of the zenith and nadir values, taken together they confirm a phase-shifted seasonal rhythm of [³H]IMI binding and 5-HT uptake in the depressed subjects. It seems therefore that alterations in the circadian and/or infradian rhythms may play an important role in the etiopathogenesis of major depression as well as in the action of antidepressant drugs and/or phototherapy.[1,2,4,6]

The purpose of our study was to investigate if similar seasonal and circadian changes are present in the central nervous system and may be mimicked by accustoming rats to different light-dark schedules; therefore we have measured the kinetic properties of [³H]IMI binding and 5-HT uptake in the hypothalamus and the cerebral cortex from rats exposed to a long-day photoperiod (LD 14:10), a short-day photoperiod (LD 8:16), or a light-dark reverted photoperiod (DL 10:14).

Adult male rats of the Sprague-Dawley strain were caged under standard conditions and accustomed for 3–4 weeks to one of the following light-dark schedules:

1. LD 14:10 (light on 6.00 a.m. to 8.00 p.m.)
2. LD 8:16 (light on 8.00 a.m. to 4.00 p.m.)
3. DL 10:14 (light on 5.00 p.m. to 7.00 a.m.)

Rats were sacrificed by decapitation 6 h after the beginning of the light period (i.e., 12 a.m. for LD 14:10 and 2 p.m. for LD 8:16) or the dark period (i.e., 1 p.m. for DL 10:14). For binding studies the brains were rapidly excised, and selected brain areas were isolated and frozen on dry ice. [^{3}H]IMI binding kinetics were studied in saturation curves (1–10 nM [^{3}H]IMI) performed at 0–4°C according to Langer et al.[8] Nonspecific binding was defined in the presence of 10^{-4} M desmethylimipramine. Kinetic constants (Kd and Bmax) were obtained by computerized nonlinear fitting analysis.

High affinity 5-HT uptake was measured by incubating cerebrocortical or hypothalamic slices (300 μm) at 37°C in the presence of [^{3}H]5-HT (0.05–2.00 μM), according to Baumann et al.[15] Blanks were obtained at 0–4°C. Km and Vmax values were evaluated by the method of Lineweaver and Burk.

Table 20.1 shows the effects of short-day (LD 8:16) or long-day (LD 14:10) photoperiods on [^{3}H]IMI binding and 5-HT uptake in the rat hypothalamus and cerebral cortex. A significant increase in the density (Bmax) of [^{3}H]IMI binding sites and in the maximal velocity (Vmax) of [^{3}H]5-HT uptake was found in the hypothalamus of LD 8:16 exposed rats with respect to LD 14:10 exposed rats. On the contrary, no significant changes in the affinity constants (Kd and Km) were detected. No analogous modifications were observed, under the same conditions, in the cerebral cortex, thus indicating that a seasonal rhythm of [^{3}H]IMI binding sites and 5-HT uptake possibly exists only in certain brain areas, such as the hypothalamus, which receives visual stimuli directly. These findings are in agreement with reports in the literature concerning circadian changes in the density of α_1- and β-adrenergic receptors in the rat hypothalamus but not in the cerebral cortex.[6,16] However, it has been suggested that circadian rhythms exist in discrete areas of the brain and may be diluted or even canceled out when a large region such as the whole cerebral cortex is assayed.[16] Under our experimental conditions the different photoperiods seem to affect only presynaptic serotonergic sites, as no difference was found when comparing the kinetic properties of postsynaptic

TABLE 20.1. Kinetic properties of [^{3}H]imipramine binding and 5-HT uptake in the hypothalamus and cerebral cortex of rats exposed to long-day (LD 14:10) or short-day (LD 8:16) photoperiods.

Exposure	[^{3}H]Imipramine binding		5-HT uptake	
	K_d (nM)	B_{max} (fmol/mg protein)	K_m (μM)	V_{max} (pmol/mg protein)
Cerebral cortex				
LD 14:10	6.40 ± 0.09	505 ± 52	0.10 ± 0.03	7.5 ± 0.6
LD 8:16	4.70 ± 0.52	519 ± 45	0.20 ± 0.03	11.5 ± 1.2
Hypothalamus				
LD 14:10	7.40 ± 0.31	733 ± 65	0.14 ± 0.01	19.9 ± 1.3
LD 8:16	6.90 ± 0.20	1014 ± 83[a]	0.20 ± 0.01	31.0 ± 1.8[a]

[a]$p < 0.05$ versus LD 14:10 (Student's t test).

TABLE 20.2. Kinetic properties of [^{3}H]imipramine binding and 5-HT uptake in the hypothalamus and cerebral cortex of rats exposed to LD 14:10 or light-dark reverted (DL 14:10) cycles and sacrificed during the light or the dark phase.

Exposure	[^{3}H]Imipramine binding		5-HT uptake	
	K_d (nM)	B_{max} (fmol/mg protein)	K_m (μM)	V_{max} (pmol/mg protein)
Cerebral cortex				
LD 14:10	6.44 ± 0.51	718 ± 53	0.20 ± 0.01	9.7 ± 0.7
DL 10:14	6.50 ± 0.42	665 ± 37	0.20 ± 0.02	9.2 ± 0.8
Hypothalamus				
LD 14:10	5.95 ± 0.61	728 ± 65	0.20 ± 0.01	15.6 ± 0.3
DL 10:14	4.89 ± 0.47	1141 ± 93[a]	0.20 ± 0.01	20.2 ± 0.1[a]

[a] $p < 0.05$ versus LD 14:10.

5-HT receptors labeled with [^{3}H]ketanserin in the hypothalamus of LD 14:10 and LD 8:16 exposed rats (unpublished results).

Table 20.2 shows that a similar increase in [^{3}H]IMI binding and 5-HT uptake was present in the hypothalamus of rats accustomed to a light-dark reverted cycle (DL 14:10) and sacrificed 6 h after stopping of lighting in comparison to rats exposed to LD 14:10 cycles and sacrificed 6 h after beginning of lighting. Therefore a circadian modification of the serotonergic presynaptic sites studied seems to be also present and related to light-dark exposure. As observed in the previous study, no light-dark difference was detected in the cerebral cortex.

The 5-HT uptake molecular complex is among the primary sites of action for antidepressant drugs[17,18] and seems to be allosterically coupled to [^{3}H]IMI binding sites, which may function as a regulatory mechanism for the 5- HT transporter.[19] The data herein presented clearly indicate that under physiological conditions, e.g., light-dark cycles or the various photoperiods, parallel modifications occur in the two sites, whereas pharmacological treatments with antidepressants[18] or aging processes[10] result in concomitant but unparallel changes in the biochemical properties of [^{3}H]IMI binding and 5-HT uptake. Therefore the functional coupling between these two sites may be basic in the etiology of depression and/or the action of antidepressant drugs. Physiological changes such as circadian variation of the 5- HT molecular complex could affect the biochemical action of antidepressants, thus modifying their therapeutic efficacy.[3] Our data therefore could be relevant to a deeper understanding of the mechanisms of action of antidepressant drugs in relation to clinical efficacy and protocol of treatment.

Moreover, because photoperiodic changes themselves seem to play an important role in the pathophysiology of affective disorders[1,2,12–14] studies on the circadian and seasonal rhythms of brain targets for antidepressants may be fruitful to a better knowledge of the biochemistry of depressive illness.

References

1. Wehr TA, Wirz-Justice A. Circadian rhythm mechanisms in affective illness and in antidepressant drug action. Pharmacopsychiatry 1982;15:31–39.
2. Goodwin FK, Wirz-Justice A, Wehr TA. Evidence that the pathology of depression and the mechanism of action of antidepressant drugs involve alterations in circadian rhythms. Adv Biochem Psychopharmacol 1982;32:1–11.

3. Herrmann L. Circadian rhythm, depression, antidepressants, single dose. Pharmaco-psychiatry 1984;17:69–70.
4. Lewy AJ, Sack RL, Miller LS, et al. Antidepressant and circadian phase-shifting effects of light. Science 1987;235:352–354.
5. Leonard BE. Neurotransmitter receptors, endocrine responses and the biological substrates of depression: a review. Hum Psychopharmacol 1986;1:3–21.
6. Wirz-Justice A, Kafka MS, Naber D, et al. Circadian rhythms in rat brain alpha- and beta-adrenergic receptors are modified by chronic imipramine. Life Sci 1980;27:341–347.
7. Langer SZ, Zarifian E, Briley M, et al. High affinity binding of ^{3}H-imipramine in brain and platelets and its relevance to the biochemistry of affective disorders. Life Sci 1981;29:211–220.
8. Langer SZ, Moret C, Raisman R, et al. High affinity ^{3}H-imipramine binding in rat hypothalamus: association with uptake of serotonin but not of norepinephrine. Science 1980;210:1133–1135.
9. Mocchetti I, Brunello N, Racagni G. Ontogenetic study of ^{3}H-imipramine binding sites and serotonin uptake system: indication of possible interdependence. Eur J Pharmacol 1982;83:151–152.
10. Brunello N, Riva M, Volterra A, et al. Age-related changes in 5-HT uptake and [^{3}H]imipramine binding sites in rat cerebral cortex. Eur J Pharmacol 1985;110:393–394.
11. Langer SZ, Raisman R. Binding of ^{3}H-imipramine and ^{3}H-desipramine as biochemical tools for studies in depression. Neuropharmacology 1983;22:407–413.
12. Arora RC, Kregel L, Meltzer HY. Seasonal variation of serotonin uptake in normal controls and depressed patients. Biol Psychiatry 1984;19:795–804.
13. Whitaker PM, Warsh JJ, Stancer HC, et al. Seasonal variation in platelet ^{3}H-imipramine binding: comparable values in control and depressed populations. Psychiatr Res 1984;11:127–131.
14. Egrise D, Rubistein M, Schoutens A. Seasonal variation of platelet serotonin uptake and ^{3}H-imipramine binding in normal and depressed subjects. Biol Psychiatry 1986;21:283–292.
15. Baumann PA, Maitre L. Blockade of presynaptic alpha-receptors and of amine uptake in the rat brain by the antidepressant mianserin. Naunyn Schmiedebergs Arch Pharmacol 1977;300:31–37.
16. Campbell IC, Durcan MJ, Wirz-Justice A, et al. Circadian rhythms in brain adrenergic receptors and the influence of mood-modifying drugs. In Schou JS, Geisler A, Norn S (eds): Drug Receptors and Dynamic processes in Cells. Copenhagen: Munksgaard, 1986;269–285.
17. Brunello N, Rovescalli AC, Riva M, et al. Lack of serotonergic modulation on ^{3}H-imipramine binding sites in basal conditions and during prolonged treatment with desmethylimipramine. Psychopharmacol Bull 1986;22:931–936.
18. Brunello N, Riva M, Volterra A, et al. Effect of some tricyclic antidepressants on ^{3}H-imipramine binding and serotonin uptake in rat cerebral cortex after prolonged treatment. Fundam Clin Pharmacol 1987;1:327–333.
19. Habert E, Graham D, Langer SZ. Solubilization and characterization of the 5-hydroxytryptamine transporter complex from rat cerebral cortical membranes. Eur J Pharmacol 1986;122:197–204.

21. Role of Serotonin (and Coexisting Peptides) in the Action Mechanism of Antidepressant Drugs

S.O. ÖGREN, K. FUXE, I. KITAYAMA, J.T. CUMMINS,
G. VON EULER, A.M. JANSSON, AND L.F. AGNATI

Much evidence suggests that serotonergic (5-hydroxytryptamine, 5-HT) neurons are important targets for the action of antidepressant drugs.[1] Thus treatment with various classes of antidepressant drugs produces multiple effects on 5-HT neurons and receptors in the brain. The implications of these changes for the mechanism of action of antidepressant drugs are presently not clear. Knowledge regarding the effects of antidepressant drugs is based on studies using gross biochemical techniques, e.g., biochemical binding studies, in large areas of the brain. It is likely that important information is missed by these methods, as selective changes in identified neurons are not detected. Morphometric and microdensitometric methods to analyze the effects of psychoactive drugs on transmitter-identified neurons, especially on the central monoamine neurons, have been developed.[2] The procedures include techniques for the quantitative evaluation of coexistence in nerve cell bodies and nerve terminals[2] as well as analysis of different receptors using quantitative receptor autoradiography in identified neurons in the brain. In this chapter we have used these methods to study the effects of acute and chronic oral treatment with imipramine.

Repeated (2×10 μmol/kg p.o. for 14 days) but not acute (10 μmol/kg p.o.) treatment with imipramine produced a 35% reduction of ^{125}I-LSD (a radioligand for 5-HT$_2$ receptors) binding in layer IV in the frontal cortex and a 37% reduction in the occipital cortex.[3] On the other hand, the binding of ^{125}I-neuropeptide Y, a new important neuropeptide, was not changed in these regions. Interestingly, in other areas of the cortex (using a different way of cutting the brain) no changes in 5-HT$_2$ receptor binding were observed. These results suggest that imipramine produces selective changes in specific receptor populations in defined areas of the brain. It is notable that receptor autoradiographic studies have shown that most of the 5-HT$_2$ receptors in the cerebral cortex labeled by ^{125}I-LSD are localized within layer IV. Layer IV is the major target for the specific afferent input to the cerebral cortex. The present data, if shown to be valid for other types of antidepressant drugs, suggest that antidepressant drugs may have an important modulatory influence on specific sensory input to the cerebral cortex.

The question arises whether such changes in 5-HT receptors, caused by chronic antidepressant treatment, are reflected in altered release or receptor activity of

5-HT and peptides known to coexist with 5-HT. Because coexistence presently is established only in the descending bulbospinal pathways, we have used the spinal cord as our model. Coexistence of at least three putative neurotransmitters— substance P (SP), thyrotropin-releasing hormone (TRH), and 5-HT—has been demonstrated in the spinal cord using immunohistochemical methods.[4] The functional significance of the coexistence has not been clarified. However, chronic treatment with antidepressant drugs with monoamine uptake blocking properties has been shown to change the tissue levels of coexisting peptides.[5] Because the radioimmunoassay (RIA) methods (analyzing large areas of the spinal cord) can give only indirect evidence that the observed changes occur in neurons with coexistence, the effect of acute and chronic imipramine treatment was studied using morphometric and microdensitometric techniques.

The microdensitometric studies showed that chronic but not acute imipramine treatment selectively increased SP immunoreactivity in the 5-HT/SP co-storing nerve terminals of the medial part of the ventral horn in both the cervical and the lumbar enlargements[6] (Fig. 21.1). In contrast, the TRH immunoreactivity appeared to be unaltered in the 5-HT nerve terminal systems of the ventral horn by chronic imipramine treatment at the dose level used in this study (2 × 10 μmol/kg p.o.). Quantitative analysis of the entity of coexistence in the 5-HT nerve terminal networks of these areas showed that all the 5-HT nerve terminals in the medial part of the ventral horn of the cervical and lumbar enlargements contained SP and TRH immunoreactivities and that this phenomenon was not changed by acute and chronic treatment with imipramine. The biochemical studies demonstrated that chronic imipramine treatment selectively reduced 5-HT utilization in the ventral horn of the spinal cord as evidenced by a reduced 5-hydroxyindoleacetic acid (5-HIAA/5-HT) ratio in the rats treated chronically with imipramine (Fig. 21.1). It is possible that the selective increases of SP immunoreactivity following chronic imipramine treatment reflect a reduced release of SP from the co-storing nerve terminals secondary to a reduced firing rate in the bulbospinal 5-HT neurons.

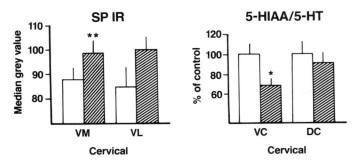

FIGURE 21.1. Effects of chronic imipramine treatment (2 × 10 μmol/kg p.o. for 14 days) on SP immunoreactivity (IR) in nerve terminal profiles of the cervical enlargement of the spinal cord in the male rat. SP was analyzed in the medial (VM) and lateral (VL) parts of the ventral horn. Means ± SEM are shown (n = 5 rats). In addition, 5-HT and 5-HIAA levels were determined by HPLC in the ventral (VC) and dorsal (DC) horns of the cervical enlargement of the spinal cord. Means ± SEM are shown (n = 7–8 rats). *$p < 0.05$. **$p < 0.01$. (Data are modified from ref. 6.)

Conclusion

The results suggest reduced activity in the 5-HT and SP transmission of the 5-HT, SP, and TRH co-storing neurons of the ventral horn after chronic imipramine treatment. Effects on 5-HT co-modulators should therefore be considered when discussing actions of antidepressant drugs also in the ascending 5-HT pathways. Effects on co-modulators may partly explain the adaptive changes in 5-HT receptors after chronic antidepressant treatment due to receptor–receptor interactions between the peptidergic co-modulator receptor (e.g., SP) and the 5-HT receptor.[7]

The functional concequences of these changes suggest interactions at both pre- and postsynaptic levels involving 5-HT and several peptides. At the presynaptic level chronic treatment of antidepressant drugs may therefore influence the release of the monoamine neurotransmitter 5-HT and the neuropeptide neurotransmitter SP by influencing mechanisms for autoregulation as well as cross-regulation of the monoamine and the peptide. The differential changes in tissue levels of the coexisting SP and 5-HT following chronic antidepressant treatment indicate that there may exist a differential sensitivity of the biosynthesis of the coexisting 5-HT and the individual peptide neurotransmitter probably due to a different coupling to the neuronal activity.

References

1. Ögren SO, Fuxe K. Effects of antidepressant drugs on serotonin receptor mechanisms. In Green R (ed): Neuropharmacology of Serotonin. Oxford: Oxford University Press, 1985;131–180.
2. Fuxe K, Agnati LF, Andersson K, et al. Quantitative microfluorimetry and semiquantitative immunocytochemistry as tools in the analysis of transmitter identified neurons. In Agnati LF, Fuxe K (eds): Quantitative Neuroanatomy in Transmitter Research. Vol 42. Hampshire: Macmillan Press, 1985;331–348.
3. Cummins JT, von Euler G, Fuxe K, et al. Chronic imipramine treatment reduces (+)2-(^{125}I)iodolysergic acid, diethylamide but not ^{125}I-neuropeptide Y binding in layer IV of rat cerebral cortex. Neurosci Lett 1987;75:152–156.
4. Hökfelt T, Ljungdahl A, Steinbusch H, et al. Immunohistochemical evidence of substance P-like immunoreactivity in some 5-hydroxytryptamine-containing neurons in the rat central nervous system. Neuroscience 1978;3:517–538.
5. Brodin E, Peterson L-L, Ogren SO, et al. Chronic treatment with the serotonin uptake inhibitor zimelidine elevates substance P levels in rat spinal cord. Acta Physiol Scand 1984;122:209–211.
6. Kitayama I, Janson AM, Fuxe K, et al. Effects of acute and chronic treatment with imipramine on 5-hydroxytryptamine nerve cell groups and on bulbospinal 5-hydroxytryptamine/substance P/thyrotropin releasing hormone immunoreactive neurons in the rat: a morphometric and microdensitometric analysis. J. Neural Transm 1987;70:251–285.
7. Fuxe K, Agnati LF. Receptor–receptor interactions in the central nervous system: a new integrative mechanism in synapses. Med Res Rev 1985;5:441–482.

22. GABA$_B$ Receptors and Antidepressant Drugs

K.G. LLOYD, P. PICHAT, AND D.J. SANGER

The molecular mechanism(s) of action of antidepressant drugs are still far from understood, although monoaminergic actions are a central theme for most tri- and tetracyclic antidepressants and monoamine oxidase inhibitors. The limitations in relating acute drug effects on monoaminergic mechanisms to chronic clinical effects are well known. Although upon repeated administration many antidepressant compounds and electroconvulsive shock (ECS) down-regulate the β-adrenergic receptor–adenylate cyclase unit,[1] it is not known if this molecular mechanism is the most relevant for the clinical antidepressant effect. Thus the search continues for other neurotransmitter-mediated mechanisms that are common to, and relevant for, antidepressant activity.

Among other neurotransmitters, this search has included a study of the synaptic indices of γ-aminobutyric acid (GABA)-mediated neurotransmission. In terms of presynaptic aspects, most antidepressants do not alter GABA levels or synthesis at doses relevant to their pharmacological activity, although repeated ECS is associated with increased GABA levels (see refs. 2–4 for bibliography). A potentially interesting observation is that some antidepressant drugs inhibit GABA uptake[5] at concentrations that may be attained upon repeated administration in man (e.g., IC$_{50}$ for imipramine at 120 μM; 10–200 μM for desmethylimipramine, iprindole, amitriptyline; brain levels for desipramine in the range of 80–100 μM at therapeutic doses[6]).

Postsynaptic indices of GABAergic transmission have also been investigated. In vitro, antidepressants do not alter the binding at either GABA$_A$ or GABA$_B$ receptors. Upon acute administration GABA receptor function (A or B type sites) is unaltered by most antidepressants. After repeated administration of antidepressants, GABA$_A$ binding ex vivo is unaltered at pharmacologically relevant doses.[2-4] This finding is in good agreement with the observation that after chronic tricyclics the neurophysiological response to iontophoretic GABA is unaltered, whereas the responses to norepinephrine and serotonin are decreased.[7]

In contrast to GABA$_A$ receptors, GABA$_B$ receptors seem to be receptive to repeated administration of antidepressants and ECS. This receptivity has been demonstrated at both the membrane level (binding, interaction with adenylate cyclase) and a behavioral level.

It was initially demonstrated that, after 18 days of subcutaneous treatment to rats, amitriptyline, desipramine, viloxazine, and citalopram significantly increased GABA$_B$ binding in the frontal cortex.[4] The number of antidepressants studied has been greatly increased and now includes a cross section of chemical classes and ECS (Table 22.1). From this list it is clear that the only point in common for these compounds is their antidepressant activity. Furthermore, this activity appears to be "exclusive" in that all compounds tested to date with antidepressant properties up-regulate GABA$_B$ binding, whereas compounds without positive actions in affective disorders do not. The latter group includes amphetamine, which is not antidepressant, although it is a monoamine uptake inhibitor. It demonstrates that inhibition of monoamine uptake per se is insufficient for either clinical antidepressant activity or for up-regulation of GABA$_B$ sites. The association of GABA$_B$ up-regulation–clinical antidepressant effect and their independence of monoamine uptake inhibition is further underlined by the observation that antidepressants with mechanisms unrelated to monoamine uptake inhibition (e.g., fengabine,[8] ECS) are associated with enhanced GABA$_B$ binding to rat cortical membranes.

These binding data have been reproduced using repeated imipramine treatment in the mouse.[9] Furthermore, the effect of repeated administration of antidepressants on GABA$_B$ receptors is not limited to a binding phenomenon. The GABA$_B$ receptor that modulates the β-adrenergic receptor-linked adenylate cyclase activity[5,10,11] is up-regulated by repeated antidepressant administration[9] (Lloyd and Pichat, unpublished results).

Other neurotransmitter interactions that involve GABA$_B$ receptors are also modified by chronic antidepressant treatment in a manner consistent with GABA$_B$ receptor up-regulation. Thus potassium-stimulated serotonin release from mouse frontal cortex is inhibited by GABA$_B$ receptor stimulation. Upon repeated administration of either ECS or various antidepressants (amitriptyline, zimelidine, mianserin) this GABA$_B$ effect is considerably enhanced.[12]

TABLE 22.1. Effect on GABA$_B$ binding to rat frontal cortex membranes of various psychotropic compounds after repeated administration.

Action	Compounds	Therapeutic class
Enhanced GABA$_B$ binding	Amitriptyline, desipramine, maprotiline, viloxazine, nomifensine, buproprion, citalopram, fluoxetine, zimelidine, pargyline, fengabine, trazodone, idazoxan, iprindole, mianserine	Antidepressant
	Progabide, valproate	Antiepileptic with clear effects on affective disorders
Unaltered GABA$_B$ binding	Diazepam	Anxiolytic
	Haloperidol, chlorpromazine	Neuroleptic
	Oxotremorine	Cholinomimetic
	Amphetamine	Psychostimulant
Decreased GABA$_B$ binding	Phenobarbital, diphenylhydantoin	Antiepileptic without positive effects on mood
	Reserpine	Neuroleptic/antihypertensive

Data from refs. 2 and 3.

These biochemical alterations in GABA$_B$ receptor activity, upon repeated antidepressant treatment, have behavioral correlates. Thus in olfactory bulbectomized rats the decreased levels of GABA$_B$ binding to frontal cortex membranes[13] is reversed by 14-day imipramine treatment *only* for those animals in which the deficit in passive avoidance learning is reversed, demonstrating a close parallel between the behavioral and biochemical phenomena.[14] Furthermore, the decrease in locomotor activity and hypothermia following a single administration of baclofen to mice is enhanced upon repeated administration of imipramine (A. R. Green, personal communication), consistent with an up-regulation of GABA$_B$ receptors.

Thus there is a large body of evidence supporting the hypothesis that a GABA$_B$ receptor up-regulation is integral to the behavioral action of antidepressants and ECS in animals, and it is likely related to antidepressant activity in man. However, it should not be considered that the GABA hypothesis is exclusive; more likely there is an interaction between GABA$_B$ and β-adrenergic receptor-mediated events at the cell membrane level. Thus repeated ECS and a wide range of antidepressants consistently up-regulate GABA$_B$ receptors and down-regulate the β-adrenergic receptor–adenylate cyclase complex; effects at other receptors or recognition sites are much less consistent.[15] The overall result on cell function of such an interaction is still under investigation as the up-regulation of GABA$_B$ receptors modulates the β-receptor-linked cyclase in the reverse sense (i.e., increased effect) to the action of antidepressants on the β-receptor complex in the absence of GABA (down-regulation). Results to date indicate a net increase in adenylate cyclase activation in the presence of isoproterenol + GABA (or baclofen) after repeated imipramine administration[9] (Pichat and Lloyd, unpublished results).

References

1. Sulser F. Functional aspects of the norepinephrine receptor coupled adenylate cyclase system in the limbic forebrain and its modification by drugs which precipitate or alleviate depression: molecular approaches to an understanding of affective disorders. Pharmacopsychiatry 1978;11:43–52.
2. Lloyd KG, Thuret F, Pilc A. Upregulation of gamma-aminobutyric acid (GABA) "B" binding sites in rat frontal cortex: a common action of repeated administration of different classes of antidepressants and electroshock. J Pharmacol Exp Ther 1985;235:191–199.
3. Lloyd KG, Pichat P. GABA synapses, depression and antidepressant drugs. In Dahl SG, Gram LF, Paul SM, et al. (eds): Clinical Pharmacology in Psychiatry (Psychopharmacology, Series 3). Berlin: Springer-Verlag, 1987;113–126.
4. Pilc A, Lloyd KG. Chronic antidepressants and GABA "B" receptors: a GABA hypothesis of antidepressant drug action. Life Sci 1984;35:2149–2154.
5. Harris M, Hopkin JM, Neal MH. Effect of centrally acting drugs on the uptake of gamma-aminobutyric acid (GABA) by slices of rat cerebral cortex. Br J Pharmacol 1973;47:229–239.
6. Hrdina PD, Dubas TC, Riva E. Brain distribution and pharmacokinetics of psychotropic drugs: desipramine. In Deniker P, Raduco-Thomas C, Villeneuve A (eds): Neuropsychopharmacology. New York: Pergamon, 1978;841–848.
7. De Montigny C, Aghajanian GK. Tricyclic antidepressants: long term treatment increases responsivity of rat forebrain neurons to serotonin. Science 1978;202:1303–1306.
8. Lloyd KG, Zivkovic B, Sanger DJ, et al. Fengabine, a novel antidepressant GABAergic agent. I. Activity in models for antidepressant drugs and psychopharmacological profile. J Pharmacol Exp Ther 1987;241:245–250.
9. Suzdak PD, Gianutsos G. Effect of chronic imipramine or baclofen on GABA-B binding and cyclic AMP production in cerebral cortex. Eur J Pharmacol 1986;131:129–133.
10. Karbon EW, Dunman RS, Enna SJ. GABA$_B$ receptors and norepinephrine-stimulated cAMP production in rat brain cortex. Brain Res 1984;306:327–332.

11. Hill DR. GABA$_B$ receptor modulation of adenylate cyclase activity in rat brain slices. Br J Pharmacol 1985;84:249–257.
12. Gray JA, Green AR. Evidence for increased GABA$_B$ receptor function in mouse frontal cotex following antidepressant administration. Br J Pharmacol 1986;89:799P.
13. Lloyd KG, Pichat P. Decrease in GABA$_B$ binding in the frontal cortex of bulbectomized rats. Br J Pharmacol 1985;87:36P.
14. Joly D, Lloyd KG, Pichat P, et al. Correlation between the behavioral effect of desipramine and GABA$_B$ receptor regulation in the olfactory bulbectomized rat. Br J Pharmacol 1987;90:125P.
15. Enna SJ, Mann E, Kendall D, et al. Effect of chronic antidepressant administration on brain neurotransmitter receptor binding. In Enna SL, Kuhar M, Coyle J (eds). Antidepressants: Neurochemical, Behavioral and Clinical Perspectives. New York: Raven Press, 1981;91–105.

23. Antidepressants and Phospholipid Metabolism: β-Adrenoceptor Regulation in Cultured Human Cells

U.E. HONEGGER

Despite 30 years of widespread use of antidepressant drugs and more than 20 years of extensive research efforts, the mode of action of these drugs has not yet been fully elucidated. Current theories on the mechanism of action of antidepressants include reduction in β-adrenoceptor density, α_1-adrenoceptor up-regulation and α_2-adrenoceptor down-regulation. Serotoninergic, $GABA_A$- and $GABA_B$ergic, cholinergic, dopaminergic, and histaminergic receptor changes have also been reported, but results have been less conclusive.

The functional consequences of neurotransmitter changes are poorly understood, especially because of the lag between the beginning of antidepressant therapy and the onset of clinical effectiveness. Another unresolved issue of antidepressant therapy is whether these mainly postsynaptic alterations are necessarily adaptive to presynaptic drug actions or whether there is a primary postsynaptic component of antidepressant drug action.[1]

Despite of the increasing number of neurotransmitter and drug receptors implicated in the action of the antidepressants, leading to confusion, the down-regulation of β-adrenoceptors seems to hold true even after treatments with tetracyclic, atypical, and monoamine oxidase (MAO) inhibitor type antidepressants and electroconvulsive shock therapy (ECT). Thus down-regulation of β-adrenoceptors remains the most consistent finding in research of antidepressant drug actions.

The question whether effects observed after long-term treatment are primary or secondary to drug actions is difficult to answer by means of in vivo experiments due to the complexity of the interactions of neurotransmitter systems in brain as well as to the difficulty of discriminating the sequence of events. As a result of looking for new means to localize the site of the drug action as well as for a simple model system that allows us to answer simple questions, we have chosen culture systems with peripheral human cells as a model for antidepressant drug research.

Cell Culture Models

Human diploid skin and embryonic lung fibroblasts are easy to maintain in culture. They can be subcultured and kept as stationary monolayers for several weeks, which allows us to perform long-term drug experiments. Fibroblasts possess a functional β-adrenergic system and were found to be suitable for the investigation of drug effects on β-adrenoceptors and norepinephrine-sensitive adenosine 3':5'-cyclic phosphate (cAMP) formation. Human spontaneously transformed macrophages were obtained from a peripheral blood sample cultured in our laboratory. In comparison to skin fibroblasts these macrophages have a five times higher density of β-adrenoceptors.

All cultures were grown in Eagle's minimum essential medium supplemented with 10% fetal calf serum. The monolayers were kept at pH 7.4, 37°C, and 5% CO_2 in air. The cells were exposed to the tricyclic antidepressant desipramine (DMI) and to other psychotropic drugs in concentrations of $5 \times 10^{-6} M$ for periods of 2 h (short term) to 12 days (long term). Using these culture models we expected to answer questions that might help us perform more relevant in vivo experiments at a later date.

Drug Effects

Cells chronically exposed to 1–10 μM DMI and other psychotropic drugs showed intracellular granular bodies similar to those described by Lüllmann-Rauch[2] in various cells and organs of cultures and animals after chronic treatments with cationic amphiphilic drugs. DMI and most of the psychotropic drugs belong to this class of amphiphilic compounds.

These drugs enter lysosomes in their nonprotonated, lipophilic form. At the low pH value of the lysosomal contents, the weakly basic drugs become protonated and accumulate within these cellular organelles. This phenomenon is referred to as lysosomotropism. The trapped drugs interfere with lysosomal functions such as phospholipid degradation, which leads to phospholipid accumulation and the formation of granular inclusions, a phenomenon known as acquired phospholipidosis.

Studies of uptake and release of radiolabeled DMI and other psychotropic drugs in short-term and chronic exposure of cultured cells to the drugs showed that the kinetics were characteristic for lysosomotropic behavior.[3] For DMI the cellular uptake was rapid and proportional to the extracellular DMI concentrations. No saturation was reached between 10^{-8} and $5 \times 10^{-4} M$ DMI. The uptake was linearly related to the extracellular pH value, as it is driven by the pH gradient. At a pH value of 7.4 in the medium the equilibrium concentration ratio between cellular and extracellular DMI was about 800:1. After subcellular fractionation of short-term and chronically drug-exposed cells, most of the DMI was found in the acidic contents of pinosomes and lysosomes.[4] The drug that accumulated after a 2-h uptake was easily released into fresh, drug-free medium. However, only a minor fraction of chronically accumulated ^{3}H-DMI could be recovered in drug-free medium, supporting the idea that the drug may be stored in a nonaccessible form eventually as complexes.

Changes in Phospholipid Metabolism and Drug Specificity

Chronic but not short-term exposures of cultured cells to DMI and other psychotropic drugs in therapeutic concentrations led to dose-dependent accumulations of total phospholipids. The extent of phospholipid storage, however, was different for the various drugs investigated.

Drug-specific changes in the relative amounts of individual phospholipids were analyzed. After extraction of the cellular phospholipids by the method of Folch et al.,[5] individual phospholipids were separated by one-dimensional, high-performance thin-layer chromatography (HPTLC) by means of a method developed in our laboratory. The spots were visualized and then quantified by reflexion densitometry.

Chronic exposure of cells to 5μM DMI induced profound changes in the cellular phospholipid composition. The alterations were characterized by overproportionate increases in phosphatidylinositol (PI) and phosphatidylethanolamine (PE) and by overproportionate decreases in sphingomyelin (SM) and phosphatidylserine (PS). Qualitatively identical changes were also seen following chronic exposure of cells to the antidepressants mianserine and iprindole. In order to test the specificity of these effects, cells were treated with neuroleptic and anxiolytic drugs. Chronic exposures of fibroblasts or macrophages to 5μM concentrations of chlorpromazine and haloperidol led to changes in the phospholipid pattern that were distinct from those seen after antidepressants. In particular, there were consistent and overproportionate increases in PI and PS and significant decreases in SM and phosphatidylcholine (PC).

Chronic exposure of cells to the benzodiazepine drugs diazepam and alprazolam caused only minor changes in the phospholipid composition. A small decrease in PS was consistently observed, whereas the proportions of the other phospholipids remained unchanged.

Desensitization of β-Adrenoceptors

Direct binding studies on intact cells were performed with the radioligand ^{3}H-CGP 12177, a hydrophilic β-adrenergic antagonist. Confluent fibroblast and macrophage cell cultures, chronically exposed to DMI, showed a dose-dependent decrease in the number of receptor binding sites.[6] This β-adrenoceptor desensitization was seen only after long-term drug exposure. The extent of receptor down-regulation was comparable to that seen in brain following chronic treatment of rats with DMI (Table 23.1). The affinity of the binding sites for CGP 12177 was not affected by the drug exposure.

TABLE 23.1. Effects of chronic desipramine application on β-adrenoceptor densities (Bmax) on cultured human cells and in rat brain.

	Bmax (fmol/mg protein)		
		Desipramine-exposed	
Cells/tissue	Controls	2 μM	5 μM
Human skin fibroblasts	6.0 ± 0.4	3.8 ± 0.3[a]	2.1 ± 0.4[a]
Human lung fibroblasts	9.3 ± 0.2	8.6 ± 0.5[b]	5.7 ± 0.9[a]
Human macrophages	49.0 ± 4.2	38.7 ± 6.7[a]	28.5 ± 4.7[a]
		10 mg/kg/day	
Rat brain	92.0 + 8.7	65.1 ± 8.9	

Values are means ± SD.
[a] $p < 0.01$.
[b] $p < 0.02$.

The drug-induced reduction in the number of β-adrenoceptor sites was also reflected in a diminished isoproterenol-sensitive cAMP response of drug-exposed cells. Effects on β-adrenergic transmission, comparable to those of DMI, were also seen after chronic cell exposure to the antidepressants mianserine and iprindole.

The fact that receptor desensitization occurred in the absence of presynaptic structures and events, and was thus independent of changing neurotransmitter levels, suggests that β-adrenoceptor desensitization in brain may be at least in part a direct postsynaptic drug action. From the in vitro findings following long-term exposure of human cell lines to therapeutic concentrations of DMI and other psychotropic drugs, it appears that psychotropic drugs specifically affect the cellular phospholipid-metabolism and the number of functional β-adrenoceptors.

An increase in the relative amount of PI is consistently accompanied by a receptor desensitization. This observation is in agreement with the finding of McOsker et al.,[7] who have described desensitization of β-adrenergic transmission following incorporation of PI into the membranes of turkey erythrocytes. The extent of receptor down-regulation seems to be further controlled by the ratios between the individual phospholipids, in particular between PS and SM and others. The effects on phospholipid composition as well as on the density of β-adrenoceptor sites seem to be similar between drugs of the same therapeutic group.

In order to verify these in vitro findings in vivo, rats were chronically treated with daily injections of DMI 10 mg/kg i.p. for 21 days.[8] A 30% decrease in the number of β-adrenoceptors was observed in brain. Receptor desensitization of similar extent was noted in submaxillary glands and lung. No change in β-adrenoceptor number was seen in heart. The total phospholipid content was not altered in these organs after chronic treatment. However, organ-specific changes were found in the phospholipid composition of submaxillary glands, lung, and liver but not in brain and heart. The changes were variable, but an increase in PI and decreases in SM and PE were consistent findings. Alterations in the phospholipid composition of the brain might have been masked by the large and stable phospholipid pool of the myelin.

Changes in membrane phospholipid composition and reduction in β-adrenoceptor density are found in both cultured cells and rats following chronic DMI administration. Thus the two drug-induced effects not only may be coincidental but could be causally related. Furthermore, the accordance of chronic DMI effects in vivo and in vitro underlines the usefulness of cell culture models for the study of drug actions.

References

1. Sulser F. Molecular mechanisms in antidepressant action. Psychopharmacol Bull 1983;19:300–304.
2. Lüllmann-Rauch R. Drug induced lysosomal storage disorders. In Dingle JT, Jacques PJ, Shaw IH (eds): Lysosomes in Applied Biology and Therapeutics. Amsterdam: North Holland, 1979;49–130.
3. Honegger U, Roscher A, Wiesmann U. Evidence for lysosomotropic action of desipramine in cultured fibroblasts. J Pharmacol Exp Ther 1983;225:436–441.
4. Stoffel P, Burkart T, Honegger UE, et al. Subcellular distribution of the antidepressant drug desipramine in cultured human fibroblasts after chronic administraiton. Biochem Pharmacol 1987;5:655–662.
5. Folch J, Lees M, Sloane-Stanley GH. A simple method for the isolation of total lipids from animal tissues. J Biol Chem 1957;226:497–509.

6. Honegger UE, Disler B, Wiesmann UN. Chronic exposure of human cells in culture to the tricyclic antidepressant desipramine reduces the number of beta-adrenoceptors. Biochem Pharmacol 1986;35:1899–1902.
7. McOsker CC, Weiland GA, Zilversmit DB. Inhibition of hormone-stimulated adenylate cyclase activity after altering turkey erythrocyte phospholipid-composition with a non-specific lipid transfer protein. J Biol Chem 1983;258:13017–13026.
8. Moor M, Honegger UE, Wiesmann UN. Organspecific, qualitative changes in the phospholipid composition of rats after chronic administration of the antidepressant drug desipramine. Biochem Pharmacol 1988;37:2035–2039.

24. Nicotinic Effects of Antidepressants

STEVEN C. DILSAVER AND M. HARIHARAN

Tricyclic antidepressants (TCAs) bind to muscarinic cholinergic receptors (mAChRs) and produce biochemical and physiological evidence of the blockade of muscarinic mechanisms.[1] Supersensitization of these mechanisms is a regularly occurring effect of agents that directly block access of acetylcholine to the post-synaptic mAChR or inhibit its release from presynaptic cholinergic neurons.[2] Treatment with amitriptyline (AMI) 10 mg/kg i.p. twice daily for 7 days or more enhances sensitivity to the hypothermic effects of oxotremorine.[3] Although the muscarinic effects of TCAs have been investigated, the influences of these and other antidepressants on parameters influenced by nicotinic mechanisms have received minimal attention.

The effects of antidepressants on nicotinic mechanisms has not been the subject of systematic study. However, Schofield et al.[4] presented evidence that a TCA binds to the ionic channel of the nicotinic receptor (nAChR). We studied the effects of AMI, desipramine (DMI), phenelzine, and bright artificial light[5] on a nicotinic mechanism involved in the regulation of core temperature.

Methods

Core temperature was telemetrically measured using the Model VM Mini-Mitter.[3] The devices were implanted into the peritoneal cavity. A transistor radio served as a receiver.

The initial nicotine challenge occurred prior to treatment with an antidepressant. Subsequent challenges occurred the morning after the previous evening's dose of antidepressant or in the course of treatment with bright light. Temperature was measured prior to and every 10 min after the injection of nicotine 1 mg/kg i.p. Baseline temperature for a given challenge was defined as the temperature immediately prior to the injection of nicotine.

Amitriptyline HCl, DMI HCl, phenelzine sulfate, and nicotine (base) were purchased from Sigma Chemical Company. Fluoxetine HCl was obtained from Lilly Pharmaceuticals. Doses of nicotine refer to the base form. Doses of the antidepressants refer to the salt. Agents were administered intraperitoneally on a milligram per-kilogram basis.

Plasma levels of nicotine and cotinine were determined by a high performance liquid chromotography (HPLC) method using a an ultraviolet detector (262 nm) with 2-phenylimadizole as an internal standard. Details of the assay are reported elsewhere.[6]

Data were analyzed using Student's paired t test. Measures of variance refer to the standard error of the mean (SEM).

Results

Amitriptyline

One week of treatment with AMI 10 mg/kg i.p. at 9 a.m. and 9 p.m. was associated with an increase in the mean maximum hypothermic response of $1.21 \pm 0.12°C$ ($p < 0.001$, $n = 10$). The mean maximum hypothermic response ($1.31 \pm 0.23°C$) remained elevated 1 week ($p < 0.001$) and 2 weeks ($1.00 \pm 0.35°C$; $p < 0.02$) after the discontinuation of AMI. The mean reduction in core temperature after 7 days of treatment with AMI relative to the pre-AMI baseline was $0.46 \pm 0.15°C$ ($p < 0.02$), after 7.5 days of abstinence $0.54 \pm 0.2°C$ ($p < 0.05$), and after 14.5 days of abstinence $0.19 \pm 0.19°C$. These results were confirmed in a second experiment.[7]

Fluoxetine

Prior to the first nicotine challenge these animals were challenged with saline 1 ml/kg i.p. The thermic response to saline was $0.22 \pm 0.10°C$. The sample ($n = 9$) exhibited a change in core temperature of $-1.41 \pm 0.24°C$ in response to the first nicotine challenge. The thermic response to nicotine after 1 week of treatment with fluoxetine 10 mg/kg i.p. at 9 a.m. and 5 p.m. was $-0.44 \pm 0.26°C$ ($p < 0.002$). The thermic response to nicotine was $0.16 \pm 0.14°C$ after 2 weeks of treatment. This response did not differ from that of saline ($p > 0.70$). The thermic response to nicotine after 1 week of withdrawal from fluoxetine was $-0.91 \pm 0.25°C$, which did not differ from baseline ($p > 0.15$).

Desipramine

The mean thermic response to saline was $+0.23 \pm 0.12°C$ ($n = 12$). The sample exhibited a change in core temperature of $-1.43 \pm 0.18°C$ in response to the first nicotine challenge. This difference was highly significant from the response to saline ($p < 0.00003$). After 1 week of treatment the sample exhibited a thermic response of $-0.58 \pm 0.22°C$. This response differed from that at baseline ($p < 0.015$). After 2 weeks of treatment the sample exhibited a decrease in temperature of $-0.8 \pm 0.21°C$, which also differed from the baseline response ($p < 0.005$). The thermic response to nicotine did not differ after 1 and 2 weeks of treatment ($p > 0.35$).

We assessed the possibility that DMI might accelerate the metabolism of nicotine. Rats were treated with saline 1 mg/kg i.p. twice daily or DMI 10 ml/kg i.p. twice daily. The animals received nicotine (base) 1 mg/kg i.p. 19–20 h after the last dose of saline ($n = 10$) or DMI ($n = 10$). Blood was collected by cardiac puncture 30 min after the injection. The mean nicotine levels in the DMI and control groups were 318.2 ± 10.4 and 220.3 ± 14.0 ng/ml, respectively ($p < 0.00003$). Thus the animals treated with DMI had higher levels of nicotine. The mean cotinine levels were 87.0 ± 10.1 and 232.1 ± 25.9 ng/ml, respectively ($p < 0.000006$). The elevated levels of cotinine in the control sample suggests that DMI retarded the metabolism of nicotine.

Phenelzine

Ten adult male rats weighing 265.5 ± 8.5 g were challenged with nicotine 1 mg/kg i.p. prior to treatment with phenelzine. Change in core temperature was determined as described above. The animals were then treated with phenelzine 15 mg/kg i.p. every other day at 4 p.m. They were rechallenged with nicotine after 14 days of treatment. Nine of ten animals exhibited significant blunting of the hypothermic response to nicotine at $\alpha < 0.005$. The hypothermic response of the sample was 1.43 ± 0.18°C at baseline and 0.55 ± 0.13°C after 14 days of treatment ($p < 0.0035$).

The ten experimental animals and eight control animals (mean weight 267.5 ± 7.1 g) received nicotine 1 mg/kg i.p. for the determination of plasma nicotine and cotinine levels as described above. The experimental and control groups exhibited mean nicotine and cotinine levels of 447 ± 27 and 230 ± 21 ng/ml compared to 394 ± 9.0 ng/ml ($p > 0.20$, $t = 1.15$, df = 11) and 289 ± 40 ng/ml ($p > 0.10$, $t = 1.47$, df = 16), respectively.

Treatment with Bright Artificial Light

Eleven rats (mean weight 312.7 ± 7.8 g) were exposed to full-spectrum bright artificial light (7,400 lux) for two consecutive weeks. The thermic response to nicotine was measured prior to light exposure and after 1 and 2 weeks of treatment. The thermic response to nicotine at baseline was −1.69 ± 0.25°C. The thermic response to nicotine was −0.66 ± 0.12°C ($p < 0.002$) after 1 week and −0.31 ± 0.14°C ($p < 0.000025$) after 2 weeks of light exposure. The difference in responsiveness between weeks 1 and 2 was significant ($p < 0.00025$).

Multiple Injections of Nicotine Do Not Account for Blunting

We assessed the possibility that multiple injections of nicotine could produce subsensitivity to the hypothermic effect of this cholinergic agonist. Eight adult male Sprague-Dawley rats were injected with nicotine 1 mg/kg i.p. at 7-day intervals. Each animal received four doses. The mean hypothermic response to nicotine was 1.37 ± 0.23°C when the sample was first challenged with nicotine and 1.32 ± 0.20°C after the fourth challenge ($p > 0.50$).

Discussion

Treatment with AMI, DMI, fluoxetine, phenelzine, and bright artificial light altered sensitivity to nicotine. We demonstrated that in the cases of DMI and phenelzine it was not due to a pharmacokinetic factor. Thus drugs from two chemical classes and bright light blunt the response to nicotine, whereas AMI enhances it. This finding suggests that nicotinic effects may be related to mechanism of action.

Nicotine promotes the release of norepinephrine in the hypothalamus and dopamine within the mesolimbic and nigrostriatal tracts.[8] It is conceivable that sub-sensitization of the hypothermic response to nicotine is an epiphenomenon. That is, should treatment with antidepressants enhance noradrenegic and dopaminergic neurotransmission, the related nicotinic mechanism, which may serve a compensatory role when these networks are defective, may become subsensitive following treatments that correct the abnormalities. The array of treatments that produce this effect highlights its possible importance.

References

1. Dilsaver SC. Pharmacologic induction of cholinergic system up-regulation and supersensitivity in affective disorders research. J Clin Psychopharmacol 1986;6:65–74.
2. Dilsaver SC. Pathophysiology of affective disorders and substance abuse: An integrative model. J Clin Psychopharmacol 1987;7:1–10.
3. Dilsaver SC, Alessi NE, Snider RM. Amitriptyline produces supersensitivity of a central muscarinic mechanism. Biol Psychiatry 1987;22:495–507.
4. Schofield GG, Witop B, Wernick JE, et al. Differentiation of the open and closed states of the ionic channels of nicotinic acetylcholine receptors by tricyclic antidepressants. Proc Natl Acad Sci USA 1981;78:5240–5244.
5. Wehr TA, Jacobsen FM, Sack DA, et al. Phototherapy of seasonal affective disorder. Arch Gen Psychiatry 1986;43:870–875.
6. Dilsaver SC, Hariharan M, Davidson RK. Phenelzine produces subsensitivity to nicotine. Prog Neuropsychopharmacol Biol Psychiatry, 1988;23:109–175.
7. Dilsaver SC, Alessi NE, Majchrzak KJ. Amitriptyline produces supersensitivity to the hypothermic effects of nicotine. Biol Psychiatry, 1988;23:169–175.
8. Dilsaver SC. Cholinergic-monoaminergic interaction in the pathophysiology of affective disorders. Int Psychopharmacol 1986;1:181–198.

25. Molecular Sites of Anxiolytic Action

JOHN F. TALLMAN

Studies of the molecular properties of high affinity receptors for the benzodiazepines have clarified many of the actions of drugs that work at these receptor proteins in experimental animals and in human brain. The original biochemical and pharmacological studies indicated that the receptor for these drugs was a part of the receptor for the transmitter γ-aminobutyric acid (GABA).[1] More recent studies have involved the purification of these proteins and intense study of their molecular and immunological properties. Some of these studies are briefly outlined here.

Purification of GABA-linked Benzodiazepine Receptors

Solubilization of the GABA[2] was caried out in the presence of nonionic detergent. The soluble receptor was then purified with a flurazepam affinity gel. Approximately 1,000-fold purification of the receptor was obtained through this procedure. Analysis of this preparation indicated the presence of several protein bands that adsorb to and are eluted from the affinity column. The major band (50 kilodaltons, kD) obtained is that which migrates with the photolabeled receptor protein in both one and two dimensions. A somewhat higher molecular weight band (55 kD) was also seen. In addition, a number of minor protein bands were seen with molecular sizes of more than 60 kD as well as at 47 kD. The purification of a protein band that has a molecular size of 45–50 kD has been seen by others and attributed to proteolysis of the subunits of the GABA–receptor complex. From our proteolytic digestion experiments of the purified separated proteins and the ability to remove this substance from the preparation by gel filtration, this possibility does not appear to be likely. The purified preparations contained similar amounts of high affinity (<10 nM) binding sites for both benzodiazepine agonists and antagonists. In addition, a small enhancement of flunitrazepam binding by 10^{-4} M GABA was noted; no pentobarbital shift was observed. Two affinity states of the GABA receptor are observed in these preparations. The high affinity state is present in numbers similar to the number of benzodiazepine receptors. In contrast, there were more lower affinity GABA sites than benzodiazepine sites. Purified benzodiazepine preparations from rat and human cerebellum also consist of a major protein with a molecular of 50 kD, as determined by sodium dodecyl sulfate polyacrylamide gel electrophoresis (SDS-PAGE). This band co-migrates with the photolabeled receptor on one- and two-dimensional gel electrophoresis. In one dimension, the protein banding pattern of receptor preparations from rat cortex and cerebellum were virtually identical on two dimensions: a major band at 50 kD and a minor band at 55 kD. Benzodiazepine receptors were purified from three nonidentical human cerebellar preparations; two of them were similiar to the rat cerebellar preparations and were used in subsequent studies. The third preparation had several other major proteins. Although other explanations for the multiple forms (e.g.) multiple alleles) are possible, a major factor in the nonuniformity seen in the human preparations may be the inability to precisely control the time until autopsy and the condition in which the tissue is received.

Peptide Mapping of the Receptor Subunits

Receptor protein can be peptide-mapped (fingerprinted) following photoaffinity labeling, phosphorylation, or iodination of the purified receptor's subunits. The method for iodination and mapping were developed in our laboratory to examine the similarities in the purified receptors. Prior to iodination the benzodiazepine receptor preparation was further purified by gel filtration on a Sephadex G-200 column. Samples enriched in the benzodiazepine receptor were pooled and lyophilized. This step has the effect of removing the 47-kD band.

Iodination of the purified receptor was carried out and to the ^{125}I-benzodiazepine receptor was added sufficient carrier receptor to enable visualization by Coomassie staining. This mixed preparation was subjected to gel electrophoresis, and protein staining bands were cut from the slab gel. The gel pieces were then applied to the wells of a long SDS gel. Varing amounts of the *Staphylococcus aureus* protease were layered on top and the proteins subjected to electrophoresis overnight. This method resulted in a characteristic pattern of peptides for the 50- and 55-kD bands, which indicates that there is fairly good conservation of structure of these proteins. Their nonidentity with the other contaminating proteins in the purified receptor was also shown.

Amino Acid Sequence of the Purified Photolabeled Fragments

A limit peptide fragment[3] was obtained by the treatment of photolabeled benzodiazepine receptors with a combination of trypsin and chymotrypsin. These fragments were isolated by a combination of gel filtration and HPLC. Preliminary amino acid sequence analysis of the fragments isolated to date have been carried out by automated Edman degradation. The analyzed sample was more than 95% a single peptide by end-group analysis and contained the entire radioactivity of the major isolated fraction.

This site that is photolabeled appears to be intimately involved in the active site of the benzodiazepine receptor and is near or at the site of action of this widely used group of anxiolytics and hypnotics. Thus important information about the site of action of these drugs in rats has been obtained, and a sequence to which antibodies are to be prepared has been obtained. Such antibodies have the potential of interaction with the active site of this receptor and may be important phar-macological tools. Knowledge of the rat sequence has allowed us to identify a region of the benzodiazepine receptor that is involved in the binding of the ben-zodiazepine molecule. This region is almost identical to a region particularly found in an *Escherichia coli* ATPase; such a coincidence may point to a phylogenetic origin for this part of the benzodiazepine receptor or indicate an interesting con-vergent evolution. The region of the ATPase containing this sequence in *E. coli* is a region involved in the binding of purines. In the past, a number of purines have been implicated as possible endogenous ligands for the benzodiazepine re-ceptor, and the ability of purines to displace benzodiazepine binding may reflect the persistence of this purine-recognizing region in the receptor. An anxiogenic peptide modulator of this receptor has been isolated and sequenced by Costa and associates[4]; perhaps the regions of the receptor we are isolating interacts with such a peptide modulator.

Because of the fourfold degeneracy of proline and the number of proteins in which this sequence has been found, the tentative sequence for the photolabeled fragment has not been that useful for those interested in receptor cloning. However, a similar structure is contained in the sequence of the bovine *a*-subunit of the cloned benzodiazepine receptor. Thus these data may assist in the ultimate proof that the sequence cloned is the correct one and indicate outside and internal regions.

Preparation of Anti-receptor Monoclonal Antibodies

Using the purified preparation described above, we prepared monoclonal antibodies against the purified receptor preparations.[5] Splenic lymphocytes were prepared from antibody-positive animals and fused with a nonsecreting myeloma line; cell suspensions were then plated in 96-well microtiter plates from which hybridoma lines were selected. Cell lines that tested positively to the receptor preparation in a solid-phase radioimmunoassay were expanded and cloned at limiting dilution. Each monoclonal line was then passed into pristane primed BALB/c exbreeders for the production of high-titer ascites. Ascites was harvested by intraperitoneal puncture 1–2 weeks later, aliquoted, and stored frozen at −80°C.

SDS, Two-Dimensional Electrophoresis, and Immunoblot

The molecular weights of the photoaffinity labeled rat cortical and cerebellar and human cerebellar benzodiazepine receptor were determined by combining SDS-PAGE and either autoradiography or gel slice techniques. The major photolabeled band has an apparent molecular weight of 50 kD. Minor photolabeled bands, in-corporating less than 5% total label, with molecular weights of 55 kD were detected by autoradiography. However, the low percentage of incorporated label makes clear detection of these bands difficult. After photolabeling the membranes were incubated at 4°C for 48 h prior to the standard extensive washing regimen. This procedure did not increase the amount of label in the 47-kD protein band, also supporting the hypothesis that this protein is not an artifact of the photolabeling procedure. The presence of only minor labeling of a 55-kD protein is consistent with most laboratories' inability to incorporate significant levels of label into this particular protein in the rat cerebellum.

Similarities between rat cortex and cerebellar and human cerebellar benzodiazepine receptors were seen in immunoblots of membrane preparations. Several monoclonal lines developed as above were used in this study. One line, E9, recognizes only the *a*-subunit, whereas another, H10, recognizes both *a*- and *B*-subunits in partially purified receptor preparation from rat brain. These immunoreactive patterns were seen in both human and rat cerebellar membrane preparations. The ability to immunologically detect but not photolabel the 55-kD protein in the cerebellum is not understood at the present time. The distinctive immunoreactive patterns displayed by both lines suggest that each recognizes a separate antigenic determinant of the receptor. The common determinant on the *a*- and *B*-subunit is recognized by H10, whereas the determinant recognized by E9 appears to be associated with only the *a*-subunit.

Posttranslational Modifications of GABA/Benzodiazepine Receptors

We found that benzodiazepine receptors,[6] like many cell surface proteins, are glycosylated. The manner in which the receptor is glycosylated, i.e., types of carbohydrate moiety, appears to vary among brain regions. In cortex and hippocampus, significant amounts of the carbohydrates are removed by neuraminidase or endoglycosidase H. In the rat cerebellum only a small percentage of the molecular weight is contributed by either sialic acids or asparagine-linked carbohydrate chains, as determined by treatment with neuraminidase and endoglycosidase H. The binding of the benzodiazepine receptor ligands and muscimol are altered in cortical regions of rat brain, whereas these treatments do not alter binding of agonists and antagonists in the rat cerebellum. These findings do not, however, suggest that the cerebellar benzodiazepine receptor is not glycosylated, as ^{125}I-concanavalin A recognizes the partially purified cerebellar receptor. Some microheterogeneity in iodinated 55-kD protein but not 50-kD protein was also seen in two dimensions.

Immunocytochemical Results with Monoclonal Antibodies

The E9 antibody was used in histochemical studies of substantia nigra (SN) in experimental animals and parallel experiments in tissue from patients with Parkinson's or Huntington's disease.[7] In the rat, E9 staining paralleled the distribution of the receptor determined autoradiographically. In primate SN (and to some extent in rat SN), staining was observed in both axons innervating the SN (particularly the dorsal and medial reticulata) and in the perikarya of the reticulata. In primate brain little staining of the cellular elements was observed in the reticulata, although in the dorsal raphe and periaqueductal gray matter perikarya staining was dense. In the SN of a Huntington's disease patient, there is a marked reduction of the GABA receptor imunoreactivity in the reticulata; staining of the melanin-containing dopamine neurons in the SN is normal, as is the density of the thalamic GABA receptors. In contrast, in Parkinson's patients most of the reticulata is intact, but the medial SN and ventral tegmental areas are lost.

Conclusions

With sophisticated molecular probes we have been able to identify the proteins involved in the action of the benzodiazepines. The study of these proteins in humans and further investigation with probes of the gene structure should allow examination of whether genetically determined changes in the receptor underlie neurological and psychiatric disorders.

References

1. Tallman J, Gallager, D. The GABAergic system: a locus of benzodiazepine action. Annu Rev Neurosci. 1985;8:21–44.
2. Duman R, Sweetnam P, Gallombardo P, Tallman J. Molecular biology of inhibitory amino acid receptors. Mol Neurobiol 1987;1:155–189.
3. Klotz K, Bochetta A, Neale J, et al. Proteolytic degradation of neuronal benzodiazepine receptors. Life Sci 1984;34:293–299.
4. Costa E, Guidotti A. Endogenous ligands for benzodiazepine recognition sites. Biochem Pharmacol 1985;34:3399–3403.
5. Sweetnam P, Nestler E, Gallombardo P, et al. Comparison of the molecular structure of human and rat GABA/benzodiazepine receptors. Mol Brain Res 1987;2:223–233.
6. Sweetnam P, Tallman J. Regional differences in brain benzodiazepine receptor carbohydrates. Mol Pharmacol 1986;29:299–306.
7. Deutch A, Sweetnam P, Gallombardo P, et al. Immunocytochemical study of the GABA/benzodiazepine receptors in neurological disorders. Presented at the Annual Meeting of the American College of Neuropsychophamacology, Puerto Rico, 1987.

26. Modulation of the Benzodiazepine/GABA Receptor Chloride Ionophore Complex: Evidence for an Asymmetrical Response of GABA-Gated Chloride Channels to Stress

Todd McIntyre, Ramon Trullas, and
Phil Skolnick

Direct and correlative evidence strongly suggests that the benzodiazepine/GABA receptor chloride ionophore complex ("supramolecular complex") mediates the principal pharmacological actions of benzodiazepines, barbiturates, and other chemically unrelated structures that can mimic (or antagonize) one or more of these actions. In contrast, it has been more difficult to evince the physiological function(s) of this supramolecular complex.

We have shown that subjecting rats to different stressors (e.g., a brief, ambient temperature swim [1,2] or sequential removal of cohorts from a common cage [3,4]) produces rapid and robust changes in the binding of a picrotoxinin-like "cage" convulsant, $[^{35}S]t$-butylbicyclophosphorothionate (TBPS),[5] to brain membranes. Thus exposure to such stressors elicited significant increases in both the apparent affinity (decreased Kd) of this radioligand and the maximum number of binding sites (Bmax) in well washed membranes of cerebral cortex. In contrast, we did not observe significant, stress-induced changes in either benzodiazepine receptors or that population of GABA receptors linked to benzodiazepine receptors [1-4] in identically prepared tissues.

While investigating these phenomena, a marked asymmetry in the characteristics of $[^{35}S]$TBPS binding was found in the right and left cerebral hemispheres of naive rats. This asymmetry was manifest as both a significantly higher apparent affinity (~24.5% reduction in Kd) and number (~42% higher Bmax) of binding sites in membranes prepared from right cortex compared to membranes from left cortex (Table 26.1, Fig. 26.1). Asymmetry in $[^{35}S]$TBPS binding was *not* observed in a number of other brain regions including cerebellum, hippocampus, and striatum.[6] Furthermore, no asymmetry of radioligand binding to benzodiazepine receptors was observed in cerebral cortex. Regional dissection of cerebral cortex revealed that the apparent asymmetrical distribution of $[^{35}S]$TBPS binding sites was present in the occipital and (combined) entorhinal/piriform cortex but was not observed in frontal, temporal, or parietal cortices (Fig. 26.1).

TABLE 26.1. Asymmetry of [^{35}S] TBPS binding to left and right cerebral cortex.[a]

Parameter	Naive rats		Restraint-stressed rats	
	Left cortex	Right cortex	Left cortex	Right cortex
Kd	44.6 ± 2.4	34.1 ± 2.3[b]	23.1 ± 1.2[d]	21.9 ± 1.4[d]
Bmax	1,263 ± 96	1,794 ± 68[c]	2,264 ± 122[d]	2,220 ± 165[e]

[a]Cerebral cortices were obtained and prepared from naive or restraint-stressed (10 min) Sprague-Dawley rats as previously described.[3,4] Values represent the means ± SEM of five animals per group. The values obtained for Kd and Bmax were obtained from Scatchard plots ($r \geqslant 0.985$) constructed as previously described.[1–4]
[b]$p < 0.001$, [c] $p < 0.02$: right cortex significantly different from left, paired t test. [d]$p < 0.01$, [e]$p < 0.05$, significantly different from corresponding area in naive rats (Student's t test). No significant differences in the characteristics of [^{35}S] TBPS binding between left and right cortex were apparent after stress.

Anatomical lateralization of both neurotransmitters (e.g., dopamine) and enzymes involved in neurotransmitter biosynthesis (e.g., choline acetyltransferase) has been reported in the mammalian central nervous system.[7,8] However, to our knowledge, a similar lateralization of either neurotransmitter-linked recognition sites or effector systems has not been documented. Although the cortical asymmetry in [^{35}S]TBPS binding sites observed could be attributable to an anatomical lateralization of GABA-gated chloride channels, studies from our laboratory have shown[3,4] that changes in these channels can be evoked by sequential removal of cohorts from a common cage, a process requiring less than 15 s. Thus the asymmetry in [^{35}S]TBPS binding observed in "naive" animals could represent a differential activation of the two hemispheres in response to removal of a rat from

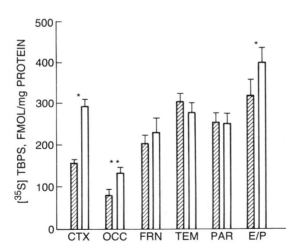

FIGURE 26.1. [^{35}S] TBPS binding in left (hatched bars) and right (open bars) areas of cerebral cortex. Values are expressed in femtomoles per milligram of protein and represent the mean ±SEM of six experiments. No more than one animal was removed from a cage per experiment to avoid variability due to an effect of cohort removal.[3,4] *$p<0.05$, **$p<0.01$ using paired comparisons made with dependent t tests. CTX = whole (pooled) cortex. OCC = occipital cortex. FRN = frontal cortex. TEM = temporal cortex. PAR = parietal cortex. E/P = pooled entorhinal/piriform cortex.

its home cage environment rather than a true anatomical lateralization. This hypothesis was examined by immobilizing (restraint) rats for 10 min prior to sacrifice. Because a brief stress produces significant increases in both the apparent affinity of [^{35}S]TBPS and number of binding sites for this radioligand,[1-4] the presence of a cortical asymmetry in stressed rats suggests an anatomical lateralization of GABA-gated chloride channels. However, if the asymmetry was no longer present following stress, it may be inferred that these differences represent the response of GABA-gated chloride channnels to changes in the environment prior to sacrifice (i.e., a process that requires less than 10 s). Table 26.1 demonstrates that although restraint stress significantly increased [^{35}S]TBPS binding in both left and right cerebral cortex compared to values obtained in naive animals, the left/right differences in both Kd and Bmax found in naive rats *were no longer manifest in the stressed animals*. These data suggest that the cortical asymmetry observed in "naive" animals may reflect the differential processing of information between hemispheres. This hypothesis is supported by the prominent differences in [^{35}S]TBPS binding found in both the occipital and the entorhinal/piriform cortices (Fig. 26.1), areas important for processing visual and olfactory cues, respectively. These observations suggest a robust response of the supramolecular complex to even "subtle" perturbation of the environment (i.e., removal of a single animal from the home cage) with a rapid response *preceding* complete activation of both the hypothalamic-pituitary-adrenocortical (HPA) axis and other neurotransmitter/modulator systems previously implicated in stress.[3,4] Because anxiety may be an essential component for the development of some forms of depression[9] and benzodiazepine receptor ligands can modify the development of learned helplessness[10] (which is considered an animal model of depression), a putative role of the supramolecular complex in the development of affective disorders such as depression appears to be an area for future studies.

References

1. Havoundjian H, Paul S, Skolnick P. Rapid, stress induced modification of the benzodiazepine receptor coupled chloride ionophore. Brain Res 1986;375:403–408.
2. Havoundjian H, Paul S, Skolnick P. Acute, stress-induced changes in the benzodiazepine/GABA receptor complex are confined to the chloride ionophore. J. Pharmacol Exp Ther 1986;237:787–793.
3. Trullas R, Havoundjian H, Zamir N, et al. Environmentally-induced modification of the benzodiazepine/GABA receptor coupled chloride ionophore. Psychopharmacology 1987;91:384–390.
4. Trullas R, Havoundjian H, Skolnick P. Is the benzodiazepine receptor complex involved in physical and emotional stress? In: Mechanisms of Physical and Emotional Stress (Ed.) G.P. Chrousos, D.L. Loriaux and P.W. Gold. Plenum: New York, pp. 183–200.
5. Squires R, Casida J, Richardson M, et al. [^{35}S]t-Butylbicyclophosphorothionate binds with high affinity to brain specific sites coupled to gamma-aminobutyric acid-A and ion recognition sites. Mol Pharmacol 1983;23:326–336.
6. McIntyre TD, Trullas R, Skolnick P. Asymmetrical Activation of GABA-gated chloride channels in cerebral cortex. Pharm Biochem Behav 1988;30:911–916.
7. Zimmerberg B, Glick S, Jerussi T. Neurochemical correlate of a spatial preference in rats. Science 1974;185:623–625.
8. Glick S, Ross D, Hough L. Lateral asymmetry of neurotransmitters in human brain. Brain Res 1982;234:53–63.
9. Roth M, Gurney C, Garside R, et al. Studies in the classification of affective disorders. Br J Psychiatry 1972;121:147–156.
10. Drugan R, Maier S, Skolnick P, et al. An anxiogenic benzodiazepine receptor ligand induces learned helplessness. Eur J Pharmacol 1985;113:453–457.

I. E. BASIC MECHANISMS OF LITHIUM ACTION

27. Lithium Inhibition of Adenylate Cyclase Activity: Site of Action and Interaction with Divalent Cations

A. MØRK AND A. GEISLER

Several studies in man and experimental animals have demonstrated that acute and chronic lithium administration inhibits various stimulated adenylate cyclase activities. Thus lithium inhibits renal antidiuretic hormone (ADH)-stimulated adenylate cyclase activity and thyroid-stimulating hormone (TSH)-stimulated enzyme activity in the thyroid. Other peripheral tissues are also affected by lithium, e.g., platelet and lymphocyte adenylate cyclase. Studies on this enzyme in the central nervous system (CNS) have elucidated that lithium in vitro inhibits the adenylate cyclase in cerebral cortex, corpus striatum, neurohypophysis, hippocampus, pineal gland, and retina. It has been assumed that this inhibition of the adenylate cyclase activity, resulting in dampening of the transmission of neurotransmitter signals, may be of relevance for the mechanism of action of lithium in the treatment of manic-depressive disorders.

Lithium and Ca^{2+} have similar hydrated ionic radii and charge densities; furthermore, lithium and Mg^{2+} possess almost the same size atomic radius, and both ions coordinate with nitrogen. Physicochemical studies have demonstrated that an interaction of lithium with Ca^{2+} and Mg^{2+} may be of importance. Fossel et al.[1] have demonstrated that lithium, at therapeutic plasma levels, competes effectively with both Ca^{2+} and Mg^{2+} for their membrane-binding sites, even at extracellular Ca^{2+} and Mg^{2+} concentrations. Such observations indicate that a certain degree of Ca^{2+} and Mg^{2+} displacement may occur from neuronal membranes during chronic lithium treatment. The action of lithium can thus be exerted by two potential mechanisms: (a) By acting as an antagonist lithium may inhibit cation-dependent enzymes by displacing divalent cations from their binding sites; and (b) by mimicking the action of divalent cations lithium may usurp the function of these cations and activate or prevent deactivation of the cation-regulated systems. Both actions interfere with the effect of divalent cations on enzymatic processes.

Research has revealed that the structure of the adenylate cyclase is complex. This messenger system consists of three essential components (Fig. 27.1): a hormone receptor (R); the catalytic unit (C), which catalyzes the formation of cyclic AMP from $MgATP^{2-}$; and a guanine nucleotide binding protein (N), which transmits the hormonal stimulus from R to the C unit. Following the binding of a hormone to its receptor, the hormone–receptor complex interacts with the N protein,

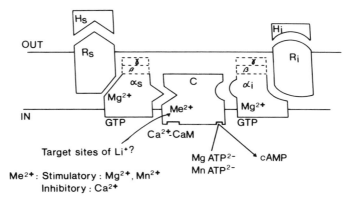

FIGURE 27.1. Basic components of the adenylate cyclase system. See text for a detailed description. (*s, i*) Stimulatory and inhibitory components, respectively. (Me^{2+}) a site on the catalytic unit sensitive to divalent cations.

which subsequently binds GTP. The binding of GTP to the α-subunit of the N protein leads to a Mg^{2+}-dependent dissociation of the N protein into α- and βγ-subunits, and the hormone–receptor affinity is reduced. The activated conformation of the α-subunit, containing GTP, stimulates the C unit so long as GTP is bound to the subunit. Upon hydrolysis of GTP by an intrinsic GTPase, the α- and βγ-subunits reassociate. The activity of the C unit is subject to stimulatory and inhibitory regulation via the R$_s$-N$_s$ and R$_i$-N$_i$ pathways, respectively.

Magnesium is essential for adenylate cyclase activity, as Mg^{2+} complexes with ATP to form the enzyme substrate. Furthermore, free Mg^{2+} is considered to modulate the enzyme activity through two independent cation sites. One Mg^{2+} site on N regulates both the agonist affinity for the hormone receptor and the activity of the N protein itself. The second Mg^{2+} site located on the C unit is responsible for the Mg^{2+} activation of the enzyme. Presumably activators of the adenylate cyclase stimulate the activity by enhancing the affinity for free Mg^{2+} to the cation site(s), whereas the affinity for MgATP^{2-} remains unaltered.[2]

The Ca^{2+} ion exerts a bimodal effect on the enzyme. Submicromolar concentrations of Ca^{2+} stimulate and higher concentrations inhibit its activity. The stimulatory effect of Ca^{2+} is mediated by calmodulin, and the inhibitory action is assumed to be mediated by interference of Ca^{2+} with the divalent cation site(s) on the enzyme.

Table 27.1 summarizes some effects of lithium in vitro and ex vivo on the adenylate cyclase activity stimulated through the individual components of the system. It is noteworthy that lithium ex vivo affects neurotransmitter-stimulated cAMP accumulation differently. Thus lithium ex vivo reduces the effect of norepinephrine, exerts no effect on dopamine, and enhances serotonin-stimulated enzyme activity. It is unknown whether these observations are due to a selective action of lithium or to differences in assay conditions. Several studies have shown that lithium inhibits the noradrenergic adenylate cyclase activity in cerebral cortex whether stimulated through the receptor, the N protein, or the C unit.[3, 6–9] Lithium in vitro and ex vivo has been shown to reduce Ca^{2+}-stimulated adenylate cyclase,[6,9] but this inhibition does not affect the binding of Ca^{2+} to calmodulin.

TABLE 27.1. Influence of lithium in vitro and ex vivo on stimulated activities of the components of brain adenylate cyclase measured as cyclic AMP accumulation.

Components	Activators	In vitro	Ex vivo	Ref.
Receptor	Norepinephrine	↓	↓	3
	Dopamine	↓	–	4
	Serotonin	n.d.	↑	5
N_s	GTP	↓	–	6
	Gpp(NH)p	↓	↓	7
	Fluoride	↓	–	8
C unit	Forskolin	↓	↓	8
	Ca^{2+}-CaM	↓	↓	6
	Mn^{2+}-CaM	↓	↓ [a]	6

(N_s) stimulatory guanine nucleotide binding protein. (CaM) calmodulin. (C unit) catalytic unit. (↓) inhibition. (↑) stimulation. (–) no effect. (n.d.) not determined.
[a] Unpublished observation.

It has been suggested that lithium inhibits stimulated adenylate cyclase activities by interfering with the regulatory role of Mg^{2+}, and a lithium–Mg^{2+} antagonism has been demonstrated in membrane preparations.[6,7] It has been suggested that lithium in vitro inhibits the adenylate cyclase activity by displacing Mg^{2+} from its allosteric binding site on the C unit of the adenylate cyclase system[9] (Fig. 27.1).

It should be emphasized that at present the mode of action of lithium is still unclarified, but studies on the mechanism by which lithium influences neurotransmission are considered to be of significance in the search for the basis of the therapeutic effect of lithium. Thus the influence of lithium on the adenylate cyclase may be involved in the mode of action of lithium in the treatment of manic-depressive disorder.

References

1. Fossel ET, Sarasua MM, Koehler KA. A lithium-7 NMR investigation of the lithium ion interaction with phosphatidylcholine-phosphatidylglycerol membranes: observation of calcium and magnesium ion competition. J Magnet Reson 1985;64:536–540.
2. Cech SY, Broaddus WC, Maguire ME. Adenylate cyclase: the role of magnesium and other divalent cations. Mol Cell Biochem 1980;33:67–92.
3. Ebstein RP, Hermoni M, Belmaker RH. The effect of lithium on noradrenaline-induced cyclic AMP accumulation in rat brain; inhibition after chronic treatment and absence of supersensitivity. J Pharmacol Exp Ther 1980;213:161–167.
4. Geisler A, Klysner R. The effect of lithium in vitro and in vivo on dopamine-sensitive adenylate cyclase activity in dopaminergic areas of the rat brain. Acta Pharmacol Toxicol (Copenh) 1985;56:1–5.
5. Hotta I, Yamawaki S. Lithium decreases 5-HT₁ receptors but increases 5-HT-sensitive adenylate cyclase activity in rat hippocampus. Biol Psychiatry 1986;21:1382–1390.
6. Mørk A, Geisler A. Effects of lithium on calmodulin-stimulated adenylate cyclase activity in cortical membranes from rat brain. Pharmacol Toxicol 1987;60:17–23.
7. Newman ME, Belmaker RH. Effects of lithium in vitro and ex vivo on components of the adenylate cyclase system in membranes from the cerebral cortex of the rat. Neuropharmacology 1987;26:211–217.
8. Andersen PH, Geisler A. Lithium inhibition of forskolin-stimulated adenylate cyclase. Neuropsychobiology 1984;12:1–3.
9. Mørk A, Geisler A. Mode of action of lithium on the catalytic unit of adenylate cyclase from rat brain. Pharmacol Toxicol 1987;60:241–248.

28. Comparison of the Effects of Lithium and Antidepressant Drugs on Second Messenger Systems in Rat Brain

MICHAEL E. NEWMAN AND BERNARD LERER

Lithium is an effective therapeutic agent in the treatment of both mania and depression. Of the various theories put forward to explain its therapeutic efficacy, those based on lithuim's actions on neurotransmitter receptors and second messengers are of special interest in that similar theories have been offered to explain the therapeutic actions of a wide variety of antidepressant drugs, including tricyclic antidepressants, monoamine oxidase inhibitors, and electroconvulsive therapy. In this chapter the effects of lithium on the neurotransmitter-stimulated processes of cyclic AMP and inositol phosphate (IP) formation in rat brain are compared with the effects of antidepressants, as exemplified by electroconvulsive shock (ECS) and desipramine (DMI), on these processes.

β-Adrenoceptors and Cyclic AMP Formation in Rat Cortical Slices

Vetulani et al.[1] first showed a reduction in β-adrenoceptor number and norepinephrine-stimulated cyclic AMP formation in the rat cortical slice preparation after chronic administration of a wide variety of antidepressant treatments. This finding has since been replicated in several laboratories. We have shown that the reduction in the degree of stimulation is also observed when the agent forskolin, which activates adenylate cyclase by direct interaction with the catalytic (C) unit of the enzyme, is used to stimulate cyclic AMP in rat cortical slices. This effect was observed after both chronic ECS and chronic DMI[2,3] and indicates that the β-adrenoceptor desensitization induced by antidepressant treatment is of the heterologous type. When membranes were prepared from rats administered the above agents, however, forskolin-stimulated adenylate cyclase activity as well as activities stimulated by sodium fluoride (NaF) or the nonhydrolyzable GTP analogue GppNHp were found to be increased relative to the activity in membranes prepared from control animals.

Lithium in vitro has been shown to reduce brain adenylate cyclase activity, and chronic administration of lithium to rats resulted in a reduction in norepinephrine-stimulated cyclic AMP formation.[4] Both Andersen and Geisler[5] and our group[6] have shown a reduction of forskolin-stimulated adenylate cyclase after lithium in vitro or administered chronically in rat cerebral cortex membranes. This finding contrasts with the results of chronic antidepressant treatment and indicates that the primary action of lithium is on the C unit of the enzyme. In the case of ECS and DMI, desensitization of β-adrenoceptors, which is the primary action of these agents, may result in a compensatory increase in postreceptor-mediated activity in the membrane preparation in which the degree of receptor–cyclase coupling is low. It is of interest that reductions in forskolin and NaF-stimulated adenylate cyclase activity were also found in platelets from a group of manic-depressive patients receiving lithium treatment compared to normal controls.[7]

Adenylate Cyclase Activity in Rat Caudate Nucleus and Hippocampus

The dopaminergic and endogenous opiate systems of the brain have both been considered to be involved in the mechanism of action of lithium and antidepressants. Dopamine stimulates adenylate cyclase via D_1 receptors and inhibits adenylate cyclase via D_2 receptors in rat striatum, whereas the receptors for endogenous opiates of the delta subtype are negatively coupled to adenylate cyclase in this brain area. Staunton et al.[8] found no effect of chronic lithium on dopamine-stimulated adenylate cyclase in rat striatum, results that were confirmed in our laboratory.[6] Chronic ECS or DMI similarly had no effect on this parameter.[9] Both chronic ECS and chronic DMI have been reported to have variable effects on opiate receptor number in rat brain (for references see ref. 9), whereas two groups[10,11] found a reduction in opiate receptor binding after chronic lithium in rat cortex, hippocampus, and striatum. Measurement of adenylate cyclase activity, however, showed no effect of any of these treatments on met-enkephalin-induced inhibition of forskolin-stimulated activity in rat caudate nucleus membranes.[6,9]

In membranes from adult rat hippocampus, serotonin (5-hydroxytryptamine, 5-HT) has been shown to stimulate adenylate cyclase by interaction with 5-HT_{1a} receptors. Hotta and Yamawaki[12] have reported that chronic lithium decreased 5-HT receptors in rat hippocampus, whereas 5-HT-sensitive adenylate cyclase was increased. These observations are of interest in view of findings that chronic lithium enhanced the serotonin syndrome produced by administration of the selective 5-HT_{1a} agonist 8-hydroxy-2-(di-*n*-propylamino)tetralin [8-OH-DPAT] to rats.[13] Both chronic ECS and chronic DMI have been shown to have no effect on 5-HT_1 receptor number as measured by ^3H-5-HT binding in rat hippocampal membranes. However, results from our laboratory showed that although neither of these treatments affected the degree of stimulation of adenylate cyclase in hippocampal membranes by 100 μM 5-HT the degree of inhibition of forskolin-stimulated activity by 5-HT, an effect also mediated by 5-HT_{1a} receptors, was reduced by both treatments. This finding parallels the reduction in 8-OH-DPAT-induced hypothermia and behavioral syndrome observed in mice after several antidepressant treatments.[14] The 5-HT_{1a} receptor may thus be a candidate for a common site of action of lithium, tricyclics, and ECS.

Phosphatidylinositol Turnover and IP Formation

The introduction by Berridge et al.[15] of lithium to potentiate agonist-induced PIP_2 breakdown and IP formation has led to the development of this assay to provide a functional measure of activity at α_1-adrenoceptors, muscarinic cholinergic receptors, and serotonin 5-HT$_2$ receptors, which are coupled to this mechanism. Kendall and Nahorski[16] showed a reduction in 5-HT-stimulated IP formation in rat cerebral cortical slices after chronic treatment of animals with the antidepressants imipramine and iprindole, a finding confirmed in our laboratory with DMI and in keeping with reported effects of antidepressants on 5-HT$_2$ receptor number. Chronic ECS had no effect on 5-HT-stimulated IP formation in cortical slices[17] but increased norepinephrine-stimulated activity in cortical slices and decreased carbachol-stimulated activity in hippocampal slices, again in keeping with reported effects on receptor number.

Three groups have investigated the effects of lithium administered in vivo on IP formation in rat cortex. Acute lithium (4 mEq/kg s.c. 24 h prior to sacrifice) was found in experiments from our laboratory to potentiate norepinephrine-stimulated IP formation in cortical slices, whereas chronic lithium resulted in a reduction in this response, without any effect on the responses to carbachol or 5-HT in either case. Kendall and Nahorski,[18] however, showed a reduction in the IP response to carbachol, elevated K$^+$, histamine, and 5-HT after both acute lithium (6.75 mEq/kg 18 h before sacrifice) and chronic lithium, whereas the norepinephrine effect was not reduced after chronic lithium administration. Casebolt and Jope[19] have, however, also reported a reduction in norepinephrine-stimulated IP formation in rat cortex, in keeping with our findings. The reasons for the discrepancies between Kendall and Nahorski's results and the others are unknown. It seems unlikely, however, that depletion of inositol levels as a result of lithium inhibition of myoinositol phosphatase, leading in turn to depletion of the membrane-bound PIP$_2$ pool, the mechanism proposed by Berridge et al.[15] for the action of lithium, can account for these results. This mechanism would envisage a ubiquitous increase in IP formation on acute lithium administration, regardless of the agonist used to stimulate PIP$_2$ breakdown, whereas after chronic lithium all activities would similarly be reduced. The compensatory increase of inositol phosphatase activity observed by Renshaw et al.[20] in rat cerebral cortex homogenates after chronic lithium administration may in part explain why the actions of lithium on IP formation observed in vitro are not reproduced in animals receiving lithium in vivo. The fact that chronic lithium, ECS, and tricyclics have all been found to affect the PIP$_2$ hydrolysis/IP formation system indicate that this system may be of considerable importance in transducing extracellular hormonal signals and mediating the modification of these signals by antidepressant treatments.

References

1. Vetulani J, Stawarz RJ, Dingell JV, et al. A possible common mechanism of action of antidepressant treatments. Naunyn Schmiedebergs Arch Pharmacol 1976;293:109–114.
2. Newman ME, Salomon H, Lerer B. Electroconvulsive shock and cyclic AMP signal transduction: effects distal to the receptor. J Neurochem 1986;46:1667–1669.
3. Newman ME, Lipot M, Lerer B. Differential effects of chronic desipramine administration on the cyclic AMP response in rat cortical slices and membranes. Neuropharmacology 1987;26:1127–1130.
4. Ebstein RP, Hermoni M, Belmaker RH. The effect of lithium on noradrenaline-induced cyclic AMP accumulation in rat brain; inhibition after chronic treatment and absence of supersensitivity. J Pharmacol Exp Ther 1980;213:161–167.
5. Andersen PH, Geisler A. Lithium inhibition of forskolin-stimulated adenylate cyclase. Neuropsychobiology 1984;12:1–3.
6. Newman ME, Belmaker RH. Effects of lithium in vitro and ex vivo on components of the adenylate cyclase system in membranes from the cerebral cortex of the rat. Neuropharmacology 1987;26:211–217.

7. Ebstein RP, Lerer B, Bennett ER, et al. Lithium modification of second messenger signal amplification in man: inhibition of phosphatidylinositol-specific phospholipase C and adenylate cyclase activity. Psychiatr Res 1988;24:45–52.
8. Staunton DA, Magistretti PJ, Shoemaker WJ, et al. Effects of chronic lithium treatment on dopamine receptors in the rat corpus striatum. Brain Res 1982;232:401–412.
9. Newman ME, Lerer B. Post-receptor mediated increases in adenylate cyclase activity after chronic antidepressant treatment: relationship to receptor desensitization. Eur J Pharmacol, 1989, in press.
10. Stengaard-Pedersen K, Schou M. In vitro and in vivo inhibition by lithium of enkephalin binding to opiate receptors in rat brain. Neuropharmacology 1982;21:817–823.
11. Wajda IJ, Banay-Schwartz M, Manigault I, et al. Effect of lithium and sodium ions on opiate- and dopamine-receptor binding. Neurochem Res 1981;6:321–331.
12. Hotta I, Yamawaki S. Lithium decreases 5-HT$_1$ receptors but increases 5-HT sensitive adenylate cyclase activity in rat hippocampus. Biol Psychiatry 1986;21:1382–1390.
13. Goodwin GM, de Souza RJ, Wood AJ, et al. The enhancement by lithium of the 5-HT$_{1a}$ mediated serotonin syndrome produced by 8-OH-DPAT in the rat: evidence for a postsynaptic mechanism. Psychopharmacology 1986;90:488–493.
14. Goodwin GM, de Souza RJ, Green AR. Presynaptic serotonin receptor-mediated response in mice attenuated by antidepressant drugs and electroconvulsive shock. Nature 1985;317:531–533.
15. Berridge MJ, Downes CP, Hanley MR. Lithium amplifies agonist-dependent phosphatidylinositol responses in brain and salivary glands. Biochem J 1982;206:587–595.
16. Kendall DA, Nahorski SR. 5-Hydroxytryptamine stimulated inositol phospholipid hydrolysis in rat cerebral cortex slices; pharmacological characterization and effects of antidepressants. J Pharmacol Exp Ther 1985;223:473–479.
17. Newman ME, Miskin I, Lerer B. Effects of single and repeated electroconvulsive shock administration on inositol phosphate accumulation in rat brain slices. J Neurochem 1987;49:19–23.
18. Kendall DA, Nahorski SR. Acute and chronic lithium treatments influence agonist and depolarization-stimulated inositol phospholipid hydrolysis in rat cerebral cortex. J Pharmacol Exp Ther 1987;241:1023–1027.
19. Casebolt TL, Jope RS. Chronic lithium treatment reduces norepinephrine-stimulated inositol phospholipid hydrolysis in rat cortex. Eur J Pharmacol 1987;140:245.
20. Renshaw PF, Joseph NE, Leigh JS. Chronic dietary lithium induces increased levels of myo-inositol-1-phosphatase activity in rat cerebral cortex homogenates. Brain Res 1986;380:401–404.

29. Effects of Lithium Ions on the Metabolism of Phosphoinositides

D. van Calker and W. Greil

The possibility that the therapeutic and prophylactic properties of lithium ions may be explained at least in part by their unique effects on the metabolism of phosphoinositides has attracted much attention. A decrease in the inositol content and a concomitant increase in the inositol-monophosphate concentration in the brain of lithium-treated animals was identified during the 1970s.[1,2] However, only the elucidation of the pivotal role of phosphoinositide-derived second messenger molecules has allowed us to realize the significance of these findings (for reviews see refs. 3–6).

Metabolism of Phosphoinositides

The metabolism of phosphoinositides is outlined in Figure 29.1 (phosphatidyl-inositol cycle). The stimulation by certain hormonal agonists of various receptors (Fig. 29.1: "receptor stimulation"), e.g., α_1-adrenergic-, muscarinic-, histamine-H_1 and various peptide receptors, leads to a phospholipase C-induced breakdown of phosphoinositides.

The hydrolysis of phosphoinositides results in the formation of diacylglycerol (DAG) and inositolphosphates. Inositol-1,4,5-trisphosphate [$(1,4,5)IP_3$], one of the inositolphosphates formed, is metabolized via two pathways. It can be dephosphorylated to inositolbisphosphate (IP_2), inositolmonophosphate (IP_1), and eventually to inositol, which is used for the resynthesis of phosphoinositides (Fig. 29.1).

A second metabolic pathway of $(1,4,5)IP_3$ involves phosphorylation to inositol-1,3,4,5-tetrakisphosphate [$(1,3,4,5)IP_4$], which in turn is dephosphorylated to $(1,3,4)IP_3$. This latter compound is metabolized by stepwise dephosphorylation to inositol (Fig. 29.1). The details of this process remain to be clarified.

Both products [DAG and I$(1,4,5)IP_3$] formed by the phospholipase C-induced hydrolysis of phosphoinositides act as intracellular messengers. DAG activates protein kinase C, an enzyme known to influence many cellular functions including processes of utmost importance in the brain such as the regulation of ion channels and neurotransmitter release (for review see ref. 7). $(1,4,5)IP_3$ promotes the release of Ca^{2+} ions from intracellular stores.

The second messenger function of these two compounds, DAG and (1,4,5)IP$_3$, is now firmly established. Evidence indicates that the products of the second metabolic pathway of (1,4,5)IP$_3$ may also have functions in the regulation of intracellular Ca^{2+} concentration.

(1,3,4,5)IP$_4$ promotes, at least in sea urchin eggs, the entry of Ca^{2+} ions from the external medium into the cells.[8] Moreover, (1,3,4)IP$_3$, although only at higher concentrations than (1,4,5)IP$_3$, stimulates the release of Ca^{2+} from intracellular stores.[9] It has therefore been suggested that this compound, which in most cells accumulates only after a time lag and at a slower rate than (1,4,5)IP$_3$, may keep the Ca^{2+} stores empty and hand over the acute control of Ca^{2+} to the plasma membrane.[9]

The interaction of these various second messengers appears to regulate, via the activation and/or inhibition of various protein kinases (e.g., protein kinase C, calmodulin-protein kinase) and other enzymes (e.g., phospholipase A$_2$), processes responsible for cellular growth and differentiation as well as neuronal (and glial?) activities.

Effects of Lithium Ions on Inositol Lipid Signaling

Lithium ions are now known to inhibit several phosphatases that promote the hydrolysis of various inositolphosphates (Fig. 29.1) (for review see ref. 6). One of these enzymes, IP$_1$ phosphatase, is inhibited at lithium concentrations well within the therapeutically active range.[10] These findings have explained the increase evoked by lithium salts of the level of IP$_1$ and the decrease in the level of inositol in the brain of experimental animals.[1,2]

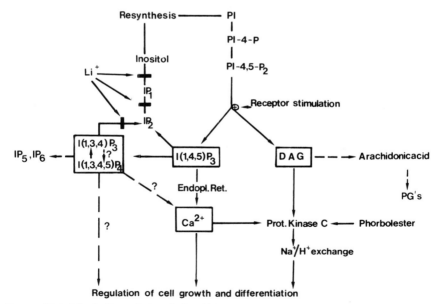

FIGURE 29.1. Metabolism of phosphoinositides: effects of lithium ions. (PI) phosphatidylinositol. (PI, PI-4-P, PI-4,5-P$_2$) phosphoinositides. (IP$_1$, IP$_2$, IP$_3$, IP$_4$) inositolphosphates. (DAG) diacylglycerol. (PG's) prostaglandins.

Lithium ions potentiate in various cells not only the agonist-induced accumulation of IP_1 but also of IP_2 and IP_3. This effect of lithium ions was demonstrated by us in rat pheochromocytoma cells (PC-12 cells).[11,12] Furthermore, we found that Li^+ ions selectively increase the agonist-induced accumulation of only the IP_3 isomer $(1,3,4)IP_3$ but do not alter the increase in $(1,4,5)IP_3$ and $(1,3,4,5)IP_4$.[12] Similar results were reported for pancreatic acinar cells[13] and liver cells.[14]

How might these lithium-induced changes relate to its mechanism of action in the treatment of affective psychoses? Berridge and his colleagues[15] proposed that the lithium-induced decrease in the cellular content of inositol in nerve cells, which do not have access to plasma inositol, might be pronounced enough to attenuate the resynthesis of phosphoinositides. This action would result in a reduced response of the nerve cell to neurotransmitters that use the phosphoinositide pathway for intracellular signaling. This mechanism should be most pronounced for nerve cells that are subject to pathologically intense stimulation. Thus with this theory lithium would selectively attenuate neuronal transmission in pathways that show a pathologically high impulse propagation.

However, supporting evidence for mechanisms such as those outlined above is not yet available. Alternatively, or in addition, the other effects of lithium on the metabolism of phosphoinositides might also be important for their therapeutic effects. The increased and prolonged accumulation of $(1,3,4)IP_3$ in the presence of lithium[12] might profoundly alter the regulation of Ca^{2+} release and sequestration by intracellular stores.[9]

Furthermore, lithium ions, by unknown mechanisms, also greatly increase the cellular content of DAG, the other second messenger formed by the hydrolysis of inositolphospholipids,[16,17] which might profoundly alter the activity of protein kinase C.

This effect might be connected with the finding that the IP_1 accumulation in the brain of lithium-treated animals is predominantly evoked by the hydrolysis of phosphatidylinositol and not by the hydrolysis of phosphatidylinositol-4,5-bisphosphate, the putative primal substrate of phospholipase C after hormonal stimulation.[18] Thus lithium might in some unknown way modify the substrate specificity of phospholipase C, at least in the brain, which would lead to an imbalance of the two limbs of the bifurcating signal pathway, such that activation of protein kinase C is favored.

Connection to Other Hypotheses

Two other theories regarding the mechanism of lithium's therapeutic action have been advocated in the past: inhibition of adenylate cyclase and modulation of receptor sensitivity (for review see ref. 19). The mechanisms outlined above can be expected to profoundly alter the balance between the various second messengers (IP_3, Ca^{2+}, DAG) generated by phosphoinositide breakdown. The protein kinases regulated by these second messengers (e.g., protein kinase C) can regulate both the number of hormone receptors and their coupling to second messenger generating systems, e.g., adenylate cyclase (for review see refs. 20–22).

Thus a complex network of feed-back and feed-forward mechanisms appears to exist that connects the various types of hormone receptor and their particular second messenger generating systems. The various theories of lithium's mechanism of action may therefore not be mutually exclusive. They might, rather, image different aspects of the functioning of a highly cooperative regulatory network, which is set in the presence of lithium to a new working point more compatible with environmental demands.

References

1. Allison JH, Stewart MA. Reduced brain inositol in lithium-treated rats. Nature 1971;233:267–268.
2. Allison JH, Blisner ME, Holland WH, et al. Increased brain myo-inositol 1-phosphate in lithium-treated rats. Biochem Biophys Res Commun 1976;71:664–670.
3. Majerus PW, Conolly TM, Deckmyn H, et al. The metabolism of phosphoinositide-derived messenger molecules. Science 1986;234:1519–1526.
4. Nahorski SR, Kendall DA, Batty I. Receptors and phosphoinositide metabolism in the central nervous system. Biochem Pharmacol 1986;35:2447–2453.
5. Marx JL. Polyphosphoinositide research updated. Science 1987;235:974–976.
6. Drummond AH. Lithium and inositol lipid-linked signalling mechanisms. Trends Pharm Sci 1987;8:129–133.
7. Kaczmarek LK. The role of protein kinase C in the regulation of ion channels and neurotransmitter release. Trends Neurosci 1987;10:30–34.
8. Irvine RF, Moor RM. Micro-injection of inositol 1,3,4,5-tetrakisphosphate activates sea urchin eggs by a mechanism dependent on external Ca^{2+}. Biochem J 1986;240:917–920.
9. Irvine RF, Letcher AJ, Lander DJ, et al. Specificity of inositol phosphate-stimulated Ca^{2+} mobilization from Swiss-mouse 3T3 cells. Biochem J 1986;240:301–304.
10. Hallcher LM, Sherman WR. The effect of lithium ion and other agents on the activity of myo-inositol-1-phosphatase from bovine brain. J Biol Chem 1980;255:10896–10901.
11. Van Calker D, Greil W. Effects of lithium ions on the metabolism of phosphoinositides: studies with rat pheochromocytoma cells (PC-12 cells). Pharmacopsychiatry 1986;19:276–277.
12. Van Calker D, Assmann K, Greil W. Stimulation by bradykinin, angiotensin II and carbachol of the accumulation of inositolphosphates in PC-12 pheochromocytoma cells: differential effects of lithium ions on inositol mono- and polyphosphates. J Neurochem 1987;49:1379–1385.
13. Burgess GM, McKinney JS, Irvine RF, et al. Inositol 1,4,5-triphosphate and inositol 1,3,4-triphosphate formation in Ca^{2+}-mobilizing-hormone-activated cells. Biochem J 1985;232:237–243.
14. Hansen CA, Mah S, Williamson JR. Formation and metabolism of inositol 1,3,4,5-tetrakisphosphate in liver. J Biol Chem 1986;261:8100–8103.
15. Berridge MJ, Downes CP, Hanley MR. Lithium amplifies agonist-dependent phosphatidylinositol responses in brain and salivary glands. Biochem J 1982;206:587–595.
16. Drummond AH, Raeburn CA. The interaction of lithium with thyrotropin-releasing hormone-stimulated lipid metabolism in GH3 pituitary tumor cells. Biochem J 1984;224:129–136.
17. Downes CP, Stone MA. Lithium-induced reduction in intracellular inositol supply in cholinergically stimulated parotid gland. Biochem J 1986;234:199–204.
18. Ackermann KE, Gish BG, Honchar MP, et al. Evidence that inositol 1-phosphate in brain of lithium-treated rats results mainly from phosphatidylinositol metabolism. Biochem J 1987;242:517–524.
19. Van Calker D, Greil W. Biochemische und zellphysiologische Effekte von Lithiumionen. In: Müller-Oerlinghausen B, Greil W (eds): Die Lithiumtherapie. Berlin: Springer Press, 1986;5–34.
20. Kikkawa U, Nishizuka Y. The role of protein kinase C in transmembrane signalling. Annu Rev Cell Biol 1986;2:149–178.
21. Sibley DR, Lefkowitz RJ. Molecular mechanisms of receptor desensitization using the β-adrenergic receptor-coupled adenylate cyclase system as a model. Nature 1985;317:124–129.
22. Enna SJ, Karbon EW. Receptor regulation: evidence for a relationship between phospholipid metabolism and neurotransmitter receptor-mediated cAMP formation in brain. Trends Pharm Sci 1987;8:21–24.

30. Comparison of Theories of Lithium Action Based on Phosphatidylinositol Metabolism with Theories Based on Cyclic AMP

R.H. BELMAKER, J. BENJAMIN, Z. KAPLAN, AND G. ROITMAN

The discovery by Berridge et al.[1] that lithium inhibits myoinositol-1-phosphatase has led to a flood of excellent empirical work. Moreover, lithium is now routinely used as a tool in the study of phosphatidylinositol metabolism, as lithium inhibition of myoinositol-1-phosphatase leads to a buildup of myoinositol-1-phosphate in response to hormone or neurotransmitter-induced breakdown of phosphatidylinositol.[2] This increase in myoinositol-1-phosphate can be used as a measure of phosphatidylinositol breakdown or neurotransmitter stimulation in many systems. Lithium is now a "key word" in many biochemistry articles; however, we argue that it does not mean that the mechanism of lithium action in manic-depressive illness is clearly or most likely related to myoinositol-1-phosphatase inhibition.

Berridge et al.[1] suggested that lithium inhibition of myoinositol-1-phosphatase in vivo leads to depletion of inositol, the product of the enzyme. This inositol is normally recycled into the cell membrane for resynthesis to phosphatidylinositol. Berridge et al.[1] suggested that lithium treatment would lead to a reduction in available phosphatidylinositol and thereby effectively inhibit receptor function. Moreover, and tantalizingly, they suggested that overactive neurotransmitter systems would use up phosphatidylinositol reserves rapidly under conditions of myoinositol-1-phosphatase inhibition; systems under less stimulation might find adequate sources of inositol from breakdown of lipids other than myoinositol. Thus Berridge and co-workers[1] suggested that manic overreactivity might respond to lithium treatment, whereas normal behavior might be little affected.

What problems exist for this attractive theory of lithium action?

1. The most widespread receptor linked to phosphatidylinositol metabolism is the M-1 muscarinic cholinergic receptor, and lithium is not thought to have in vivo anticholinergic side effects. It has been suggested, in reply, that peripherally inositol is so readily available from the bloodstream that myoinositol-1-phosphatase inhibition is not physiologically significant, and thus peripheral anticholinergic side effects are not noted.

2. Whereas lithium clearly inhibits myoinositol-1-phosphatase at therapeutic lithium concentrations of 0.8–1.0 mM, no clear changes in phosphatidylinositol turnover have been demonstrated in rat brain as a result.[3]

3. Chronic lithium for 3 weeks given in vivo to rats leads to a significant increase in myoinositol-1-phosphatase activity, suggesting that this system may compensate for lithium inhibition in a manner that contrasts with lithium's long-term clinical effects.[4]

4. Behavioral correlates of the lithium effect on myoinositol-1-phosphatase are contradictory. Honchar et al.[5] reported a dramatic syndrome of seizures and death in rats pretreated with a single injection of LiCl 3 mEq/kg and then administered pilocarpine 50 mg/kg 24 h later. Honchar et al.[5] suggested that buildup of active second messengers proximal to myoinositol-1-phosphatase inhibition might mediate this effect, which could be blocked by atropine. However, this phenomenon suggests that lithium is *procholinergic*, not anticholinergic as suggested by Berridge et al.[1] Z. Kaplan in our laboratory has shown that pilocarpine–lithium interactional toxicity is limited to rats and *does not occur in mice.* Such species-specific effects are often not generalizable to man. Indeed, several years ago we[6] gave physostigmine 1.25 mg i.v. to five manic-depressive patients with therapeutic serum levels of lithium and five control normals with no lithium treatment. Our hypothesis was that lithium treatment would block the well known physostigmine syndrome of psychomotor retardation and apathy, which lasts less than an hour. We found no such lithium inhibition of physostigmine, but (gratefully, in retrospect) we observed no unusual toxicity (and certainly no seizures or death) in the five long-term lithium patients who received intravenous physostigmine.

In summary, inhibition of myoinositol-1-phosphatase by lithium at therapeutic concentrations is an exciting finding but has yet to be shown to have clear effects on phosphatidylinositol metabolism or specific behaviors.

Inhibition of Noradrenergic Adenylate Cyclase

Another viable theory of lithium action studied by our group is based on the inhibition by lithium of norepinephrine (NE)-sensitive adenylate cyclase at central noradrenergic synapses.[7] Adenylate cyclase inhibition by lithium may also explain certain common side effects of lithium therapy, e.g., nephrogenic diabetes insipidus, which may be related to lithium inhibition of the adenylate cyclase sensitive to antidiuretic hormone (ADH) in the kidney.[8] Other hormone-sensitive adenylate cyclases, such as the glucagon-sensitive adenylate cyclase in humans, are not inhibited by lithium at therapeutic blood levels,[9] suggesting a relative specificity for lithium action on adenylate cyclases.

A drug that shares the adenylate cyclase inhibiting properties of lithium may well be a potential antimanic agent. Demeclocycline (DMC, demethylchlortetracycline) is an effective, widely used tetracycline derivative with an antibiotic spectrum similar to that of the other tetracyclines. DMC, at therapeutic dosages, can cause a dose-related, reversible, nephrogenic diabetes insipidus in normal persons without changes in other tubular or glomerular functions.[10] This diminished concentrating ability of the kidney is thought to be due to interference by DMC with the action of ADH on the distal nephron.[11] Evidence from studies on isolated human renal medulla suggests that DMC interferes with the cellular action of ADH

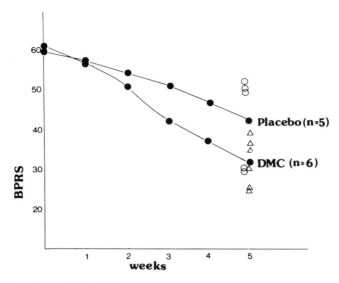

Figure 30.1. Effect of DMC addition to haloperidol in the treatment of excited psychoses. (○) Placebo patients. (△) DMC patients.

by inhibition of ADH-dependent adenylate cyclase.[12] The action of lithium on the kidney is associated with a similar decrease in ADH-dependent cyclic AMP formation in the renal medulla.[13] This effect on renal concentrating ability, common to both lithium and DMC, has prompted the use of both drugs in the treatment of excessive water retention associated with the syndrome of inappropriate ADH secretion.[14] Preliminary studies suggest that DMC may, like lithium, also inhibit the NE-sensitive adenylate cyclase in rat brain.[15] Moreover, DMC, like lithium, has been shown to inhibit the hyperactivity induced in rats by injections of amphetamine, an animal model of mania.[15]

It is suggested that DMC may share lithium's therapeutic efficacy in mania with the effect on NE-sensitive adenylate cyclase at central NE synapses underlying the therapeutic mechanism of both drugs.

To test this concept, we are conducting a double-blind controlled trial of DMC plus haloperidol versus placebo plus haloperidol in excited manic and schizoaffective patients. The design is similar to that of previous controlled studies from our group of lithium plus haloperidol versus placebo plus haloperidol[16] and carbamazepine plus haloperidol versus placebo plus haloperidol.[17] Patients are accepted for our protocol only if their history suggests lack of clinical response to lithium or lack of ability to tolerate its side effects. Patients are treated with haloperidol in doses determined freely by the treating physician. DMC or placebo is added after physical examination and blood chemistry studies are completed. The Brief Psychiatric Rating Scale (BPRS) is rated on entry into the study and once weekly for 5 weeks by an experienced clinician (G.R.) blind to whether the patient is on DMC or placebo. Preliminary results are shown in Figure 30.1. Although results are clearly not yet significant in only 11 patients, DMC shows a marked trend for greater improvement compared with placebo. The trend does not depend on one or two patients, but the six DMC-treated patients appear to do generally better than the five placebo-treated patients. It is noteworthy that the curve of DMC-treated patients diverges from that of placebo-treated patients after 3 weeks of treatment and not before, similar to what has been reported in previous studies of the addition of lithium[16] or carbamazepine[17] to haloperidol in excited schizoaffective disorder.

If these results are confirmed as we enlarge our sample size, DMC could be shown to have "lithium-like" properties in mania. Prediction of psychoactive effects from the biochemical effect on noradrenergic adenylate cyclase could provide strong evidence for the effect on adenylate cyclase as the mode of lithium action.

Acknowledgment. This study was supported by a grant from Mr. Harry Stern of Melrose Park, Pennsylvania.

References

1. Berridge Mj, Downes CP, Hanley MR. Lithium amplifies agonist-dependent phosphatidylinositol responses in brain and salivary glands. Biochem J 1982;206:587–595.
2. Hokin LE. Receptors and phosphoinositide generated second messengers. Annu Rev Biochem 1985;54:205–235.
3. Sherman WR, Munsell LY, Gish BG, et al. Effects of systemically administered lithium on phosphoinositide metabolism in rat brain, kidney and testis. J Neurochem 1985;44:798–807.
4. Renshaw PF, Joseph NE, Leigh JS Jr. Chronic dietary lithium induces increased levels of myoinositol-1-phosphatase activity in rat cerebral cortex homogenates. Brain Res 1986;380:401–404.
5. Honchar MP, Olney JW, Sherman WR. Systemic cholinergic agents induce seizures and brain damage in lithium-treated rats. Science 1983;220:323–325.
6. Oppenheim G, Ebstein RP, Belmaker RH. The effect of lithium on physostigmine-induced behavioral syndrome and plasma cyclic GMP. J Psychiatr Res 1979;15:133–139.
7. Belmaker RH. Receptors, adenylate cyclase, depression and lithium. Biol Psychiatry 1981;16:333–350.
8. Geisler A, Wraae O, Olesen OV. Adenyl cyclase activity in kidneys of rats with lithium-induced polyuria. Acta Pharmacol Toxicol (Copenh) 1972;31–203.
9. Ebstein RP, Kara T, Belmaker RH. The effects of lithium on the glucagon-sensitive adenylate cyclase in vivo in man. Acta Pharmacol Toxicol (Copenh) 1977;41:80.
10. Singer I, Rotenberg D. Demeclocycline-induced nephrogenic diabetes insipidus in vivo and in vitro studies. Ann Interm Med 1973;79:679–683.
11. Orloff J, Handler JS. The role of adenosine 3',5'-phosphate in the action of antidiuretic hormone. Am J Med 1967;42:757–768.
12. Dousa TP, Wilson DM. Effects of demethylchlortetracycline on cellular action of antidiuretic hormone in vitro. Kidney Int 1974;5:279–284.
13. Dousa T, Hechter O. The effect of NaCl and LiCl on vasopressin-sensitive adenyl cyclase. Life Sci 1970;9:765–770.
14. Forrest JN Jr, Cox M, Hong C, et al. Superiority of demeclocycline over lithium in the treatment of chronic syndrome of inappropriate secretion of antidiuretic hormone. N Engl J Med 1978;298:173–177.
15. Belmaker RH. Adenylate cyclase and the search for new compounds with the clinical profile of lithium. Pharmacopsychiatry 1984;17:9–15.
16. Biederman J, Lerner Y, Belmaker RH. Combination of lithium carbonate and haloperidol in schizoaffective disorder: a controlled study. Arch Gen Psychiatry 1979;36:327–333.
17. Klein E, Bental E, Lerer B, et al. Carbamazepine and haloperidol versus placebo and haloperidol in excited psychoses: a controlled study. Arch Gen Psychiatry 1984;41:165–170.

31. Serotonin and Catecholamines in Lithium Treatment

PAUL J. GOODNICK

The mechanism of lithium's action in treating and preventing relapse of bipolar affective disorder is not yet fully determined. There have been numerous laboratory projects that have shed light on the basic science background of lithium action that have been reviewed elsewhere.[1] However, the completion of controlled biological studies in human subjects is essential to understanding the basis of lithium action. This section highlights such studies' results concerning serotonin and catecholamines. The review separates results by duration of lithium treatment: short term and long term.

Serotonin (5-hydroxytryptamine, 5-HT) depletion has been hypothesized to be a cause of vulnerability to the onset of manic-depressive disorder.[2] Linnoila et al.[3] found that short-term lithium administration reduced urinary turnover of 5-HT and 5-hydroxyindoleacetic acid (5-HIAA), the primary metabolite of 5-HT, in depressed patients[3]; it was not true in controls.[4] There have been no studies of effects of long-term lithium treatment on urinary 5-HT.

In contrast, there have been numerous reports focusing on lithium's effect on blood 5-HT parameters. Two reports have found that platelet 5-HT uptake is reduced during initial lithium therapy of mania and depression.[5,6] Wood et al.[7] showed that long-term lithium prophylaxis gradually shifts platelet uptake toward normal control levels.[7] Several studies[5,8,9] have shown that long-term lithium prophylaxis (6 months or more) induces an increase in platelet 5-HT uptake. Short-term lithium administration has been reported to lead to increases in platelet 5-HT content,[10] but other evidence is consistent with long-term induction of reductions in platelet 5-HT content.[11]

Neuroendocrine studies have also indicated a possible dichotomy of short-term versus long-term lithium influences on 5-HT. The 5-hydroxytryptophan (5-HTP)-stimulated increase in blood cortisol may be increased during both mania and depression; Meltzer et al.[12] proposed that this finding may indicate a state of postsynaptic supersensitivity. Acute lithium treatment of mania appears to further accentuate this response,[13] but other evidence is consistent with reductions in this response toward control levels following long-term prophylaxis.[14,15] Another study found a significant effect of long-term lithium therapy on the cortisol response to fenfluramine, a 5-HT agonist.[16]

The proposed contrast of effects of short-term and long-term lithium administration on 5-HT falters in application to measurement of cerebrospinal fluid (CSF) 5-HIAA. Study results of protocols on acute[17] and prophylactic[18] administration agree on lithium-induced increases in CSF 5-HIAA.

Further work appears needed to clarify if lithium can acutely reverse mood change by increasing the efficiency of synaptic 5-HT. This change might occur by the combination of a reduction in 5-HT uptake with an increase in postsynaptic sensitivity. When given prophylactically, lithium might act to specifically reverse the 5-HT abnormality. The above results are summarized in Table 31.1; further details of individual studies may be found elsewhere.[19]

There are numerous studies linking abnormalities in norepinephrine (NE) and dopamine (DA) to mania and depression. Yet there are far fewer studies on lithium's effect on catecholamines in human subjects. Linnoila et al.[20] found that acute lithium administration reduces urinary output of homovanillic acid (HVA), the primary metabolite of DA, and reduces whole body urinary DA turnover in depressed patients; this result was not found in normal controls.[4] There have not been any studies of effects of long-term lithium on urinary DA. There have been a multitude of studies of effects of acute lithium treatment on urinary NE and its primary metabolite methylhydroxyphenylglycol (MHPG). Older studies[21–23] appear to show that when lithium treatment is successful it decreases urinary MHPG in mania and increases urinary MHPG in depression. In contrast, another report found lithium-induced reductions in urinary NE turnover in depression.[24] No effect on urinary MHPG was found following lithium administration to normal controls.[4] In the only study of long-term lithium, Schildkraut[23] indicated its lack of influence on urinary MHPG.

Acute lithium therapy may decrease some measures of α_2 functions[25,26] but has no effect on lymphocyte β-receptors.[27] Study results conflict regarding the influence of long-term lithium prophylaxis on α_2 receptors: Whereas one study reported reductions,[26] the other reported a lack of effect on net receptor density.[7] Short-term lithium may lead to increases in CSF HVA[17]; discontinuation of long-term prophylaxis has not been followed by significant changes in concentrations of CSF HVA or MHPG.[18] Short-term lithium therapy may reduce the apomorphine-induced fall in blood prolactin, a DA parameter,[28] as well as the methylphenidate-induced rise in blood growth hormone,[29] an NE parameter. Discontinuation of lithium prophylaxis has led to some increases in the degree of hypotension but has had no effect on net increase in blood growth hormone following clonidine, an α_2 agonist.[15,30] These results are shown in Table 31.2.

TABLE 31.1. Lithium effects on serotonin.

Parameter	Short term	Long term
Urine 5HT	Decreased[3]	Unknown
Blood platelet 5-HT		
Content	Increased[10]	Decreased[11]
Uptake	Decreased[5,6]	Increased[5,8,9,11]
CSF 5-HIAA	Increased[17]	Increased[18]
Neuroendocrine sites		
5-HTP-induced cortisol response	Increased[13]	Decreased[14,15]
Fenfluramine-induced cortisol response	Unknown	Increased[16]

TABLE 31.2. Lithium effects on catecholamines.

Parameter	Short term	Long term
Urine		
HVA	Decreased[20]	Unknown
MHPG	Mood-determined[21–24]	None[23]
Blood		
α_2 Receptors	Decreased[25,26]	Possibly decreased[7,26]
β Receptors	None[27]	Unknown
CSF		
HVA	Possibly increased[17]	None[18]
MHPG	Unknown	None[18]
Neuroendocrine sites		
Ampomorphine-induced prolactin response	Slight Decrease[28]	Unknown
Methylphenidate-induced growth hormone response	Decrease[29]	Unknown
Clonidine-induced hypotension and growth hormone response	Unknown	Hypotension: possibly decreased[15,30] Growth hormone response: none[15]

Thus acute lithium treatment may exert some influence on measures of NE and DA, but there is little documented effect of long-term lithium prophylaxis. In summary, acute lithium effects on mood disorders may be exerted through a combination of effects on NE, DA, and 5-HT, among major neurochemicals. However, chronic lithium therapy may exert a prophylactic effect predominantly via 5-HT pathways.

References

1. Goodnick PJ, Gershon S. Lithium. In Lajtha A (ed): Handbook of Neurochemistry. Vol. 9. New York: Plenum Press, 1985;103–149.
2. Prange AJ Jr, Sisk JL, Wilson IC, et al. Balance, permission, and discrimination among amines: a theoretical consideration of the actions of 1-tryptophan in disorders of movements and affects. In Barchas J, Usdin E (eds): Serotonin in Affective Disorders. New York: Academic Press, 1973;539–548.
3. Linnoila M, Miller TL, Bartko J, et al. Five antidepressant treatments in depressed patients. Arch Gen Psychiatry 1984;41:688–692.
4. Rudorfer MV, Karoum F, Ross RJ, et al. Differences in lithium effects in depressed and healthy subjects. Clin Pharmacol Ther 1985;37:66–71.
5. Meltzer HY, Arora RC, Goodnick PJ. Effect of lithium carbonate on serotonin uptake in blood platelets of patients with affective disorders. J Affective Disord 1983;5:215–221.
6. Rausch JL, Janowsky DS, Huey LY. Treatment effect of lithium carbonate on platelet serotonin uptake. Abstracts of Panels & Posters, A.C.N.P. Annual Meeting, 1984;123.
7. Wood K, Swade C, Abou-Saleh M, et al. Drug plasma levels and platelet 5HT uptake inhibition during long-term treatment with fluvoxamine or lithium in patients with affective disorder. Br J Clin Pharmacol 1983;15:365S–368S.
8. Born GVR, Grignani G, Martin K. Long-term effect of lithium on the uptake of 5-hydroxytryptamine by human platelets. Br J Clin Pharmacol 1980;9:321–325.
9. Coppen A, Swade C, Wood K. Lithium restores abnormal 5HT transport in patients with affective disorders. Br J Psychiatry 1980;136:235–238.
10. Corona GL, Cucchi ML, Santagostino G, et al. Blood noradrenaline and 5HT levels in depressed women during amitriptyline or lithium treatment. Psychopharmacology 1982;77:236–241.

11. Goodnick PJ, Arora RC, Jackman H, et al. Neurochemical changes during discontinuation of lithium prophylaxis. II. Alterations in platelet serotonin function. Biol Psychiatry 1984;19:891–898.
12. Meltzer HY, Umberkoman-Witta B, Robertson A, et al. Effect of 5-hydroxytryptophan on serum cortisol levels in major affective disorders. I. Enhanced response in depression and mania. Arch Gen Psychiatry 1984;41:366–374.
13. Meltzer HY, Lowy M, Robertson A, Goodnick PJ, et al. Effect of 5-hydroxytryptophan on serum cortisol levels in major affective disorders. III. Effect of antidepressants and lithium carbonate. Arch Gen Psychiatry 1984;41:391–397.
14. Goodnick PJ. Effect of long term lithium on the 5HTP-induced cortisol response in bipolar patients. Abstracts of the 40th Society of Biological Psychiatry Annual Meeting, Dallas, 1985;135.
15. Goodnick PJ, Fieve RR, Schlegel A. Clinical, biochemical, and neuroendocrine effects of lithium discontinuation. Psychopharmacol Bull 1987;23:510–513.
16. Muhlbauer HD, Muller-Oerlinghausen B. Fenfluramine stimulation of serum cortisol in patients with major affective disorders and healthy controls: further evidence for a central serotonergic action of lithium in man. J Neural Transm 1985;61:81–94.
17. Bowers MB Jr, Heninger GR. Lithium: clinical effects and cerebrospinal fluid acid monoamine metabolites. Commun Psychopharmacol 1977;1:135–145.
18. Berrettini WH, Nurnberger JI Jr, Scheinin M, et al. Cerebrospinal fluid amines and their metabolites in euthymic bipolar patients. Biol Psychiatry 1985;20:257–269.
19. Goodnick PJ. Serotonergic mechanisms of lithium action. Mt Sinai J Med (NY) 1987;54:182–187.
20. Linnoila M, Karoum F, Potter WZ. Effects of antidepressant treatments on dopamine turnover in depressed patients. Arch Gen Psychiatry 1983;40:1015–1017.
21. Greenspan K, Schildkraut JJ, Gordon EK, et al. Catecholamine metabolism in affective disorders. III. MHPG and other catecholamine metabolites in patients treated with lithium carbonate. J Psychiatr Res 1970;7:171–183.
22. Beckmann H, St-Laurent J, Goodwin FK. The effect of lithium on urinary MHPG in unipolar and bipolar depressed patients. Psychopharmacology (Berlin) 1975;42:277–282.
23. Schildkraut JJ. Pharmacology—the effects of lithium on biogenic amines. In Gershon S, Shopsin B (eds): Lithium: Its Role in Psychiatric Research and Treatment. New York: Plenum Press, 1973;51–73.
24. Linnoila M, Karoum F, Rosenthal N, et al. Electroconvulsive treatment and lithium carbonate. Arch Gen Psychiatry 1983;40:677–680.
25. Hollingsworth PJ, Smith CB, Cameron OC, et al. Platelet alpha$_2$ adrenergic receptors in psychiatric and nonpsychiatric patients before and after treatment. Abstracts of Panels & Posters, A.C.N.P. Annual Meeting, 1983;101.
26. Garcia-Sevilla JA, Guimon J, Garcia-Vallejo P, et al. Biochemical and functional evidence of supersensitive platelet α_2-adrenoceptors in major affective disorder. Arch Gen Psychiatry 1986;43:51–57.
27. Extein I, Tallman J, Smith CC, et al. Changes in lymphocyte beta-adrenergic receptors in depression and mania. Psychiatry Res 1979;1:191–197.
28. Goodnick PJ, Meltzer HY. Effect of subchronic lithium treatment on apomorphine-induced change in prolactin and growth hormone secretion. J Clin Psychopharmacol 1983;3:239–243.
29. Huey LY, Janowsky DS, Judd LL, et al. Effects of lithium carbonate on methylphenidate-induced mood, behavior, and cognitive processes. Psychopharmacology 1981;73:161–164.
30. Goodnick PJ, Meltzer HY. Neurochemical changes during discontinuation of lithium prophylaxis. I. Increases in clonidine-induced hypotension. Biol Psychiatry 1984;19:883–889.

32. Lithium and Calcium Antagonists: Do They Act on One Neuronal Function?

J.B. ALDENHOFF

Slowing of cellular calcium (Ca) regulation is one action of lithium[1] with particular relevance for neuronal function. During excitation the intracellular Ca concentration (Ca_i) increases; after which it decreases to the resting level.[2] Lithium slows this reequilibration of Ca_i, as observed in snail neurons.[1] Thus under maintained Ca influx, a higher equilibrium of Ca_i could be established due to lithium.[1] This action may correspond to the lithium effects on inositoltriphosphate[3] and could explain several side effects of clinical lithium therapy.[4] However, consideration of the involvement of this mechanism in the therapeutic actions of lithium requires more detailed knowledge on the possible role of Ca in normal and disturbed nervous function.

In neurons, Ca-dependent processes represent an intrinsic, nonsynaptic feedback system that provides the competence for adaptation to different functional tasks. Ca ions pass the membrane through more or less specific channels regulated by changes of membrane potential or transmitter binding.[5] This Ca influx lasts until Ca_i reaches a critical level in the submembranal compartment; then a potassium current is activated that repolarizes the membrane.[2] This Ca-dependent potassium current represents a strong inhibitory mechanism of the single neuron itself without synaptic input. Its attractiveness for psychiatry lies in its sensitivity to modulatory influences: many amines, peptides, or drugs with relevance for theories on the origin of psychic disorders (e.g., norepinephrine,[6] dopamine,[7] corticotropin-releasing factor (CRF),[8] caffeine,[9] neuroleptics[10]) modify (i.e., increase or decrease) this potassium current. When it is decreased, the capacity for negative feedback after excitation becomes impaired and the neuron switches to a state of higher activation, coincidentally with increased Ca influx. Such an overdrive in Ca currents and discharge activity could be a functional prerequisite for states of pathological activity, possibly underlying neuropsychiatric symptoms such as epilepsy, mania, or depression.

When lithium interacts with this system in the above-described way, the following effects may occur. Slowing of the Ca regulation with a concomitant increase in Ca_i supposedly enhances the inhibitory potassium current, thereby increasing the capacity for negative feedback. The neuron might then be less susceptible to excitatory influences. In rats a reduction of neuronal discharge activity based on putative Ca conductance has been reported due to lithium.[11]

A less complicated pharmacological access to the same system might be provided by the Ca antagonists. Their interaction with Ca channels is well established.[12] However, differently than in smooth or heart muscle, the findings on functional relevance of Ca antagonistic effects on the various types of neuronal Ca channel are still equivocal. Whereas it is unclear if Ca antagonists act on normal neuronal function at all, overactivity has been shown to be regulated down by Ca antagonists. This reaction has been observed in hippocampal neurons excited by the action of CRF[13] as well as in experimental epilepsy.[14] In both models the reduction of potassium currents plays the central role in the generation of overactivity. Supposedly, Ca antagonists reduce overactivity by regulating back the overdrive of Ca influx.

Pharmacologically induced behavioral overactivity is modulated by Ca antagonists in a way that supports the principle discussed above.[15,16] From open studies in clinical psychiatry, Ca antagonists have been claimed to be effective on the manic syndrome.[17,18] In a double-blind study on patients with mania, gallopamil has been shown to reduce mainly the excitability of these patients.[19] Normal volunteers, however, did not report any marked effects on mood or on motor abilities.[19] Thus in their clinical actions, a similarity between lithium and Ca antagonists is obvious.

Considering the basic actions of both substances, the following hypothetical model is proposed: Lithium enhances a basic negative feedback system that acts functionally as a "physiological Ca antagonist." It may stabilize the system internally against disturbing influences. Its sensitivity for dysequilibration by many neuromodulators represents an important physiological basis for overactivity: Instead of feed-back regulation, feed-forward phenomena might be generated by Ca overdrive. Increased Ca currents could be promoted by a reduction of hyperpolarizing potassium currents[6,8,9] or even by activation of new or as yet inactive Ca channels.[20] In such a state of overactivity, neuronal function becomes sensitive to the pharmacological modification by Ca antagonists.

Preclinical as well as clinical evidence for this theory is still weak and needs further confirmation. Indeed, this model exceeds the methodological limitations of various attempts, biochemical or electrophysiological. Furthermore, it supports the idea that modification of the action of one substance by another substance must not happen exclusively at the same receptor but might occur by interactions on the common pathway of both substances from neuron to behavior.

References

1. Aldenhofff JB, Lux HD. Lithium slows neuronal calcium regulation in the snail Helix pomatia. Neurosci Lett 1985;54:103–108.
2. Gorman ALF, Hermann A, Thomas MV. Ionic requirements for membrane oscillations and their dependence on the calcium concentration in a mollusacan pace-maker neuron. J Physiol (Lond) 1982;327:185–217.
3. Berridge MJ. Inositol trisphosphate and diacylglycerol as second messengers. Biophys J 1984;222:345–360.
4. Aldenhoff JB, Lux HD. Lithium und kalziumabhängige Zellfunktionen: der Beitrag eines membranphysiologischen Untersuchungsansatzes zur Erklärung therapeutischer Lithium Wirkungen. Fortschr Neurol 1984;52:152–163.
5. Miller R. Multiple calcium channels and neuronal function. Science 1987;235:46–52.
6. Haas L, Konnerth A. Histamine and noradrenaline decrease calcium-activated potassium conductance in hippocampal pyramidal cells. Nature 1983;302:432–434.
7. Benardo LS, Prince DA. Dopamine action on hippocampal pyramidal cells. J Neurosci 1982;2:415–423.

8. Aldenhoff JB, Gruol DL, Rivier J, et al. CRF decreases post burst hyperpolarizations and excited hippocampal pyramidal neurons. Science 1983;221:875–877.
9. Greene RW, Haas ML. Adenosine actions on CA1 pyramidal neurons in rat hippocampal slices. J Physiol (Lond) 1985;366:119–127.
10. Dinan TG, Crunelli V, Kelly JS. Neuroleptic decrease calcium-activated potassium conductance in hippocampal pyramidal cells. Brain Res 1987;407:159–162.
11. Bloom FE, Henriksen SJ, Newlin SA, et al. Neuronal discharge patterns: index of chronic lithium treatments. In Olsen RW, Yamamura HI (eds): Psychopharmacology and Biochemistry of Neurotransmitter Receptors. New York: Elsevier/North Holland, 1980;203–220.
12. Nowycky MC, Fox AP, Tsien RW. Three types of neuronal calcium channel with different calcium agonist sensitivity. Nature 1985;316:440–443.
13. Aldenhoff JB. Does CRF act via a calcium-dependent mechanism? Psychoneuroendocrinology 1986;11:231–236.
14. Walden J, Speckmann EJ, Witte OW. Suppression of focal epileptiform discharges by intraventricular perfusion of a calcium antagonist. Electroencephalography Clin Neurophysiol 1985;61:299–309.
15. Grebb J, Ellsworth K, Freed W. Calcium channel inhibitors differentially affect phencyclidine- and amphetamine-induced behavioral stimulation in mice. Abstr Soc Neurosci 1984;10:1095.
16. Swerdlow NR, Koob GF, Aldenhoff JB. The effects of verapamil on the locomotor-activating properties of CRF in the rat. Psychoneuroendocrinology 1986;11:237–240.
17. Dose M, Emrich HM, Cording-Tömmel C, Zerssen Dv. Use of calcium antagonists in mania. Psychoneuroendocrinology 1986;11:241–243.
18. Dubovsky SL, Franks RD, Lifschitz M, et al. Effectiveness of verapamil in the treatment of a manic patient. Am J Psychiatry 1982;139:502–504.
19. Aldenhoff JB, Schlegel S, Heuser I, et al. Antimanic effects of the calcium anntagonist D 600: a double-blind placebo-controlled study. Clin Neuropharmacol 1986;9(suppl 4):553–555.
20. Dolin S, Little H, Hudspith M, et al. Increased dihydropyridine-sensitive calcium channels in rat brain may underlie ethanol physical dependence. Neuropharmacology 1987;26:275–279.

33. Red Blood Cell Lithium Transport in Affective Illness: A Possible Mechanism of Action of Lithium

GHANSHYAM N. PANDEY AND JOHN M. DAVIS

Lithium (Li) is a monovalent cation that has been shown to be effective in the treatment of bipolar illness. It has been observed in patients that during Li treatment, Li distributes unevenly between red blood cells and plasma, such that red blood cell concentrations of Li are significantly lower than those of plasma. This distribution of Li, which appears to be similar to the sodium (Na) distribution, suggests active transport or extrusion of Li from the red blood cells. Wide variations in the Li distribution ratio between red blood cells and plasma (commonly referred to as the Li ratio) have been observed in patients during Li treatment. The Li ratio has been related to diagnosis and to long- and short-term treatment response, as well as to the side effects of Li therapy. An important observation that may be related to the mode of action of Li is that patients who respond to Li therapy have a significantly higher Li ratio than patients who do not respond.[1] In our study of schizoaffective patients we observed that those patients who responded to Li treatment had a significantly higher Li ratio than those patients who did not respond.[2] These observations suggested a relation between the transport of Li across the red blood cell membrane and its mode of action. In order to examine the mode of action of Li in relation to its transport across the red cell membrane, we studied the mechanism of Li transport in human red blood cells.

Pathways of Lithium Transport in Human Red Blood Cells

As a result of studies conducted by us and other groups of investigators,[3,4] at least four distinct pathways of Li transport in human red blood cells have been identified and characterized (Fig. 33.1): (a) ouabain-sensitive Li transport pathway; (b) Na-dependent, ouabain-insensitive, Li–Na countertransport (LSC) pathway; (c) anion-exchange pathway; and (d) passive leak diffusion pathway. Ouabain-sensitive Li transport in human red blood cells appears to be mediated by the Na-K pump. Li can be transported in either direction under certain given conditions mediated by this pathway. Both Na and K competitively inhibit Li transport mediated by this pathway. Li transport mediated by the LSC system is insensitive to ouabain and can drive Li against its electrochemical gradient by an oppositely directed

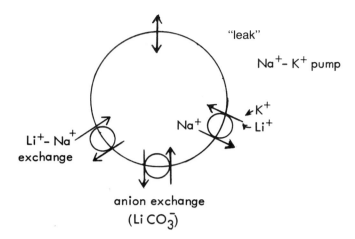

FIGURE 33.1. Pathways of lithium transport in human red blood cells.
[Reproduced from *The Journal of General Physiology* 1987; 72:233–247, by copyright permission of the Rockefeller University Press.]

electrochemical gradient. The transport of Li mediated by this pathway can be inhibited by phloretin, quinine, and quinidine. It does not require ATP and is stimulated by the presence of Na on the opposite side of the membrane. However, no other cation tested was found to promote Li movement by this pathway. Li can be transported in either direction through this pathway. It has been suggested that the phloretin-sensitive LSC system is mediated by a carrier molecule through a tightly coupled Li-Na exchange mechanism. The presence of bicarbonate in the medium results in another pathway by which Li is transported across the red blood cell membrane as a result of anion pairing with bicarbonate ions. However, this pathway cannot move Li against its gradient.

In theory, all of the above pathways described for Li transport allow Li movement in both directions across the red blood cell membrane. However, because of the presence of high concentrations of both Na and K in plasma and red blood cells, the transport of Li mediated by the Na-K pump in either direction is negligible. Therefore under in vivo conditions Li is transported into red blood cells by passive leak diffusion and the anion exchange system, whereas Li is extruded out of red blood cells primarily by the LSC system. The steady-state Li distribution between red blood cells and plasma is thus determined by a balance between the relative rates of the uphill Li influx mediated by the LSC system and the downhill Li influx mediated by the passive leak diffusion and anion-exchange mechanism.

Lithium Transport In Vitro and Lithium Ratio In Vivo

In order to examine which moities of Li transport are responsible for the observed interindividual variations in the Li ratio in vivo, we determined Li transport mediated by the various pathways in patients before the start of Li therapy and the Li ratio in vivo during the course of Li treatment.[5]

We observed a significant negative correlation between the Li ratio in vivo and Na-dependent and phloretin-sensitive Li efflux as well as a significant positive correlation between the Li ratio in vivo and in vitro. We did not find any significant correlation between the Li ratio in vivo and the ouabain-sensitive Li influx or Li efflux mediated by passive leak diffusion. These results indicated that the interindividual variations in the Li ratio under in vivo conditions observed in patients during Li treatment are caused by interindividual differences in the Li transport mediated by the LSC system.

Lithium Transport in Bipolar Illness

We studied Li transport in bipolar patients admitted to our research ward at the Illinois State Psychiatric Institute and normal control volunteers with no history of a psychiatric disorder.[5] The various Li transport measurements were (a) total downhill and Na-dependent Li efflux, (b) net uphill Li efflux, (c) Li efflux in Na-free media, and (d) Li ratio in vitro. In an earlier study we also measured ouabain-sensitive Li influx.[6] The results of our studies are shown in Table 33.1. We observed that the uphill Li efflux (Li-Na counterflow) in bipolar patients was significantly lower than that in normal controls. We also observed that total downhill Li efflux and the mean Na-dependent efflux in bipolar patients were substantially lower than the means of normal controls, although the variances did not differ. There was no significant difference between the passive leak diffusion between bipolar patients and normal controls. We also observed that the net in vitro Li ratio in bipolar patients was significantly higher than that in normal controls. These determinations of Li transport, with the exception of passive leak diffusion, are either direct or indirect measures of the LSC system. Bipolar patients were significantly different from normal controls on all measures of Li-Na exchange except for the Na-stimulated Li efflux, suggesting that bipolar patients have a deficiency in Li transport mediated by Li-Na exchange. Our results also indicate that there is not a 1:1 relation between bipolar illness and abnormalities of Li transport. That is, not all bipolar patients have high Li ratios or abnormal LSC. It appears that only a subgroup of bipolar patients shows a defect in the LSC system.

Effect of Lithium Treatment on Lithium Transport in Human Red Blood Cells

We also studied Li transport in patients during the course of Li therapy and observed that the Li transport mediated by the LSC mechanism was significantly decreased during Li treatment.[6] We also observed that the Li ratio determined in

TABLE 33.1. Lithium transport measurements in RBCs: bipolar patients and normal controls.

| Subjects | Li^+ ratio | | Uphill Li efflux (mEq/l RBCs $\times$ 4 h) | | Downhill Li^+ Efflux (mEq/l RBCs $\times$ 1h) | |
	In vivo	In vitro	Li^+-Na^+ counterflow	Total	Passive leak diffusion	Na^+ dependents
Bipolar patients	0.55 ± 0.19 ($n = 21$)	0.29 ± 0.13 ($n = 22$)	0.40 ± 0.16 ($n = 22$)	0.20 ± 0.04 ($n = 21$)	0.06 ± 0.02 ($n = 15$)	0.13 ± 0.05 ($n = 15$)
Normal controls	—	0.23 ± 0.07 ($n = 88$)	0.46 ± 0.09 ($n = 42$)	0.23 ± 0.03 ($n = 15$)	0.07 ± 0.02 ($n = 15$)	0.16 ± 0.03 ($n = 15$)
Values	—	< 0.01	0.05	<0.02	NS	$= 0.06$

Results are the mean $\pm$ SD.

[Reprinted from ref. 5, with permission. Copyright 1979, American Medical Association.]

vitro during Li treatment[7] in 18 patients (0.40 ± 0.03) was significantly higher than the Li ratio determined during baseline pretreatment (0.29 ± 0.02). Several other investigators have also reported that Li treatment causes significant inhibition of LSC during the early phases of Li treatment. It is not clear at this time if the inhibition of LSC as a result of Li treatment is related to the subsequent response to Li treatment.

Genetic Aspects of Lithium Transport

Using the twin study method, we found evidence of genetic control of the Li ratio under both in vitro and in vivo conditions.[5] Because the twin study method provides limited information on the degree of genetic control of a quantitative trait, we investigated the Li ratio in vitro in adult members of families in which there was no history of major psychosis.[5] The parent–offspring and sibling–sibling correlations suggested that genetic factors account for a substantial portion of the variance in the Li ratio. We also studied the Li ratio in families of bipolar patients and observed that in family members of bipolar patients who had a history of affective illness the Li ratio was significantly higher than in those relatives who did not have such a history.[8] Segregation analysis indicated polymorphism at an autosomal gene locus.[9] These results suggested an association between bipolar illness and the Li ratio.

Lithium Transport and the Mode of Action of Lithium

There are two related questions: (a) What is the relation between abnormal red blood cell Li transport and bipolar illness? and (b) How is Li transport related to the mode of action of Li?[7] We and several other groups of investigators have observed a decreased LSC in bipolar illness. We have also shown that first-degree relatives of bipolar patients who have a history of affective disorders are more likely to have a defect in the LSC system than first-degree relatives who do not have such a history. It is unlikely that a defective LSC system in red blood cells is a causative factor for bipolar illness. However, it is possible that a defect in the LSC system in red blood cells may be related to a similar defect in the central nervous system (CNS). The presence of an LSC system has been reported in the cells of the CNS.[10] It is likely that the LSC system in the CNS may be slightly different from that in red blood cells, such that it may be involved in the transport of other physiologically active cations such as calcium or positively charged neurotransmitters. If it is true, a defective LSC system may alter the distribution and hence the effect of physiologically active cations that may be related to the bipolar illness.

The second question concerns the relation between the LSC system and the mode of action of Li. Two important observations suggest that a relation may exist. Some investigators reported that patients who respond to Li therapy have a higher Li ratio in vivo than those who do not respond. Also, the observation that treatment with Li causes inhibition of the LSC system in human red blood cells suggests a relation between altered Li transport and response to Li therapy. If such a relation does exist, it is possible that Li might produce its therapeutic effect by altering the transport of physiologically active cations such as a calcium and other positively charged neurotransmitters in the brain. Alternatively, Li may compete with neurotransmitters for their receptors or for activation of adenylate cyclase and thus alter the effects of neurotransmitters.

References

1. Mendels J, Frazer A: Intracellular Li concentration and clinical response: towards a membrane theory of depression. J Psychiatr Res 1973;10:9–18.
2. Casper RC, Pandey G, Gosenfeld L, et al: Intracellular Li and clinical response. Lancet 1976;2:418.
3. Pandey GN, Sarkadi B, Haas M, et al: Lithium transport pathways in human red blood cells. J Gen Physiol 1987;72:233–247.
4. Duhm J: Lithium transport pathways in erythrocytes. In Emrich HM, Aldenhoff JB, Lux HD (eds): Basic Mechanism in the Action of Lithium. Amsterdam: Excerpt Medica, 1982;1–20.
5. Pandey GN, Dorus E, Davis JM, et al: Lithium transport in human red blood cells: genetic and clinical aspects. Arch Gen Psychiatry 1979;36:902–908.
6. Ostrow DG, Pandey GN, Davis JM, et al: A heritable disorder of Li transport in erythrocytes of a subpopulation of manic depressive patients. Am J Psychiatry 1978;135:1070–1078.
7. Pandey GN, Baker J, Chang S, et al: Prediction of red cell-plasma Li$^+$ ratio in vivo by in vitro methods. Clin Pharmacol Ther 1978;24:343–347.
8. Dorus E, Pandey GN, Shaughnessy R, et al: Lithium transport across red cell membrane: a cell membrane abnormality in manic depressive illness. Science 1979;205:932–934.
9. Dorus E, Cox NJ, Gibbons RD, et al: Lithium ion transport and affective disorders within families of bipolar patients: identification of a major gene locus. Arch Gen Psychiatry 1983;40:532–545.
10. Reiser G, Duhm J: Transport pathways for Li ions in neuroblastoma glioma by hybrid cells at therapeutic concentrations of Li. Brain Res 1982;252:247–258.

I.F. MONOAMINE OXIDASE INHIBITORS

34. Selective Localization and Selective Inhibition of Monoamine Oxidase in Human Brain

ANNE-MARIE O'CARROLL, JAMES P. SULLIVAN, CHRISTOPHER J. FOWLER, AND KEITH F. TIPTON

The enzyme monoamine oxidase (EC 1.4.3.4; MAO) exists in two forms, the A and B forms, which differ in their inhibitor sensitivities and substrate specificities (see refs. 1,2 for reviews). The A form of the enzyme (MAO-A) is sensitive to inhibition by low concentrations of clorgyline, whereas the B form (MAO-B) is inhibited by low concentrations of ($-$)-deprenyl (selegiline). Inhibitors selective toward the A form of the enzyme have been shown to be effective antidepressants, whereas those that are selective toward the B form are not generally effective, although it has been suggested that they may be of value in the treatment of some forms of the disease.[3] MAO-B inhibitors have also been shown to be useful as adjuncts in the treatment of Parkinson's disease.[4]

The two forms of MAO are rather similarly distributed in human brain. Studies on their specificities in this tissue have indicated epinephrine, norepinephrine, and dopamine to be substrates for both forms of the enzyme.[5,6] The Km values and maximum velocities of each of these substrates are similar with each enzyme form. As has been found in other tissues,[1,2] 5-hydroxytryptamine (5-HT) and, at low concentrations, 2-phenethylamine are specific substrates for the A and B forms, respectively.

Studies on the activities of the two forms of MAO in homogenates prepared from brain may, however, give values that do not reflect their contributions to the metabolism of amines in vivo. The existence of high-affinity systems for the transport of specific amines into the nerve terminals might be expected to result in metabolism occurring predominantly in those organelles with glial cell metabolism, becoming important only at higher amine concentrations. Thus Demerest et al.[7] reported that, in rat brain, low concentrations of dopamine were largely metabolized in the nerve terminals, and similar conclusions were reached in studies on the effects of hemitransection on dopamine metabolism.[8] In contrast, the contribution of compartments other than serotonergic nerve terminals was found to be significant in studies on the effects of the specific uptake inhibitor norzimelidine on the metabolism of low concentrations of 5-HT by preparations from mouse brain.[9]

In order to assess the forms of monoamine oxidase present in nerve terminals, we have used intact synaptosomal fractions, prepared from postmortem human hypothalamus and caudatus by the method of Hardy et al.,[10] in combination with the specific uptake inhibitors—amfonelic acid for dopamine, citalopram for 5-HT, and maprotiline for norepinephrine—to study the intrasynaptosomal metabolism of low concentrations of these amines. The selective inhibitor clorgyline was used in this system to determine the proportions of the two forms of MAO present.[11] The results obtained in these studies are summarized in Table 34.1.

The observation that dopaminergic nerve terminals from human caudatus contain little MAO-B suggests that the dopamine-sparing action of l-deprenyl, which has been advanced to explain its efficacy in the treatment of Parkinson's disease,[12] results from inhibition of the enzyme in structures outside the dopaminergic nerve terminals. This finding also has relevance to the mode of action of the dopaminergic neurotoxin 1-methyl-4-phenyl-1,2,3,6-tetrahydropyridine (MPTP). This compound has been shown to be converted to the 1-methyl-4-phenylpyridinium ion (MPP$^+$), which is the active neurotoxin, by the action of MAO-B.[13] The absence of significant amounts of that form of the enzyme in caudatal dopaminergic synaptosomes indicates that this conversion must occur outside the susceptible nerve endings. This conclusion is consistent with the demonstration that MPP$^+$ is actively transported into dopaminergic neurons by the dopamine transport system[14] and that inhibitors of this uptake protect against the toxic effects of MPTP.[15]

The observation that both forms of MAO are present in noradrenergic synaptosomes suggests that MPTP could be oxidized within these structures to form the toxic MPP$^+$. However, MPTP was found to be a relatively poor inhibitor of MAO-A activity in intact synaptosomes, with an I_{50} value greatly in excess of 100 μM. Because the sensitivity increased greatly on disruption of the synaptosomal membranes these results indicate that MPTP does not readily penetrate the nerve terminals. This may be a contributing factor to the relative insensitivity of noradrenergic neurons to MPTP toxicity.

Because of the specificty of 5-HT as a substrate for MAO-A, the methods used here cannot be used to determine the presence of the B-form of the enzyme in human brain nerve terminals. Studies with monoclonal antibodies have indicated that these terminals contain mainly MAO-B.[16] The results of the present study, however, indicate the presence of some MAO-A within these terminals, which is consistent with the results obtained with mouse brain, where a fall in activity toward 5-HT was seen when a synaptosomal preparation was treated with norzimelidine.[9]

TABLE 34.1. Intra- and extra-neuronal MAO activities in human brain.

Substrate	Intrasynaptosomal oxidation (%)		
	Total	Due to MAO-A	Due to MAO-B
Dopamine	27 ± 8	< 95	> 5
Norepinehrine	35 ± 8	39 ± 10	61 ± 10
5-Hydroxytrptamine	25 ± 3	—	—

Activities toward dopamine, norepinephrine (each at 0.25 μM) and 5-HT (at 0.1 μM) were determined radiochemically in crude synaptosomal fractions from the caudatus for dopamine and from the hypothalamus for 5-HT and norepinephrine. Extraneuronal activities were determined in the presence of inhibitory concentrations of amfonelic acid, citalopram, and maprotiline; and the activity in each specific synaptosomal type was then calculated from the results obtained in the absence of the one of these uptake inhibitors that was selective for each specific amine.

MAO-A inhibitors would thus be expected to elevate the concentrations of 5-HT and, to a lesser extent, those of norepinephrine and dopamine. These increases may contribute to the greater antidepressant effects of these agents than the MAO-B inhibitors, which have little effect on 5-HT oxidation.

References

1. Tipton KF. Enzymology of monoamine oxidase. Cell Biochem Funct 1987;4:79–87.
2. Fowler CJ, Tipton KF. On the substrate specificities of the two forms of monoamine oxidase. J Pharm Pharmacol 1984;36:111–115.
3. Pare CMB. Clinical studies with monoamine oxidase inhibitors and tricyclic antidepressants. In Tipton KF, Dostert P, Strolin Benedetti M (eds): Monoamine Oxidase and Disease. New York: Academic Press, 1984;469–478.
4. Birkmeyer W, Riederer P, Ambrozi L, et al. Implications of combined treatment with Mardopa and l-deprenyl in Parkinson's disease. Lancet 1977;2:439–443.
5. O'Carroll A-M, Fowler CJ, Phillips JP, et al. The deamination of dopamine by human brain monoamine oxidase: specificity for the two enzyme forms in seven brain regions. Naunyn Schmiedebergs Arch Pharmacol 1983;322:198–202.
6. O'Carroll A-M, Bradsley ME, Tipton KF. The oxidation of adrenaline and noradrenaline by the two forms of monoamine oxidase from human and rat brain. Neurochem Int 1986;8:493–500.
7. Demerest KT, Smith DJ, Azzaro AJ. The presence of the type A form of monoamine oxidase within nigrostriatal dopamine-containing neurones. J Pharmacol Exp Ther 1980; 215:461–468.
8. Stenström A, Arai Y, Oreland L. Intra- and extra-neuronal monoamine oxidase-A and -B activities after central axotomy (hemitransection) on rats. J Neural Transm. 1985;65:105–113.
9. Ross SB, Ask A-L. Structural requirements for uptake into serotonergic neurone. Acta Pharmacol Toxicol (Copenh) 1980;46:270–277.
10. Hardy JA, Doff PR, Oakely AE, et al. Metabolically active synaptosomes can be prepared from frozen rat and human brain. J Neurochem 1983;40:608–614.
11. O'Carroll AM, Tipton KF, Sullivan JP, et al. Intra- and extrasynaptosomal deamination of dopamine and noradrenaline by the two forms of human brain monoamine oxidase. Biogenic Amines 1987;4:47–60.
12. Riederer P, Reynolds GP. Deprenyl is a selective inhibitor of brain MAO-B in the long-term treatment of Parkinson's disease. Br J Pharmacol 1980;9:98–99.
13. Heikkila RE, Manzino L, Cabbat FS, et al. Protection against the dopaminergic neurotoxicity of 1-methyl-4-phenyl-1,2,3,6-tetrahydropyridine by monoamine oxidase inhibitors. Nature 1984;311:467–469.
14. Javitch JA, Snyder SH. Uptake of MPP (+) by dopamine neurones explains selectivity of parkisonism-inducing neurotoxin, MPTP. Eur J Pharmacol 1985;106:455–456.
15. Sundström E, Jonsson G. Pharmacological interference with the neurotoxic actions of 1-methyl-4-phenyl-1,2,3,6-tetrahydropyridine (MPTP) on catecholaminergic neurons in the mouse. Eur J Pharmacol 1985;110:293–299.
16. Thorpe LW, Westlund KN, Kochersperger LM, et al. Immunocytochemical localization of monoamine oxidase in human peripheral tissues and brain. J Histochem Cytochem 1987;35:23–32.

35. Effect of Selective Monoamine Oxidase Substrates and Inhibitors on Lipid Peroxidation and Their Possible Involvement in Affective Disorders

M. STROLIN BENEDETTI AND P. DOSTERT

The purpose of this chapter is to examine how the oxidative deamination of mono-amines by monoamine oxidase (MAO) and its inhibition can affect lipid peroxidation (LPO) and the physiopathological processes in mental diseases related to this phenomenon. MAO exists in two forms, termed MAO-A and MAO-B. Serotonin (5-HT) and norepinephrine (NE) are regarded as specific substrates for MAO-A, dopamine (DA) is considered a substrate for both forms, and 2-phenylethylamine (PEA), benzylamine (Bz), and n-pentylamine (n-P) substrates for MAO-B. MAO-A and MAO-B can be selectively inhibited by clorgyline and l-deprenyl respectively, whereas nialamide inhibits both forms of the enzyme.

Oxidative deamination of monoamines by MAO produces NH_3, aldehydes, and H_2O_2, agents with established or potential neurotoxicity. H_2O_2 in particular has been invoked as a damaging agent in neurons. Through the Fenton or the Haber-Weiss reaction, H_2O_2 generates highly reactive hydroxyl radicals ($OH^{\cdot}$) and can start LPO.

Peroxidative Damage by Biogenic Amines and the Pentose Phosphate Pathway

As the metabolism of biogenic amines produces reactive oxidative species, brain damage can result from LPO at specific sites or in pathological conditions, e.g., when NADPH is in poor supply. H_2O_2 generated by MAO in the brain appears to be detoxified mainly by glutathione peroxidase (GSHP), but glutathione reductase (GSHR) is also important, as it regenerates reduced glutathione for GSHP. GSHR needs NADPH, which is also necessary for detoxication of the aldehydes produced by the metabolism of biogenic amines. NADPH is produced by the pentose phosphate pathway (PPP) operating in the brain.[1] The PPP produces NADPH through two enzymatic steps during the transformation of glucose-6-phosphate to ribose-5-phosphate. A convenient marker of PPP is $^{14}CO_2$ released from 1-^{14}C-glucose. 5-HT, NE, and DA stimulate the formation of $^{14}CO_2$ from 1-^{14}C-glucose by rat brain synaptosomes, and this stimulation is totally abolished by nialamide. The effect of monoamine transmitters in enhancing the PPP's activity could be mediated by a number of mechanisms, but detoxication of H_2O_2 and reduction of the aldehydes are probably the main ones.[1]

Malondialdehyde, MAO, and H_2O_2 Detoxifying Enzymes

H_2O_2 produced by MAO can give origin to $OH^.$ and start LPO. Superoxide radical $O_2^{.-}$ produced within cells by enzymatic and spontaneous autoxidation of various molecules is generally assumed to be weakly toxic by itself, but it is toxic indirectly, as it participates in the formation of $OH^.$. As a result of LPO, malondialdehyde (MDA) is formed, a compound known to be toxic to a variety of biological systems. MDA can condense with thiobarbituric acid (TBA), and the product of the reaction absorbs at 535nm. LPO is generally evaluated by following TBA-reactive material. Comparative data on the production of TBA-reactive material in the various structures of the human brain and on the activities of MAO and H_2O_2-detoxifying enzymes in the same structures would form a basis for assessing the extent to which MAO is involved in LPO in different physiopathological situations. Data from the literature are reported below, although they are in fact incomplete and not comparable.

Young or Old Normal Subjects

Boehme et al.[2] described a distinct regional distribution of TBA-reactive material in normal human brain, with high levels in the cerebellum vermis and low levels in the pons and putamen; thalamus, cortex, substantia nigra, caudate nucleus, and hypothalamus gave intermediate values. Reznikoff et al.[3] studied the distribution of MAO in human brain from men with no known neurological or psychiatric disease by determining the distribution of ^{3}H-pargyline-binding sites. Levels of binding sites were high in hypothalamus and low in cerebellar cortex, thalamus pons, and frontal cortex; structures such as substantia nigra, caudate nucleus, and putamen gave intermediate values. Concerning the H_2O_2-detoxifying enzymes, the highest peroxidase activity is in the substantia nigra of nonneurological control brains, whereas there is less regional variation for catalase.[4] In normal subjects serum lipid peroxide levels, evaluated in terms of TBA-reactive material, tend to increase with age up to 70 years and then to decline. Brain, platelet, and lymphocyte MAO-B activities increase with normal aging. Ambani et al.[4] found lower peroxidase and catalase activities in most of the brain structures in old healthy subjects than in young controls, although for peroxidase the decrease was significant only in the globus pallidus and for catalase only in the cerebellar, occipital, and temporal cortical regions.

Subjects with Mental or Neurological Diseases

In patients with Down's syndrome GSHP activity is significantly higher in erythrocytes and MAO activity is lower in platelets. In Down's syndrome fetal brain, LPO as well as Cu/Zn-dependent superoxide dismutase (SOD) are significantly elevated in the cerebral cortex with no rise in GSHP in the same structure. No information is available on brain MAO, so it is impossible to say if MAO contributes further to the peroxidative stress produced by the increased SOD activity in this illness.

In parkinsonian patients data on MAO activity are contradictory, while the activities of catalase and peroxidase[4] and the selenium content are decreased in the brain, especially in the substantia nigra. In Alzheimer's disease an increase in brain and platelet MAO-B has been clearly established. Published findings on the activity of GSHP in Alzheimer's disease resemble those in subjects with Down's syndrome. In patients with Alzheimer's disease the activity of the selenium-dependent enzyme GSHP is increased or unchanged in erythrocytes. No significant alterations in this enzyme activity were observed in autopsied brain regions from patients with Alzheimer's disease.

Lipofuscin

Malondialdehyde formed as a result of LPO may react with amino groups in proteins and in certain phospholipids giving lipofuscin by polymerization. Lipofuscin accumulates in various tissues, including the central nervous system. It has been shown that it increases with age in normal individuals and in at least three dementia syndromes: Alzheimer's, Parkinson's, and Batten's diseases.[5] In Batten's disease peroxidation also seems to play a pathogenic role. Biochemically it is characterized by low cellular GSHP activity and low selenium content in blood. The clinical symptoms might be related to lipofuscin deposition as a consequence of low GSHP activity. It would be useful to know if MAO-A or MAO-B activity is modified in Batten's disease.

Dopamine, Norepinephrine, 6-Hydroxydopamine, Neuromelanin

The effect of DA on LPO is complex, as it can play either a toxic or a beneficial role. DA can be converted to 6-hydroxydopamine (6-OHDA), which is highly neurotoxic mainly through the production of toxic oxidative species, such as H_2O_2, $O_2 \cdot$ and therefore OH^-.[6] DA can also play a direct toxic role in LPO. Autoxidation of DA yields the oxidative species produced by 6-OHDA autoxidation, but an o-quinone is also formed, which probably contributes to the cytotoxicity. The cytotoxicity of DA, which is greater than that of NE or epinephrine, appears to derive from two major factors. DA undergoes autoxidation more readily than the other catecholamines. Moreover, the oxidation of epinephrine or NE to o-quinones is followed by faster cyclization than with DA.[6,7]

Neuromelanin is a product of catecholamine metabolism. It is formed by polymerization of cyclic derivatives produced by autoxidation of catecholamines. Unlike the melanin of skin, neuromelanin is deposited in association with lipofuscin, rather than in melanosomes, and is not the product of the enzyme tyrosinase. The fact that neuromelanin is deposited progressively with time within the cytoplasm of catecholamine neurons does not necessarily indicate that it is a toxic phenomenon, although neurotoxins might bind to neuromelanin, be stored, and then be released gradually. DA is more toxic than NE as it is more easily autoxidized and the corresponding o-quinone forms cyclization products less easily. Moreover neuromelanin accumulates more rapidly in the noradrenergic neurons, which could explain why dopaminergic neurons degenerate faster than noradrenergic neurons during old age.

Dopamine and NE can both act as radical scavengers of O_2^- and OH^-. Thus in vivo experiments have shown that NE protects axon terminals from 6-OHDA toxicity.[8]

Selective MAO Substrates and LPO

The effects of selective MAO substrates on LPO have been studied by measuring MDA in rat brain homogenates.[9] LPO was inhibited by DA ($IC_{50} = 8 \times 10^{-6} M$), NE ($IC_{50} = 1.2 \times 10^{-5} M$), and 5-HT ($IC_{50} = 2.8 \times 10^{-5} M$). Selective inhibition of MAO-A slightly reduced but did not abolish the inhibition of LPO by 5-HT, whereas selective inhibition of MAO-B had no effect. The effects of pyrogallol, catechol, and hydroquinone on LPO inhibition were also studied. The IC_{50} values— $2.1 \times 10^{-6} M$, $1.3 \times 10^{-5} M$, and $2.6 \times 10^{-4} M$, respectively—are in agreement with the results of Kappus et al.,[10] who studied the effect of catechol and pyrogallol derivatives on LPO in liver microsomal fraction. Therefore, although DA, NE, and 5-HT may induce LPO by production of H_2O_2, they seem to act as radical scavengers rather than as LPO inducers, at least in vitro.

Lipid peroxidation was induced by 2-PEA, Bz, and n-P ($10^{-5} M$ to $10^{-3} M$).[9] This induction was completely abolished by selective inhibition of MAO-B, whereas selective inhibition of MAO-A had no effect. With liver mitochondrial membranes Kagan et al.[11] found induction of LPO by 2-PEA and Bz and inhibition by 5-HT, in agreement with the results of Guffroy et al.[9] Therefore the inhibition of MAO-B, rather than MAO-A, should protect against LPO.

Selective MAO Inhibitors and LPO

In addition to MDA, alkanes of low molecular weight are produced during LPO. The most reliable way to determine LPO in vivo is to measure exhaled alkanes. They appear in the breath of rats after intraperitoneal CCl_4 and are also formed in small amounts endogenously. As pentane is metabolized five to ten times faster than ethane and is species- and strain-dependent, it is recommended that ethane rather than pentane be monitored for evaluating LPO in vivo. The free radical producing LPO after administration of CCl_4 is trichlormethyl radical.

As MAO produces H_2O_2, the effect of MAO inhibitors on in vivo LPO was studied.[12] Groups of rats received either CCl_4 (1 ml/kg i.p.) or CCl_4 1 h after l-deprenyl (10 mg/kg p.o.) or clorgyline (10 mg/kg p.o.). The amount of ethane exhaled by rats pretreated with l-deprenyl was 66% of that exhaled by CCl_4-treated rats, whereas the pretreatment with clorgyline had no effect. It is interesting that another MAO-B inhibitor, RO 19-6327 (10 mg/kg p.o.), has also shown some protection against in vivo LPO under the same experimental conditions (Da Prada et al., personal communication).

Affective disorders, such as unipolar depression, have been related to high MAO activity. It should therefore be useful to investigate phenomena related to LPO in these disorders so as to better understand the possible roles of MAO-A and MAO-B and the therapy with selective inhibitors.

References

1. Hothersall JS, Greenbaum AL, McLean P. The functional significance of the pentose phosphate pathway in synaptosomes: protection against peroxidative damage by catecholamines and oxidants. J Neurochem 1982;39:1325–1332.

2. Boehme DH, Kosecki R, Carson S, et al. Lipoperoxidation in human and rat brain tissue: developmental and regional studies. Brain Res 1977;136;11–21.
3. Reznikoff G, Manaker S, Parsons B, et al. Similar distribution of monoamine oxidase (MAO) and parkinsonian toxin (MPTP) binding sites in human brain. Neurology 1985;35:1415–1419.
4. Ambani LM, Van Woert MH, Murphy S. Brain peroxidase and catalase in Parkinson disease. Arch Neurol 1975;32:114–118.
5. Clausen J. Demential syndromes and the lipid metabolism. Acta Neurol Scand 1984;70:345–355.
6. Graham DG, Tiffany SM, Bell WR, et al. Autoxidation versus covalent binding of quinones as the mechanism of toxicity of dopamine, 6-hydroxydopamine and related compounds toward C 1300 neuroblastoma cells in vitro. Mol Pharmacol 1978;14:644–653.
7. Graham DG. Oxidative pathways for catecholamines in the genesis of neuromelanin and cytotoxic quinones. Mol Pharmacol 1978;14:633–643.
8. Sachs C, Jonsson G, Heikkila R, et al. Control of the neurotoxicity of 6-hydroxydopamine by intraneuronal noradrenaline in rat iris. Acta Physiol Scand 1975;93:345–351.
9. Guffroy C, Strolin Benedetti M, Dostert P. Induction or inhibition of lipid peroxidation in rat brain homogenates by biogenic and other amines. Abstracts of the 6th General Meeting of the ESN, Prague, 1986;369.
10. Kappus H, Kieczka H, Scheulen M, et al. Molecular aspects of catechol and pyrogallol inhibition of liver microsomal lipid peroxidation stimulated by ferrous ion-ADP-complexes or by carbon tetrachloride. Naunyn Schmiedeberg's Arch Pharmacol 1977;300:179–187.
11. Kagan VE, Smirnov AV, Savov VM, et al. Lipid peroxidation in mitochondrial membranes induced by enzymatic deamination of biogenic amines. Acta Physiol Pharmacol Bulg 1983;9:3–12.
12. Richard C, Guichard JP, Strolin Benedetti M, et al. Effect of MAO inhibitors on in vivo lipid peroxidation. Pharmacol Toxicol 1987;60(suppl 1):38.

36. Pharmacology of Monoamine Oxidase Inhibitors

JOHN P.M. FINBERG

The clinical use of monoamine oxidase (MAO) inhibitors for depression was curtailed because of cases of hypertensive crisis following ingestion of tyramine-containing foods ("cheese effect"), potentiation of other indirectly acting amines, and interaction with a variety of other drugs.[1,2] Realization of the existence of isoenzymes of MAO, termed MAO-A and MAO-B, led to the hope that selective inhibitors of those enzyme forms may have clinical effectiveness without causing these side effects, as tyramine is a substrate for both enzyme forms.[3] However, clorgyline, a selective inhibitor of MAO-A, did cause the "cheese effect," whereas (−)-deprenyl (selective MAO-B inhibitor) did not.[4,5] This difference could be explained by the fact that MAO-A is the predominant enzyme form found in sympathetic nerves[6] and the gastrointestinal tract.[7] Knoll[8] claimed that (−)-deprenyl possesses an additional property that selectively antagonizes tyramine responses by inhibiting both neuronal amine uptake and norepinephrine (NE) release.

Studies in our group led to the discovery of the selective MAO-B inhibitory property of AGN 1135.[9] We were therefore interested to see if this inhibitor also did not cause tyramine potentiation.

Studies Using Isolated Rat Vas Deferens as a Model System to Investigate Tyramine Potentiation

Selective inhibition of MAO type A by 80% or more using clorgyline or LY 51641 was associated with significant tyramine potentiation, whereas selective inhibition of MAO-B by 60% using (−)-deprenyl was not.[10] When (−)-deprenyl or AGN 1135 was added to the organ bath at concentrations of 20 μM or more, tyramine responses were suppressed in the presence of the inhibitor but were potentiated following washout[11] These higher concentrations produced inhibition of both type A and type B MAO. The initial suppression of the tyramine response could not be explained by inhibition of neuronal amine uptake, as parallel determination of uptake by the vas deferens of ^{3}H-metaraminol and ^{3}H-tyramine showed no marked effect by high concentrations of (−)-deprenyl and AGN 1135. Using denervated vasa deferentia, all the MAO inhibitors mentioned above were found to possess reversible α-adrenoceptor antagonistic properties at concentrations of 10 μM or more, which could explain the initial suppression of tyramine response. Glover et al.[12] have reported that (−)-deprenyl inhibits tyramine-induced efflux of ^{3}H-NE, following prior inhibition of MAO-A with clorgyline, in isolated rat brain slices. This finding indicates that (−)-deprenyl may possess some specific action on tyramine-induced release of NE in addition to the properties described above in the vas deferens.

Studies in Anesthetized Cats

Using chloralose-anesthetized cats, we investigated the modification of pressor and nictitating membrane responses to tyramine and β-phenylethylamine by clorgyline, (−)-deprenyl, and AGN 1135.[13] An intravenous dose of AGN 1135 (1.5 mg/kg) produced potentiation of the contractile response to β-phenylethylamine on the nictitating membrane without affecting pressor responses to tyramine. Biochemical determination of MAO activity in liver and brain confirmed the selective inhibition of MAO-B by this dose of AGN 1135, whereas a higher dose of the inhibitor (5 mg/kg) inhibited both MAO forms and caused potentiation of tyramine pressor responses.

The studies described above indicate that selective inhibition of MAO type A is associated with tyramine potentiation, whereas selective inhibition of MAO type B can be achieved without tyramine potentiation, and is not an exclusive property of (−)-deprenyl. The lack of cheese effect with MAO-B inhibitors is of clinical importance, as (−)-deprenyl has been reported to possess antidepressant properties. However, studies have shown that doses of 30 mg or more may be required in depressed patients,[14] which may also result in extensive inhibition of MAO-A and potentiation of tyramine pressor responses.[15]

Effect of Chronic MAO Inhibition on Norepinephrine Release

Acute inhibition of MAO has no detectable effect on postsynaptic response to stimulation of sympathetic nerves. Very large doses of MAO inhibitors have been reported to possess adrenergic neuron blocking properties, but these large doses may cause pharmacological effects not seen in clinically relevant doses. Because prolonged MAO inhibition has been reported to cause down-regulation of cerebral cortical β- and α$_2$-adrenoceptors, the effect of chronic MAO inhibition on NE release from sympathetic nerves has been studied using isolated vas deferens and pithed rat preparations.

Following chronic treatment of rats with either clorgyline (1 mg/kg) or nialamide (50 mg/kg) daily for 3 weeks, there was a decrease in the fractional release of ^{3}H-NE from the isolated vas deferens by electrical field stimulation.[16] On the other hand, release of NE and epinephrine into the blood following electrical stimulation of the sympathetic nervous system was increased in pithed rats treated chronically with clorgyline.[17] Production of a similar degree of MAO inhibition and similar increase in arterial tissue NE concentration by acute MAO inhibition was not accompanied by increased catecholamine release in response to stimulation.

Conclusions

Chronic MAO-A inhibition results in redistribution of releasable NE pools in sympathetic nerve endings such that more NE is available for release by nerve stimulation. In tissues such as the vas deferens, where the synaptic cleft is extremely narrow and presynaptic inhibitory adrenoceptor control is effective, net release of NE may be decreased by a higher degree of presynaptic α_2-adrenoceptor stimulation. In blood vessels with wide synaptic clefts, net release of NE is enhanced. Such a difference in amine release between various types of synapse may exist also in the central nervous system.

References

1. Blackwell B, Marley E. Interactions of cheese and of its constituents with monoamine oxidase inhibitors. Br J Pharmacol 1966;26:120–141.
2. Stockley IH. Monoamine oxidase inhibitors. Part 2. Inter-actions with antihypertensive agents, hypoglycaemics, CNS depressants, narcotics and antiparkinsonian agents. Pharmaceutical J 1973;211:95–98.
3. Johnston JP. Some observations upon a new inhibitor of monoamine oxidase in brain tissue. Biochem Pharmacol 1968;17:1285–1297.
4. Lader MH, Sakalis G, Tansella M. Interactions between sympathomimetic amines and a new monoamine oxidase inhibitor. Psychopharmacology 1970;18:118–123.
5. Elsworth JD, Glover V, Reynolds GP, et al. Deprenyl administration in man: a selective monoamine oxidase B inhibitor without the "cheese effect." Psychopharmacology 1978;57:33–38.
6. Jarrott B. Occurrence and properties of monoamine oxidase in adrenergic neurons. J Neurochem 1971;18:7–16.
7. Strolin-Benedetti M, Boucher T, Carlsson A, et al. Intestinal metabolism of tyramine by both forms of monoamine oxidase in the rat. Biochem Pharmacol 1983;32:57–52.
8. Knoll J. The possible mechanisms of action of (−)-deprenyl in Parkinson's disease. J Neural Transm 1978;43:177–198.
9. Kalir A, Sabbagh A, Youdim MBH. Selective acetylenic "suicide" inhibitors of monoamine oxidase types A and B. Br J Pharmacol 1981;73:55–64.
10. Finberg JPM, Tenne M. Relationship between tyramine potentiation and selective inhibition of monoamine oxidase types A and B in the rat vas deferens. Br J Pharmacol 1982;77:13–21.
11. Finberg JPM, Tenne M, Youdim MBH. Tyramine antagonistic properties of AGN 1135, an irreversible inhibitor of monoamine oxidase type B. Br J Pharmacol 1981;7365–7374.
12. Glover V, Pycock CJ, Sandler M. Tyramine-induced noradrenaline release from rat brain slices: prevention by (−)-deprenyl. Br J Pharmacol 1983;80:141–148.
13. Finberg JPM, Youdim MBH. Modification of blood pressure and nictitating membrane response to sympathetic amines by selective monoamine oxidase inhibitors, types A and B, in the cat. Br J Pharmacol 1985;85:541–546.
14. Quitkin FM, Liebowitz MR, Stewart JW, et al. 1-Deprenyl in atypical depressives. Arch Gen Psychiatry 1984;120:777–781.
15. Sunderland T, Mueller EA, Cohen RM, et al. Tyramine pressor sensitivity changes during deprenyl treatment. Psychopharmacology 1985;86:432–437.
16. Hovevey-Sion D. Effect of acute and chronic treatment with antidepressants on presynaptic alpha$_2$ adrenoceptors and [^{3}H]noradrenaline release from sympathetic neurons. DSc thesis, Technion, Haifa, Israel, 1986.
17. Finberg JPM, Kopin IJ. Chronic clorgyline treatment enhances release of norepinephrine following sympathetic stimulation in the rat. Naunyn Schmiedebergs Arch Pharmacol 1986;332:236–242.

37. Regulation of Functional Cytoplasmic Pool of Serotonin by MAO-A and MAO-B: Implications for Antidepressant Therapy

Moussa B.H. Youdim

Abnormalities in serotonin (5-HT) metabolism (synthesis, release, and oxidation) and function have been implicated in the pathogenesis of neuropsychiatric diseases, especially depressive illness.[1] Understanding the mechanism of 5-HT release so it can "function" and regulation of the latter appear to be important for any rational therapeutic approach to depression.[2] The general acceptance that 5-HT in the presynaptic neuron is stored in two pools, a large (vesicular) one and a smaller one,[3] prompted us to examine which of the two compartments is the "functional" pool. It has been generally assumed that the smaller pool contains the newly synthesized 5-HT, which is preferentially released.[4] In order to identify the functional pool of 5-HT, we have linked neurotransmitter release to the occurrence of the characteristic 5-HT behavioral syndrome in reserpinized rats.[5] This method is valid as almost all the previous studies have used normal animals, where the 5-HT vesicular compartment is intact.

Results and Discussion

In non-reserpine-treated (normal) rats the 5-HT behavioral syndrome can be elicited by (a) inhibition of monoamine oxidase (MAO) followed by l-tryptophan or 5-hydroxytryptophan treatment; (b) use of direct 5-HT receptor agonists such as 5-methoxy-N,N-dimethyltryptamine and an MAO inhibitor; (c) drugs that release 5-HT from the presynaptic neuron (e.g., p-chloroamphetamine, PCA); (d) a combination of selective MAO-A inhibition (clorgyline); and (e) selective 5-HT uptake inhibitors (indalpine or fluoxetine)[5-7] (Fig. 37.1).

Investigation of the functional pool of 5-HT in vivo in reserpinized rats was initiated, as the vesicular content of 5-HT is largely eliminated leaving only the small, newly synthesized neurotransmitter pool intact. Furthermore, tryptophan hydroxylase, the rate-limiting enzyme of 5-HT synthesis, remains unchanged and postsynaptic 5-HT receptors binding sites are not altered.[5]

Reserpine (5 mg/kg) treatment of rats, in order to disrupt vesicular amine storage, reduces 5-HT in hypothalamus striatum and spinal cord by 90% and in the raphe nucleus by 75%. Despite this fact, the 5-HT-releasing drug PCA[8] produces a be-

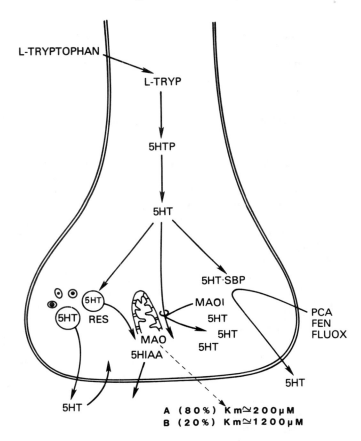

FIGURE 37.1. Dynamics of a serotonergic nerve ending. (L-TRYP) L-tryptophan. (5HTP) 5-hydroxytryptophan. (5HT) serotonin. (RES) reserpine. (SBP) serotonin-binding protein. (MAOI) monoamine oxidase inhibitor. (PCA) p-chloroamphetamine. (FEN) fenfluramine. (FLUOX) fluoxetine. (5HIAA) 5-hydroxyindoleacetic acid. Note the Km values of MAO-A and MAO-B for serotonin.

havioral syndrome in these rats that is no different from the one observed in normal unreserpinized animals given PCA.[9] The behavioral effect of PCA is dose-dependent (2.5–10.0 mg/kg), and the MAO inhibitors pargyline and clorgyline, but not l-deprenyl, potentiate this effect and shift the dose-response curve to the left.[5] These data indicate that PCA-initiated 5-HT release, a non-Ca^{2+}-dependent or exocytotic-dependent event,[8] is governed by the state of intraneuronal MAO-A activity. Support for this hypothesis has come from experiments where selective inhibition of MAO-A by clorgyline, and not selective MAO-B inactivation, causes a significant increase in brain 5-HT as measured in hypothalamus and raphe nuclei of normal and reserpine-treated rats.[10] Although MAO-B inhibition by itself has no influence on brain 5-HT, in combination with MAO-A inhibition the increase in 5-HT level is significantly greater than that observed with clorgyline alone. These contradictory results, originally described by Green and Youdim,[11] were explained by the relative proportions of MAO-A and MAO-B within the central 5-HT neurons and their affinities for 5-HT when each enzyme is selectively inactivated (Fig 37.1). It is now apparent that, contrary to previous notions but supporting the findings of Green and Youdim,[11] a significant portion (20%) of MAO activity in the 5-HT neuron (raphe nuclei) is type B, as identified by antibody and monoclonal antibody developed to this enzyme.[12,13]

Fowler and Tipton[14] have already shown that the apparent Km values of MAO-A and MAO-B for 5-HT are 200 and 1,200 μM, respectively. Thus when MAO-A is inhibited in vivo, brain 5-HT concentration rises to a level that would satisfy its affinity for MAO-B and be oxidized by it. This fact would explain why brain 5-HT levels are not as high after clorgyline treatment compared to the use of a nonselective MAO inhibitor or the combination of selective MAO-A and MAO-B inhibitors.[10,11] The lower affinity of MAO-B for 5-HT would not result in 5-HT accumulation after inhibition of MAO-B (Fig. 37.1).

That the 5-HT behavioral responses are mediated by 5-HT at postsynaptic receptor sites is supported by the antagonistic action of 5-HT receptor blocker methergoline. Furthermore, the irreversible tryptophan hydroxylase inhibitor p-chlorophenylalanine, which inhibits the synthesis of new 5-HT, prevents the PCA-induced behavior in reserpinized rats. Indications are therefore that newly formed 5-HT is released into function in the absence of vesicular storage sites.[5]

The question remains as to whether in the absence of vesicular storage sites, as is the case after reserpine treatment, the release of newly formed functional 5-HT compound is governed by other mechanisms. Neither selective MAO-A or MAO-B inhibitors nor selective 5-HT uptake blockers (fluoxetine or indalpine) alone can bring about the 5-HT behavioral syndrome in normal or reserpine-treated animals.[7,10] By contrast, the combination of clorgyline (but not l-deprenyl) and a 5-HT uptake blocker (indalpine or fluoxetine) produces a behavioral syndrome indistinguishable from that initiated by PCA that is blocked by methergoline. In the absence fo 5-HT oxidation by MAO-A and the reuptake process, the neurotransmitter concentration within the synaptic cleft would be sufficiently high to initiate postsynaptic events. By contrast, if reuptake is intact, 5-HT would be available for oxidation by intact MAO-B within the presynaptic 5-HT neuron after reuptake (Fig. 37.1).

It is apparent that release of cytoplasmic newly synthesized 5-HT clearly participates in the 5-HT behavioral syndrome.[5] The selective 5-HT uptake blockers fluoxetine and indalpine can protect normal and reserpine-treated rats from the 5-HT-depleting and behavioral actions of low doses of PCA. They do not, however, prevent the 5-HT behavioral syndrome after higher doses of PCA.[5] In the experiments where high doses of PCA are combined with fluoxetine, brain (striatum, hypothalamus, raphe nuclei, spinal cord) 5-HT levels are, in fact, increased. At first glance the latter data are contradictory to the modes of actions of PCA and fluoxetine. Fluoxetine may also act as a weak inhibitor of 5-HT release, which would overcome MAO inhibitory activity of higher doses of PCA.[5]

The increase in brain 5-HT after higher doses of PCA could result in the inhibition of MAO-A and MAO-B. MAO inhibition is thought to be a significant part of the overall in vivo pharmacological activity of amphetamines and their derivatives. D-Amphetamine and its derivatives inhibit MAO-A in vitro and in vivo.[15] PCA has Ki values of 2 and 9 μM for MAO-A and MAO-B, respectively, in rat brain. These values indicate that similar concentrations can be reached in the brain with doses used to elicit the 5-HT behavioral syndrome.[15,16] It may also explain the powerful psychotropic activity of PCA as being dependent on a combination of MAO inhibition and 5-HT release. The ability of PCA to inhibit MAO supports this conclusion, as at a high PCA concentration pargyline does not potentiate its 5-HT behavioral syndrome.[5]

Conclusion

Our studies indicate that the "functional" pool of serotonin released into synapses represents a small fraction of cytoplasmic nonvesicular compartments. Its size is governed by the rate of synthesis and oxidation by MAO-A and MAO-B.

References

1. Van Praag HM. Serotonin precursors in the treatment of depression. In Ho BT, Schoolar JC, Usdin E (eds): Serotonin in Biological Psychiatry. New York: Raven Press, 1982;259–286.
2. Kuhn DM, Wolf WA, Youdim MBH. Serotonin neurochemistry revisted: a new look at some old axioms. Neurochem Int 1986;8:141–154.
3. Glowinski J. Properties and functions of intraneuronal monoamine compartments in central aminergic neurons. In Iversen LC, Iversen SD, Snyder SH (eds): Handbook of Psychopharmacology. New York: Plenum Press, 1978;136–167.
4. Shields PJ, Eccleston D. Evidence for the synthesis and storage of 5-hydroxytryptamine in two separate pools in the brain. J Neurochem 1973;220:881–888.
5. Kuhn DM, Wolf WA, Youdim MBH. Serotonin release in vivo from a cytoplasmic pool: studies on the serotonin behavioral syndrome in reserpinized rat. Br J Pharmacol 1985;84:121–129.
6. Grahame-Smith DG. Studies in vivo on the relationship between brain tryptophan, 5-HT synthesis and hyperactivity in rats treated with a monoamine oxidase inhibitor and l-trytophan. J Neurochem 1971;18:1053–1066.
7. Ashkenazi R, Finberg JPM, Youdim MBH. Behavioural hyperactivity in rats treated with selective monoamine oxidase inhibitors and LM 5008, a selective 5-hydroxytryptamine uptake blocker. Br J Pharmacol 1983;79:765–770.
8. Sanders-Bush E. Regulation of serotonin storage and release. In Ho BT, Schoolar JC, Usdin E (eds): Serotonin in Biological Psychiatry. New York: Raven Press, 1982;17–34.
9. Trulson ME, Jacobs B. Behavioural evidence for the rapid release of CNS serotonin by PCA and fenfluramine. Eur J Pharmacol 1976;36:149–154.
10. Wolf WA, Youdim MBH, Kuhn DM. Does brain 5-HIAA indicate serotonin release or monoamine oxidase activity? Eur J Pharmacol 1985;109:381–387.
11. Green AR, Youdim MBH. Effect of monoamine oxidase inhibition by clorgyline, deprenyl or tranylcypromine on 5-HT concentration in rat brain and hyperactivity following subsequent tryptophan administration. Br J Pharmacol 1975;55:415–417.
12. Levitt P, Pintar J, Breakefield X. Immunocytochemical demonstration of monoamine oxidase B in brains astrocytes and serotonergic neurons. Proc Natl Acad Sci USA 1982;79:6385–6389.
13. Westlund K, Denney R, Kochersperger L, et al. Distinct monoamine oxidase A and B populations in primate brain. Science 1985;230:181–183.
14. Fowler C, Tipton KF. Deamination of 5-hydroxytryptamine by both forms of monoamine oxidase in the rat brain. J Neurochem 1982;38:733–739.
15. Youdim MBH, Finberg JPM. Monoamine oxidase inhibitor antidepressants. In Grahame-Smith DG, Cowen PJ (eds): Psychopharmacology 2. Part 1. Preclinical Psychopharmacology. Amsterdam: Elsevier, 1985;35–70.
16. Fuller RM, Hemrick-Luecke DK. Influence of ring and side chain substituents on the selectivity of amphetamine as a monoamine oxidase inhibitor. Res Commun Substance Abuse 1982;3:159–165.

38. Neurochemical Profile of the Antidepressant Moclobemide, a Reversible Type A Monoamine Oxidase Inhibitor with Minimal Tyramine Potentiating Activity in Rats

W.P. BURKARD, R. KETTLER, M. DA PRADA, AND W.E. HAEFELY

Moclobemide [p-chloro-N-(2-morpholinoethyl)-benzamide HCl; Ro 11-1163] is a short-acting, reversible, preferential type A monoamine oxidase inhibitor (MAOI).[1,2] This benzamide derivative is nontoxic and chemically unrelated to any of the irreversible MAOIs of the first generation. Accordingly, in contrast to iproniazid, moclobemide did not show hepatotoxic effects in rats.[3]

Moclobemide was shown to be a rather weak inhibitor of MAO-A and MAO-B in vitro in the rat brain, with IC_{50} values of 3 and more than 1,000 μM, respectively. However, preferential inhibition of MAO-A was attained in the rat brain 2 h after oral administration with an ED_{50} of 3.2 mg/kg: the value for MAO-B was 26 mg/kg. This ex vivo inhibition characterizes moclobemide as a relatively potent inhibitor of MAO-A in comparison with other reversible MAOIs with a morpholino group.[1,4]

We present here results obtained with moclobemide in three series of experiments: potentiation of the tyramine pressure effects; moclobemide-induced downregulation of β-adrenoceptors; and interaction of moclobemide at various uptake and receptor sites.

It is generally accepted that tyramine acts on sympathetic noradrenergic neurons by releasing norepinephrine (NE), which in turn increases blood pressure by stimulating postjunctional α-adrenoceptors. MAO-A inhibitors potentiate the tyramine pressor response by (a) presystemic inhibition of the breakdown of tyramine in liver and gut, thereby allowing more amine to reach the systemic circulation: (b) inhibiting metabolic inactivation of tyramine taken up into sympathetic nerve endings: and (c) preventing the deamination of the released NE by intra- and extraneuronal MAO inhibition.

The pressor effect of tyramine administered orally 1 h after moclobemide was investigated in freely moving rats.[5] As shown in Figure 38.1 in animals pretreated with tranylcypromine, a usually subthreshold dose of tyramine (5 mg/kg p.o.) pro-

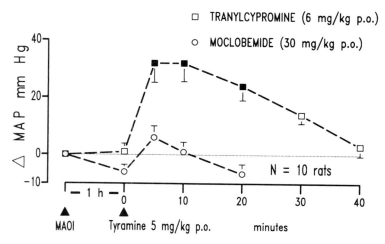

□ TRANYLCYPROMINE (6 mg/kg p.o.)

○ MOCLOBEMIDE (30 mg/kg p.o.)

N = 10 rats

MAOI   Tyramine 5 mg/kg p.o.   minutes

FIGURE 38.1. Potentiation by moclobemide or tranylcypromine of tyramine pressor responses in conscious, unrestrained rats. The predrug values of the mean arterial blood pressure (MAP) ranged between 108 and 127 mm Hg. The values shown are mean changes in MAP ± SEM. The MAOIs were administered orally 1 h before tyramine. Tyramine 5 mg/kg p.o. was given at time 0. Ten animals per dose were used. Filled symbols indicate statistical significance $p < 0.05$ versus the control.

duced a marked increase (32 mm Hg) in the mean arterial blood pressure (MAP) as early as 5 min after administration. Moclobemide, however, did not significantly modify the blood pressure effect of tyramine. Similar results were obtained after simultaneous application of tyramine and moclobemide (not shown). These and previous results in rats[5] agree well with the observation that negligible hypertensive reactions were observed in volunteers treated with moclobemide and ingesting tyramine alone or together with a meal.[6]

A decrease in the binding of β-adrenoceptor ligands (down-regulation) is a common but not indispensible response to repeated administration of various classes of antidepressant drugs, including MAO inhibitors.[7] In the present experiments moclobemide was injected nine times over 4 days, and the rats were decapitated 4 h after the last intraperitoneal administration. Moclobemide (50 mg/kg) decreased the Bmax (176 fmol/mg protein) of DHA binding significantly—by more than 20%—without changing the Kd (0.79 nM) or the Hill coefficient (0.985) (Fig. 38.2).

Overall, the adaptive changes of β-adrenoceptors that occur following repeated administration of moclobemide are similar to those obtained with clinically established antidepressants. Similar results were obtained with other MAO-A inhibitors, e.g., amiflamine, cimoxatone, or brofaremine.

In other experiments, moclobemide was tested for its ability to inhibit high-affinity uptake of monoamines into synaptosomes prepared from either striatum [dopamine (DA) uptake], hypothalamus [norepinephrine (NE) uptake], or forebrain [5-hydroxytryptamine (5-HT) uptake]. In vitro moclobemide did not influence amine uptake in concentrations up to $10^{-4} M$, and ex vivo in doses up to 300 mg/kg it only weakly (less than 50%) inhibited the uptake of either DA, NE, or 5-HT. In addition, moclobemide ($10^{-5} M$) did not interact with a variety of neu-

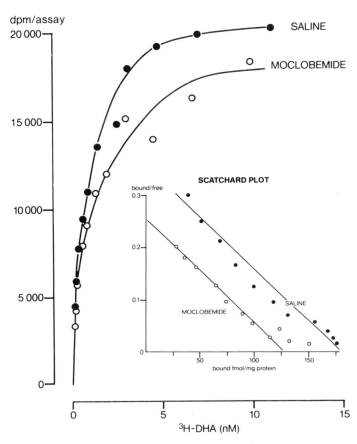

Figure 38.2. Saturation of specific [³H]dihydroalprenolol (³H-DHA) binding in membrane preparations from rat cortex. *Inset:* Corresponding Scatchard transformation. Points are means of duplicate determinations differing by less than 5%. The determinations were replicated twice.

rotransmitters or drug-binding sites, including: (a) dopamine D1 and D2 receptors; (b) α_1-, α_2-, and β-adrenoceptors; (c) serotonergic receptors 5-HT 1, 5-HT 1A, 5-HT 2; (d) histamine H1, muscarinic cholinoceptors; (e) opioid μ, δ, and κ receptors; and (f) benzodiazepine receptors. The binding studies indicate that this benzamide derivative did not affect dopamine receptors. In line with this study, moclobemide did not alter the prolactin level in human plasma.[8]

In summary, moclobemide only minimally enhanced the pressor effect of oral tyramine in rats, produced a down-regulation of β-adrenoceptor binding sites, and failed to interact with the uptake of NE, DA, and 5-HT or with various receptor binding sites for monoamines and histamine.

References

1. Da Prada M, Keller HH, Kettler R, et al. Ro 11-1163, a specific and short acting MAO inhibitor with antidepressant properties. In Kamijo K, Usdin E, Nagatsu T (eds): Monoamine Oxidase. Basic and Clinical Frontiers. Amsterdam: Excerpta Medica, 1981;182.
2. Keller HH, Kettler R, Keller G, et al. Short-acting novel MAO inhibitors: in vitro evidence for the reversibility of MAO inhibition by moclobemide and Ro 16-6491. Naunyn Schmiedebergs Arch Pharmacol 1987;335:12.
3. Schläppi B. The lack of hepatotoxicity in the rat with the new and reversible MAO-A inhibitor moclobemide in contrast to iproniazid. Drug Res 1985;35:800.
4. Kan J-P, Steinberg R, Mouget-Goniot C, et al. SR95191, a selective inhibitor of type A monoamine oxidase with dopaminergic properties. II. Biochemical characterization of monoamine oxidase inhibition. J Pharmacol Exp Ther 1987;240:251.
5. Da Prada M, Kettler R, Burkard WP, et al. Moclobemide, an antidepressant with short-lasting MAO-A inhibition: brain catecholamines and tyramine pressor effects in rats. In Tipton KF, Dostert P, Strolin-Benedetti M (eds): Monoamine Oxidase and Disease. New York: Academic Press, 1984;137.
6. Korn A, Da Prada M, Raffesberg W, et al. Effect of moclobemide, a new reversible monoamine oxidase inhibitor, on absorption and pressor effect of tyramine. J Cardiovasc Pharmacol 1988;11:17.
7. Sulser F, Janowsky AJ, Okada F, et al. Regulation of recognition and action function of the norepinephrine (NE) receptor-coupled adenylate cyclase system in brain: implication for the therapy of depression. Neuropharmacology 1983;22:425.
8. Stefanis CN. Personal communication, 1987.

II NEUROBIOLOGY OF AFFECTIVE DISORDERS

II.A. NEW GENETIC FINDINGS

39. Power of Genetic Linkage Studies for Heterogeneous Disorders

LYNN R. GOLDIN AND ELLIOT S. GERSHON

There is substantial evidence from family, twin, and adoption studies that the major psychiatric disorders (affective disorders and schizophrenia) each have significant genetic components of etiology.[1] Although the mode of genetic transmission is not known, it is possible that single genetic loci cause susceptibility to psychiatric disorders in a proportion of cases. Advances in molecular genetics now make it possible to screen nearly the entire human genome with genetic marker loci in order to locate a particular disease gene. In 1987 a large Amish pedigree with many cases of bipolar illness (and a few cases of unipolar illness) showed strong evidence of linkage of the illness to the insulin gene-*HRAS1* region of chromosome 11,[2] indicating that a major gene for the illness was likely to be located in this region. However, two other studies[3,4] did not find this linkage in families from other populations with similar patterns of illness. This finding suggests that other causes of familial bipolar illness must exist.

It is clear that molecular genetic techniques will be widely used to find genes for psychiatric disorders in the near future. However, several questions are relevant in terms of the application of these methods to behavioral disorders. What types of familial sample should be collected: large pedigrees, small pedigrees, affected sib-pairs? How many individuals are needed? What assumptions should be made about the mode of inheritance, heterogeneity, and population prevalence in order to determine the best linkage strategy?

We have considered the power of the affected-sib-pair (ASP) method and pedigree lod score method when genetic heterogeneity is present, allowing for a range of assumptions with regard to the population prevalence, genetic model, recombination fraction, and proportion of families linked. With respect to bipolar illness, we consider how the linkage finding in the Amish population can be tested in more representative population samples.

Methods

ASP Analyses

The method of linkage analysis using ASPs is based on the fact that, by chance alone, sib-pairs share 2, 1, or 0 marker alleles identical by descent (IBD) with probabilities of 25%, 50%, and 25%, respectively. If *affected*-sib-pairs share two marker alleles significantly more frequently than 25% of the time, it suggests that the disease locus is linked to the marker locus. This method was used to demonstrate linkage of various diseases to the HLA region. Blackwelder and Elston[5] calculated the power of different sib-pair statistics for finding linkage. We have adapted their procedure to calculate the sample size of ASPs needed to find linkage in the presence of heterogeneity. This method assumes that some proportion of ASPs are linked and the remainder are not linked to the marker locus. We have assumed that whether a sib-pair share 2, 1, or 0 alleles IBD is known exactly. We have examined dominant and recessive models with reduced penetrance for disorders with both 1% and 7% population prevalence. These prevalences correspond to those for schizophrenia (or bipolar illness) and major affective disorder (including both bipolar and unipolar), respectively.

Lod Score Analyses

In order to calculate the number of families needed to find linkage under different assumptions, a defined pedigree structure consisting of 17 individuals in three generations, 8 of them designated affected, was used. Simulation was then used to assign marker allele phenotypes to all individuals based on the likelihood of the family given the disease gene parameters, the recombination fraction, and the probability that the family was of the "linked" type. The marker locus was assumed to be maximally informative; that is, all unrelated individuals were heterozygous and different from their mates. Different numbers of families were simulated. For each set of parameters and number of families, ten replicate samples were generated. The hypotheses of linkage and heterogeneity were evaluated for each sample using the admixture test of Smith[6] as described by Ott.[7] We examined two genetic models: a dominant gene with high penetrance (85%) corresponding to the parameters found in the Amish pedigree[2] and a dominant gene with reduced (50%) penetrance. For each model we varied the recombination fraction and the proportion of families linked.

Results and Discussion

Affected-Sib-Pairs

Table 39.1 shows the number of ASPs required to detect linkage with 80% power for several sets of assumptions. A larger sample size is needed if the disorder is dominant (rather than recessive). This result is expected because a recessive disease always leads to a more skewed IBD distribution in ASPs. For a disorder with 1%

TABLE 39.1. Number of Affected-sib-pairs required to find linkage with 80% power.

Model	Recombination fraction	100% Linked	50% Linked
Recessive	0.01	7	29
	0.05	11	40
	0.10	19	63
Dominant	0.01	7	50
	0.05	15	72
	0.10	27	120

Population prevalence: 1%.

prevalence, linkage is not difficult to detect when there is no heterogeneity. A maximum of 30 ASPs would be required when transmission of the disease is dominant. However, when only 50% of families are linked, the sample size increases as much as fivefold. For example, if schizophrenia were dominantly inherited, 120 ASPs would be sufficient to find linkage up to 10% recombination and 50% heterogeneity. However, if only 25% of families were linked, 200 ASPs would be needed (results not shown) if linkage were close (1% recombination). In the case of a disorder with 7% population prevalence, the results (not shown) are nearly the same as with 1% prevalence when the transmission is recessive. However, a sample size approximately one-third larger is needed to detect linkage under the dominant case because, with a higher population frequency, an unaffected parent would be more likely to carry the disease gene, causing the IBD distribution to be less skewed. We have also considered the case of Alzheimer's disease, which is hypothesized to be transmitted as an autosomal dominant trait with nearly complete penetrance by age 85–90.[8] This fact is especially relevant because of the finding of linkage to chromosome 21 markers in familial, early-onset cases. If this linkage were present in a large proportion of late-onset cases, the ASP method would offer a good alternative to test this hypothesis. Approximately 60 ASPs would be sufficient to find close linkage if only 50% of cases were linked.

It should be remembered that these calculations assume that the marker is highly polymorphic and that the sharing of marker alleles is known exactly in each ASP. In most cases, it would require sampling the parents of each sib-pair. However, other methods of ASP analysis could make the test more efficient, such as sampling more than two affected per family.

Lod Score Analyses

Table 39.2 shows the approximate number of families needed to detect linkage in at least 80% of the generated samples under the two models of dominant inheritance that we tested. These results are approximate because only a few sample sizes were tested and the results are based on only ten replicate samples. Nonetheless, several trends are evident. When there is no heterogeneity or very close linkage, linkage is not difficult to detect. Ten families are sufficient up to 50% heterogeneity. As expected, increasing numbers of families are needed as heterogeneity increases and as either penetrance is reduced or recombination increases. Thus if the number of families in an actual study were limited, in order to have a high probability of detecting a true linkage the investigator would have to screen more of the genome in order to reduce the maximum recombination fraction between the disease and marker loci.

TABLE 39.2. Approximate number of moderate sized families needed to detect linkage in at least 80% of generated samples.

Penetrance	Recombination fraction	100% Linked	50% Linked	25% Linked
High (85%)	0.01	< 10	< 10	20
	0.05	< 10	10	20
	0.10	< 10	10	> 30
Reduced (50%)	0.01	< 10	< 10	20
	0.05	< 10	10–20	> 30
	0.10	< 10	20	> 30

Conclusions

It is clear that the ASP and pedigree lod score method each have their advantages and disadvantages. The lod score method appears generally more efficient, but the ASP method may be preferable in cases where intact pedigrees are difficult to obtain. In either case, to be able to rigorously test linkage hypotheses, allowing for heterogeneity and a variety of modes of genetic transmission, relatively large samples are needed, which emphasizes the need to design large, multicenter collaborative studies.

References

1. Nurnberger JI Jr, Goldin LR, Gershon ES. Genetics of psychiatric disorders. In Winokur G, Clayton P (eds): Medical Basis of Psychiatry. Philadelphia: Saunders, 1986;486–521.
2. Egeland JA, Gerhard DS, Pauls DL, et al. Bipolar affective disorders linked to DNA markers on chromosome 11. Nature 1987;325:797–801.
3. Detera-Wadleigh S, Berrettini WH, Goldin LR, et al. Close linkage of c-Harvey-ras-1 and insulin to affective disorder is ruled out in 3 North American pedigrees. Nature 1987;325:806–808.
4. Hodgkinson S, Sherrington R, Gurling H, et al. Molecular genetic evidence for heterogeneity in manic depression. Nature 1987;325:805–806.
5. Blackwelder WC, Elston RC. A comparison of sib-pair linkage tests for disease susceptibility loci. Genet Epidemiol 1985;2:85–97.
6. Smith CAB. Testing for heterogeneity of recombination fraction values in human genetics. Ann Hum Genet 1963;27:175–182.
7. Ott J. Analysis of Human Genetic Linkage. Baltimore: Johns Hopkins University Press, 1985.
8. Breitner JCS, Murphy EA, Folstein MF. Familial aggregation in Alzheimer's disease. I. A model for age-dependent expression of an autosomal dominant gene. J Psychiatr Res 1986;20:31–43.

40. Single Locus Markers in Affective Disorders

ELLIOT S. GERSHON

In the affective disorders, the fact that multifactorial models are consistent with some studies and single locus models are usually rejected does not necessarily rule out single locus inheritance. The power of these methods to detect major loci in complex diseases may be low. Goldin et al.[1] found by simulation that a single locus for a disease could not be identified for certain modes of inheritance, especially "quasirecessive" inheritance, where the heterozygote individuals have low, but not zero, penetrance. In addition, if affective disorders are genetically heterogeneous, the detection of single locus genetic mechanisms may require a valid linkage marker or single-gene vulnerability factor.

The importance of finding a genetic marker, whether as an inherited vulnerability factor or as a chromosomal linkage marker, is self-evident. It would provide important information on the inherited pathophysiological event and have immediate application to prevention and treatment.

Gene mapping provides a general approach to locating single locus markers. One can systematically study all genes active in the central nervous system, specific to the central nervous system, or active in specific chromosomal regions about which one has a hypothesis. With the advent of molecular genetic methods, mapping of the entire human genome with respect to an illness is now close to a practical possibility. The gene mapping approach using restriction fragment length polymorphisms (RFLPs) of genomic DNA has proved valuable in several studies in neurological and psychiatric disorders, including the affective disorders.

The power of a linkage demonstration is that it unequivocally ties the transmission of illness to a particular gene region, although it does not actually specify which gene within that region is responsible for the illness. Linkage also aids greatly in resolving genetic heterogeneity once it is established, although it should be noted that the presence of heterogeneity makes linkage more difficult to detect.

Restriction Fragment Length Polymorphisms on Chromosome 11

The use of large pedigrees in linkage studies is based on the assumption that even in an illness that is genetically heterogeneous there will be genetic homogeneity within pedigrees. It is questionable for a common disease in a large population, where persons marrying into the pedigree may bring in different forms of illness; but in a population isolate, homogeneity may be considered more likely, at least within a pedigree. The Amish population studied by Egeland is an isolate in which several large pedigrees segregating for affective illness have been identified. In one pedigree Egeland et al.[2] found autosomal dominant transmission and linkage of bipolar and unipolar illness to the insulin-*ras* oncogene region of the short arm of chromosome 11. In Bethesda we have found this linkage not to be present in three smaller pedigrees,[3] and Hodgkinson et al.[4] did not find this linkage in three Icelandic pedigrees. It is difficult to find methodological fault with the Amish study, as the pedigrees were cultured, with the diagnoses and cells available to interested scientists, before the chromosome 11 markers were applied to it. The nonreplication seems to be due to genetic heterogeneity in this case, with the implication that the Amish form of manic-depressive illness is genetically uncommon in the other populations studied.

Color Blindness Region of X Chromosome

Between 1969 and 1974 Winokur and his colleagues, and shortly afterward Mendlewicz and co-workers, reported that bipolar illness is linked to the X-chromosome markers Xg blood group and protan-deutan color blindness.[5-9] At the time of the initial reports, it was not known that these results were inconsistent with each other because linkage of bipolar illness to both Xg and to protan and deutan color blindness is not compatible with the known large chromosomal map distance between the Xg locus (on the short arm) and the protan-deutan region (at the tip of the long arm).

We were unable to replicate either of these linkages in our own data. For both Xg and protan-deutan color blindness, close linkage to affective illness was ruled out.[10,11] Our pedigrees were not heterogeneous with respect to each other, and there were no single pedigrees strongly suggesting linkage to either marker. Mendlewicz and associates,[12] on the other hand, reported eight new families in Belgium and suggested linkage to color blindness in at least one.

It has been argued[8] that there is linkage to color blindness but not Xg blood group, and that heterogeneity accounts for differences among investigators. This proposal is difficult to accept when the initial series was so strikingly positive and the replication series so negative, and in view of the inconsistency of the intial finding that both Xg and color blindness were linked to bipolar illness. If methodological errors in diagnostic or ascertainment procedures produced the unique homogeneity of the 1972–1974 pedigree series of Mendlewicz and colleagues, it would explain why the strikingly positive results are not replicated in either our series or the later series of Mendlewicz et al.[12]

Strongly positive, multigenerational pedigrees for the red-green color blindness linkage have since been reported by Baron and co-workers,[13] and Mendlewicz and co-workers have reported linkage to the glucose-6-phosphate dehydrogenase (G6PD) locus (a marker on the X chromosome close to the red-green color blindness loci)[14] and to the blood clotting factor IX, which is within 15–30 centiMorgans of the red-green color blindness region.[15]

DNA probes for this region of the X chromosome now exist, and their use may make virtually all pedigrees informative for linkage and lead to a resolution of the controversy of whether there is a generally reproducible finding of linkage to the color-blindness region in a portion of manic-depressives. My colleagues (Berrettini, Gelernter, Detera-Wadleigh) and I have applied the St14 probe of Oberle et al.,[16] which marks the color blindness of the X chromosome to new manic-depressive pedigrees, and we continue to find linkage to be excluded; further pedigrees will be studied before these results are published.

References

1. Goldin LR, Cox NJ, Pauls DL, et al: The detection of major loci by segregation and linkage analysis: a simulation study. Genet Epidemiol 1984;1:285–296.
2. Egeland JA, Gerhard DS, Pauls DL, et al. Bipolar affective disorders linked to DNA markers on chromosome 11. Nature 1987;325:783–787.
3. Detera-Wadleigh SD, Berrettini WH, Goldin LR, et al. Close linkage of c-Harvey-ras-1 and the insulin gene to affective disorder is ruled out in three North American pedigrees. Nature 1987;325:806–808.
4. Hodgkinson S, Sherrington R, Gurling H, et al. Molecular genetic evidence for heterogeneity in manic depression. Nature 1987;325:804–806.
5. Reich T, Clayton PJ, Winokur G: Family history studies. V. The genetics of mania. Am J Psychiatry 1969;125:1358–1369.
6. Baron M, Rainer JD, Risch N. X-linkage in bipolar affective illness. J Affective Dis 1981;3:141–157.
7. Winokur G, Tanna VL: Possible role of X-linked dominant factor in manic-depressive disease. Dis Nerv Sys 1969;30:87–94.
8. Risch N, Baron M. X-linkage and genetic heterogeneity in bipolar-related major affective illness: reanalysis of linkage data. Ann Hum Genet 1982;46:153–166.
9. Mendlewicz J, Fleiss JL: Linkage studies with X-chromosome markers in bipolar (manic-depressive) and unipolar (depressive) illnesses. Biol Psychiatry 1974;9:261–294.
10. Leckman JF, Gershon ES, McGinniss MH, et al. New data do not suggest linkage between the Xg blood group and bipolar illness. Arch Gen Psychiatry 1979;36:1435–1441.
11. Gershon ES, Targum SD, Matthysse S, et al. Color blindness not closely linked to bipolar illness. Arch Gen Psychiatry 1979;36:1423–1430.
12. Mendlewicz J, Linkowski P, Guroff JJ, et al. Color blindness linkage to bipolar manic-depressive illness: new evidence. Arch Gen Psychiatry 1987;36:1442–1447.
13. Baron M, Risch N, Hamburger R, et al. Genetic linkage between X-chromosome markers and bipolar affective illness. Nature 1987;326:289–292.
14. Mendlewicz J, Linkowski P, Wilmotte J. Linkage between glucose-6-phosphate dehydrogenase deficiency and manic-depressive psychosis. Br J Psychiatry 1980;137:337–342.
15. Mendlewicz J, Sevy S, Brocas H, et al. Polymorphic DNA marker on X chromosome and manic depression. Lancet 1987;30:1230–1232.
16. Oberle I, Drayna D, Camerino G, et al. The telomeric region of the human X chromosome long arm: presence of a highly polymorphic DNA marker and analysis of recombination frequency. Proc Natl Acad Sci USA 1985;82:2824–2828.

41. One Form of Bipolar Affective Disorder is Mapped to Chromosome 11

KENNETH K. KIDD, JANICE A. EGELAND,
DANIELA S. GERHARD, DAVID L. PAULS,
JAMES N. SUSSEX, CLEONA R. ALLEN,
ABRAM M. HOSTETTER, JUDITH R. KIDD,
ANDREW J. PAKSTIS, AND DAVID E. HOUSMAN

Geneticists have long recognized the power of genetic linkage as a tool in understanding complex traits, but lack of adequate numbers of genetic markers in humans has been a barrier to the use of genetic linkage to understand complex human disorders. The discovery of large numbers of genetic markers identifiable directly in the DNA—the restriction fragment length polymorphisms (RFLPs)—and the rapidly developing international effort to map the human genome have removed that barrier. Genetic linkage can now be used routinely to identify major loci responsible for complex human disorders as the first step toward understanding the etiology and pathogenesis of a disorder. Here we briefly review the evidence for a major locus causing bipolar affective disorder and discuss some of the implications of the finding.

The families of manic depressive probands in the Old Order Amish have a combination of characteristics making them especially suitable for genetic linkage studies.[1-3] One particular family was chosen in the early 1980s for initial attempts at linkage using RFLPs. Among the first markers tested were several on the short arm of chromosome 11: *HBBC*, *D11S12*, *INS*, and *HRAS1*. These loci were chosen because they were among the first very polymorphic markers that were all on the same chromosome arm. Unexpectedly, when linkage analyses were run between these markers and a hypothesized locus for manic depressive illness, the results were positive, favoring linkage to the *INS-HRAS1* region with odds of 50:1.[2,4] That result could not be considered significant but was sufficiently suggestive to warrant studies of additional family members focused on those markers. While those studies were being pursued, many other markers on other chromosomes were being studied[5] and provided evidence against linkage to many parts of the genome (Table 41.1). The linkage result on chromosome 11 is now highly significant evidence for linkage.[3]

The curve in Figure 41.1 summarizes the evidence for linkage of the postulated locus for affective disorders to the *INS* and *HRAS1* locus. The maximum point occurs 2 centiMorgans (cM) distal to *HRAS1* with a lod score of 4.96, indicating

TABLE 41.1. Distribution of lod scores for 41 RFLP loci[a].

Model	No. of loci with lod scores in each interval at $\theta = 0$			
	< -2	-2 to -1	-1 to 0	0 to $+1$
M	9	17	11	4
H	20	13	3	5

[a]The distribution of the lod scores for the RFLPs segregating in pedigree OOA110 gave evidence that the locus for affective disorders either was not located nearby (lod < -1) or it was uninformative (lod betwen -1 and $+1$).[5] The two models used were based on analyses presented in Egeland et al.[3]

odds of greater than 90,000:1 favoring linkage over chance as the explanation for the data. However, the curve is broad, and the 95% confidence interval encompasses the region from 17 cM proximal to *INS* to more than 25 cM distal to *HRAS1*. (*HRAS1* is near the end of the chromosome so that statistical distance on the distal side may have no biological meaning.) Testing of additional loci may narrow the confidence interval; one of those loci is the gene for tyrosine hydroxylase *(TH)*, as discussed below.

We find these results convincing. They indicate that a locus exists near *INS* and *HRAS1* and that a variant allele at this locus predisposes individuals carrying it to develop an affective disorder, primarily manic depressive illness. However,

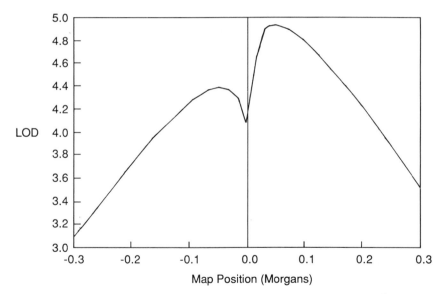

FIGURE 41.1. Results of multipoint linkage analyses of the data of Egeland et al.[3] Each point on the curve gives the relative odds for the locus for affective disorders being at that position on the genetic map defined by the *INS* (O.OM) and *HRAS1* (0.031M) loci. This figure differs from that in Egeland et al.[3] only in that lod scores have been calculated for additional points; the data, parameter values, and statistical methods are as described in that report.
[Reprinted by permission from *Nature* 1987; 325:783–787. Copyright (C) 1987 MacMillan Journals Limited.]

this predisposing allele does not necessarily exist in other families with bipolar affective disorder. As shown by Hodgkinson et al.,[6] Detera-Wadleigh et al.,[7] and Baron et al.,[8] there are definitely families in which manic depressive illness is caused by a predisposing allele at some other locus elsewhere in the genome, an unidentified autosomal locus in some cases and an X-linked locus in others. The existence of genetic heterogeneity for manic depressive illness seemed *a priori* likely to human geneticists and has now been confirmed. Although research continues toward identifying the actual genes for the chromosome 11 form and the X-linked form, the search for the other autosomal form(s) goes on.

Given the very speculative state on the chromosome 11 linkage of affective disorders when *TH* was first shown to be somewhere on chromosome 11,[9] linkage provided only minimal scientific support for hypotheses relating *TH* to bipolar affective disorder. By the end of 1986 the situation had changed dramatically. *TH* was mapped to the tip of 11p by *in situ* hybridization[10] and placed on the linkage maps just 3 cM distal to *HRAS1*.[11] Can it be mere chance that a neuropsychiatric disorder and a known gene of fundamental relevance to all catecholamine synthesis map to the identical small region, or has the map indicated what the etiological defect is for one form of affective disorder? Although there are many relevant caveats, hypotheses relating the two loci are certainly strengthened by the linkage result. The major caveat is that the predisposing gene for bipolar affective disorder and *TH* have been mapped only with wide margins of uncertainty. These two loci might easily be more than 10 cM apart based on current data. If, however, we take the most likely map position of each, they are both just distal to *HRAS1*, mapped to essentially the same place.

Can *TH*, a locus fundamentally involved in catecholamine synthesis, cause a disorder that is episodic and limited to such a narrow range of possible neuropsychiatric symptoms? At first it seems too simplistic a hypothesis. However, Grima et al.[12] have shown that TH enzyme levels have complex regulation. Because different parts of the DNA sequence are involved in the different kinds of regulation, it is possible that a mutational change in one place in the DNA could affect *TH* enzyme activity (including its regulation) in one neuronal pathway while activity in all other tissues was normal.

Even if *TH* is not the gene involved, knowing the chromosomal region provides a powerful assist to studies that should shortly provide much more understanding of the etiology and pathogenesis of one form of bipolar affective disorder.

Acknowledgments. Preparation of this chapter was supported by grants from the National Institutes of Mental Health (MH30929 and MH39239). The study of Egeland et al.[3] was also supported by grants from the National Institutes of Mental Health (MH28287, MH00508, and MH28274).

References

1. Egeland JA, Hostetter AM. Amish study I: affective disorders among the Amish, 1976–1980. Am J Psychiatry 1983;140:56–61.
2. Kidd KK, Gerhard DS, Kidd JR, et al. Recombinant DNA methods in genetic studies of affective disorders. Clin Neuropharmacol 1984;7:198–199.
3. Egeland JA, Gerhard DS, Pauls DL, et al. Bipolar affective disorders linked to DNA markers on chromosome 11. Nature 1987;325:783–787.

4. Gerhard DS, Egeland JA, Pauls DL, et al. Is a gene for affective disorder located on the short arm of chromosome 11? Am J Hum Genet 1984;36:3S.
5. Kidd JR, Egeland JA, Pakstis AJ, et al. Searching for a major genetic locus for affective disorder in the Old Order Amish. J Psychiatr Res 1987;21:577–580.
6. Hodgkinson S, Sherrington R, Gurling H, et al. Molecular genetic evidence for heterogeneity in manic depression. Nature 1987;325:805–808.
7. Detera-Wadleigh SD, Berrettini WH, Goldin LR, et al. Close linkage of c-Harvey-ras-1 and the insulin gene to affective disorder is ruled out in three North American pedigrees. Nature 1987;325:806–808.
8. Baron M, Risch N, Hamburger R, et al. Genetic linkage between X-chromosome markers and bipolar affective illness. Nature 1987;326:289–292.
9. Powell J, Bino C, Lamouroux A, et al. Assignment of the human tyrosine hyroxylase gene to chromosome 11. FEBS Lett 1984;175:37–40.
10. Craig S, Buckle V, Lamouroux A, et al. Localization of the human tyrosine hydroxylase gene to 11p15: gene duplication and evolution of metabolic pathways. Cytogenet Cell Genet 1986;42:29–32.
11. Moss PAH, Davies KE, Boni C, et al. Linkage of tyrosine hydroxylase to four other markers on the short arm of chromosome 11. Nucleic Acids Res 1986;14:9927–9932.
12. Grima B, Lamouroux A, Boni C, et al. A single human gene encoding multiple tyrosine hydroxylases with different predicted functional characteristics. Nature 1987;326:707–711.

42. X-Linkage Studies in Affective Disorders

MIRON BARON

Bipolar affective illness is a major and relatively common psychiatric condition characterized by recurrent manic and depressive episodes and variable age at onset. It has long been recognized that heredity plays an important role in the etiology of bipolar illness. This notion originated in studies of familial aggregation and was reinforced by twin and adoption data that favored a substantial genetic component in the transmission of the disorder. Yet the mode of genetic transmission and the specific genes involved remain unknown.

Genetic linkage studies offer a powerful approach to the elucidation of genetic mechanisms. Here we concern ourselves with X-chromosome polymorphisms as potential linkage markers for bipolar affective disorder. The X-linkage hypothesis is reviewed in the light of methodological developments, and new data are presented on linkage of bipolar illness to the X chromosome markers color blindness and glucose-6-phosphate dehydrogenase (G6PD) deficiency. The potential contribution of recombinant DNA techniques to linkage studies in affective disorders is discussed.

X-Linkage Hypothesis

The X-linkage hypothesis of bipolar illness has been debated for at least half a century. Women are more commonly affected than men, and in some families the disorder is seldom transmitted from father to son. Both circumstances point to the X chromosome as a possible site for the purported bipolar gene.

Segregation analysis of family data has ruled out X linkage as the exclusive mode of genetic transmission[1–3;] however, in light of the secular trend (generational differences in the rates of affective illness)[4,5] and the likely heterogeneous nature of the disorder, the results from traditional types of model fitting, e.g., segregation analysis, are difficult to interpret. To address this issue we performed logistic regression analysis incorporating generational, sex, and X-linkage effects on three major data sets obtained from North American and European populations.[5] In all three samples, the largest effect was due to X-linkage; the results also suggested genetic heterogeneity in that only a subgroup of bipolar individuals carry the X-linked gene.

Linkage studies with the X-chromosome markers color blindness, G6PD deficiency, and the Xg blood group have not yielded consistent results.[6-8] Although the discrepancy among the various studies can be ascribed to methodological issues and genetic heterogeneity,[6-8] the possibility of systematic bias in some of the earlier studies has been raised,[9] especially in the light of the claim by some investigators that bipolar illness is linked to both color blindness and Xg[10]; this claim is deemed incompatible with the X-chromosome map owing to the large distance between the loci for color vision and Xg.

The conflicting results and the methodological uncertainties have underscored the need for independent replication of the X-linkage findings. Also, the success of any genetic linkage study is greatly dependent on the quality of the family material and on the availability of a highly polymorphic genetic marker.

Most of the studies so far reported have not met these requirements. Large multigeneration pedigrees with mulitple affected cases have been in short supply; additionally, the frequency of the genetic markers color blindness and G6PD deficiency in the populations from which the bulk of the pedigrees were drawn is fairly low. These limitations have compromised the power of previous linkage studies of X-chromosome markers and, in some measure, may explain the paucity of pedigrees strongly suggestive of linkage. Clearly, more effort was needed to pin down the X-linkage relations for bipolar affective illness using suitable data.

US–Israel Binational Study

The Israeli population is particularly suitable for genetic linkage studies of affective illness owing to the high geographic concentration, the stability and accessibility of families, the availability of large pedigrees especially in the non-Ashkenazi community, the high frequency of the X-chromosome marker G6PD deficiency among certain non-Ashkenazi groups, and the low rate of alcoholism and drug use. It was for these reasons that this population was selected to extend and replicate the X-linkage data on bipolar affective disorder. The study is described in detail elsewhere.[11]

Briefly, the sample was composed of five large multigeneration pedigrees ascertained through bipolar probands. The families contained 161 adult individuals, 47 of whom were ill with bipolar illness or related affective disorder. Four pedigrees segregated for color blindness, and one pedigree segregated for G6PD deficiency. Four of the five pedigrees were non-Ashkenazi, and one pedigree was Ashkenazi. The data were analyzed for linkage of color blindness or G6PD deficiency to bipolar illness using the computer program LIPED, allowing for age-dependent penetrance. The data were also subjected to multipoint analysis for the combined lod scores for both color blindness and G6PD. The results showed close linkage of bipolar affective illness to the color blindness–G6PD region. This particular linkage was found only in the non-Ashkenazi pedigrees. The maximum lod score ranged from 7.52 (assuming homogeneity of the sample) to 9.17 (assuming heterogeneity); thus the odds in favor of linkage ranged between 30 million to 1 and 1 billion to 1.

Implications and Future Course

The ability to trace the genetic defect to a specific region of the genetic material is a major advance in our understanding of the biology of bipolar affective illness. What are the implications of this finding?

First, although the faulty genes have yet to be identified, our finding has narrowed the search to a well circumscribed region of a particular chromosome. It now appears that the gene for one form of manic-depression resides in close proximity to the DNA segments that give rise to the inherited traits of color blindness and the biochemical defect G6PD deficiency. Molecular genetic techniques can now be harnessed to examine DNA polymorphisms in the color blindness–G6PD region with the aim of replicating the X-linkage findings in different populations and estimating the fraction of the X-linked cases in the bipolar population. In addition, these methods could be used to identify and characterize the structure of the bipolar gene and to elucidate its biological function. These data, in turn, could shed light on the biochemistry of the illness and pave the way to treatment measures that are better focused and more specific than those available at this time.

Second, genes are not necessarily destiny. Not all individuals who inherit the gene get the disease. There may be biological or environmental factors that interact with the genetic disposition to prevent expression of the illness. By the same token, offensive or injurious circumstances, in conjunction with the genetic risk, can increase the likelihood of illness. Once we understand the nature of these interactions and the biological function of the gene itself, we should be able to devise specific preventive and treatment measures. This goal, however, is some distance away.

Third, the X-linked form of bipolar illness is not the only form there is. Another group of researchers[12] have reported linkage between genetic markers on chromosome 11 and bipolar disorder in the Old Order Amish population in Pennsylvania. Thus we have what appear to be two genetic types of the illness that are tied to different chromsomes. It is not unlikely that other forms, both genetic and nongenetic, will be discovered. A case in point is mental retardation, where many types, each with its own set of causes, have been revealed. The finding of different illness types may have practical implications because it could eventually help clinicians tailor treatment to different cases of bipolar illness should the underlying biochemistry vary among the different types.

Fourth, as we gather more knowledge, the discovery of genetic markers could prove helpful for detecting individuals who have this genetic endowment and are therefore at risk for the disorder. That is, they could be given genetic counseling.

Finally, by showing that some forms of the illness are strongly influenced by genetic factors, it is hoped that the social stigma attached to bipolar illness can be removed. However, the biological stigma may have its own inherent problems.

Summary

Although the most recent findings have no immediate implications for the prevention and treatment of bipolar affective illness, we believe that they constitute major steps toward achieving this goal. In conjunction with the explosion in human genetic research, these studies herald a new era in medical genetics generally and psychiatric genetics particularly.

Acknowledgments. The other participants in the US–Israel Collaborative Study were Neil Risch, Ph.D., Rahel Hamburger, Ph.D., Batsheva Mandel, Stuart Kushner, M.D., Michael Newman, Ph.D., Dov Drumer, M.D., and Robert H.

Belmaker, M.D. The study was supported by NIMH RSD Award MH00176 to Dr. Baron, NIH RCD Award HD00648 to Dr. Risch, and grants from the NIMH (MH36963) and the US–Israel Binational Science Foundation (No. 3350).

References

1. Bucher KD, Elston RC, Green R, et al. The transmission of manic-depressive illness. II. Segregation analysis of three sets of family data J Psychiatr Res 1981;16:65–78.
2. Fieve RR, Go R, Dunner DL, et al. Search for biological/genetic markers in a long-term epidemiological and morbid risk study of affective disorders. J Psychiatr Res 1984;18:425–445.
3. Tsuang MT, Bucher KD, Fleming JA, et al. Transmission of affective disorders: an application of segregation analysis to blind family study data. J Psychiatr Res 1985;19:23–30.
4. Klerman GL, Lavori PW, Rice J, et al. Birth-cohort trends in rates of major depressive disorders among relatives of patients with affective disorders. Arch Gen Psychiatry 1985;42:689–693.
5. Risch N, Baron M, Mendlewicz J. Assessing the role of X-linked inheritance in bipolar-related major affective illness. J Psychiatr Res 1986;20:275–288.
6. Gershon ES, Mendlewicz J, Castpar M, et al. A collaborative study of genetic linkage of bipolar manic-depressive illness and red/green colorblindness. Acta Psychiatr Scand 1980;61:319–338.
7. Baron M, Rainer JD, Risch N. X-linkage in bipolar affective illness: perspectives on genetic heterogeneity, pedigree analysis and the X-chromosome map. J Affective Bias 1981;3:141–157.
8. Risch N, Baron M. X-linkage and genetic heterogeneity in bipolar-related major affective illness: re-analysis of linkage data. Ann Hum Gene 1982;46:153–166.
9. Gershon ES, Bunney WE Jr. The question of X-linkage in bipolar manic-depressive illness. J Psychiatr Res 1976;13:99–117.
10. Mendlewicz J, Fleiss JL. Linkage studies with X-chromosome markers in bipolar (manic-depressive) and unipolar (depressive) illness. Biol Psychiatry 1974;9:261–294.
11. Baron M, Risch N, Hamburger R, et al: Genetic linkage between X-chromosome markers and bipolar affective illness. Nature 1987;326:289–292.
12. Egeland JA, Gerhard DS, Pauls DL, et al: Bipolar affective disorders linked to DNA markers on chromosome 11. Nature 1987;325:783–787.

43. Recombinant DNA Studies of X Linkage in Affective Disorders

JULIEN MENDLEWICZ

Heredity is an important contributing factor in the vulnerability to manic-depressive illness. Family, twin, and adoption studies corroborate the genetic diathesis for the illness, but these studies do not elucidate the mode of transmission of manic-depressive psychosis.[1-4] The use of linkage analysis has become widespread but has rarely been applied to psychiatric conditions. Linkage studies using color blindness and glucose-6-phosphate dehydrogenase (G6PD) deficiency as X-chromosome markers have shown that a dominant X-linked gene may be involved in the genetic transmission of a subtype of bipolar manic-depressive illness (MDI).[1,5-12] The maximal lod score reported for the MDI-G6PD linkage was 4.21 at a recombination fraction of $\theta = 0.06$.[10] However, instances of apparent father-to-son transmission of the illness have been described in family studies performed by us and by others,[2,13] and data that do not support a linkage between color blindness and bipolar illness have also been reported.[14] Genetic heterogeneity, as has been previously postulated for manic depression,[11,15,16] could account for these apparently contradictory findings. According to this model, only a subgroup of bipolar pedigrees will show close linkage to the X chromosome and thus carry the X-linked gene, but not all bipolar illness can be X-linked. The increasing number of restriction fragment length polymorphisms (RFLPs) characterized in humans makes it possible to apply new linkage analysis using selected DNA probes.

Patients and Methods

Previous linkage studies had pointed to the subterminal region of the long arm of the X chromosome as a possible site for the MDI locus.[1,5-12] Therefore a factor IX probe,[17] which is known to hybridize to the Xq27 band,[18] was used to test the hypothesis that the disease trait and a common RFLP at the F9 locus[18,19] would co-segregate in a series of informative pedigrees. The pedigrees of all consecutive admissions of unipolar or bipolar probands between April 1983 and May 1986 to the Department of Psychiatry, Erasme Hospital, the Free University of Brussels were screened for possible linkage analysis. The patients were referred by private physicians, outpatient clinics, and both state and private hospitals. The existence of secondary cases in the patient's families was not a criterion for admission to treatment. In this sample, about 30% of our patients had a family history of manic-depression.

The pedigree data were first obtained from the proband and available relatives at the time of admission. The "family study method" (i.e., personal interview with all available relatives) was used after obtaining informed consent because this method has been proved to be more reliable than the "family history method" (i.e., family data collected from the proband only[20]). Pertinent medical and social records about probands and relatives were used when available.

All probands, spouses, and available relatives were separately examined by two investigators who used the Schedule for Affective Disorders and Schizophrenia[21] according to the research diagnostic criteria of Spitzer et al.[22] Assessment of the family members was carried out in blind with respect to the proband's diagnosis. Disagreements were referred to the senior investigator (J.M.), who blindly determined the final diagnoses, using all available sources of information. All diagnoses were made independently based on DNA marker analysis.

Those subjects diagnosed as bipolar, unipolar, or cyclothymic (i.e., primary affective disorders[23]) were considered "affectively ill." Subjects with secondary depression or alcoholism were considered "well." We have previously shown that within a family unit identified by an affectively ill proband, bipolar illness, unipolar illness, and cyclothymia are genetically related phenotypes expressing the same genotype.[4–6]

DNA samples were prepared from peripheral leukocytes of probands and available relatives. They were analyzed for the presence of Taq 1 polymorphism at the F9 locus.[18,19]

Results

Among a sample of 24 families of probands with two or more affected relatives, ten pedigrees were found to be informative for linkage analysis between MDI and the F9 locus. Figure 43.1 illustrates one informative pedigree with the relevant clinical and RFLP data and the lod score curve for all pedigrees.

A statistical analysis of the pedigrees was performed using the "LINKAGE" program of Lathrope et al.[24] The resulting lod score curve displays a maximal lod score of 3.10 at $\theta = 0.11$, which is strong indication for the existence of a linkage between a MDI locus and factor IX in the Xq 27 region.

Although most pedigrees we analyzed were compatible with a full penetrance of the disease, lod score analysis was also performed using different values of the penetrance. If the considered penetrance is 0.9 or 0.8, the peak lod scores obtained were 2.75 and 2.40, respectively. Thus the results were still highly suggestive for the existence of a linkage.

Discussion

Our findings do not support the report of a possible linkage between MDI and a locus on chromosome 11 in one Amish family,[25] which was also not replicated in three Icelandic and three North American families.[26,27] Our results with the DNA recombinant method confirmed early and more recent linkage studies in manic-depression using color blindness and G6PD deficiency as genetic markers.[1,5–12,28]

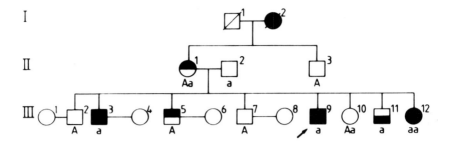

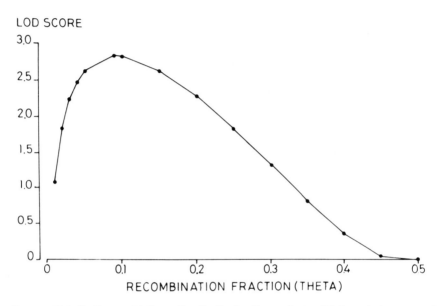

FIGURE 43.1. Pedigree of informative family for the analysis of linkage between manic depression and a Taq I polymorphism at the factor IX locus and lod score curve. Circles represent female members; squares represent male members. A black symbol indicates subjects with bipolar (full) or unipolar (half) illness. A slashed symbol indicates deceased individuals. The arrow identifies the propositus.

The known heterogeneity of MDI together with the high degree of inbreeding in the Amish may provide some explanation for this apparent discrepancy. The localization of an MDI locus in the subterminal region of the long arm of the X chromosome may have important implications for the mapping of gene loci in this region of the human X chromosome and raises a number of interesting possibilities, among which are the banking of DNA samples form high-risk persons and ultimately the isolation and sequencing of the gene responsible for the disease.

References

1. Winokur G, Clayton P, Reich T. Manic Depressive Illness. St. Louis: Mosby, 1969.
2. Mendlewicz J, Rainer JD. Morbidity risk and genetic transmission in manic-depressive illness. Am J Hum Genet 1974;25:692–701.

3. Kallmann FJ. Genetic principles in manic-depressive psychoses. In Hoch P, Zubin J (eds): Depression. New York: Grune & Stratton, 1954;1–24.
4. Mendlewicz J, Rainer JD. Adoption study supporting genetic transmission in manic-depressive illness. Nature 1977;268:327–329.
5. Mendlewicz J, Fleiss JL, Fieve RR. Evidence for X-linkage in the transmission in manic-depressive illness. JAMA 1972;222:1624–1627.
6. Mendlewicz J, Fleiss JL. Linkage studies with X-chromosome markers in bipolar (manic-depressive) and unipolar depressive illness. Biol Psychiatry 1974;9:261–294.
7. Belmaker RH, Wyatt RJ. Possible X-linkage in a family with varied psychoses. Isr Ann Psychiatry 1976;14:345–353.
8. Baron M. Linkage between an X-chromosome marker (deutan color blindness) and bipolar affective illness. Arch Gen Psychiatry 1977;24:721–727.
9. Mendlewicz J, Linkowski P, Guroff JJ, et al. Color blindness linkage to bipolar manic-depressive illness: new evidence. Arch Gen Psychiatry 1979;36:1442–1447.
10. Mendlewicz J, Linkowski P, Wilmotte J. Linkage between glucose-6-phosphate dehydrogenase deficiency and manic-depressive psychoses. Br J Psychiatry 1980;137:337–342.
11. Gershon ES, Mendlewicz J, Gaspar M. A collaborative study of genetic linkage of bipolar manic-depressive illness and red/green color blindness. Acta Psychiatr Scand 1980;61:319–338.
12. Del Zompo M, Bocochetta A, Goldin LR, et al. Linkage between X-chromosome markers and mani-depressive illness, two Sardinian pedigrees. Acta Psychiatr Scand 1984;70:282–287.
13. Johnson GPS, Leeman MM. Analysis of familial factors in bipolar affective illness. Arch Gen Psychiatry 1977;24:1074–1983.
14. Gershon ES, Targum SD, Matthysse S, et al. Color blindness not closely linked to bipolar illness. Arch Gen Psychiatry 1979;36:1423–1430.
15. Mendlewicz J. Le concept d'hétérogénéité dans la psychose maniaco-depressive: l'inform. Psychiatrique 1974;2:411–416.
16. Risch N, Baron M. X-linkage and genetic heterogeneity in bipolar related major affective illness: re-analysis of linkage data. Ann Hum Genet 1982;46:153–166.
17. Choo KH, Gould KG, Rees DJG, et al. Molecular cloning of the gene for human anti-haemophilia IX. Nature 1982;299:178–180.
18. Camerino G, Grezeschif KH, Jaye M, et al. Regional localization on the human X chromosome and polymorphism of the coagulation factor IX gene (haemophilia B locus). Proc Natl Acad Sci USA 1984;81:498–502.
19. Gianelli F, Choo KH, Winship PR, et al. Characterisation and use of an intragenic polymorphic marker for detection of carriers of haemophilia B (factor IX deficiency). Lancet 1984;239–241.
20. Mendlewicz J, Fleiss JL, Cataldo M, et al. The accuracy of the family history method in family studies of affective illness. Arch Gen Psychiatry 1975;32:309–314.
21. Spitzer RL, Endicott J. Schedule for Affective Disorders and Schizophrenia. New York: New York State Psychiatric Institute, 1978.
22. Spitzer RL, Endicott J, Robins E. Research diagnostic criteria: rationale and reliability. Arch Gen Psychiatry 1978;35:773–782.
23. Robins E, Guze SB. Classification of affective disorders: the primary-secondary, the endogenous-reactive, and the neurotic-psychotic concepts. In Williams TA, Katz MM, Shields JAS (eds): Recent Advances in the Psychobiology of the Depressive Illness. U.S. Department of Health, Education and Welfare publication (HSM) 70-0953. Washington DC: US Government Printing Office, 1972;283.
24. Lathrope GM, Lalouel JM, Julier C, et al. Multilocus linkage analysis in humans: detection of linkage and estimation of recombination. Am J Hum Genet 1985;37:482–498.
25. Egeland JA, Gerhard DS, Pauls DL, et al. Bipolar affective disorders linked to DNA markers on chromosome 11. Nature 1987;325:783–787.
26. Hodgkinson S, Sherrington R, Gurling H, et al. Molecular genetic evidence of heterogeneity in manic depression. Nature 1987;325:805–806.
27. Detera-Wadleigh SD, Berrettini WH, Goldin LR, et al. Close linkage of C-Harvey-ras-1 and the insulin gene to affective disorder is ruled out in three North American pedigrees. Nature 1987;325:806–808.
28. Baron M, Risch N, Hamburger R, et al. Genetic linkage between X-chromosome markers and bipolar affective illness. Nature 1987;326:289–292.

44. Segregation Analysis in Families of Affective Patients Subdivided According to Treatment Outcome and Personality Disorders

E. Smeraldi, M. Gasperini, F. Macciardi, A. Orsini, M. Provenza, and G. Sciuto

The aim of biological research in psychiatric genetics has been focused on discriminating among hypothetically and etiologically different forms of disease using different partitioning criteria to identify unequivocal phenotypes strictly related to well shaped genetic structure or, using an opposite approach, to validate, with formal genetic methodologies, identifiable phenotypic criteria. In previous studies[1] we developed strategies to generate subgroups of families as homogeneous as possible, aiming to detect the possible mode of transmission of affective disorders. The biological criterion of outcome on lithium treatment appeared to differentiate subgroups of familial segregation structures, but not yet in a sufficiently unequivocal way.

Moreover, because experimental data[2,3] showed that diagnostic classes that include dysthymic disorder, cyclothymic disorder and atypical depression, when occurring in informative families, could be incomplete forms (intermediate phenotypes) of the same disease, we took into account the broader clinical spectrum of diseases, hypothesizing that they may be specifically linked to the same genetic susceptibility that leads to affective disorders. In fact, using spectrum disorders to detect secondary cases of depressive disease greatly modified the familial segregation patterns of our affective probands and indicated the great importance of using intermediate phenotypes to have more precise indications of susceptibility to use in segregation studies.[4] In a previous study[5] we tested the relation between the familial susceptibility segregation and the possible genetic mechanism underlying the outcome of affective probands on antidepressant treatments. We found two Single Major Locus (SML) hypotheses more suitable for good and nonresponder groups, whereas the model that best fits the group of poor responders was the polygenic one. These findings confirmed how the pharmacological criterion of antidepressant tricyclic drug treatment outcome identifies different, even not conclusive, familial segregation structures of affective disorders. Moreover, they suggested that we redefine the group of families of the poor responder probands carefully and restrictively partition these patients into "good responders" or "nonresponders" from the point of view of the clinical improvement.

Other investigations pointed out how personality traits and disorders were of great interest in affecting the clinical picture and course of the affective illness as well as in influencing pharmacological treatment outcomes. With regard to the latter, it is important to underline how the presence of a specific personality disorder[6] could affect the outcome of antidepressant treatment in terms of reduced improvement of the symptomatological picture. In other words, the coexistence of a *DSM-III* axis II diagnosis and an axis I affective disorder induces a lesser degree of recovery from major depression. A preliminary study about the relation between affective and personality disorders in the Italian population reported that the presence or absence of a given personality disorder in the proband predicted differential affective risks in families; it appeared also to be significantly related to different classes of age at onset of disease[7] thus agreeing with the previous report[8] of increased familial risks in groups of patients with the earliest age at onset. All these reports could be consistent with the hypothesis that personality disorders may influence the severity of the form, under the hypothesis of a genetic etiological process. For this reason we performed segregation analyses, taking into account, in addition to the pharmacological criteria (the outcome on tricyclic agents), the characteristic diagnosed on axis II of having or not having personality disorders, aiming to elicit hypothetically homogeneous study groups of affective patients.

Materials and Methods

We collected information on first-, second-, and third-degree relatives (when available) of 75 subjects (52 female and 23 male) diagnosed as having major depression, recurrent disorders (43 subjects), and bipolar disorders (32 subjects) according to *DSM-III* criteria.[9] Diagnosis of a personality disorder (PD) was assessed using the PDE scale when the patient was normothymic.[10] The demographic and clinical information on the families of our patients, e.g., sex, present age, presence of secondary cases of affective disorders, and age at onset, was collected by direct interviews with the patients and their relatives. We considered as affected the relatives who met the *DSM-III* criteria for: (a) major depression; (b) recurrent, bipolar, dysthymic, or cyclothymic disorders; or (c) atypical depression.

We submitted our data to segregation analyses, performed by means of the POINTER program.[11] The threshold model requires population prevalences so that liability thresholds can be defined. We incorporated separate prevalences for male and female subjects. The total population prevalence of the disorder was then subdivided according to the proportion of onset in these five ages groups ranging between 10 and 50 years. The analyses were performed on the Sperry UNIVAC 1100/90 computer at the University of Milan.

Results and Comments

Table 44.1 shows the estimated likelihood values obtained. First we ruled out the hypothesis of no genetic transmission for all the groups. For the group of tricyclic responders with PD (good-R with PD), the SML dominant model appears to be the most suitable. The models that best fit the group of "non-R with PD" are the dominant and the additive SML and the mendelian without any valuable differences among them. Moreover, we cannot rule out the polygenic model. It can easily be seen that the exact mode of transmission for these subjects is still unclear and that, conversely, the amount of heterogeneity is even high.

Table 44.1. Goodnesses of fit for groups of families according to alternative hypotheses of disorder transmission.

	With personality disorders		Without personality disorders	
Hypothesis	Tricyclic responders ($n = 26$)	Tricyclic nonresponders ($n = 17$)	Tricyclic responders ($n = 29$)	Tricyclic nonresponders ($n = 3$)
No transmission	1,092.47	462.07	1343.4	61.03
Polygenic	648.11	223.25	580.07	31.52
Mixed	617.57		517.14	
Recessive SML	686.01	278.27	603.99	33.98
Dominant SML	466.37[a]	221.35[a]	486.03	17.74
Additive SML	467.40	221.35[a]	656.17	17.73
Mendelian SML	467.37	221.35[a]	486.64	34.37
Tau 1	467.39		173.29[a]	
Tau 2	488.71	232.13	496.19	17.42[a]

SML = Single Major Locus.
[a] = Best fit value.

A good fit has been obtained for the group of "good-R without PD" under the SML hypothesis with transmission probability estimate, i.e., with a penetrance defect in the homozygous condition, whereas the group of "non-R without PD" shows a best fit for an SML hypothesis with reduced penetrance for heterozygous subjects. Thus there are some considerations that must be emphasized. First, the dychotomic subdivision presence/absence of PD seems directly related to different genetic structures, the patients with PD fitting a saturated model of transmission in contrast to subjects without PD whose segregation pattern appears to be best described by models characterized by a penetrance defect. We should also re-member that, up to now, we cannot say what the penetrance defect might be. Moreover, this phenotypic characterization appears more important than the out-come on tricyclics in eliciting homogeneous subgroups of disease. The criterion of pharmacological outcome in detecting the heterogeneity of affective disorders seems to be confirmed, even though the presence of PD has been found to affect the frequency of affective disease in families more markedly, thus conditioning a differential mode of transmission of susceptibility. Nevertheless, because we con-sidered the presence of PD as a whole, we failed to identify specific clusters of PD truly linked to the susceptibility structure of affective disorders. For example, previous epidemiological reports[7] supported clusters of specific PD diagnoses (avoidant, compulsive, passive-aggressive, dependent) in unipolar probands.

The segregation model shows that subjects with a PD diagnosis are best described by the dominant SML or intermediate forms of SML, the only variant parameter being the dominance value (d). Accordingly, we can hypothesize different fre-quencies of heterozygous subjects to be affected, leading to theoretical multiple threshold models. An indirect confirmation can be derived from the diagnosis of spectrum disorders that are not homogeneously distributed, as we found an excess of dysthymic disorder, cyclothymic disorder and atypical depression among the relatives of the good tricyclic responders independently from the existence of a particular PD in the probands (Table 44.2). These so-called intermediate phenotypes could also be incomplete or have a milder expression of the underlying genetic structures, suggesting the extreme importance of a careful evaluation of the whole phenotype in its constituents.

TABLE 44.2. Illness distribution in groups of families: typical affective disorders vs. atypical and spectrum affective disorders in relatives

Affective disorder	Presence of personality disorders (%)		Absence of personality disorders (%)	
	Responders	Nonresponders	Responders	Nonresponders
Morbidity risks in relatives for:				
Typical	5.4	6.2	7.1	4.5
Atypical and "spectrum"	1.8	1	2.5	
Total	7.2	7.2	9.6	4.5

In any case, the responder/nonresponder dichotomy alone is not enough to set up a particular segregation structure when conditioned by a PD. This finding could have its own specific meaning, taking into account what several authors have pointed out and focusing on the complex relation between the two variables. The presence of a PD is not identifiable with the concept of premorbid personality, but it could even correspond to an incomplete recovery under tricyclic therapy.

Finally, our experimental findings suggest the reliability of SML hypothesis of transmission for clearly defined subgroups of affective disorders. This choice appears to be of great interest when considering its suitability for linkage studies, supported by the identification of a linkage with a marker locus on chromosome 11.[12]

References

1. Smeraldi E, Petroccione A, Gasperini M, et al. The search for genetic homogeneity in affective disorders. J Affective Dis 1984;7:99–107.
2. Perris C, Perris H, Ericsson U, et al. The genetics of depressions: a family study of unipolar and neurotic reactive depressed patients. Arch Psychiatr Nervenkr 1982;232:137–155.
3. Gasperini M, Orsini A, Bussoleni C, et al. Genetic approach to the study of the heterogeneity of affective disorders. J Affective Dis 1987;12:105–113.
4. Goldin LR, Gershon ES, Targum SD, et al. Segregation and linkage studies in families of patients with bipolar, unipolar and schizoaffective mood disorders. Am Hum Genet 1983;35:274–287.
5. Orsini A. Antidepressant responses and segregation analyses in affective families. Presented at the Workshop on Anxiety and Depression: Assessment and Treatment. Milan, 22–23 September 1986.
6. Roose SP, Glassman AH, Walsh BT, et al. Tricyclic nonresponders, phenomenology and treatment. Am J Psychiatry 1986;143:373–374.
7. Gasperini M, Provenza M. The relationship between affective illness and personality disorders: preliminary reports. Paper presented at the Workshop on Anxiety and Depression: Assessment and Treatment. Milan, 22–23 September 1986.
8. Weissman MM, Gershon ES, Kidd KK, et al. Onset of major depression in early adult: increased familial loading and specificity. Arch Gen Psychiatry 1984;41:13–21.
9. American Psychiatric Association. Diagnostic and Statistical Manual of Mental Disorders. 3rd Ed. Washington DC: APA, 1980.
10. Loranger AW, Susman VL, Oldham JM, et al. Personality Disorder Examination (PDE): A Structured Interview for DSM-III-R and ICD-9 Personality Disorders. WHO/ADA-MAHA Pilot Version. White Plains, NY: The New York Hospital–Cornell Medical Center, Westchester Division, 1985.
11. Lalouel JM, Rao DC, Morton NE, et al. A unified model for complex segregation analysis. Am J Hum Genet 1983;35:816–826.
12. Egeland JA, Gerhard DS, Pauls DL, et al. Bipolar affective disorders linked to DNA markers on chromosome 11. Nature 1987;325:783–787.

II.B. BIOLOGICAL MARKERS

45. Peripheral Blood Cell Biological Markers in Depression

J. John Mann, James P. Halper,
Richard P. Brown, P. Anne McBride,
John A. Sweeney, Ann Peters,
and Philip J. Wilner

The classical monoamine hypotheses of depressive illness have postulated a deficiency of norepinephrine and/or serotonin at functionally important receptors in the central nervous system (CNS).[1,2] An alternative "receptor hypothesis" would explain reduced transmission by a deficiency in signal amplification by the receptor complex. This focus on the receptor gained impetus from studies showing that virtually all effective somatic antidepressant treatment modalities shared the common effect of down-regulation and/or desensitization of β-adrenergic receptor complexes.[3,4] Moreover, a significant number of antidepressants down-regulate 5-HT$_2$ (serotonin; 5-hydroxytryptamine) receptors, although, in contrast, electroconvulsive shock up-regulates 5-HT$_2$ receptors.[4,5]

The α$_2$- and α$_1$-receptors have also been reported to be altered by antidepressants.[4,6] Because of the difficulty of studying the noradrenergic system and, to a lesser degree, the serotonergic system in the brain of human subjects, investigators have turned to peripheral blood elements, where components of monoaminergic systems can be studied more readily. A large series of studies of platelet monoamine oxidase in schizophrenia and depression[7,8] was followed by measurement in psychiatric patients of platelet 5-HT uptake,[9,10] platelet imipramine binding,[11] platelet 5-HT content,[12] platelet α$_2$-receptor binding,[6] and leukocyte and lymphocyte β-adrenergic indices.[13] Our laboratory has developed a method for studying the platelet 5-HT$_2$ receptor complex.[14]

In addition to accessibility, these receptor complexes can be studied in isolation from the modulating effects of presynaptic elements. It is an advantage if the problem is due to a primary defect in the receptor complex because such a defect would be manifest systemically if genetically mediated. Alternately, if the peripheral receptor complex is normal, the focus should shift to the presynaptic elements of the system. Details of platelet markers are discussed elsewhere in this volume, so that this chapter concentrates on selected lymphocyte β-adrenergic indices and platelet serotonergic indices.

Lymphocyte β-Adrenergic Indices

We and other laboratories have reported that inpatients with endogenous depression have a blunted maximal lymphocyte cyclic AMP response to isoproterenol.[13] Dose-response studies with isoproterenol indicate no alteration in β-adrenergic receptor affinity.[15] Results of binding studies are less clear. Antagonist binding studies in intact lymphocytes indicate no change in binding indices,[13] although studies in membrane preparations of leukocytes have reported a reduced number of binding sites (Bmax).[16] Whether these differences are due to the white blood cell type (polymorphonuclear cells versus monocytes), technical factors (assay of whole cell versus membrane preparation), or the patient population (endogenous versus nonendogenous or unipolar versus bipolar) remains to be determined.

Lymphocytes have β_2-adrenergic receptors, yet antidepressants mainly affect β_1-adrenergic receptors in the brain.[4] Therefore the question is raised as to whether β_1-adrenergic receptors are also altered in depressive illness. Data from our laboratory and others[17,18] indicate that there is an excessive release of norepinephrine and epinephrine after an orthostatic challenge test in depressed patients compared to controls. However, the heart rate response to the catecholamine release is blunted, a finding that is consistent with the presence of blunted cardiac β-adrenergic receptors. Atrial β-adrenergic receptors mediating a chronotropic effect are largely of the β_1-receptor subtype. Therefore it seems that in depressive illness, as had also been reported in cardiac disease, the lymphocyte β_2-adrenergic receptor changes reflect changes in peripheral β_1-adrenergic receptors.[17]

Treatment of depressed patients with tricyclic antidepressants results in a normalization of lymphoctyte β-adrenergic cyclic AMP responsiveness,[19] suggesting that the blunted responsiveness is state-dependent.

Other Lymphocyte Receptors in Depressive Illness

Prostaglandin Receptors

Cyclic AMP responses to prostaglandin E_1 (PGE_1) in lymphocytes have been reported to be normal in depressed patients.[20] This finding, if confirmed, suggests homologous (receptor specific) desensitization of β-adrenergic receptor complexes. However, there is evidence of a blunted cyclic AMP response to PGE_1 in platelets of depressed patients.[21] Thus, either prostaglandin receptors behave differently in lymphocytes versus platelets, or methodological or technical factors are responsible for these differences in results.

Corticosteroid Receptors

Less blunting of mitogen-induced lymphocyte proliferation by corticosteroids in vitro has been reported by some but not all laboratories in depressed patients exhibiting dexamethasone resistance compared to depressed patients whose plasma cortisol levels suppressed normally.[22] This reduced corticosteroid suppression of mitogen-induced lymphocyte proliferation correlated with the presence of fewer corticosteroid binding sites on lymphocytes from dexamethasone-resistant depressed patients.[23] It is hypothesized that the relative resistance to dexamethasone suppression of cortisol levels observed in some depressed patients may be due to a generalized loss of corticosteroid binding sites, including those in the pituitary and hypothalamus that are involved in feedback inhibition of corticotropin-releasing factor (CRF) and ACTH.

Platelet Receptor Studies

Platelet Serotonin Transporter

It may not be possible to directly assay the binding site for the transporter, but serotonin uptake kinetics have been studied in depressed patients for 10 years. Briefly, serotonin uptake (Vmax) appears to be reduced in drug-free patients with endogenous depression but not in patients with nonendogenous depression.[9,10] The abnormality persists into the euthymic state, suggesting that it is a biochemical trait.

Imipramine Binding Studies

The imipramine binding studies are reviewed in detail elsewhere. Most studies[11] have found that patients with major depressive disorders (MDDs) have fewer platelet imipramine binding sites than healthy controls. Whether these findings can be generalized to brain tissue is not certain because, although there are reports[24] of fewer imipramine binding sites in the brains of suicide victims (which include a significant proportion of depressed patients), other studies[25] of depressed patients who have died of causes other than suicide have produced conflicting results. A systemic reduction in the number of imipramine binding sites might be a consequence of a genetically induced abnormality. Such an effect would not be state-dependent. Although the effect of antidepressant medication treatment of depression on platelet imipramine binding is unclear, electroconvulsive treatment does not alter imipramine binding. Thus platelet imipramine binding, like serotonin uptake, appears to be a state-independent measure. This observation would be consistent with a genetic basis for the altered binding.

Platelet α_2-Adrenergic Receptors

An increase in platelet α_2-receptor binding sites has been reported in depressed patients,[6] an increase that is apparently state-dependent. In contrast, the central α_2-receptor mediated response of clonidine-induced growth hormone release is blunted in depressive illness during the acute illness and in remission. It may therefore be a trait-dependent abnormality.[26,27] Whether these apparently conflicting results in platelet versus brain α_2-receptor indices reflect differences between pre- and postsynaptic α_2-receptors, platelet and CNS α_2-receptors, or patient populations is unclear. We are therefore currently uncertain as to how to interpret the platelet changes in terms of potential central dysfunction involving brain α_2-receptors.

Platelet Prostaglandin Receptors

As mentioned above, cyclic AMP responses to PGE are blunted in platelets of depressed patients.[20] Whether these changes are state- or trait-dependent remains to be established.

Platelet Monoamine Oxidase Activity

We and others have shown that depressed bipolar patients have lower platelet monoamine oxidase (MAO) activity than unipolar patients with an endogenous depression.[8] It also appears that control subjects' levels of MAO activity fall somewhere between those of unipolar and bipolar subjects, but the differences in individual studies are not always statistically significant. The differences in MAO activity are trait-dependent because they are found in the euthymic as well as the depressed state.[8]

Red Blood Cell Markers

Increased ratios of intracellular lithium versus extracellular lithium concentrations in red blood cells have been reported in patients with bipolar disorders.[28] Evidence from twin and family stuides indicate that lithium ion ratios are under genetic control via regulation of a lithium–sodium ion counterflow mechanism. The allele at this autosomal major gene locus that results in increased lithium ion ratios is also associated with increased risk of affective disorders.[29]

Diagnostic Power of Biological Markers

Diagnostic power is a complex subject that has been reviewed elsewhere.[30] Briefly, the diagnostic power of biological markers depends on their specificity, sensitivity, and the base rate of the illness in the study population. Biological markers often perform well in a clinic population where the disease of interest comprises, for example, half the total number of patients; however, they perform poorly in the general population where the rate may be 1–10% of the total. Imagine a hypothetical super biological marker with a sensitivity of 90% and specificity of 90%. In a research clinic with a rate of 50% for the illness of interest, the correlation coefficient ϕ is 0.799 and the chance-corrected proportion of agreement (κ) is 0.8. However, with a base rate of 10% (much closer to reality for depressive illness in the population) the κ value falls to 0.59; and for a base rate of 25% (closer to a general psychiatric clinic rate), the κ value is 0.75.

If the performance of the biological marker is closer to currently available markers (i.e., 50% sensitivity and 90% specificity), for an illness base rate of 25% the κ is 0.428. It is clear that without a major breakthrough, our current available biological markers lack the diagnostic power necessary for routine clinical application.

Etiological Significance of Abnormal Monoamine Indices in Peripheral Blood Elements

Because these biological markers do not have sufficient diagnostic power for routine clinical use, their main value lies in clarifying the pathophysiology of depressive illness. Peripheral blood cell studies offer the following advantages: (a) easy access to tissue for repeat sampling in vivo; (b) the ability to study neurochemical components such as enzymes, receptors, and uptake systems in isolation; (c) evaluation of direct effects of hormones and other relevant humoral factors on neurobiological components in vivo and in vitro; and (d) detection of genetically mediated protein abnormalities that manifest systemically. The blood elements may ultimately prove most valuable in the event of a genetic abnormality because they can be a source of the abnormal protein and can lead to a breakthrough in terms of etiology as well as development of a diagnostic test.

Acknowledgments. This work was supported by USPHS grants MH37907 and MH40695, an Irma T. Hirschl Trust Research Scientist Award to Dr. Mann, and a Mallinckrodt Scholar Award to Dr. Brown.

References

1. Schildkraut JJ. The catecholamine hypothesis of affective disorders: a review of supporting evidence. Am J Psychiatry 1965;122:509–522.
2. Potter WZ. Psychotherapeutic drugs and biogenic amines: current concepts and therapeutic implications. Drugs 1984;28:127–143.
3. Sulser F, Vetulani J, Mobley PL. Mode of action of antidepressant drugs. Biochem Pharmacol 1978;27:257–261.
4. Charney DS, Menkes DB, Heninger GR. Receptor sensitivity and the mechanisms of action of antidepressant treatment. Arch Gen Psychiatry 1981;38:1160–1180.
5. Costain DW, Green AR, Grahame-Smith DG. Enhanced 5-hydroxytryptamine-mediated behavioral responses in rats following repeated electroconvulsive shock: relevance to the mechanism of the antidepressive effect of electroconvulsive therapy. Psychopharmacology 1979;61:167–170.
6. Garcia-Sevilla JA, Zis AP, Hollingsworth PJ, et al. Platelet alpha$_2$-adrenergic receptors in major depressive disorders. Arch Gen Psychiatry 1981;38:1327–1333.
7. Wyoh RJ, Murphy DL, Low platelet monoamine oxidase activity and schizophrenia. Schizoph Bull 1976;2:77–89.
8. Mann JJ. Altered platelet monoamine oxidase activity in affective disorders. Psychol Med 1979;9:729–736.
9. Meltzer HY, Arora RC, Bober R, et al. Serotonin uptake in blood platelets of psychiatric patients. Arch Gen Psychiatry 1981;38:1322–1326.
10. Kaplan RD, Mann JJ. Altered platelet serotonin uptake in schizophrenia and melancholia. Life Sci 1982;31:583–588.
11. Briley MS, Langer SZ, Raisman R, et al. ^{3}H-Imipramine binding sites are decreased in platelets of untreated depressed patients. Science 1980;209:303–305.
12. Quan-Bui KHL, Plaisant LO, Leboyer M, et al. Reduced platelet serotonin in depression. Psychiatry Res 1984;13:129–139.
13. Mann JJ, Brown RP, Halper JP, et al. Reduced sensitivity of lymphocyte beta-adrenergic receptors in patients with endogenous depression and psychomotor agitation. N Engl J Med 1985;313:715–720.
14. McBride PA, Mann JJ, Polley MJ, et al. Assessment of binding indices and physiological responsiveness of the 5-HT$_2$ receptor on human platelets. Life Sci 1987;40:1799–1908.
15. Halper JP, Mann JJ, Brown RP, et al. Blunted beta-adrenergic responsivity of peripheral blood mononuclear cells in endogenous depression: isoproterenol dose response studies. Arch Gen Psychiatry 1988;45:241–244.
16. Extein I, Tallman J, Smith CC, et al. Changes in lymphocyte beta-adrenergic receptors in depression and mania. Psychiatry Res 1979;1:191–197.
17. Wilner PJ, Brown RP, Sweeney JA, et al. Blunted orthostatic response in major depressives. In: New Research Abstracts. 140th Annual Meeting. Chicago: American Psychiatric Association, 1987.
18. Rudorfer MV, Ross RJ, Linnoila M, et al. Exaggerated orthostatic responsivity of plasma norepinephrine in depression. Arch Gen Psychiatry 1985;42:1186–1192.
19. Mann JJ, Brown RP, Sweeney JA, et al. State-dependent dysregulation of beta-adrenergic responsivity in endogenous depression. In: Abstracts, 25th Annual Meeting American College of Neuropsychopharmacology. Washington, DC, 1986;187.

20. Pandey GN, Dysken MW, Garver DL, et al. Beta-adrenergic function in affective illness. Am J Psychiatry 1979;136:675–678.
21. Kafka MS, Siever LJ, Nurnberger JI, et al. Platelet alpha-adrenergic receptor function in affective disorders and schizophrenia. Psychopharmacol Bull 1985;21:599–602.
22. Kronfol Z, House JD, Silva J, et al. Depression, urinary free cortisol excretion and lymphocyte function. Br J Psychiatry 1986;148:70–73.
23. Gormley CJ, Lowry MT, Reder AT, et al. Glucocorticoid receptors in depression: relationship to the dexamethasone suppression test. Am J Psychiatry 1985;142:1278–1284.
24. Stanley M, Virgilio J, Gershon S. Tritiated imipramine binding sites are decreased in the frontal cortex of suicides. Science 1982;216:1337–1339.
25. Ferrier IN, McKeith IG, Cross AJ, et al. Postmortem neurochemical studies in depression. Ann NY Acad Sci 1986;487:128–142.
26. Langer G, Heinze G, Reim B, et al. Reduced growth hormone responses to amphetamine in endogenous depressive patients: studies in normal "reactive" and "endogenous" depressive, schizophrenic and chronic alcholic subjects. Arch Gen Psychiatry 1970;33:1471–1475.
27. Checkley SA, Slade AP, Shur E. Growth hormone and other responses to clonidine in patients with endogenous depression. Br J Psychiatry 1981;138:51–55.
28. Pandey GN, Dorus E, David JM, et al. Lithium transport in human red blood cells: genetic and clinical aspects. Arch Gen Psychiatry 1979;36:902–908.
29. Dorus E, Cox NJ, Gibbons RD, et al. Lithium ion transport and affective disorders within families of bipolar patients: identification of a major gene locus. Arch Gen Psychiatry 1983;40:545–552.
30. Cohen J. Statistical approaches to suicidal risk factor analysis. Ann NY Acad Sci 1986;487:34–41.

46. α_2-Adrenoceptors and Associated Functional Responses in Endogenous Depression

JESÚS A. GARCÍA-SEVILLA

Modulation of neurotransmitter receptors by antidepressant drugs has been related to their clinical mechanisms of action; consequently, possible abnormalities of such receptors have been postulated in the etiology of depressive illness. In recent years much interest in this field has focused on inhibitory α_2-adrenoceptors that regulate the release of norepinephrine in the central nervous system. Human platelets also possess inhibitory α_2-adrenoceptors, which have been used as a model system to study possible dysfunctions of this receptor in depression.[1,2] This chapter reviews data supporting the hypothesis that depression is related to α_2-adrenoceptor supersensitivity.

Radioligand Binding to α_2-adrenoceptors in Platelets and Brain During Depression

The density and affinity of α_2-adrenoceptors were quantitated by means of the binding of selective [³H]agonists and [³H]antagonists. In drug-free depressed patients the specific binding of the partial agonist [³H]clonidine to platelet membranes was significantly increased (Bmax 40% greater) with respect to control subjects,[3,4] as seen in Table 46.1, which shows the combined results from two studies. The mean Kd value for the radioligand was also increased (affinity for the receptor was decreased). In another study[5] the specific binding of the full agonist [³H] ($-$)epinephrine to platelets of depressed patients with melancholia was also found to be increased (Bmax 48% greater) without significant changes in the Kd value for the radioligand (Table 46.1). In contrast, the specific binding of the antagonist [³H]yohimbine is not altered in depressed patients (Table 46.1).

These results are similar to those reported in other studies and indicate that [³H]agonist binding to α_2-adrenoceptors is increased in platelets of depressed patients, whereas [³H]antagonist binding appears to be unchanged (for review of these studies see García-Sevilla et al.,[4] Kafka and Paul,[2] and Piletz et al.[1]). Moreover, Piletz et al.,[1] using a statistical test (meta-analysis) to combine results from representative binding studies with agonist and antagonist radioligands, have concluded that platelet α_2-adrenoceptor density is increased in depressed patients.

TABLE 46.1. [³H]Agonist and [³H]antagonist binding to α_2-adrenoceptors in platelets of depressed patients and brain of depressed suicide victims.

Radioligand and group	Blood platelets binding parameters		Frontal cortex binding parameters	
	Kd (nM)	Bmax (fmol/mg P)	Kd (nM)	Bmax (fmol/mg P)
[³H]Clonidine				
Control	6.0 ± 0.5	35 ± 2 (41)	1.2 ± 0.2	60 ± 8 (10)
Depressed	9.1 ± 1.3[a]	49 ± 2[b] (30)	1.5 ± 0.2	103 ± 17[a] (5)
[³H] (−)Epinephrine				
Control	2.4 ± 0.2	46 ± 3 (23)	—	—
Depressed	3.4 ± 0.6	68 ± 6[c] (14)		
[³H] Yohimbine				
Control	4.0 ± 0.5	165 ± 12 (16)	—	—
Depressed	5.2 ± 0.8	183 ± 9 (18)		

Each value is the mean ± SEM of (n) subjects per group.
[a]$p < 0.05$; [c]$p < 0.005$; [b]$p < 0.001$ compared with the corresponding control value (two-tailed student's t-test.)
Data for the blood platelets are from García-Sevilla et al.[3-5] and Smith et al.[8]
[Data from ref. 5 is reprinted with permission of Munksgaard International Publishers Ltd, Copenhagen, Denmark. Data from ref. 8 is reprinted with permission from Pergamon Journals Ltd, copyright 1983.]

Taken together these results indicate that depression is associated with a defect of the high-affinity state of the α_2-adrenoceptor that preferentially recognizes agonists.[4,5]

In suicide victims with a previous diagnosis of depression the specific binding of [³H]clonidine to cortical membranes was increased (Bmax 72% greater) compared to that in control subjects (Table 46.1). A similar increase was observed in the hypothalamus (Bmax 58% greater, $p<0.05$) but not in the amygdala and caudate nucleus. These preliminary results indicate that α_2-adrenoceptor density is also increased in certain brain regions of depressed suicide victims.

Functional Responses of Platelet α_2-adrenoceptors in Depressed and Euthymic Patients

Activation of platelet α_2-adrenoceptors causes both inhibition of the enzyme adenylate cyclase and induction of aggregation, although it has been questioned that a single receptor mediates both responses.[6] The inhibition of adenylate cyclase activity induced by epinephrine was used as a biochemical index of receptor activation. Also, the primary aggregation response induced by epinephrine and UK 14304 and its selective inhibition by yohimbine were used as functional indexes of receptor sensitivity.

In drug-free depressed patients the inhibitory effect induced by epinephrine on basal and forskolin-stimulated adenylate cyclase activity was not different from that in controls (Table 46.2). Moreover, forskolin activated basal activity to the same extent in both groups of subjects (Table 46.2), which indicated that the catalytic unit of the enzyme is also normal in depression. These results are at variance with other studies,[7] which have found that this biochemical response of the platelet α_2-adrenoceptor is subsensitive in depression. (See Piletz et al.[1] and Kafka and Paul[2] for other studies on this controversial topic.)

TABLE 46.2. Inhibition of the enzyme adenylate cyclase and induction of aggregation by α_2-adrenoceptor agonists in platelets of depressed and euthymic patients.

Group	Inhibition of basal adenylate cyclase		Induction of primary phase of aggregation	
	Epinephrine EC_{50} (μM)	Maximum (%)	Epinephrine EC_{50} (μM)	UK14304 EC_{50} (μM)
Control	0.82 ± 0.11	54 ± 2 (10)	0.72 ± 0.07 (42)	0.25 ± 0.02 (38)
Depressed	0.81 ± 0.13	49 ± 3 (10)	0.49 ± 0.06^a (13)	0.13 ± 0.01^b (15)
Euthymic (lithium-treated)	—	—	0.38 ± 0.05^b (12)	—
Euthymic (untreated)	—	—	—	0.12 ± 0.01^b (6)

Each value is the mean $\pm$ SEM of (n) subjects per group.
Basal adenylate cyclase activity (pmol/min/mg P): 5.72 ± 0.30 (control) and 4.89 ± 0.55 (depressed). Forskolin (10 μM) was equally effective in stimulating basal enzyme activity in both groups: 256 ± 7 (control) and 205 ± 18 (depressed).
UK 14304: 5-bromo-6[2-imidazolin-2-ylamino]-quinoxaline.
The euthymic-treated group had received lithium carbonate (400–1400 mg/day) for 3–24 months.
$^a p < 0.02$; $^b p < 0.001$ compared with the corresponding control value (two-tailed Student's t-test).
Data for the epinephrine-induced aggregation are from García-Sevilla et al.[4] [Copyright 1986, American Medical Association.]

In drug-free depressed patients, however, epinephrine- and UK 14304-induced platelet aggregation were potentiated (EC_{50} decreased by 32–48%), which indicated increased α_2-adrenoceptor sensitivity (Table 46.2). In contrast, the selective inhibition by yohimbine of the epinephrine-induced aggregation was unchanged in the same patients.[4] These results are consistent with [^{3}H]agonist and [^{3}H]antagonist binding studies reported above. In fact, in depressed patients there was a negative correlation ($r -0.70$; $p<0.01$) between functional responses (EC_{50} values for epinephrine-induced aggregation) and the densities of platelet α_2-adrenoceptors (Bmax for [^{3}H]clonidine binding),[4] indicating that depression is associated with true supersensitive platelet α_2-adrenoceptors. In euthymic patients (lithium-treated or untreated) an enhanced sensitivity to epinephrine or UK 14304 in promoting aggregation was also found (Table 46.2), suggesting further that α_2-adrenoceptor supersensitivity could represent a trait marker for depression.

These results suggest that α_2-adrenoceptor-mediated aggregation is a better marker than inhibition of adenylate cyclase for assessing functional changes of the receptor in depressed patients. The dissociation between inhibition of adenylate cyclase and induction of aggregation also suggest that the two functional responses represent different phenomena of the same receptor activation.[6]

Acknowledgments. The author wishes to thank P. Areso, T. Giralt, J. Guimón, J.J. Meana, D. Padró, and C. Udina for their invaluable collaboration. These studies were supported by CAICYT grants 1018/81 and 1244/84 and by the U.S.–Spanish Joint Committee grant CCB84/007.

References

1. Piletz JE, Schubert DSP, Halaris A. Evaluation of studies on platelet alpha$_2$ adrenoreceptors in depressive illness. Life Sci 1986;39:1589–1616.
2. Kafka MS, Paul SM. Platelet α_2-adrenergic receptor in depression. Arch Gen Psychiatry 1986;43:91–95.

3. García-Sevilla JA, Zis AP, Hollingsworth PJ, et al. Platelet α_2-adrenergic receptors in major depressive disorder. Arch Gen Psychiatry 1981;38:1327–1333.
4. García-Sevilla JA, Guimón J, García-Vallejo P, et al. Biochemical and functional evidence of supersensitive platelet α_2-adrenoceptors in major affective disorder. Arch Gen Psychiatry 1986;43:51–57.
5. García-Sevilla JA, Udina C, Fuster MJ, et al. Enhanced binding of [^{3}H](−)adrenaline to platelets of depressed patients with melancholia: effect of long-term clomipramine treatment. Acta Psychiatr Scand 1987;75:150–157.
6. Clare KA, Scrutton MC, Thompson NT. Effects of α_2-adrenoceptor agonists and of related compounds on aggregation of, and on adenylate cyclase activity in, human platelets. Br J Pharmacol 1984;82:467–476.
7. Siever LJ, Kafka MS, Targum S, et al. Platelet α-adrenergic binding and biochemical responsiveness in depressed patients and controls. Psychiatry Res 1984;11:287–302.
8. Smith CB, Hollingsworth PJ, García-Sevilla JA, et al. Prog Neuropsychopharmacol Biol Psychiatry 1983;7:241–247.

47. Neurotransmitters and Their Metabolites in CSF in Depression and Under the Influence of Antidepressant Drugs

ANNETTE GJERRIS AND OLE J. RAFAELSEN

In the search for a possible deficiency in the monoaminergic systems in depressive illness, most interest has been concentrated on the amine metabolites 5-hydroxyindoleacetic acid (5-HIAA), 3-hydroxy-4-methoxyphenylglycol (MHPG), and to a lesser extent homovanillic acid (HVA) in cerebrospinal fluid (CSF). The reason for measuring the metabolites and not the amines themselves has been the lack of proper analytical methods.

Amine Metabolites in CSF

As described in a review by Post et al.,[1] the results reported on CSF amine metabolites measured in depressed patients have often been inconsistent. Low, normal, or even high concentrations of CSF 5-HIAA, MHPG, and HVA have been described in melancholia and in subgroups of depressed patients when compared with controls.[2-7]

"Parent" Amines in CSF

As methods have now been developed that enable us to measure the amines themselves in tissue and CSF, we have at last acquired the tools for a more exact and also more dynamic investigation of possible amine dysfunctions in depression. Post et al.,[8] Christensen et al.,[9] and Gjerris et al.[10] found no differences in CSF concentrations of norepinephrine (NE) when comparing depressed patients with controls. Christensen et al.[9] and Gjerris et al.[10] described a significant reduction in CSF epinephrine in depressed patients. Moreover, supporting the study by Berger et al.,[11] Gjerris et al.[10] found significantly negative correlations between single items on the Hamilton Depression Scale (HDS), "somatic anxiety" and "somatization," and CSF epinephrine levels.

Until now CSF concentrations of serotonin (5-hydroxytryptamine, 5-HT) in depressive patients have been reported in only one study.[12] In this study patients with endogenous depression classified according to the Newcastle Rating Scale for Depression had significantly higher concentrations of CSF 5-HT than controls.

This finding does not contradict the possible reduction in CSF 5-HIAA in depression described in some studies,[7] as high levels of the amine itself and low levels of the main metabolite may express a decrease in rate of metabolism. Our finding[13] of increased levels of total CSF dopamine (DA) and some reports of reduced levels of CSF HVA in depression[7] may be explained in the same way. Supporting the findings by King et al.,[14] who measured free CSF DA in depressed patients, we found a relation between "acceptable social function" and high levels of CSF DA.

Antidepressant Treatment: Influence on CSF Amines

A rather consistent finding, contradicting the logic of low CSF 5-HIAA being causal for depression, is that tricyclic antidepressants as well as monoamine oxidase inhibitors (MAOIs) further reduce the level of 5-HIAA in CSF.[15–17] Not less confusing is the finding that clinical recovery from depression occurred independently of whether CSF concentrations of 5-HT were increased (MAOI treatment) or decreased (amitriptyline) after clinical recovery. The 5-HIAA/5-HT ratio, evaluated before and after treatment, showed that isocarboxazide and electroconvulsive shock treatment (ECT) reduced the ratio, whereas amitriptyline increased it.[12]

In the study by Christensen et al.[9] patients who recovered had significantly higher levels of CSF epinephrine after depression than during depression. The character of antidepressant treatment was not standardized in the above-mentioned report. In the study by Gjerris et al.[10] CSF epinephrine was not measured after clinical recovery, but the finding of low CSF epinephrine in "somatizing depression" brings up the question of whether this type of depression responds specifically to treatment with MAOI (isocarboxazide), which has been shown to induce a marked increase in CSF epinephrine in rats, also after long-term treatment.[18]

Amine Turnover

As an expression of amine turnover, the 5-HIAA/5-HT, HVA/DA, and MHPG/NE ratios have been calculated; there were no differences in the ratios when depressed patients were compared with controls. The negative finding might be explained by possible differences in the ventriculolumbar gradient between the "parent" amine and its metabolite.

Methodological Problems

Interpretation of results from CSF concentration studies is problematical. First, the origin of the substances measured in CSF is not clear.[1] Thus a ventricular lumbar gradient influencing the concentrations measured at the lumbar level has been described for 5-HIAA, HVA, NE, and DA, [19–21] but results from such gradient studies have not yet been reported for epinephrine and 5-HT.

Second, other factors such as diurnal and seasonal variation have been described for some of the transmitters, although a consensus has not yet been obtained.[7,19] Third, physical activity, food intake, and level of anxiety have been noted to influence the amine concentrations measured in CSF.[1] Finally, the differences in the statistical methods applied might add to the lack of agreement in the results obtained in different studies: Some authors use parametric statistics that sometimes include corrections for nonspecific variable and sometimes do not, whereas other groups use nonparametric statistics.

Conclusion

The simplest formulation of the amine hypothesis in depression—that the biological background for development of a depressive state is a deficiency in either the noradrenergic or the serotoninergic system, expressed in low concentrations of 5-HIAA or MHPG—should be rejected. Instead, several amines and peptides seem to be involved, and hence the depressive state might be considered the result of an imbalance between different transmitter systems and changes in turnover within these systems. Furthermore, much more attention should be paid to the origin of the transmitter substances measured and the influence of various physiological factors. The latter may either blur the results or lead to their misinterpretation.

References

1. Post RM, Ballenger JC, Goodwin FK. Cerebrospinal fluid studies of neurotransmitter function in manic and depressive illness. In Wood JH (ed): Neurobiology of Cerebrospinal Fluid 1. New York: Plenum Press, 1980;685–717.
2. Vestergaard P, Sørensen T, Hoppe E, et al. Biogenic amine metabolites in cerebrospinal fluid of patients with affective disorders. Acta Psychiatr Scand 1978;58:88–95.
3. Ågren H. Symptom patterns in unipolar and bipolar depression correlating with mono-amine metabolites in the cerebrospinal fluid. II. Suicide. Psychiatr Res 1980;3:225–236.
4. Träskman L, Åsberg M, Bertilsson L, et al. Monoamine metabolites in CSF and suicidal behavior. Arch Gen Psychiatry 1981;38:631–636.
5. Van Praag HM. Depression, suicide and the metabolism of serotonin in the brain. J Affective Disord 1982;4:275–290.
6. Koslow SH, Maas JW, Bowden CL, et al. CSF and urinary biogenic amines and metabolites in depression and mania. Arch Gen Psychiatry 1983;40:999–1010.
7. Åsberg M, Bertilsson L, Mårtensson B, et al. CSF monoamine metabolites in melancholia. Acta Psychiatr Scand 1984;69:201–219.
8. Post RM, Lake CR, Jimerson DC, et al. Cerebrospinal fluid norepinephrine in affective illness. Am J Psychiatry 1978;135:907–912.
9. Christensen NJ, Vestergaard P, Sørensen T, et al. Cerebrospinal fluid adrenaline and noradrenaline in depressed patients. Acta Psychiatr Scand 1980;61:178–185.
10. Gjerris A, Rafaelsen OJ, Christensen NJ. CSF-adrenaline—low in "somatizing depression." Acta Psychiatr Scand 1987;75:516–520.
11. Berger PA, King R, Lemoine P, et al. Cerebrospinal fluid epinephrine concentrations: discrimination of subtypes of depression and schizophrenia. Pharmacol Bull 1984;20:412–415.
12. Gjerris A, Sørensen AS, Rafaelsen OJ, et al. 5-HT and 5-HIAA in cerebrospinal fluid in depression. J Affective Disord 1987;12:13–22.
13. Gjerris A, Werdelin L, Rafaelsen OJ, et al. CSF dopamine—increased in depression: CSF-dopamine, noradrenaline and their metabolites in depressed patients and in controls. J Affective Disord 1987;13:279–286.
14. King RJ, Mefford IN, Wang C, et al. CSF dopamine levels correlated with extraversion in depressed patients. Psychiatr Res 1986;19:305–310.
15. Post RM, Goodwin FK. Effects of amitriptyline and imipramine on amine metabolites in the cerebrospinal fluid of depressed patients. Arch Gen Psychiatry 1974;30:234–239.
16. Mendlewicz J, Pinder RM, Stulemeijer SM, et al. Monoamine metabolites in cerebrospinal fluid of depressed patients during treatment with mianserin or amitriptyline. J Affective Disord 1982;4:219–226.
17. Potter WZ, Scheinen M, Golden RW, et al. Selective antidepressants and cerebrospinal fluid. Arch Gen Psychiatry 1985;42:1171–1177.

18. Gjerris A, Barry DI, Christensen NJ, et al. Brain and cerebrospinal fluid epinephrine in isocarboxazide and zimeldine-treated rats. In Usdin E, Carlsson A, Dahlström A, et al. (eds): Catecholamines. Part C: Neuropharmacology and Central Nervous System— Therapeutic Aspects. New York: Alan R. Liss, 1984;139–142.
19. Gjerris A, Werdelin L, Gjerris F, et al. CSF-amine metabolites in depression, dementia and in controls. Acta Psychiatr Scand 1987;75:619–628.
20. Ziegler MG, Wood JH, Lake CR, et al. Norepinephrine and 3-methoxy-4-hydroxyphenyl glycol gradients in human cerebrospinal fluid. Am J Psychiatry 1977;134:565–568.
21. Gjerris A, Gjerris F, Sørensen PS, et al. Do concentrations of neurotransmitters measured in lumbar cerebrospinal fluid reflect the concentrations at brain level? Acta Neurochir (Wien) 1988;91:55–59.

Summary

Blood platelets are considered a peripheral model of the serotonergic neuron. The pharmacodynamic parameters of imipramine binding and serotonin uptake in platelets and neurons share identical characteristics. These two serotonergic markers were studied in several neuropsychiatric disorders in which an abnormal function of the serotonergic system was suspected. Our studies along with data from other laboratories indicate that only in adult major depression is there a simultaneous decrease in imipramine binding and serotonin uptake in platelets. It is suggested that a concurrent decrease in these two peripheral serotonergic parameters may serve as a reliable specific diagnostic tool in major depression.

References

1. Raisman R, Briley M, Langer SZ. Specific tricyclic antidepressant binding sites in rat brain. Nature 1979;281:148–150.
2. Rehavi M, Paul SM, Skolnick P, et al. Demonstration of specific high affinity binding sites for [^{3}H]imipramine in human brain. Life Sci 1980;26:2273–2279.
3. Paul SM, Rehavi M, Skolnick P, et al. Demonstration of specific high affinity binding sites for [^{3}H]imipramine on human platelets. Life Sci 1980;26:953–959.
4. Briley MS, Raisman R, Langer SZ. Human platelets posses high-affinity binding sites for [^{3}H]imipramine. Eur J Pharmacol 1979;58:347–348.
5. Paul SM, Rehavi M, Rice KC, et al. Does high affinity [^{3}H]imipramine binding label serotonin reuptake sites in brain and platelets? Life Sci 1981;28:2753–2760.
6. Briley MS, Langer SZ, Raisman R, Tritiated imipramine binding sites are decreased in platelets of untreated depressed patients. Science 1980;209:303–305.
7. Paul SM, Rehavi M, Skolnick P, et al. Depressed patients have decreased binding of tritiated imipramine to platelet serotonin "transporter." Arch Gen Psychiatry 1981;38: 1315–1317.
8. Langer SZ, Galzin AM, Poirier MF, et al. Association of [^{3}H]imipramine and [^{3}H]paroxetine binding with the 5HT transporter in brain and platelets: relevance to studies in depression. J Recept Res 1987;7:499–521.
9. Roy A, Everett D, Pickar D, et al. Platelet tritiated imipramine binding and serotonin uptake in depressed patients and controls. Arch Gen Psychiatry 1987;44:320–327.
10. Whitaker PM, Warsh JJ, Stancer HC, et al. Seasonal variation in platelet [^{3}H]imipramine binding, comparable values in control and depressed populations. Psychiatry Res 1984; 11:127–135.
11. Briley MS, Raisman R, Arbilla S, et al. Concomitant decrease in [^{3}H]imipramine binding in cat brain and platelets after chronic treatment with imipramine. Eur J Pharmacol 1982;81:309–314.
12. Stanley M, Virgilio J, Gershon S. Tritiated imipramine binding sites are decreased in the frontal cortex of suicides. Science 1982;216:137–139.
13. Paul SM, Rehavi M, Skolnick P, et al. High affinity binding of antidepressants to biogenic amine transport sites in human brain and platelet: studies in depression. In Post RM, Ballenger JC (eds): Neurobiology of Mood Disorders. Baltimore: Williams & Wilkins, 1984;846–853.
14. Tuomisto J, Tukiainen E. Decreased uptake of 5-hydroxytryptamine in blood platelets from depressed patients. Nature 1976;262:596–598.
15. Traskman L, Asberg M, Bertilsson L, et al. Monoamine metabolites in CSF and suicidal behavior. Arch Gen Psychiatry 1981;38:631–636.
16. Hrdina PD, Lapierre YD, Horn ER, et al. Platelet [^{3}H]imipramine binding: a possible predictor of response to antidepressant treatment. Prog Neuropsychopharmacol Biol Psychiatry 1985;9:619–623.
17. Tanimoto K, Maeda K, Terada T. Alteration of platelet [^{3}H]imipramine binding in mildly depressed patients correlates with disease severity. Biol Psychiatry 1985;20:340–343.
18. Lewis DA, McChesney C. Tritiated imipramine binding distinguishes among subtypes of depression. Arch Gen Psychiatry 1985;42:485–488.

19. Rehavi M, Weizman R, Carel C, et al. High affinity [³H]imipramine binding in platelets of children and adolescents with major affective disorders. Psychiatry Res 1984:13:31–39.
20. Targum SD, Kapodanno AE; The dexamethasone suppression test in adolescent psychiatric inpatients. Am J Psychiatry 1983;140:589–591.
21. Weizman A, Carmi M, Hermesh H, et al. High affinity imipramine binding and serotonin uptake in platelets of eight adolescent and ten adult obsessive-compulsive patients. Am J Psychiatry 1986;143:335–339.
22. Palmer AM, Francis PT, Benton JS, et al. Presynaptic serotonergic dysfunction in patients with Alzheimer's disease. J Neurochem 1987;48:8–15.
23. Weizman R, Dick J, Mosek A, et al. Unaltered platelet [³H]imipramine binding in dementia of the Alzheimer type. Neuropsychobiology 1988;19:69–72.
24. Suranyi-Cadotte BE, Gauthier S, Lafaille F, et al. Platelet [³H]imipramine binding distinguishes depression from Alzheimer dementia. Life Sci 1985;37:2305–2311.
25. Weizman A, Morgenstern H, Kaplan B, et al. Upregulatory effect of triphasic oral contraceptive on platelet [³H]imipramine binding sites. Psychiatry Res 1987;23:23–29.
26. Rehavi M, Sepcuti H, Weizman A. Upregulation of imipramine binding and serotonin uptake by estradiol in female rat brain. Brain Res 1987;410:135–139.

49. Resting EEG as a Genetic Marker

F. VOGEL

A genetic marker is a heritable trait that is present in a fraction of a population and indicates increased susceptibility to a certain disease. This susceptibility might have one of two bases.[1]

1. Carriers of this variant might have a physiological disadvantage, which might lead to an "association" between the variant and the disease.
2. The marker gene locus might be closely linked with a gene locus influencing susceptibility, and the two loci might be in *linkage disequilibrium*.

The two situations can be distinguished mainly by family studies. Associations with restriction fragment length polymorphisms (RFLPs) belong to the second category. They are used for genetic counseling as well as for identification of "major genes" in complex phenotypes and their action by "reverse genetics."[1]

When the role of the electroencephalogram (EEG) as "genetic marker" for affective disorder is discussed, the term is used in its first meaning. Only a "trait" can serve as a marker. The EEG, however, always indicates a "state," although this state represents a "trait" under many normal conditions, as shown by its stability in the same individual[2] and its concordance in monozygotic (MZ) twins for the resting EEG,[3-5] the reaction to ethanol,[6] and for averaged evoked potentials.[7] Even if it cannot serve as marker, the EEG "state" may also help in elucidating the pathogenesis of a disease, e.g., the sleeping EEG in affective disorders.

Within the genetic variation of the normal resting EEG, a few "traits" have been identified, some of them with simple mendelian modes of inheritance.[4]

1. Low-voltage EEG, which occurs in about 4% of the adult population. The mode of inheritance is autosomal-dominant.
2. EEG with "monomorphic" alpha waves. It occurs in about 4% of the adult population, and a dominant major gene appears to be involved. These EEG variants are in a certain way countertypes.
3. Alpha waves mixed diffusely with beta waves. This pattern is a more common EEG type. Such EEGs are seen more frequently in women than in men, and their frequency increases in both sexes with advancing age. The genetic basis is polygenic.

Healthy probands with these three EEG variants have been compared using many physiological and psychological parameters.[8-11] Group differences between the two "countertypes"—the low-voltage EEG and the EEG with monomorphic alpha waves—were shown for reaction time, blood dopamine beta hydroxylase (DBH) levels, amplitudes and latencies of evoked potentials, and aspects of mental performance and personality. These group differences were explained by the theory[12] that the function of the alpha rhythm is thalamic modulation and selective amplification of incoming stimuli. The EEG type with diffuse beta waves combined low performance in spatial and arithmetic scores with low working speed, long reaction time, and high error-proneness in tasks testing concentration and working speed (disturbances of thalamic-cortical function by high tonic arousal in the ARAS?).

Except for a higher mania (Ma) score on the Minnesota Multiphasic Personality Index (MMPI) in subjects with monomorphic alpha waves compared with those having a low-voltage EEG, none of these group differences suggested a relation with affective disorders. Such a relation could exist, however, with the EEGs found in some alcohol addicts. Here EEGs have been described with reduced and somewhat irregular alpha activity. As shown by twin studies,[6] alpha activity of such EEGs becomes much more active and regular after alcohol intake, and this reaction is strongly concordant in MZ twins. It might lead to a corresponding improvement in feeling tone. Family studies have proved the genetic origin of this EEG type.[13] It appears to be a true "genetic marker."

Monozygotic twin concordance was also shown for evoked potentials[7] and for the "augmenting-reducing" response.[14] "Augmenters" were found more often in patients with affective disorders and their relatives than in normal controls.[15] Psychological differences between augmenters and reducers were also described in normal subjects. For example, augmenters were found to be more often "sensation-seeking" than reducers.[16] We confirmed the augmenting–reducing dichonoty as a fairly constant personal characteristic,[8] but no associations with personality scores (MMPI and 16 PF) in the expected direction were discovered. Table 49.1 shows the data for the depression, mania, and psychopathy scores of the MMPI. The

TABLE 49.1. Augmenters and reducers among normal students in relation to "affective MMPI scores.

Subjects	Augmenters	Reducers
Depression		
Male	21.72 (75)	21.92 (37)
Female	24.03 (87)	25.88 (25)
Both	22.96 (162)	23.52 (62)
Mania		
Male	16.81 (75)	16.65 (37)
Female	16.61 (87)	18.16 (25)
Both	16.70 (162)	17.26 (62)
Psychopathy		
Male	17.65 (75)	18.65 (37)
Female	17.08 (87)	19.80[a] (25)
Both	17.35 (162)	19.11[a] (62)

Results are given as means. Numbers of subjects are in parentheses.
[a]Differences are significant ($0.05 > p > 0.01$).

only significant difference was found for the psychopathy score, but the direction was opposite to that expected if it is assumed that "sensation-seeking" individuals also have higher psychopathy scores.

Electroencephelographic studies in patients suffering from affective disorder are hampered by the fact that most patients are under treatment or have been treated with psychotropic drugs. Perris[17] reviewed the available studies, the results of which are conflicting. When increases or decreases of alpha activity or increases of slow activity were observed, in most cases it could not be decided whether they were *traits*, clinical signs of a disease *state*, or caused by drug therapy, which in itself causes various EEG alterations. Such distinction is possible using the research design of Knott et al.,[18] who compared the EEGs with sib-pairs, one of whom had suffered from bipolar disease but failed to show psychotic signs at the time of examination and the other of whom had never suffered from an affective disorder. The former patients showed "a significantly smaller percentage of time in alpha." The data of Knott et al. paralleled the alpha reduction seen in some alcoholics.[13] A certain weakness of the alpha-producing circuit between thalamus and cortex might lead to an increased vulnerability for mood swings, especially for certain types of depression. The relation between depression and alcohol addiction has often been discussed. However, two other results should warn against too-optimistic generalizations: There was no increase of depression scores in normal subjects, whether with diffuse beta waves or with a low-voltage EEG.[10,11]

Another dimension might be added to these considerations by EEG studies in relation to suicide attempts. According to Struve,[19] paroxysmal EEGs are much more common among psychiatric patients who had attempted suicide than among other patients. Such EEGs had been described earlier in patients displaying temper tantrums and aggressive behavior.

Summary

This review has been confined to the problem of whether characteristics of the EEG can be used as genetic markers (by the definition given at the beginning) that might indicate increased susceptibility for affective disorder. To date, there is little evidence to support any useful EEG markers. One possible exception is the EEG with reduced and slightly irregular alpha activity. Its carriers appear to run an increased risk of becoming alcohol addicts. Moreover, studies on the resting EEG in affective disorder point to a certain increase of this EEG type as a personal *trait* in bipolar patients. It is hoped that other EEG traits to be discovered in the future might have a better predictive value.

Acknowledgment. Supported by the Deutsche Forschungsgemeinschaft.

References

1. Vogel F, Motulsky AG. Human Genetics—Problems and Approaches. 2nd Ed. New York: Springer Verlag, 1986.
2. Stassen HH, Günter R, Bomben G. Longterm stability of EEG: computerized recognition of person by EEG spectral patterns. In: Proceedings of the 6th International Conference on Pattern Recognition, 1982;619–622.

3. Stassen HH, Bomben G, Propping P. Genetic aspects of the EEG: an investigation into the within-pair similarity of monozygotic and dizygotic twins with a new method of analysis. Electroencephalogr Clin Neurophysiol 1987;66:489–501.
4. Vogel F. The genetic basis of the normal human electroencephalogram (EEG). Humangenetik 1970;10:91–114.
5. Vogel F. Grundlagen und Bedeutung genetisch bedingter Variabilität des normalen menschlichen EEG. EEG EMG 1986;17:173–188.
6. Propping P. Genetic control of ethanol action in the central nervous system. Hum Genet 1977;33:309–334.
7. Buchsbaum MS. Average evoked response and stimulus intensity of identical and fraternal twins. Physiol Psychol 1974;2:365–370.
8. Vogel F, Krüger J, Höpp HP, et al. Visually and auditory evoked EEG potentials in carriers of four hereditary EEG variants. Hum Neurobiol 1986;5:49–58.
9. Vogel F, Schalt E, Krüger J, et al. The electroencephalogram (EEG) as a research tool in human behavior genetics: psychological examinations in healthy males with various inherited EEG variants. I. Rationale of the study, material, methods, heritability of test parameters. Hum Genet 1979;47:1–45.
10. Vogel F, Schalt E, Krüger J. II. Results. Hum Genet 1979;47:47–80.
11. Vogel F, Schalt E, III. Interpretation of the results. Hum Genet 1979;47:81–111.
12. Anderson P, Andersson SA. Physiological Basis of the Alpha-Rhythm. New York: Appleton-Century-Crofts, 1968.
13. Propping P, Krüger J, Mark N. Genetic disposition of alcoholism: an EEG study in alcoholics and their relatives. Hum. Genet 1981;59:51–59.
14. Von Knorring L, Monakhov K, Perris C. Augmenting-reducing: an adaptive switch mechanism to cope with incoming signals in healthy subjects and psychiatric patients. Neuropsychobiology 1978;4:140–179.
15. Gershon ES, Buchbaum MS. A genetic study of averaged evoked response augmentation/reduction in affective disorders. In Shagass C, Gershon S, Friedhoff AJ (eds): Psychopathology and Brain Dysfunction. New York: Raven Press, 1977.
16. Zuckerman M, Murtau T, Siegel J. Sensation-seeking and cortical augmenting-reducing. Soc Psychophysiol Res 1974;5:535–542.
17. Perris C. Central measures of depression. In van Praag H, et al. (eds): Handbook of Biological Psychiatry. Part II. Brain Mechanisms and Abnormal Behavior. New York: Marcel Dekker, 1980;183–223.
18. Knott V, Waters B, Lapierre Y, et al. Neurophysiological correlates of sibling pairs discordant for bipolar affective disorders. Am J Psychiatry 1985;142:248–250.
19. Struve FA. Clinical electroencephalography and the study of suicide behavior. Suicide Life Threat Behav 1986;16:133–165.

50. EEG Sleep Changes in Recurrent Depression

DAVID J. KUPFER AND ELLEN FRANK

A few years ago we presented data pointing to the possible role of electroencephalographic (EEG) sleep patterns as a biological correlate in affective disorders. At that time we argued that although the notion of biological markers was becoming an increasingly prominent one their definition remained unclear and their application was often inappropriate. Any discussion of biological markers should begin, therefore, with the criteria for a valid biological marker and a minimum portrait delineating two types of marker. The first, the *episodic* (so-called *state*) *marker* appears during a clinically definable episode of illness but is not apparent at the completion of an episode when the patient is in remission. It was assumed that the marker was not present before the episode, and that it will present during the course of any future episodes. The second type of marker is viewed as a *trait marker*, not a so-called marker of the present state. It may be apparent in one of several blends: premorbidly or during, between, or only at the conclusion of an episode. A final point is that the same biological marker may be incorporated in both types (episodic/trait) of marker.

Only recently have investigators become interested in studying clinical and biological parameters during clinical remission and any changes preceding a recurrence in affective disorder patients. A group of patients with definite recurrent affective disorders is likely to demonstrate biological abnormalities. Longitudinal measurements provide the best opportunity to delineate differences between state and trait correlates in depressive states and to develop a set of precise definitions for which the term "biological marker" could be used. Preliminary data are available showing residual changes in shortened rapid-eye-movement (REM) latency, increased REM activity during the first half of the night, and sleep continuity disturbances even in the remission phase.[1] Yet they may still represent, on the whole, "reversible" parameters that can be associated only with the course of the episode.

Given the longitudinal design of our maintenance study in recurrent depression, we hope to be able to disentangle episodic variables from trait variables.[2,3] Although the treatment outcome study is not yet complete, the signs to date point to REM sleep variables as correlates of early recurrence in patients discontinued from active medication after clinical recovery (within 6 months of remission).

In a sample of 19 patients assigned to long-term maintenance interpersonal psychotherapy (MIPT) alone without pill, individuals were studied prior to their treatment for an index episode for depression, during continuation therapy, and into
a maintenance period in which 12 of these 19 patients subsequently had a recurrence
of their depression. Five of these patients had a recurrence within 6 months of
their assignment to maintenance treatment, and seven of the remaining patients
suffered a recurrence after 6 months. The sample of 19 patients (5 men and 14
women) had a median age of 39 with a baseline Hamilton score of 20. Their age
at onset of the depressive disorder began at 30.4 years $\pm$ 10.8; they had had a
median number of four previous episodes; and the median duration of their index
episode was 16 weeks. As shown in Figure 50.1, we examined three subgroups
(recurrence within 6 months, recurrence after 6 months, no recurrence) of this
sample. What is most significant is that throughout the entire treatment period
those patients who had an early recurrence of their depression showed a shortened
REM latency at treatment for the index episode, during clinical remission and
prior to a recurrence. In contrast, other sleep variables did not separate out these
subgroups. Even such variables as REM percent and REM activity showed no
differences over the three time periods.

Our further interest in examining REM latency over several episodes has led
to an examination of 19 cases of depression studied during a drug-free period at
the time of their index episode and during recurrence of their episode. Using paired
techniques of analysis, we found no significant severity differences during the two
episodes, but significant alterations in several REM measures in the recurrent
episode were noted compared to sleep during the index episode: increased REM

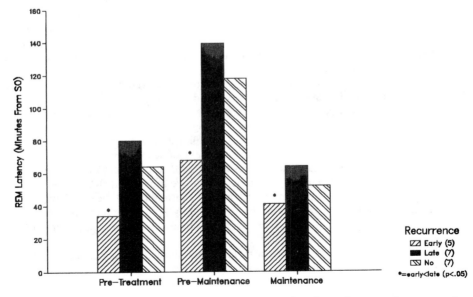

FIGURE 50.1. REM latency across time for 19 patients assigned to maintenance interpersonal
psychotherapy (MIPT) alone: pretreatment (baseline); premaintenance (active treatment);
and maintenance (no active drug).

percent and REM activity, and decreased REM latency. However, no significant changes were noted in other sleep measures, including sleep continuity and sleep architecture measures. At this time we are currently examining the distributions of REM and delta wave sleep using automated measures. Our interpretation of these findings is that during the recurrent episode patients had been depressed on the average of only 2–3 weeks, whereas during the index episode they had, on the average, been depressed at least 4 months. It appears that REM latencies, at least in this selected group of patients, are lower during the initial phase of the episodes than during a latter phase of an episode of depression.

In 1984 we concluded that there is increasing evidence that patients with recurrent depression may continue to demonstrate residual abnormalities such as shorter REM latency, increased REM activity during the first half of the night, and sleep continuation disturbances even in the clinical remission phase.[1] We thought that oscillation in REM latency may be more sensitive to the clinical course, that changes in the REM percent and sleep maintenance variables were sensitive to drug effects, and that the onset of a new episode may be associated with a redistribution in REM activity. Although it is too early to assume that there will not be a specificity of sleep variables directly related to the difference between the episode state and the clinical remission period, we are confident that there are trait-related variables that predispose the individuals who are most likely to relapse or suffer an early recurrence from those who are most likely to continue in recovery.

Earlier suggestions that REM sleep measures would represent both episode and trait correlates of disease are beginning to come true. Investigators in the United States and Europe are conducting studies along similar lines. It is still too early to conclude that neuroendocrine measures do not have the same amount of potency as do sleep measures in examining this question. One caveat with this approach is that we have examined naturalistic data rather than examining the effects of various pharmacological or nonpharmacological probes. We are confident that a profile will be developed that represents a truly psychobiological set of measures that can help us predict with accuracy those correlates for the episode and those correlates of high risk for new episodes. These data sets may represent important information concerning our attempt to understand early warning signs in the development of new episodes in depression.

A proposal on the hypothalamic peptide modulation of EEG sleep in depression may offer several advantages for dissecting out episode and trait variables: (a) It provides additional experimental tools to test the effects of neuropeptide challenge strategies on the sleep EEG, (b) It facilitates the examination of interactions among various biological rhythms. (c) Specific predictions concerning the level of dissociation among selected biological in the depressive state and in the state of clinical recovery can be made.[4]

Acknowledgment. Supported in part by National Institute of Mental Health Grant MH–29618.

References

1. Kupfer DJ. The role of EEG sleep as a biological correlate in affective disorders. In Burrows G (ed): Advances in Neuropsychopharmacology. London: Smith-Gordon John Libbey, 1984;65–71.

2. Frank E, Kupfer DJ. Maintenance treatment of recurrent unipolar depression: pharmacology and psychotherapy. In Kemali D, Racagni G (eds): Chronic Treatments in Neuropsychiatry. New York: Raven Press, 1985;139–151.
3. Kupfer DJ, Frank E, Perel JM. Biology, therapeutics and prophylaxis in recurrent depression. In Hippius H, Klerman G, Matussek N (eds): New Results in Depression Research. Heidelberg: Springer-Verlag, 1986;119–125.
4. Ehlers CL, Kupfer DJ. Hypothalamic peptide modulation of EEG sleep in depression: a further application of the S-process hypothesis. Biol Psychiatry 1987;22:513–517.

II.C. CHRONOBIOLOGY

51. Circadian and Ultradian Rhythms of 3-Methoxy-4-Hydroxyphenylglycol in Subtypes of Depressive Illness

ANGELOS HALARIS

The catecholamine hypothesis of affective disorders, as originally postulated by Bunney and Davis[1] and Schildkraut,[2] has focused on norepinephrine (NE) as the neurotransmitter intricately linked to mania and certain types of depressive illness. Although a definitive causal relation between aberrant noradrenergic transmission and affective illness has not been unequivocally established, this conceptual framework has provided the impetus for a host of innovative modifications and expansions of the original hypothesis. Some of the most intriguing hypotheses include the adrenergic receptor down-regulation hypothesis, [3–6] the phase-advance hypothesis of circadian rhythms,[7–9] and the dysregulation hypothesis introduced by Siever and Davis.[10]

Altered noradrenergic function is tantamount to the pathophysiology of affective illness.[11] Noninvasive indicators of noradrenergic activity in the central nervous system (CNS) include the measurement of 3-methoxy-4-hydroxyphenylglycol (MHPG), the principal CNS metabolite of NE,[12–14] in various body fluids. The origin and distribution of MHPG in each of the principal body fluids has been reviewed elsewhere.[15] Several studies have confirmed that MHPG levels in cerebrospinal fluid (CSF), urine, and plasma are altered with changes in mood states.[16–19] Significant elevations of MHPG levels have been associated with stressed normal subjects or manic patients.[18,20] Urinary excretion of MHPG is significantly decreased in certain types of depressed patients, especially bipolar manic-depressives[21]; moreover, altered excretion rates of MHPG may be predictive of a response to treatment with certain antidepressants.[22–24] Despite these results, however, attempts to demonstrate consistent and unequivocal decreases in MHPG in depressed patients have failed. Indeed, both decreases and increases in baseline MHPG levels have been reported, and some studies have found no significant differences between depressed patients and normal controls or other patient populations. Furthermore, successful treatment of depressed patients with tricyclic antidepressants does not produce a sustained increase in MHPG levels, as might be expected if NE activity were directly related to the depressed mood state.[25,26]

Methodological improvements during the 1970s (e.g., electron-capture gas chromatography and high-performance liquid chromatography) have permitted more frequent sampling, which led to the discovery that plasma and urinary MHPG levels follow a distinct diurnal variation.[20,27–29] Because plasma MHPG is usually determined at a single time point (typically 9 a.m.), whereas urine samples are collected over 24 h, the presence of a diurnal rhythm complicates the interpretation of data obtained with either approach. Furthermore, studies have suggested that the phase and/or period of diurnal MHPG rhythms may be altered in affective disorders.[29,30] Wehr and co-workers[30] were the first to demonstrate that urinary MHPG in manic-depressives showed a circadian rhythm that was phase-advanced (i.e., had an earlier peak) of approximately 1–3 h compared with normal subjects. This finding of a phase advance was confirmed by Giedke et al.,[31] but these authors failed to find a clear diurnal rhythm of MHPG in their depressed patients. Pflug and colleagues[32] also demonstrated this phase advance but related it to a shorter period of urinary MHPG. It is possible that these divergent results are related to the general methodological difficulties of urinary measurements, although it is clear that both central and peripheral compartments of MHPG are highly correlated,[33,34] and furthermore that the urinary and plasma compartments of MHPG also have clear and consistent interrelations.[35]

As noted above, phase advances in the rhythms of manic and depressed patients have been reported for both plasma and urine. Because blood sampling is conventionally performed at the same time of day in both control and depressed subjects, a phase advance (or delay) in the diurnal rhythm could be mistakenly interpreted as indicating an increase (or decrease) in baseline MHPG levels of depressed subjects. Following our pilot studies, in which we measured baseline plasma MHPG levels in various groups of manic-depressives,[18] and having been impressed with a greater than expected variability in values obtained from unipolar depressives, we chose to conduct diurnal measurements rather than single time point evaluations in carefully diagnosed groups of patients. It was thought that the capability to obtain instantaneous measurements of plasma MHPG levels would better define the diurnal rhythm and would more consistently delineate a pathological pattern in depressives. Initial findings using this method demonstrated that MHPG levels peaked earlier in a patient with rapidly cycling bipolar illness,[19] and the successful treatment with desipramine (DMI) caused an apparent phase delay of the phase-advanced diurnal rhythm in three endogenously depressed patients.[29]

We have demonstrated that the metabolism of NE, as reflected by levels of total plasma MHPG, undergoes diurnal variation in normal male subjects and depressed patients.[35] This finding corroborates results from previous investigations on the circadian rhythm of NE and of catecholamine metabolites in healthy volunteers[30,31] as well as in depressed patients.[30,32] Furthermore, these results complement the findings of studies by Kafka,[36] who demonstrated circadian rhythms in the densities of α_1- and β-adrenergic receptors and NE-stimulated cyclic adenosine monophosphate (cAMP) in rats, although these studies had remained unconfirmed for the α_2-adrenergic receptors[37] until recently. Kafka and co-workers[38] have now confirmed the presence of diurnal rhythmicity in α_2-receptors in discrete regions of the rat brain. A circadian MHPG rhythm in rat hippocampus and possibly in occipital cortex has also been described by Kafka and co-workers.[39] Our finding of a phase advance in the MHPG rhythm in our depressed patient population is consistent with results from previous investigations.[30–31] This abnormality was detected convincingly in our group of endogenous patients, and treatment with DMI partly corrected the phase shift. In contrast, the nonendogenous subgroup did not demonstrate such a phase abnormality.

Norepinephrine rhythms might be accounted for by sleep, level of perceived stress, or alcohol intake. Food does not appear to influence the rhythm of epinephrine or NE, and effects of posture on rhythms of NE are still controversial. Previous unpublished observations from our laboratory did not point to the need to control for food intake or feeding schedules. Additionally, the effects of posture were not controlled for in our study. It is possible that these factors may have influenced the results, but it is rather unlikely, as volunteers and patients were studied and restudied under comparable and highly consistent conditions. Nevertheless, future investigations should more carefully control for temperature rhythms, posture, level of stress, and sleep parameters in order to further elucidate the concomitants of aberrant circadian MHPG rhythms.

Depressed patients as a group exhibited a lesser degree of synchronization to the circadian cosine model than did volunteers. It was especially true in retarded depressives. Following treatment there was a partial correction of this desynchrony, which occurred significantly in retarded depressives. Nonretarded depressives did not demonstrate a correction in this parameter. Giedke and co-workers[31] obtained similar results in a group of bipolar and unipolar depressives measuring urinary MHPG, but they conducted their measurements on a mixed sample of medicated and drug-free patients. It may have somewhat distorted their results because the effects of the drugs were shown to lengthen the MHPG period. Pflug and colleagues[32] demonstrated that the MHPG rhythm was dissociated from the temperature rhythm during the depression stage of a bipolar patient. During her well state the rhythms were resynchronized. It is possible that the level of desynchrony demonstrated in our patient population represents a shifting of one internal zeitgeber from another or, alternatively, an inability of the internal zeitgeber to adjust to external cues such as dawn or dusk. Demonstration of ultradian periodicity in these MHPG rhythms would be supporting evidence for either of the above hypotheses.

The detection of an ultradian MHPG rhythm in at least a subpopulation of our depressed patients is an intriguing finding. The ultradian rhythm may be partially or fully responsible for the apparent phase advance and the poor fit of the MHPG circadian rhythm by the cosine model in the group of depressed patients. Neither the cause nor the mechanism by which such a rhythm emerges is understood. Even less well understood is the possible relevance to the pathophysiology of depressive illness. The fact that the amplitude of the ultradian MHPG rhythm diminishes with successful antidepressant drug treatment may be unrelated to the reversal of depressive symptomatology.

Like other investigators,[8,32] we did find that subsequent to antidepressant drug treatment patients demonstrated a longer period length than that of volunteers. It was especially true in patients who responded to treatment and in the endogenous subgroup. It is possible that the corrective effects of tricyclic antidepressants may be related, at least in part, to the increasing circadian period length caused by these drugs. As period length increases, phase is delayed. Although we could not demonstrate on repeated measures ANOVA a significant change in our patients with respect to period length, we were able to show that period and acrophase were highly correlated in the depressives, whereas in the normal volunteers they were not. It is hypothesized that period and phase are distinctly related, and that this relation does not appear in volunteers because of the degree of synchronization of their zeitgebers.

Clearly, these findings can be viewed only as preliminary. Nevertheless, they are sufficiently intriguing to warrant additional studies that are more rigorously designed and include well defined subtypes of affective disorders.

Acknowledgment. I gratefully acknowledge the significant contributions of Edward M. DeMet, Ph.D., Harry Gwirtsman, M.D., John Piletz, Ph.D., and Abraham Wolf, Ph.D..

References

1. Bunney WE Jr, Davis JM. Norepinephrine in depressive reactions: a review. Arch Gen Psychiatry 1965;13:483–494.
2. Schildkraut JJ. The catecholamine hypothesis of affective disorders: a review of supporting evidence. Am J Psychiatry 1965;122:509–522.
3. Banerjee SP, Kung LS, Riggi SJ, et al. Development of β-adrenergic receptor subsensitivity by antidepressants. Nature 1977;268:455–456.
4. Sulser F, Vetulani J, Mobley PL. Mode of action of antidepressant drugs. Biochem Pharmacol 1978;27:257–261.
5. Charney DS, Menkes DB, Heninger GR. Receptor sensitivity and the mechanism of action of antidepressant treatment. Arch Gen Psychiatry 1981;38:1160–1180.
6. Charney DS, Heninger GR, Sternberg DE, et al. Presynaptic adrenergic receptor sensitivity in depression. Arch Gen Psychiatry 1981;38:1334–1340.
7. Papousek M. Chronobiological aspects of cyclothymia. Fortschr Neurol Psychiatr 1975;43:381–440.
8. Kripke DF, Mullaney DJ, Atkinson M, Wolf S. Circadian rhythm disorder in manic-depressives. Biol Psychiatry 1978;13:335–351.
9. Wehr TA, Goodwin FK. Biological rhythms and psychiatry. In Arieti S, Brodie HKH (eds): American Handbook of Psychiatry. 2nd Ed. Vol. 7. New York: Basic Books, 1981;46–74.
10. Siever LJ, Davis KL. Overview: toward a dysregulation hypothesis of depression. Am J Psychiatry 1985;142:1017–1031.
11. Schildkrut JJ. Current status of the catecholamine hypothesis of affective disorders. In Lipton MA, DiMascio A, Killam KF (eds): Psychopharmacology: A Generation of Progress. New York: Raven Press, 1978;1223–1234.
12. Axelrod J, Kopin IJ, Mann JD. 3-Methoxy-4-hydroxyphenylglycol sulfate, a new metabolite of epinephrine and norepinephrine. Biochim Biophys Acta 1959;36:576–577.
13. Maas JW, Landis DH. In vivo studies of metabolism of norepinephrine in central nervous system. J Pharmacol Exp Ther 1968;163:147–162.
14. Maas JW, Landis DH. The metabolism of circulating norepinephrine by human subjects. J Pharmacol Exp Ther 1971;177:600–612.
15. DeMet EM, Halaris AE. Origin and distribution of 3-methoxy-4-hydroxyphenylglycol in body fluids. Biochem Pharmacol 1979;28:3043–3050.
16. Schildkraut JJ, Kety SS. Biogenic amines and emotion. Science 1967;156:21–30.
17. Gordon EK, Oliver J. 3-Methoxy-4-hydroxyphenylethylene glycol in human cerebrospinal fluid. Clin Chim Acta 1971;35:145–150.
18. Halaris AE, DeMet EM. Studies of norepinephrine metabolism in manic and depressive states. In Usdin E, Kopin IJ, Barchas J (eds): Catecholamines: Basic and Clinical Frontiers. New York: Pergamon Press, 1979;1866–1868.
19. Ostrow D, Halaris A, Dysken M, et al. State dependence of noradrenergic activity in a rapidly cycling bipolar patient. J Clin Psychiatry 1984;45:306–309.
20. Cymerman A, Francesconi RF. Alteration of circadian rhythmicities of urinary 3-methoxy-4-hydroxyphenylglycol (MHGP) and vanillylmandelic acid (VMA) in man during cold exposure. Life Sci 1975;16:225–236.
21. Muscettola G, Potter WZ, Pickar D, et al. Urinary 3-methoxy-4-hydroxyphenylglycol and major affective disorders. Arch Gen Psychiatry 1984;41:337–342.
22. Fawcett JA, Maas JW, Dekirmenjian H. Depression and MHPG excretion: response to dextroamphetamine and tricyclic antidepressants. Arch Gen Psychiatry 1972;26:246–251.

23. Beckmann H, Goodwin FK. Urinary MHPG in subgroups of depressed patients and normal controls. Neuropsychobiology 1980;6:91–100.
24. Rosenbaum AH, Schatzberg AF, Maruta J, et al. MHPG as a predictor of antidepressant response to imipramine and maprotiline. Arch Gen Psychiatry 1980;137:1090–1092.
25. Beckmann H, Goodwin FK. Antidepressant response to tricyclics and urinary MHPG in unipolar patients. Arch Gen Psychiatry 1975;32:17–21.
26. Halaris AE, DeMet EM. Open trial evaluation of a pyrrolidine derivative (AHR-1118) on norepinephrine metabolism. Prog Neuropsychopharmacol 1980;4:43–49.
27. Markianos E, Beckmann H. Diurnal changes in dopamine-β-hydroxylase, homovanillic acid and 3-methoxy-4-hydroxyphenylglycol in serum in man. J Neural Transm 1976;39:79–93.
28. Hollister LE, Davis KL, Overall JE, et al. Excretion of MHPG in normal subjects. Arch Gen Psychiatry 1978;35:1410–1415.
29. DeMet EM, Halaris AE, Gwirtsman HE, et al. Effects of desipramine on diurnal rhythms of plasma 3-methoxy-4-hydroxyphenylglycol (MHPG) in depressed patients Psychopharmacol Bull 1982;18:221–223.
30. Wehr TA, Muscettola G, Goodwin FK. Urinary 3-methoxy-4-hydroxyphenylglycol circadian rhythm. Arch Gen Psychiatry 1980;37:257–263.
31. Giedke H, Gaertner HJ, Mahal A. Diurnal variation of urinary MHPG in unipolar and bipolar depressives. Acta Psychiatr Scand 1982;66:243–253.
32. Pflug B, Engelmann W, Gaertner HJ. Circadian course of body temperature and the excretion of MHPG and VMA in a patient with bipolar depression. J Neural Transm 1982;53:213–215.
33. Lingjaerde O. The biochemistry of depression. Acta Psychiatr Scand 1983;302:36–51.
34. Maas JW, Kocsis JH, Bowden CL, et al. Pretreatment neurotransmitter metabolites and response to imipramine or amitriptyline treatment. Psychol Med 1982;12:37–43.
35. DeMet EM, Halaris AE, Gwirtsman HE, et al. Diurnal rhythm of 3-methoxy-4-hydroxyphenylglycol (MHPG): relationship between plasma and urinary levels. Life Sci 1985;37:1731–1741.
36. Kafka MS. The effect of antidepressants on circadian rhythms in brain neurotransmitter receptors. Acta Pharmacol Toxicol [Suppl 1] (Copenh) 1985;56:162–164.
37. Jones SB, Bylund DB, Reiser CA, et al. Alpha$_2$ adrenergic receptor binding in human platelets: alterations during the menstrual cycle. Clin Pharmacol Ther 1983;34:90–96.
38. Kafka MS, Benedito MA, Blendy JA, et al. Circadian rhythms in neurotransmitter receptors in discrete rat brain regions. Chronobiol Int 1986;3:91–100.
39. Kafka MS, Benedito MA, Roth RH, et al. Circadian rhythms in catecholamine metabolites and cyclic nucleotide production. Chronobiol Int 1986;3:101–115.

52. Chronobiological Dysregulation of the Noradrenergic System in Depression

LARRY J. SIEVER, EMIL F. COCCARO,
STUART SILVERMAN, STEVEN GREENWALD, AND
KENNETH L. DAVIS

Whereas models of abnormal noradrenergic activity in depression initially posited a deficiency or excess in noradrenergic activity in depression and mania, respectively, more recent formulations of abnormal adrenergic activity in the affective disorders have focused on the temporal regulation of noradrenergic activity.[1] It has been suggested that there is a phase advance of noradrenergic activity in depression, and an earlier peak of urinary 3-methoxy-4-hydroxyphenylglycol (MHPG) excretion has been demonstrated in one study of major depressive disorder.[2] However, other studies suggest that a better characterization of the noradrenergic and related systems in the affective disorders is that it is dysregulated, i.e., more erratic and variable in its activity.[3] Evidence for such a formulation derives from studies of the basal rhythmicity of the noradrenergic system and responses of this system to naturalistic and pharmacological studies. These studies suggest that an impairment in the regulation (e.g., feedback control) of the noradrenergic system may result in a poorly buffered output of this system.[1]

Several studies have suggested that diurnal rhythms of the noradrenergic metabolite MHPG in depression are desynchronized and highly variable among individual patients, with multiple, erratic peaks.[3] Studies of the chronobiology of body temperature and onset of rapid-eye-movement (REM) sleep, which may be partially regulated by noradrenergic function, are more disorganized with suggestions of higher frequency rhythms.[3] Cortisol secretion, which is indirectly regulated by the noradrenergic system at the suprahypothalamic level, is also increased and erratic.[4] The apparently erratic, disorganized quality of these chronobiological patterns may be attributable to the superimposition of higher frequency harmonics of the predominant rhythm. The shift to higher frequency harmonics is indicative of a destablized system, as has been postulated in the case of the noradrenergic system in depression.[3]

The etiology of poorly regulated output of the noradrenergic system is not known but could reside in one or more of the many regulatory processors that impinge on noradrenergic release, e.g., regulation of tyrosine hydroxylase activity, regulation of exocytotic release, and feedback control of release by the α_2-adrenergic receptor. Some evidence suggests that there may be functional impairment in presynaptic α_2-adrenergic function. Impairment in the efficiency of a regulatory site such as the α_2-adrenergic receptor might contribute to dysregulated norad-renergic output in response to increased demand or stress. Whereas the diminished efficiency of the regulatory site would be expected to persist beyond the acute phase of depression, the overt dysregulation in response to stress would be expected to be state-related, e.g., associated with the acute state of depression, and to partially remit when the system was no longer stressed.[1]

Preliminary data are consistent with such a model. In one case study, urinary MHPG concentrations measured at intervals during the day and averaged were characterized chronobiologically by multiple, erratic peaks in a bipolar patient in the depressed state, whereas the same patient in the remitted state evidenced the normal single afternoon peak.[5] Apparently disordered rhythms of plasma MHPG, characterized by the appearance of a 12-h rhythm largely replacing the expected 24-h rhythm, observed in the acute state of depression seems to normalize in patients treated with antidepressants.[6] Preliminary results of a study in our laboratory of the daytime rhythms of plasma MHPG and pituitary hormones suggest that erratic increased concentrations of MHPG and cortisol associated with suggestions of higher frequency ultradian rhythms in these systems may be found in

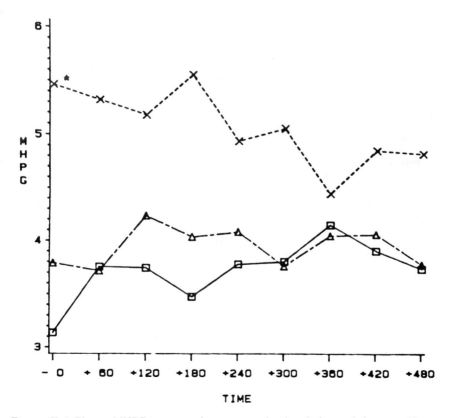

FIGURE 52.1. Plasma MHPG concentrations measured at hourly intervals between 10 a.m. and 6 p.m. in supine, acute depressed patients, remitted depressed patients, and normal controls. (×) acute depressed patients. (△) remitted depressed patients. (□) normal controls.

acute depressives but partially normalize in the remitted state (Fig. 52.1). These results contrast with the persistence of receptor-mediated abnormalities, e.g., the blunted growth hormone response to clonidine mediated by the α_2-adrenergic receptor, observable in both the acute and the remitted state.[7]

Summary

A growing body of evidence suggests that the chronobiology of the noradrenergic system may be destabilized or dysregulated. The destabilization may manifest as erratic peaks, perhaps reflecting higher-frequency harmonics of the predominant 24-h rhythm. There are suggestions that the overt chronobiological destabilization associated with depression is state-dependent and may partially normalize with remission. Reductions in efficiency of regulatory sites, such as the α_2-adrenergic receptor, might contribute to the stress-induced overt destabilization of the depressive state. Further exploration of these hypotheses may be helpful in elucidating the character of the trait vulnerability to depression and how it interacts with precipitants to depression, e.g., stress, to lead to the overt psychobiological destabilization associated with the acute depressive episode.

References

1. Siever LJ, Davis KL. Overview: towards a dysregulation hypothesis of depression. Am J Psychiatry 1985;142:1017–1031.
2. Wehr TA, Muscettola G, Goodwin FK. Urinary MHPG circadian rhythm: early timing (phase advance) in manic-depressives compared with normal subjects. Arch Gen Psychiatry 1980;37:257–263.
3. Siever LJ, Coccaro EF, Davis KL. Chronobiologic instability of the noradrenergic system in depression. In Halaris A (ed): Chronobiology and Neuropsychiatric Disorders. New York: Pergamon Press, 1987;1–22.
4. Sachar EJ, Hellman L, Roffwarg HP, et al. Disrupted 24-hour patterns of cortisol secretion in psychotic depression. Arch Gen Psychiatry 1973;28:19–24.
5. Pflug B, Engelmann W, Gaertner HJ. Circadian course of body temperature and the excretion of MHPG and VMA in a patient with bipolar depression. J Neural Transm 1982;53:213–215.
6. Halaris A. Circadian and ultradian rhythms of 3-methoxy-4-hydroxyphenylglycol in subtypes of depressive illness. In: New Directions in Affective Disorders. New York: Springer Verlag, Ch. 51 (this volume).
7. Siever LJ, Coccaro EF, Friedman R, et al. Noradrenergic and serotonergic dysfunction in the affective disorders. In: New Directions in Affective Disorders, New York: Springer-Verlag, Ch. 10 (this volume).

53. Diurnal Rhythm of Cortisol in Depression: What Is Normal and What Is Not

URIEL HALBREICH, GREGORY ASNIS,
RICHARD SHINDLEDECKER, AND R. SWAMI NATHAN

Abnormalities of the hypothalamic-pituitary-adrenal (HPA) system in depression have been reported in numerous studies. It has been suggested that patients with major depressive disorder—endogenous subtype (MDD-ED) have increased basal levels of cortisol (in plasma and urine) and nonsuppressibility of cortisol in response to dexamethasone, i.e., an abnormal dexamethasone suppression test (DST). A plethora of disturbances in the rhythm of cortisol secretion have been reported, mainly a "flattened curve" and a phase advance of cortisol, meaning that levels of plasma cortisol in MDD-ED patients peak earlier and they do not decrease in the early afternoon and evening, as is the case with the normal plasma cortisol curve. It has also been suggested that MDD-ED patients have a larger number of secretory episodes per 24 h, and that the amount of cortisol secreted during each episode is higher than normal.[1-5] In most reports it has also been assumed than an abnormality of one of the functions of the HPA means that the entire system is abnormal; in particular, an abnormal DST is often reported as "abnormal HPA system" or "cortisol hypersecretion."

In this chapter we concentrate on the rhythm functions of the HPA system, comparing 32 patients diagnosed as having MDD-ED to 72 normal subjects.[6-8]

Shape of the 24-Hour Curve: Its Amplitude and Acrophase

The normal 24-h pattern of cortisol secretion fits a cosinor curve with an acrophase during the late morning hours: 10 h 16 min $\pm$ 2 h 32 min. The pattern of the 24-h curve of the MDD-ED patients did not differ from that of the normals. The acrophase was at 10 h 48 min $\pm$ 1 h 48 min. There was also no difference in the amplitude (the magnitude of fluctuations from the mesor, or mean, levels) or in some other statistical parameters that might express a relative decrease of fluctuation.[8] The 24-h curve of cortisol levels has not been found to be flat in MDD-ED patients or even in those who could be defined as being hypersecretors of cortisol. This result was confirmed by two other groups[9,10] who also confirmed the lack of acrophase advance in MDD-ED patients. The fact that such an advance was found in earlier studies is probably due to two methodological weaknesses: First, blood samples were obtained infrequently, and patient groups were small.

Second, and more important, the age variable had not been taken into account, and older depressives were compared to young normals. An inverse correlation between age and acrophase has been found by us and the Iowa group,[8,10] meaning that older people tend to have earlier peaks of cortisol levels. Once age is controlled for, the acrophases of depressives and normals do not differ from each other.

Nadir, Time of First Secretory Episode, and Relation to Sleep Onset

Depressives were found to be different from normal subjects in rhythm indices that are pertinent to the quiescent early night period and the early activation of cortisol secretion. The normal nadir was at 1 h 19 min $\pm$ 1 h 47 min, whereas the MDD-ED nadir was found to be significantly earlier: 0 h 38 min $\pm$ 47 min (t = 2.091, p = 0.039). This difference was mainly due to age (F = 4.00, p = 0.049, ANCOVA), and when age was controlled for there was only a nonsignificant trend (p = 0.151) toward such a difference.

Even though the time of minimal levels of cortisol is only slightly abnormal in MDD-ED patients, it might be suggested that the HPA system is activated earlier in endogenous depression. Normally the active secretion of cortisol starts about 2 h after sleep onset. In MDD-ED patients the first secretory episode of cortisol following the night nadir was at 1 h 45 min $\pm$ 1 h 54 min, whereas in the normals it occurred at 2 h 49 min $\pm$ 1 h 30 min (t = 3.042, p = 0.0031). As is the case with other parameters of rhythm, age has a significant effect on time of first episode (F = 11.20, p = 0.0014), and a negative correlation between the two variables has been demonstrated. Nonetheless, when age was controlled for, the difference between the two groups was still significant (F = 7.24, p = 0.0089).

As was mentioned earlier, there is normally an association between time of sleep onset and the beginning of cortisol secretion. This association is probably different in MDD-ED patients. Not only is the clock-time of the first secretory episode earlier, the time lag between sleep onset and that episode is shorter. As is demonstrated in Figure 53.1, cortisol levels of depressives start to climb earlier after sleep onset. The figure shows that it is true only in MDD-ED patients who have relatively higher levels of cortisol but not in those who have normal levels; hence this phenomenon is not universal in ED patients (as is the case with most functions of the HPA system).

The possible dissociation between sleep onset and the beginning of active secretion of cortisol might be of heuristic significance. It may point to a possibility that the two oscillators are dissociated from each other in at least some MDD-ED patients. The dissociation, or imbalance between various time-related functions, might be of importance in the pathophysiology of depressions and not necessarily only an abnormality of each of them in isolation.

Secretory Episodes: Their Number and Magnitude

It has been suggested[2] that MDD-ED patients have more secretory episodes during the 24-h period and each episode is of higher magnitude than those in normals. By application of Fourier's analysis (spectral analysis) we have demonstrated that as a group ED patients had increased 4-h variance density (higher magnitude of cortisol secretory episodes), but they did not have a larger number of episodes

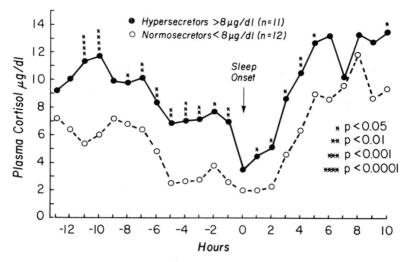

FIGURE 53.1. Mean hourly plasma cortisol levels in hypersecreting and normosecreting endogenously depressed patients according to time of sleep onset. (Definition of hypo- and normosecretion here is arbitrary. Patients were divided into two almost equal groups according to cortisol levels higher or lower than 1 SD of the normal mean.)

per 24 h (higher frequency). If any, the opposite may exist (6.5 episodes/24 h in the ED patients versus 8.8 episodes/24 h in the normal group). We concluded that MDD-ED patients have an abnormal ultradian rhythm (rhythm shorter than 24 h) that is manifested in fewer secretory episodes, but during each episode more cortisol is secreted. The abnormal ultradian rhythm in ED patients is further confirmed by a nonsignificant circadian fluctuation (tA) and a lower-than-normal (though still significant) fitness of the cosinor curve. As is the case with other parameters of the HPA system, only a subgroup of MDD-ED patients have abnormal ultradian rhythm, and some others have a perfectly normal rhythm.

Conclusion

A detailed examination of the 24-h and ultradian rhythms of cortisol in endogenous depressives reveals that as a group MDD-ED patients did not differ from normals in the general pattern of the 24-h cortisol curve, which is not "flat," nor were there any differences in the acrophase and amplitude. Depressives do differ from normals in the timing of the first secretory episode and its relation to sleep onset as well as the magnitude of secretory episodes, but probably not in their frequency. Age plays an important role in time-related variables of the HPA system. For each of the variables only a subgroup of MDD-ED patients are abnormal, and abnormality in one variable does not imply that other variables are abnormal as well: They might be only partially associated with each other.

Acknowledgment. The reported studies were supported in part by NIMH grants R01-37111, R01-41423, and R01-29841; GCRC grants RR50 and RR53; and the Ritter's Foundation.

References

1. Gibbons JL, McHugh PR. Plasma cortisol in depressive illness. J Psychiatr Res 1962;1:162–171.
2. Sachar EJ, Hellman L, Roffwarg HP, et al. Disrupted 24-hour patterns of cortisol secretion in psychotic depression. Arch Gen Psychiatry 1973;28:19–24.
3. Carroll BJ, Curtis GC, Mendels J. Neuroendocrine regulation of depression. I. Limbic system-adrenocortical dysfunction. Arch Gen Psychiatry 1976;33:1039–1044.
4. Carroll BJ, Curtis GC, Mendels J. Neuroendocrine regulation in depression. II. Discrimination of depressed from nondepressed patients. Arch Gen Psychiatry 1976;33:1051–1058.
5. Carroll BJ, Feinberg M, Greden JF, et al. A specific laboratory test for the diagnosis of melancholia: standardization, validation, and clinical utility. Arch Gen Psychiatry 1981;38:15–22.
6. Halbreich U, Zumoff B, Kream J, et al. The mean 1300–1600h plasma cortisol concentration as a diagnostic test for hypercortisolism. J Clin Endocrinol Metab 1982;54:1262–1264.
7. Halbreich U, Asnis GM, Shindledecker R, et al. Cortisol secretion in endogenous depression. I. Basal plasma levels. Arch Gen Psychiatry 1985;42:904–908.
8. Halbreich U, Asnis GM, Shindledecker R, et al. Cortisol secretion in endogenous depression. II. Time-related functions. Arch Gen Psychiatry 1985; 42:909–914.
9. Linkowski P, Mendlewicz J, Leclercq R, et al. The 24-hour profile of adrenocorticotropin and cortisol in major depressive illness. J Clin Endocrinol Metab 1985;61:429.
10. Sherman B, Wysham B, Phohl B. Age-related changes in the circadian rhythm of plasma cortisol in man. J Clin Endocrinol Metab 1985;61:439.

54. Circadian Rhythm Disturbances in Affective Disorders: Facts and Fictions

D. VON ZERSSEN, G. DIRLICH, AND J. ZULLEY

The cycling nature of affective disorders has put these psychopathological conditions into the focus of medical chronobiology. However, our knowledge is still rather limited in this respect, and too often casual observations and theoretical speculations are accepted as proving profound disturbances of biological (above all, circadian) rhythms in these disorders. It is our intention to evaluate critically the present state of knowledge in this field in order to disentangle proved facts from mere fictions. Particular reference is made to carefully designed observations of affectively ill patients in a time-cue-free environment, as they provide the only solid basis for conclusions regarding the endogenous component of biological rhythms. Only those hypotheses are discussed that have drawn most attention in chronobiological research to affective disorders.

Assumed Disturbances of Circadian Rhythms

Period

Rapid cycling in bipolar affective illness was explained by Halberg[1] as a beat phenomenon due to the interaction of circadian rhythms entrained to the 24-h routine of daily life with a free-running rhythm of, for example, adrenocortical activity. The cycle length of psychopathology should then be predictable from the period of this nonentrained and the entrained (24-h) rhythm—or vice versa: The period of the free-running circadian rhythm should be predictable from the 24-h period of entrained circadian rhythms and the period of the cycles of the mental disorder.

This concept was demonstrated rather than validated on the basis of data from a single case study in a rapid cycler.[2] Later it was supported by self-assessed oral temperature data in an outpatient suffering from rapidly cycling bipolar affective illness.[3] The same authors also reported the occurrence of free-running biological rhythms in other outpatients with rapidly cycling manic-depressive disease who had taken the measurements themselves during the illness. Unfortunately, it cannot be excluded that the abnormalities were entirely caused by unreliable data due to the mental state in which the patients took the measurements.

Some light is thrown on this problem by case reports from another group of researchers. They had found a 22.5-h component in addition to the 24-h component in the periodogram of oral temperature during an episode of a bipolar II depression when the patient was hospitalized. This component did not appear in a data set obtained by the patient herself after clinical recovery and during subsequent episodes.[4] Nevertheless, the finding was interpreted by the authors as reflecting a free-running period rather than problems in taking the measurements. Because of the lengthening of the free-running circadian period in plants and lower animals by lithium it was even inferred that the prophylactic effect of this compound in recurrent affective disorders was caused by a normalization of an abnormally fast endogenous rhythm in afflicted human subjects.[5] However, in five other depressives subsequently studied by Pflug et al.,[6] no such abnormality could be detected in the circadian rhythm of oral temperature. In our own investigation of a larger number of depressives,[7,8] no free-running period could be ascertained in the power spectrum of rectal temperature, urinary free cortisol, or any other variable.

Phase

Despite the mainly negative findings regarding free-running circadian periods in depressives living in an environment with a 24-h routine, the idea of an abnormally fast endogenous rhythm of the main circadian clock was not given up. It was argued that the clock might be reset every day by external time cues; the phase of circadian rhythms, however, would then be advanced owing to the driving force of the main circadian pacemaker that tended to go faster than in a state of mental health.[9,10] Such a phase-advance of circadian rhythms was indeed described for several variables, e.g., cortisol and core body temperature.[9,10] The early timing of the first rapid-eye-movement (REM) period during night sleep[11] was, in this context, considered as reflecting a phase-advance of the REM propensity cycle. However, subjects with early REM episodes at the beginning of night sleep also tend to have a shortened REM latency after awakenings in the middle of the night[12] or during daytime naps,[13–15] thus indicating that it is a sleep onset phenomenon unrelated to the circadian REM propensity cycle.

Furthermore, the findings of a phase-advance of biological rhythms are far from being consistent.[16–18] For example, if rectal temperature is continuously measured at night over a period of several days[19] or more[20] in depressives and control subjects of similar sex and age distribution, no difference with respect to the circadian phase position can be ascertained. With respect to the cortisol rhythm, an early timing of either the circadian maximum[21] or, more often, the circadian minimum,[22–25] but never of both the maximum and the minimum together, was described, the most consistent finding being an early timing of cortisol secretion after the evening trough.[26] Because this finding may well be related to the patients' sleep disorder[17] it is indispensable to study this relation in more depth before speculating about an underlying dysfunction of circadian clocks.

The phase-advance hypothesis has received some support from studies concerning therapeutic interventions. Thus advancing the sleep time by several hours alleviated the clinical condition in some depressives, either as the only therapeutic measure[27] or in combination with preceding partial sleep deprivation.[28] The interpretation of this effect, however, is difficult, as the sleep advance implies a sleep deprivation during the second half of the night, which in itself seems to be of therapeutic value.[29] It is therefore doubtful whether it is this effect or that of the early timing of sleep as such (or some kind of placebo effect?) that induces the clinical improvement. Other evidence for the phase-advance hypothesis is seen in the property of some antidepressants to delay the phases of circadian rhythm in animals.[30] Investigations regarding classical antidepressants are still scarce, however, and the respective results are inconsistent.[31] Furthermore, there is no evidence of a phase delay of hormonal rhythms (melatonin as well as cortisol) during a 3-week trial with the tricyclic antidepressant desipramine in human subjects; rather, there is a trend in the opposite direction.[32]

Amplitude

The amplitude of several circadian rhythms was reported to be diminished during episodes of depression. Because this finding was found not only in the average educed waveform derived from a series of cycles but also in individual cycles of, for example, the cortisol rhythm,[33] it cannot, at least not exclusively, be explained by the intraindividual variation of the temporal location of the maxima and minima.[6] However, in carefully designed studies no change or even an increase in amplitude of the cortisol rhythm[7] was ascertained, and in core body temperature only the decrease during night sleep was found to be attenuated.[19,20] Because it may well be related to stress and sleep disturbances experienced by the patients,[16,17] it does not seem justified to draw conclusions regarding circadian clocks.

Circadian Sleep Parameters

As is well known from everyday life experience and experimental sleep research,[34] sleep propensity exhibits a circadian rhythm. Some authors[35,36] believe that it can be ascribed to the influence of the circadian pacemaker governing the rhythmicity of other circadian functions (e.g., adrenocortical activity, renal excretion of water and electrolytes, core body temperature). Others[37,38] postulated the existence of a separate internal clock for the circadian modulation of sleep propensity. Although sleep disturbances are prominent in affective disorders and early morning awakening is one of the core symptoms of melancholia,[11] dysfunctions of this hypothetical clock for the sleep-wake cycle have rarely been suggested as causing or accompanying episodes of affective disorders. An exception is the hypothesis of a lengthening of the internal period of this clock in manic episodes, particularly at the time of switch from depression to mania.[39] This fact should explain the occurrence of 48-h sleep-wake cycles at this stage of a bipolar illness. However, an alternative explanation of this phenomenon, which does not assume any change in the period of a circadian clock, is based on Borbély's[35] two-process model of sleep regulation: During a state of hyperactivity with severe hyposomnia, total sleep loss during one night is compensated for the next night, and so forth.[16]

The two-process model was also used to explain the typical sleep pattern in depressives.[40] It was suggested that a deficiency of a hypothetical sleep factor caused early morning awakening, as the low amount of this factor accumulated until the beginning of night sleep was inactivated much earlier than a normal amount. This finding leads to the prediction of a lengthening of the sleep-wake cycle under free-running conditions.

Findings in Patients Isolated from External Time Cues

Subjects

Up to now, observations of circadian rhythms in five affectively ill patients investigated in an environment without external time cues have been published: One was a 66-year-old man studied by our group in Munich[41–43]; the four others, all of them women within the age range 36–56 years, were studied by Wehr et al.[44] at the U.S. National Institute of Mental Health (NIMH). The five patients cover a wide range of affective psychopathologies and courses. With the exception of case 5, they were free of drugs before and during the investigation. Two were unipolar depressives; one of them (our case 1) exhibited regular 48-h cycles of the disorder for 12 years, and the other (case 2) suffered from a typical episode of unipolar major depression. Of the three bipolar patients, one (case 3) had developed rapid cycling with an average cycle length of 6 days, one (case 4) was suffering from a typical bipolar manic-depressive psychosis, being in a depressive episode when the experiment started; the last one (case 5) had been hypomanic for several weeks after antidepressive medication with a selective type A monoamine oxidase inhibitor (MAOI), which she continued to take during the study. (It should be noted that, due to the inclusion of our Munich patient, the number of patients studied at the NIMH has increased by one compared with those in the study by Wehr et al.[44])

Predictions

From the above-mentioned hypotheses the following predictions for these subjects during temporal isolation can be inferred.

1. If the basis of 48-h rhythms of depression is an interaction of a free-running rhythm (with a period length of 16 h) with the entrained 24-h rhythm, the first subject studied should either exhibit a 16-h component in one circadian rhythm that might have been obscured in a 24-h regimen or he should switch to a 16-h period with all his rhythms.[43] In the latter case, the depression should disappear, as there would no longer occur a state of internal desynchronization of biological rhythms assumed to be at the origin of rapid cycling.

2. If the internal clock had a tendency toward a shorter than 24-h period, this tendency should become obvious in the nonentrained state. If a deficiency of a sleep factor was present, however, the sleep-wake cycle should free-run with an abnormally long period, i.e., much longer than the usual 24-h period in the state of free-run.[37] It should also alleviate the sleep disturbances of this patient including the early occurrence of REM episodes.

3. If Halberg's hypothesis[1] were valid for this case of rapid cycling, a period of 20 or 28 h should become apparent in the nonentrained state; and if no other period occurred, the cycles of psychopathology should be abolished—analogous to the predictions for case 1.

4. As long as he is depressed, this patient should display a shortening of circadian rhythms (similar to case 2). In case of a switch to mania, this shortening should be reversed, at least with respect to the sleep-wake cycle, which then should adopt a period much longer than 25 h, probably around 50 h.

5. Except for a possible lengthening of the sleep-wake cycle, no definite conclusions for this hypomanic patient can be drawn. In fact, according to the literature, the slightest deviation from a normal synchronized 25-h rhythm would be expected in comparison to patients in a depressed state.

Results

In none of the five data sets were these predictions fulfilled. On the contrary, the findings were not only negative in this respect but pointed to other directions.

1. The 48-h cycles of depression persisted, and internal desynchronization occurred with irregular sleep-wake cycles varying around 19 h, whereas the biological variables such as rectal temperature, renal excretion of water, electrolytes, and free cortisol exhibited a more regular, nearly 24-h rhythm.

2. Despite only slight improvement of the depression, the circadian sleep-wake and temperature rhythms lengthened slightly to an average of around 24.5 h with a normal proportion of sleep and wakefulness (around 1:2) and the REM latency remaining short (47 min instead of 50 min in the entrained state).

3. The sleep-wake and temperature rhythms lengthened in a normal fashion to an average of 25 h per cycle with a normal percentage of sleep. No evidence of a 20- or 28-h component appeared in the sleep-wake or temperature rhythms. Nevertheless, the cycling of psychopathology persisted without any perceivable change in its temporal pattern.

4. During the experiment, a switch from depression to mania occurred. It was temporally associated with a reduction in the initially slightly increased cycle length. Because of a large scatter of the times awake or asleep during each cycle in combination with a general tendency to short sleep periods, the pattern became rather irregular.

5. Unexpectedly, a seriously disturbed circadian sleep-wake pattern and a comparable disruption of the temperature rhythm appeared in this hypomanic patient. The authors interpreted their findings as indicating repeated changes in the period of the sleep-wake rhythm and its desynchronization from the temperature rhythm. Close inspection of the data, however, reveals concordant changes in the sleep-wake and the temperature rhythms as well as irregular fluctuations of both of them around a 24-h period rather than any systematic changes in the underlying periods. As under entrained conditions, the average sleep time of this patient was remarkably short, averaging less than 20% per cycle with a broad range of variation.

Conclusions

None of the aforementioned chronobiological hypotheses of affective disorders could be substantiated by findings obtained in an environment without zeitgebers. Remarkably, in only one of the five subjects (case 1) did internal desynchronization between the sleep-wake and the temperature rhythms seem to have occurred. This subject was a rapid cycler displaying 48-h cycles of unipolar depression that persisted in isolation from external time cues. The predicted 16-h component of a free-running rhythm was not observed in his shortened sleep-wake cycle, which varied markedly around 19 h, or in any of his vegetative rhythms, which remained near 24 h. In the other rapid cycler (case 3), the sleep-wake and the temperature rhythms remained synchronized, the periods lengthening to slightly more than 24 h. This finding is well in line with findings in healthy subjects. Similarly, in one typical case of unipolar depression (case 2), no deviation of the endogenous circadian rhythm could be revealed in temporal isolation. The period became longer, not shorter, as predicted by the phase-advance hypothesis. On the other hand, the period of the sleep-wake cycle did not increase beyond the average free-running period of healthy subjects, a finding that contradicts the sleep factor deficiency hypothesis.

In a bipolar manic-depressive (case 4), the period of the sleep-wake cycle showed a tendency toward shortening when the patient switched from depression to mania, not the other way round. This finding is exactly the opposite of what was expected from the interpretation of alternating nights of sleep and sleeplessness during such switches in an entrained environment indicating a lengthening of the endogenous period of the sleep-wake cycle. However, the tendency toward hyposomnia increased in the manic state, which is concordant with the assumption that the abnormal sleep pattern during switches from depression to mania can be explained as an expression of severe hyposomnia in an otherwise undisturbed circadian system.

Finally, a severe disruption of circadian rhythms was observed during a rather stable state of hypomania, a finding that could not be predicted from any of the current chronobiological hypotheses on affective disorders outlined above.

These hypotheses should no longer serve as guidelines for chronobiological investigations in affective disorders. Rather, they should be substituted by new theoretical approaches to the circadian phenomena in these disorders. Suggestions have been made in previous reports from our group.[16-18,42,45] The available space does not allow their detailed description. They have in common that mechanisms such as masking of biological rhythms by the disease process in the brain, and vice versa, and an entrainment of this process to signals from the circadian system are at work. Findings for or against these theoretical assumptions must be obtained by further investigations of patients, control subjects, and animal models.

References

1. Halberg F. Physiologic considerations underlying rhythmometry with special reference to emotional illness. In Ajuriaguerra J de (ed): Cycles Biologique et Psychiatrie. Paris: Masson, 1968; 73–126.
2. Bryson RW, Martin DF. 17-Ketosteroid excretion in a case of manic-depressive psychosis. Lancet 1954;2:365–367.
3. Kripke DF, Mullaney DJ, Atkinson M, et al. Circadian rhythm disorders in manic-depressives. Biol Psychiatry 1978;13:335–351.
4. Pflug B, Erikson R, Johnsson A. Depression and daily temperature: a long-term study. Acta Psychiatr Scand 1976;54:254–266.
5. Engelmann W, Pflug B. Rhythmische Aspekte der Lithiumwirkung. In Heimann H, Pflug B (eds): Rhythmusprobleme in der Psychiatrie. Stuttgart: Fischer, 1978;65–74.
6. Pflug B, Johnsson A, Martin W. Alterations in the circadian temperature rhythms in depressed patients. In Wehr TA, Goodwin FK (eds): Circadian Rhythms in Psychiatry. Pacific Grove: Boxwood Press, 1983;71–76.
7. Von Zerssen D, Barthelmes H, Dirlich G, et al. Circadian rhythms in endogenous depression. Psychiatry Res 1985;16:51–63.
8. Dirlich G, Barthelmes H, von Lindern L, et al. A chronobiologic study of depression: discussion from a methodologic perspective. In Halaris A (ed): Chronobiology and Psychiatric Disorders. New York: Elsevier, 1987;133–158.
9. Wehr TA, Goodwin FK. Biological rhythms and psychiatry. In Arieti S, Brodie HKH (eds): American Handbook of Psychiatry, Vol. 7: Advances and New Directions. 2nd Ed. New York: Basic Books, 1981;46–74.
10. Wehr TA, Goodwin FK. Biological rhythms in manic-depressive illness. In Wehr TA, Goodwin FK (eds): Circadian Rhythms in Psychiatry. Pacific Grove: Boxwood Press, 1983;129–184.
11. Gillin JC, Sitaram N, Wehr T, et al. Sleep and affective illness. In Post RM, Ballenger JC (eds): Neurobiology of Mood Disorders. Baltimore: Williams & Wilkins, 1984;157–189.
12. Schulz H, Tetzlaff W. Distribution of REM latencies after sleep interruption in depressive patients and control subjects. Biol Psychiatry 1982;17:1367–1376.
13. Kupfer DJ, Gillin JC, Coble PA, et al. REM sleep, naps and depression. Psychiatry Res 1981;5:195–203.
14. Pugnetti L, Colombo A, Cazzullo CL, et al. Daytime sleep patterns of primary depressives: a morning nap study. Psychiatry Res 1982;7:287–298.

15. Elsenga S, Wiegand M, Lauer C, et al. Nocturnal sleep and napping after total sleep deprivation in depression. in prep.
16. Von Zerssen D. Chronobiology of depression. In Angst J (ed): The Origins of Depression: Current Concepts and Approaches. Berlin: Springer, 1983;253–271.
17. Von Zerssen D. What is wrong with circadian clocks in depression? In Halaris A (ed): Chronobiology and Psychiatric Disorders. New York: Elsevier, 1987;159–179.
18. Von Zerssen D, Doerr P, Emrich HM, et al. Diurnal variation of mood and the cortisol rhythm in depression and normal states of mind. Eur Arch Psychiatry Neurol Sci 1987;237:36–45.
19. Avery DH, Wildschiødtz G., Rafaelsen OJ. Nocturnal temperature in affective disorder. J Affective Disord 1982;4:61–71.
20. Lund R, Kammerloher A, Dirlich G. Body temperature in endogenously depressed patients during depression and remission. In Wehr TA, Goodwin FK (eds): Circadian Rhythms in Psychiatry. Pacific Grove: Boxwood Press, 1983;77–88.
21. Dietzel M, Saletu B, Lesch OM, et al. Light treatment in depressive illness: polysomnographic, psychometric and neuroendocrinological findings. Eur Neurol 1986;25(suppl 2):93–103.
22. Yamaguchi N, Maeda K, Kuromaru S. The effects of sleep deprivation on the circadian rhythm of plasma cortisol levels in depressive patients. Folia Psychiatr Neurol Jpn 1978;32:479–487.
23. Jarrett DB, Coble PA, Kupfer DJ. Reduced cortisol latency in depressive illness. Arch Gen Psychiatry 1983;40:506–511.
24. Linkowski P, Mendlewicz J, Leclercq R, et al. The 24-hour profile of adrenocorticotropin and cortisol in major depressive illness. J Clin Endocrinol 1985;61:429–439.
25. Sherman BM, Pfohl B. Rhythm-related changes in pituitary-adrenal function in depression. J Affective Disord 1985;9:55–61.
26. Halbreich U. The circadian rhythm of cortisol and MHPG in depressives and normals. In Halaris A (ed): Chronobiology and Psychiatric Disorders. New York: Elsevier, 1987;49–73.
27. Wehr TA, Wirz-Justice A, Goodwin FK, et al. Phase advance of the circadian sleep-wake cycle as an antidepressant. Science 1979; 206:710–713.
28. Souêtre E, Salvati E, Pringuey D, et al. Antidepressant effects of the sleep/wake cycle phase advance: preliminary report. J Affective Disord 1987;12:41–46.
29. Schilgen B, Tölle R. Partial sleep deprivation as therapy for depression. Arch Gen Psychiatry 1980;37:267–271.
30. Wehr TA, Wirz-Justice A. Circadian rhythm mechanisms in affective illness and in antidepressant drug action. Pharmacopsychiatry 1982;15:31–39.
31. Wirz-Justice A. Light and dark as a "drug." Prog Drug Res 1987;31:383–425.
32. Thompson C, Mezey G, Corn T, et al. The effect of desipramine upon melatonin and cortisol secretion in depressed and normal subjects. Br J Psychiatry 1985;147:389–393.
33. Sachar EJ, Hellman L, Roffwarg HP, et al. Disrupted 24-hour patterns of cortisol secretion in psychotic depression. Arch Gen Psychiatry 1973;28:19–24.
34. Horne J. Why We Sleep: The Functions of Sleep in Humans and Other Mammals. Oxford: Oxford University Press, 1988.
35. Borbély AA. A two process model of sleep regulation. Hum Neurobiol 1982;1:195–204.
36. Daan S, Beersma D. Circadian gating of human sleep-wake cycles. In Moore-Ede MC, Czeisler CA (eds): Mathematical Models of the Circadian Sleep-Wake Cycle. New York: Raven Press, 1984;129–158.
37. Wever RA. The Circadian System of Man. New York: Springer, 1979.
38. Kronauer RE, Czeisler CA, Pilato SF, et al. Mathematical model of the human circadian system with two interacting oscillators. Am J Physiol 1982;242:R3–R17.
39. Wehr TA, Goodwin FK, Wirz-Justice A, et al. 48-Hour sleep-wake cycles in manic-depressive illness: naturalistic observations and sleep deprivation experiments. Arch Gen Psychiatry 1982;39:559–565.
40. Borbély AA, Wirz-Justice A. Sleep, sleep deprivation and depression. Hum Neurobiol 1982;1:205–210.
41. Doerr P, Von Zerssen D, Fischler M, et al. Relationship between mood changes and adrenal cortical activity in a patient with 48-hour unipolar-depressive cycles. J Affective Disord 1979;1:93–104.

42. Dirlich G, Kammerloher A, Schulz H, et al. Temporal coordination of rest-activity cycle, body temperature, urinary free cortisol, and mood in a patient with 48-hour unipolar-depressive cycles in clinical and time-cue-free environments. Biol Psychiatry 1981;16:163–179.
43. Von Zerssen D, Dirlich G, Fischler M. Influence of an abnormal time routine and therapeutic measures on 48-hour cycles of affective disorders: chronobiological considerations. In Wehr TA, Goodwin FK (eds): Circadian Rhythms in Psychiatry. Pacific Grove: Boxwood Press, 1983;109–127.
44. Wehr TA, Sack DA, Duncan WC, et al. Sleep and circadian rhythms in affective patients isolated from external time cues. Psychiatry Res 1985;15:327–339.
45. Campbell SS, Zulley J. Induction of depressive-like sleep patterns in normal subjects. In Halaris A (ed): Chronobiology and Psychiatric Disorders. New York: Elsevier, 1987;177–132.

II.D. PSYCHONEUROENDOCRINOLOGY

55. Pathophysiology of the Limbic-Hypothalamic-Pituitary-Adrenocortex System: An Overview

F. Holsboer

Psychoneuroendocrine research over the past two decades has provided clear evidence that clinical depression is frequently associated with hypersecretion of ACTH and cortisol. As a parent abnormality of this phenomenon, the resistance of ACTH and cortisol to the suppressive effect of dexamethasone was detected. This neuroendocrine probe (dexamethasone suppression test, DST) has received considerable interest as a validator of nosological concepts, a laboratory test to monitor clinical progress, and an ancillary aid for treatment selection. More recently, the availability of corticotropin-releasing hormone (CRH) has enabled researchers to study more closely the pathophysiology underlying altered regulation of the limbic-hypothalamic-pituitary-adrenocortical (LHPA) system. This overview highlights some of these new developments.

ACTH and Cortisol Dynamics in Depression

The 24-h plasma cortisol concentration shifts to higher mean values in acute major depression. This phenomenon is produced by an approximately twofold increase of cortisol released per secretory pulse, although the frequency of pulses remains unchanged.[1] In contrast to patients with Cushing's disease in whom cortisol is elevated at all times, the secretory pulses in depression are separated by intervals without any release. Also the circadian rhythm is preserved in depression. These differences along with the intermittent nature of the disease may account for the absence of cushingoid stigmata among hypercortisolemic depressives. ACTH release is also increased in depression; this enhancement is relatively muted, however, when compared to associated cortisol responses. The most likely explanation for this dissociation is that due to the trophic nature of ACTH long-term elevation of ACTH produces increased responsiveness secondary to adrenocortical hyperplasia.[2] However, co-release of other adrenogenic N-terminal proopiomelanocortin (POMC) products may also be involved.

Dexamethasone Suppression Test

Nonsuppressed DST results were initially considered by Carroll et al.[3] to indicate the clinical state classified as endogenous, or melancholic, depression. In parallel with increasing awareness of considerable confusion about diagnostic constructs for affective disorders, the use of DST results as dependent variables has been questioned. Most centers involved in clinical neuroendocrinology now agree that DST nonsuppression is not pathognomonic for endogenous depression.[4-6] As part of the research on the DST much work was done on technical factors that may invalidate DST results. Among these intervening variables are acute hospital admission, withdrawal from drugs or alcohol, intake of anticonvulsants or birth control pills, and acute weight loss. Particular interest greeted our original finding that elevated levels of cortisol after DST covary with decreased plasma concentrations of the test drug dexamethasone.[7,8] However, the suspicion that low dexamethasone levels account for DST nonsuppression could be rejected because we showed that during the pharmacodynamically relevant early distribution phase, i.e., the first few hours after oral ingestion, plasma dexamethasone levels were indistinguishable between suppressors and nonsuppressors.[9] Furthermore, after intravenous administration of dexamethasone, plasma levels were extremely low in both suppressors and nonsuppressors.[10] These findings suggest that low plasma dexamethasone levels in nonsuppressors indicate enhanced excretion of the test drug rather than impaired gastrointestinal absorption followed by decreased bioavailability.

Attention has focused on whether DST nonsuppression normalizes in parallel with clinical remission. Most studies in this area agree that normalization of initially abnormal DST results precedes or coincides with full clinical recovery.[11,12] Thus the DST, rather than being a diagnostic aid, may serve as a laboratory test to monitor the clinical course. It may be of particular importance whenever clinical symptomatology has improved despite persistent DST nonsuppression. In these cases the DST result may indicate the impending risk for a relapse into a new depressive episode.

Clinical Studies with Corticotropin-Releasing Hormone

The ACTH response to CRH is blunted in depression.[13,14] This finding can be taken as evidence that elevated circulating levels of cortisol restrain pituitary corticotrophs to release an adequate magnitude of ACTH after specific stimulation with CRH. Thus the locus of pathology leading to hypercortisolemic depression is at a suprapituitary site, most likely in the limbic brain. To further investigate the inhibitory role of elevated cortisol levels we measured the ACTH response to CRH in depressives who were pretreated with metyrapone in order to reduce circulating cortisol. We found that stimulated net ACTH output in depressives, who were deprived of elevated cortisol, became indistinguishable from ACTH responses in normal controls (Fig. 55.1), indicating the key role of cortisol as a suppressor of releasable ACTH in depression.[15]

In normal controls, DST nonsuppression cannot be induced by exogenous CRH.[16] However, if vasopressin is co-administered, cortisol levels escape from dexamathasone suppression. A different situation was detected in patients with depression, where irrespective of DST status additional quantities of ACTH and

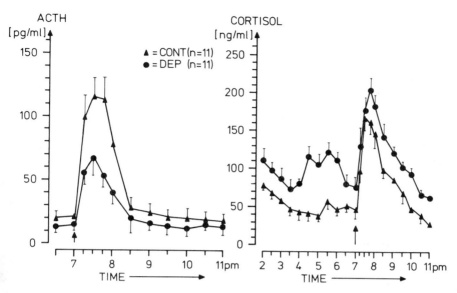

FIGURE 55.1. hCRH stimulation test in depression. After injection of 100 µg hCRH at 7 p.m. (arrow) patients with endogenous depression release significantly less ACTH than matched controls (area under curve, AUC: 3.0 ± 2.6 pg × min/ml · 10^3 versus 6.2 ± 3.4; $p < 0.01$). In contrast, the net cortisol output remains indistinguishable (11.5 ± 4.2 ng × min/ml · 10^3 versus 11.8 ± 4.6) despite significantly elevated mean cortisol secretion at baseline between 2 and 7 p.m. (95.3 ± 25.8 versus 56.6 ± 14.6 ng/ml, $p < 0.001$). [From Holsboer et al.[15], with permission.]

cortisol can be provoked by CRH. The phenomenon of ACTH and cortisol elevation after a combined dexamethasone/CRH administration is state-dependent, as it disappears in most cases after return to euthymia or a switch into mania.

The interpretation of this finding involves functional changes in the hippocampus, which is the most important central feedback element of the LHPA system. Glucocorticoid overexposure may lead to stepwise down-regulation of glucocorticoid receptors and subsequent weakening of this feedback element.[17]

After administration of dexamethasone, which binds predominantly at the anterior pituitary and deprives the circulation of endogenous corticosteroids, the hippocampus may further enhance stimulatory inputs and thus override the suppressive effect of dexamethasone. By this route a functional change in the limbic brain, and specifically the hippocampus, may account for the impaired potency of dexamethasone to suppress adequately ACTH and cortisol output, and it may facilitate ACTH and cortisol release after CRH despite dexamethasone pretreatment.

Conclusion

Neuroendocrine research devoted to the LHPA system in depression has substantiated the close linkage between altered regulation of the LHPA system and depression. In this line it has become obvious that peripherally measured ACTH and cortisol elevations are driven by central dysregulation leading to enhanced

CRH production, which mediates endocrine and probably also behavioral changes characteristic of depression.

As a corollary of this approach the neuropharmacological sequelae of exaggerated adrenocortical activity deserve particular attention in future investigations. Basic research has provided ample evidence that almost all neurotransmitter/receptor systems involved in the etiology and treatment of depression are influenced by glucocorticoids. For example, monoaminergic neurons contain strong glucocorticoid receptor immunoreactivity.[18] Moreover, suppression or activation of gene expression is strongly modulated by the corticosteroid–receptor complex for which specific response elements in the DNA structure have been identified.[19] Given the many upstream effects of glucocorticoids, it becomes apparent that these hormones may play a key role in maintenance of neuronal plasticity throughout the life-span.

References

1. Halbreich U, Asnis GM, Shindldecker R, et al: Cortisol secretion in endogenous depression. II. Time related functions. Arch Gen Psychiatry 1985;42:904–914.
2. Amsterdam JD, Maislin G, Abelman E, et al: Adrenocortical responsiveness to the ACTH stimulation test in depressed patients and healthy volunteers. J Affective Disord 1986;11:265–274.
3. Carroll BJ, Feinberg M, Greden JF, et al: A specific laboratory test for the diagnosis of melancholia. Arch Gen Psychiatry 1981;38:15–22.
4. Berger M, Pirke KM, Doerr P, et al: The limited utility of the dexamethasone suppression test for the diagnostic process in psychiatry. Br J Psychiatry 1984;145:372–382.
5. Stokes PE, Stoll PM, Koslow SH, et al: Pretreatment DST and hypothalamic-pituitary-adrenocortical function in depressed patients and comparison groups. Arch Gen Psychiatry 1984;41:257–267.
6. Holsboer F, Philipp M, Steiger A, et al: Multisteroid analysis after DST in depressed patients—a controlled study. J Affective Disord 1986;10:241–249.
7. Holsboer F, Haack D, Gerken A, et al: Plasma dexamethasone concentrations and differential glucocorticoid suppression response in depressives and controls. Biol Psychiatry 1984;19:281–291.
8. Holsboer F, Wiedemann K, Gerken A, et al: The plasma dexamethasone variable in depression—test retest studies and early biophase kinetics. Psychiatry Res 1986;17:97–103.
9. Holsboer F, Wiedemann K, Boll E: Shortened dexamethasone half-live time in depressed dexamethasone nonsuppressors. Arch Gen Psychiatry 1986;43:813–815.
10. Wiedemann K, Holsboer F: Plasma dexamethasone kinetics during the DST after oral and intravenous administration of the test drug. Biol Psychiatry 1987;22:1340–1348.
11. Holsboer F, Liebl R, Hofschuster E: Repeated dexamethasone suppression test during depressive illness: normalization of test result compared with clinical improvement. J Affective Disord 1982;4:93–101.
12. Greden JA, Gardner R, King D, et al: Dexamethasone suppression tests in antidepressant treatment of melancholia—the process of normalization and test-retest reproducibility. Arch Gen Psychiatry 1983;40:493–500.
13. Holsboer F, Gerken A, von Bardeleben U, et al: Human corticotropin-releasing hormone in depression—correlation with thyrotropin secretion following thyrotropin releasing hormone. Biol Psychiatry 1986;21:601–611.
14. Gold PW, Loriaux DL, Roy A, et al: Responses to corticotropin-releasing hormone in the hypercortisolism of depression and Cushing's disease: pathophysiologic and diagnostic implications. N Engl J Med 1986;314:1329–1335.
15. Holsboer F, von Bardeleben U, Buller R, et al: Stimulation response to corticotropin-releasing hormone (CRH) in patients with depression, alcoholism and panic disorder. Horm Metab Res 1987;16(Suppl.):80–88.
16. Von Bardeleben U, Holsboer F, Stalla GK: Combined administration of human corticotropin-releasing factor and lysine vasopressin induces cortisol escape from dexamethasone suppression in healthy subjects. Life Sci 1985;37:1613–1618.

17. Sapolsky RM, Krey LC, et al: Prolonged glucocorticoid exposure reduces hippocampal neuron number: implications for aging. J Neurosci 1985;5:1221.
18. Härfstrand A, Fuxe K, Cintra A, et al: Glucocorticoid receptor immunoreactivity in monoaminergic neurons of rat brain. Proc Na†l Acad Sci USA 1986;83:9779–9783.
19. Yamamoto KR: Steroid receptor regulated transcription of specific genes and gene networks. Annu Rev Genet 1985;19:209–252.

56. Neuroendocrine Dysfunctions in Affective Disorders: Effects of Clinical Changes

A. STEIGER, U. VON BARDELEBEN, K. WIEDEMANN,
E. HOLSBOER-TRACHSLER, AND F. HOLSBOER

It is evident from current knowledge of complex interactions between hormones and neurotransmitter–receptor systems, sleep structure, gene expression, behavior, immune function, aging, psychopathology, and neuropsychological function that hormones play a key role in all aspects of affective disorders. Longitudinal studies by serial application of neuroendocrine tests allow us to investigate changes of the behavioral complex concurrently with laboratory measures.

Serial Dexamethasone Suppression Tests

The most widely studied endocrine function test in psychiatric research is the dexamethasone suppression test (DST), which enables us to investigate the feedback circuitry of the limbic-hypothalamic-pituitary-adrenocortical (LHPA) system. Serial application of the DST in depressed patients with initially abnormal test results showed a relation between clinical course and cortisol levels after this neuroendocrine probe. Weekly monitoring of patients who were initially nonsuppressors on the DST demonstrated a gradual return of the cortisol concentration to normal. In most cases the normalization occurred 3–4 weeks prior to complete remission of the clinical symptomatology. A depressive relapse in remitted patients who were previously nonsuppressors was preceded by a switch of the DST status from suppression to nonsuppression. These results demonstrated the applicability of the DST as a laboratory test for serial monitoring of the clinical treatment of depression.[1,2]

Further studies from our laboratory, simultaneously analyzing plasma dexamethasone levels and plasma cortisol 9–24 h after oral administration of the test drug, showed an association of cortisol nonsuppression by the DST and decreased plasma dexamethasone levels.[3] A longitudinal study of DST and dexamethasone levels showed that normalization of the cortisol concentration in the test is associated with a stepwise increase of plasma dexamethasone levels.[4] The investigation of the pharmacokinetics of dexamethasone after oral DST in depressed patients illustrated that a shortened half-life of dexamethasone was secondary to enhanced elimination, and absorption and distribution during the pharmacodynamically relevant early biophase were indistinguishable.[5]

In an additional study conducted in collaboration with the University of Zürich, the DST was performed in 31 inpatients with a severe acute schizophrenic exacerbation 4 to 5 days after hospitalization and 4 weeks later or prior to discharge. Fifteen patients (48%) were nonsuppressors at the first test. When retested, DST normalization was associated with reduction of the psychopathology, although the change in the rating scale scores was only moderate. These findings question the utility of the DST as a predictor of the clinical course in schizophrenia. In line with the results in depressed patients, low dexamethasone levels were associated with an abnormal DST among schizophrenic nonsuppressors as well.[6]

Serial hCRH-Dexamethasone Tests

Further investigation of pituitary-adrenocortical dysregulation in patients with depression has been enhanced by the sequencing and synthesis of ovine (oCRH) and human (hCRH) corticotropin-releasing hormone. We demonstrated that dexamethasone-induced cortisol suppression in normal controls was resistant to hCRH administration (100 μg i.v. at 3 p.m. after 1.5 mg dexamethasone at 11 p.m. the night before).[7] We applied this combined test of dexamethasone suppression and hCRH stimulation to inpatients with depression 1–2 weeks after admission and repeated the hCRH-DST in selected patients until remission. In the follow-up patients, tricylic antidepressant medication was maintained throughout the study to avoid withdrawal effects. In a subgroup of these patients the hCRH application could induce an escape of ACTH and cortisol despite dexamethasone pretreatment.[8] This escape phenomenon was independent of DST status and appeared to be related to the clinical course of depression as it subsided with clinical recovery. In contrast to the DST, which usually normalizes before full clinical improvement, the normalization of the hCRH-DST took a longer time in most cases, particularly in aged individuals.

The inability of dexamethasone and elevated cortisol to inhibit hCRH stimulation could reflect an impairment of the negative feedback mechanism at the hippocampus during depression where a persistent hypercortisolism induced a down-regulation of glucocorticoid receptors. As there is more binding of dexamethasone in the pituitary than in the limbic brain, impaired inhibitory influence by the hippocampus in combination with dexamethasone-induced lowered levels of endogenous glucocorticoids may facilitate an ACTH and cortisol escape by hCRH stimulation.

Serial Sleep-Endocrine Investigations

Sleep-endocrine studies in depressed patients are a tool to investigate simultaneously several biological axes under physiological conditions. We examined sleep electroencephalograms (EEGs) and nocturnal secretion of cortisol and growth hormone (GH) in ten male patients with endogenous depression (a) during acute depression before treatment (t1) and (b) after clinical remission and withdrawal of the antidepressant medication (t2).

The major findings were as follows: At t1 sleep structure showed characteristics that are known in acutely depressed patients, particularly a shortened REM latency (time difference from sleep onset to the first period of rapid-eye-movement sleep), an increased number of rapid eye movements (REM density), decreased slow wave sleep (SWS; stages 3 and 4), and increased wakefulness. Between t1 and t2 there was no significant change of sleep variables, except for a decrease in the time spent in stage 4 and a decrease in the number of early morning awakenings. The pattern of cortisol secretion followed the course known from normal controls,[9] with the lowest secretion during the first hours of the night, tending to a nadir, followed by a cortisol rise, a second nadir, and a final increase. At t1 the cortisol secretion during the whole night and at the time of the first and second nadirs was significantly elevated in comparison to that at t2. After recovery the cortisol rise shifted to a later clock-time, and cortisol latency (time difference from sleep onset to the cortisol rise) was increased. The nocturnal plasma concentration of GH was relatively low during both investigations and did not show significant differences between t1 and t2 (Fig. 56.1). These results indicate that enhanced cortisol secretion and advanced cortisol rise in acute depression normalize independently of the sleep structure.

Conclusions

Abnormal DST results and enhanced cortisol secretion during sleep are frequent concomitants of the depressive state, which regularly become normalized after successful treatment. In contrast to the state-dependent markers derived from the

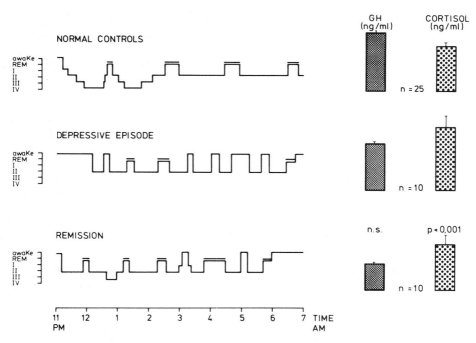

FIGURE 56.1. Clinical remission in ten initially depressed men resulted in a statistically significant ($p < 0.001$) decrease of mean cortisol secretion (101.7 ± 3.0 versus 72.4 ± 2.2 ng/ml), which comes close to values observed among normal controls (68.0 ± 3.0 ng/ml). In contrast, mean GH secretion did not change (3.75 ± 0.3 versus 2.1 ± 0.6 ng/ml), remaining markedly below levels recorded among younger controls (6.9 ± 2.3 ng/ml). No significant effect of clinical recovery on the sleep EEG was observed.

physiology of cortisol regulation, sleep architectural changes and nocturnal GH patterns remain indistinguishable between depression and euthymia if the study sample serves as its own control. These findings may rekindle the interest in biological trait markers of depression. However, it is noteworthy that monoaminergic neurons involved in the regulation of sleep and GH secretion contain glucocorticoid receptors.[10] Thus the persistent abnormalities may be regarded as long-term effects, or metabolic scars, of previous hypercortisolism. For that reason the question of whether biological abnormalities in remitted patients are trait characteristics remains unanswered so long as no data from premorbid individuals are available.

References

1. Holsboer F, Liebl R, Hofschuster E. Repeated dexamethasone suppression test during depressive illness: normalization of test result compared with clinical improvement. J Affective Disord 1982;4:93–101.
2. Greden JA, Gardner R, King D, et al. Dexamethasone suppression tests in antidepressant treatment of melancholia—the process of normalization and test-retest reproducibility. Arch Gen Psychiatry 1982;40:493–500.
3. Holsboer F, Haack D, Gerken A, et al. Plasma dexamethasone concentrations and differential glucocorticoid suppression response in depressives and controls. Biol Psychiatry 1984;19:281–291.
4. Holsboer F, Wiedemann K, Gerken A, et al. The plasma dexamethasone variable in depression—test retest studies and early biophase kinetics. Psychiatry Res 1986;17:97–103.
5. Holsboer F, Wiedemann K, Boll E. Shortened dexamethasone half-life time in depressed dexamethasone nonsuppressors. Arch Gen Psychiatry 1986;43:813–815.
6. Holsboer-Trachsler E, Buol C, Wiedemann K, et al. Dexamethasone suppression test in severe schizophrenic illness—effects of plasma dexamethasone and caffeine levels. Acta Psychiatr Scand 1987;75:608–613.
7. von Bardeleben U, Holsboer F, Stalla GK, et al. Combined administration of human corticotropin- releasing factor and lysine vasopressin induces cortisol escape from dexamethasone suppression in healthy subjects. Life Sci 1985;37:1613–1618.
8. Holsboer F, von Bardeleben U, Wiedemann K, et al. Serial assessment of corticotropin-releasing hormone response after dexamethasone in depression—implications for pathophysiology of DST nonsuppression. Biol Psychiatry 1987;22:228–234.
9. Steiger A, Herth T, Holsboer F. Sleep electroencephalography and the secretion of cortisol and human growth hormone in normal controls. Acta Endocrinol (Copenh) 1987;116:36–42.
10. Härfstrand A, Fuxe K, Cintra A, et al. Glucocorticoid receptor immunoreactivity in monoaminergic neurons of rat brain. Proc Natl Acad Sci USA 1983;83:9779–9783.

57. Preclinical and Clinical Investigations of Corticotropin-Releasing Factor: Assessment of Its Role in Depressive Disorders

CHARLES B. NEMEROFF AND MICHAEL J. OWENS

Starting with nearly a half million hypothalami, Vale and his colleagues[1] succeeded in determining the amino acid sequence of ovine corticotropin-releasing factor (CRF) in 1981. Shortly thereafter, human and rat CRF were sequenced and found to be identical; they differed from ovine CRF (oCRF) in only 7 of the 41 amino acid residues. The endocrine role of CRF as the major physiological regulator of ACTH and β-endorphin secretion from the anterior pituitary has now been well established. However, considerable data have accumulated from a variety of disciplines which indicate that this peptide plays an important neurobiological role apart from its neuroendocrine role. These findings have been comprehensively reviewed elsewhere.[2]

Immunohistochemical and radioimmunoassay studies have revealed that CRF is heterogeneously distributed throughout the mammalian central nervous system (CNS). High concentrations of CRF are found in the cerebral cortex, several brainstem nuclei associated with autonomic functioning, and limbic areas including the amygdala.[3,4] Similarly, utilizing both autoradiographic and biochemical methods, high affinity CRF binding sites, putative receptors, have been identified in the CNS.[5] These areas with a high density of binding sites generally contain substantial quantities of CRF.

Our group[6] and others[7] have shown that CRF is released from brain slices by depolarizing concentrations of potassium and that this release is calcium-dependent. Electrophysiological studies have revealed that direct microapplication of CRF alters the firing rate of several CNS neurons, including those of the locus coeruleus, the A6 noradrenergic cell group that projects to the forebrain.[8] Intraventricularly (ICV) administered CRF also produces electroencephalographic (EEG) changes indicative of increased arousal.[9]

When administered directly into the CNS, CRF produces several behavioral and physiological alterations that are not mediated by activation of the hypothalamic-pituitary-adrenal (HPA) axis and, moreover, are insensitive to glucocorticoid feedback. Many of the effects of ICV CRF are not unlike those observed when laboratory animals are exposed to stress. These effects include increases in heart rate, mean arterial pressure, oxygen consumption, blood glucose, and plasma catecholamine concentrations, all of which seem to be mediated by an increase in central sympathetic outflow or inhibition of parasympathetic activity in certain target organs.[10]

To determine whether stress alters CRF neurons, we measured the concentration of CRF in 36 rat brain regions microdissected by the method of Palkovits and Brownstein[11] following exposure to either acute or chronic stress.[12] Because stress is known to activate the HPA axis, a reduction in CRF concentrations in the median eminence of the hypothalamus was predicted. Indeed a 50% decrease in CRF concentrations was observed in both the acute and chronic stress groups. It was, as expected, associated with an increase in plasma corticosterone concentrations. Much more intriguing, however, was the observation that both acute and chronic stress produced a twofold rise in the concentration of CRF in the locus coeruleus. Although measurement of CRF concentrations alone cannot distinguish among changes in synthesis, release, and degradation, this finding is of particular interest in view of the evidence noted above that CRF excites locus coeruleus neurons. Thus CRF may modulate the major noradrenergic cell group in the CNS, an area implicated in the pathophysiology of affective disorders.

Other behavioral effects of centrally administered CRF have been reported. When administered intraventricularly in rats, CRF increases locomotor activity in a manner similar to that seen in response to a mild stressor, e.g., footshock or novelty.[13] In addition, CRF suppresses both sexual behavior in female rats[14] and food consumption (induced by either food deprivation or appetite stimulants) in rats.[15] Koob and Bloom[16] have shown in a variety of paradigms that centrally administered CRF produces behavioral alterations consistent with the hypothesis that CRF is released in the CNS in response to stress.

Taken together, the available data are concordant with the view that CRF fulfills many of the requisite criteria for consideration as a neurotransmitter and that CRF acts as a neurotransmitter in the CNS to integrate the neuroendocrine, autonomic, and behavioral responses of an organism to stress.

Because many investigators have obtained data suggesting that stress precipitates depressive episodes in genetically vulnerable individuals and because one of the most reproducible findings in biological psychiatry is the hyperactivity of the HPA axis in patients with endogenous depression,[17] we have sought to determine if hypersecretion of CRF may result in the hypercortisolemia seen in depressed patients as well as several of the signs and symptoms of this disorder. Two groups have, in pilot studies, attempted to test this hypothesis by measuring the concentrations of CRF in the plasma of depressed patients. Widerlöv et al.[18] reported that drug-free depressed patients had significantly higher plasma CRF concentrations than normal controls. However, Charlton et al.[19] were unable to replicate this finding. Better studied by Gold et al.[20] and Holsboer et al.,[21] however, is the blunted ACTH response to intravenously administered CRF in patients with major depression when compared to normal controls. Our group has confirmed these observations (Krishnan and Nemeroff, unpublished observations). This finding is most likely due either to intact negative feedback by glucocorticoids (which are, as noted above, elevated in depressed patients) or to desensitization of anterior pituitary CRF receptors after chronic CRF hypersecretion. In any case, the HPA axis hyperactivity in depression may certainly be due to chronic CRF hypersecretion. A blunted ACTH response to CRF is also observed in patients with anorexia nervosa, many of whom are hypercortisolemic.[22]

Because of the aforementioned findings, we attempted, in two studies, to directly test the hypothesis that CRF is hypersecreted in depressed patients by measuring

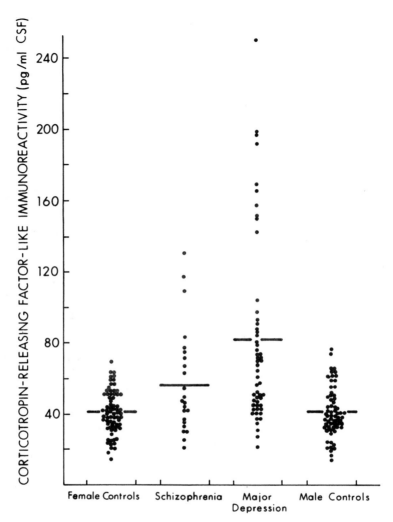

FIGURE 57.1. Concentration of CRF-like immunoreactivity in CSF of female neurological controls ($n = 73$), patients with *DSM-III* schizophrenia ($n = 23$), patients with *DSM-III* major depression ($n = 54$), and male neurological controls ($n = 65$). Respective group mean concentrations of CRF-like immunoreactivity were 40.64 ± 1.43, 57.77 ± 5.96, 80.66 ± 7.07, and 40.91 ± 1.77 pg/ml CSF. Using ANOVA and Newman-Keuls tests for statistical significance, the mean CSF concentrations of CRF-like immunoreactivity in the patients with major depression were significantly elevated ($p < 0.001$) compared to controls, and those of the schizophrenic patients were significantly elevated at the $p < 0.05$ level when compared to controls. The depressed group also had significantly elevated ($p < 0.01$) relative to the schizophrenic group. [From ref. 24. Copyright 1987, the American Psychiatric Association. Reprinted by permission.]

the concentration of this peptide in the CSF of drug- free psychiatric patients and appropriate controls. In the first study, conducted in collaboration with Widerlöv and his colleagues,[23] 11 of 23 depressed patients had CSF CRF concentrations higher than the highest normal control. As a group, the depressed patients had higher CSF CRF concentrations than the controls, whereas the schizophrenic and demented patients showed no such elevation. In a second study[24] of 54 drug-free depressed patients and 138 controls, the depressed patients exhibited, as a group, a twofold elevation in CSF CRF concentrations (Fig. 57.1). Our group has not found a correlation between CSF CRF concentrations and dexamethasone non-suppression; however, Gold and his colleagues (personal communication) have found a significant correlation between postdexamethasone plasma cortisol concentrations and CSF CRF concentrations.

Because both the preclinical and clinical findings described above are concordant with the hypothesis that CRF hypersecretion occurs in depression, we sought to determine if a reduction (down-regulation) in the number of binding sites (Bmax) for CRF occurs in the CNS of depressed individuals. It is now a well established phenomenon in neurobiology and endocrinology that chronic exposure to an agonist results in a compensatory decrease in the number of binding sites. We therefore measured the number (Bmax) and affinity (Kd) of CRF binding sites in the frontal cortex of 26 suicide victims (some of whom were certainly depressed) and 29 age- and sex-matched controls using [^{125}I]-Tyr°-oCRF. Scatchard analysis revealed no difference between the affinity of the radioligand for its receptor in the two groups. However, a 23% decrease in CRF receptor density was found in the suicide group.[25]

The findings reported here are not discordant with the suggestion that CRF systems throughout the brain are pathologically altered in depression. Further proof that CRF is hypersecreted in depression awaits current investigations that seek to determine if CRF gene expression is increased. Although unclear at this time, it is intriguing to postulate that these alterations in CRF neurons may be responsible for the much more widely studied changes in catecholaminergic and indoleaminergic circuits that have been reported to be altered in depression. The development of novel pharmacological treatments for affective disorders based on these studies, such as CRF receptor antagonists, may prove beneficial to patients who do not respond to tricyclic antidepressants, monoamine oxidase inhibitors, or electroconvulsive therapy.

Acknowledgments. We are grateful to Sheila Walker for excellent secretarial assistance. The work was supported by NIMH grants MH-42088, MH-39415, MH-40524, and MH-40159.

References

1. Vale W, Spiess J, Rivier C, et al. Characterization of a 41-residue ovine hypothalamic peptide that stimulates secretion of corticotropin and β-endorphin. Science 1981;213:1394–1397.
2. Owens MJ, Nemeroff CB. The neurobiology of corticotropin-releasing factor: implications for affective disorders. In Schatzberg AF, Nemeroff CB (eds): Hypothalamic-Pituitary-Adrenal Axis Physiology and Pathophysiology. New York: Raven Press, 1988;1–36.
3. Swanson LW, Sawchenko PE, Rivier J, et al. Organization of ovine corticotropin-releasing factor immunoreactive cells and fibers in the rat brain: an immunohistochemical study. Neuroendocrinology 1983;36:165–186.

4. Palkovits M, Brownstein MJ, Vale W. Distribution of corticotropin-releasing factor in rat brain. Fed Proc 1985;44:215–219.
5. De Souza EB, Kuhar MJ. Corticotropin-releasing factor receptors in the pituitary gland and central nervous system: methods and overview. Methods Enzymol 1986;124:560–590.
6. Smith MA, Bissette G, Slotkin TA, et al. Release of corticotropin-releasing factor from rat brain regions in vitro. Endocrinology 1986;118:1997–2001.
7. Suda T, Yajima F, Tomori N, et al. In vitro study of immunoreactive corticotropin-releasing factor release from the rat hypothalamus. Life Sci 1985;37:1499–1505.
8. Valentino RJ, Foote SL, Aston- Jones G. Corticotropin-releasing factor activates noradrenergic neurons of the locus coeruleus. Brain Res 1983;270:363–367.
9. Ehlers CL, Henriksen SJ, Wang M, et al. Corticotropin releasing factor produces increases in brain excitability and convulsive seizures in rats. Brain Res 1983;278:332–336.
10. Brown MR, Fisher LA, Spiess J, et al. Corticotropin-releasing factor: actions on the sympathetic nervous system and metabolism. Endocrinology 1982;111:928–931.
11. Palkovits M, Brownstein MJ. Microdissection of brain areas by the punch technique. In Cuello AC (ed): Brain Microdissection Techniques. New York: Wiley, 1983;1–36.
12. Chappell PB, Smith MA, Kilts CD, et al. Alterations in corticotropin-releasing factor-like immunoreactivity in discrete rat brain regions after acute and chronic stress. J Neurosci 1986;6:2908–2914.
13. Sutton RE, Koob GF, Le Moal M, et al. Corticotropin releasing factor produces behavioral activation in rats. Nature 1982;297:331–333.
14. Sirinathsinghji DJS, Rees LH, Rivier J, et al. Corticotropin-releasing factor is a potent inhibitor of sexual receptivity in the female rat. Nature 1983;305:232–235.
15. Morley JE, Levine AS. Corticotropin releasing factor, grooming and ingestive behavior. Life Sci 1982;31:1459–1464.
16. Koob GF, Bloom FE. Corticotropin-releasing factor and behavior. Fed Proc 1985;44:220–222.
17. Evans DL, Burnett GB, Nemeroff CB. The dexamethasone suppression test in the clinical setting. Am J Psychiatry 1983;140:586–589.
18. Widerlöv E, Ekman R, Wahlestedt C. Elevated corticotropin releasing factor-like immunoreactivity in plasma from major depressives. In: Abstracts of the 15th Collegium Internationale Neurd Psychopharmacologicum 1986;207.
19. Charlton BG, Leake A, Ferrier IN, et al. Corticotropin-releasing factor in plasma of depressed patients and controls. Lancet 1986;1:161–162.
20. Gold PW, Chrousos G, Kellner C, et al. Psychiatric implications of basic and clinical studies with corticotropin-releasing factor. Am J Psychiatry 1984;4:619–627.
21. Holsboer F, Müller OA, Doerr HG, et al. ACTH and multisteroid responses to corticotropin-releasing factor in depressive illness:relationship to multisteroid responses after ACTH stimulation and dexamethasone suppression. Psychoneuroendocrinology 1984;9:147–160.
22. Hotta M, Shibasaki T, Masuda A, et al. The responses of plasma adrenocorticotropin and cortisol to corticotropin-releasing hormone (CRH) and cerebrospinal fluid immunoreactive CRH in anorexia nervosa patients. J Clin Endocrinol Metab 1986;62:319–324.
23. Nemeroff CB, Widerlöv E, Bissette G, et al. Elevated concentrations of CSF corticotropin-releasing factor-like immunoreactivity in depressed patients. Science 1984;226:1342–1344.
24. Banki CM, Bissette G, Arato M, et al. Cerebrospinal fluid corticotropin- releasing factor-like immunoreactivity in depression and schizophrenia. Am J Psychiatry 1987;144:873–878.
25. Owens MJ, Stanley M, Bissette G, et al. CRF receptor number is decreased in the frontal cortex of suicide victims. In: Abstracts of the American College of Neuropsychopharmacology, 1986;189.

58. Neuroendocrine Effects of Intravenous Ovine Corticotropin-Releasing Factor and Human Growth Hormone-Releasing Factor in Affective Disorder Patients and Normal Controls

S. Craig Risch, Lewis L. Judd,
J. Christian Gillin, David S. Janowsky,
Lou Ann McAdams, and Shahkrokh Golshan

A wide variety of neuroendocrine abnormalities have been reported in affective disorder patients. Probably the most extensively studied have been hypothalamic-pituitary-adrenal (HPA) activation and dexamethasone resistance. In addition, an elevated 24-h pituitary growth hormone secretion has been reported in depressed patients. Reduced pituitary growth hormone responses to central nervous system (CNS) probes have been reported in depressed patients, particularly in response to the noradrenergic agent clonidine. The sequencing and availability of corticotropin-releasing factor (CRF) and growth hormone-releasing factor (GRF) allow direct testing of pituitary responses to these neuropeptides in affective disorder patients. Our findings to date confirm the reports by Gold and colleagues[1] and Holsboer and colleagues[2] of an attenuated ACTH response to intravenously administered ovine CRF in depressed patients. In addition, we preliminarily report an attenuated growth hormone response to intravenous human GRF in depressed patients.

Methods

Subjects were drug-free for at least 14 days prior to participation in the study, were voluntary and able to give informed consent, and were medically healthy as determined by medical history, physical examination, and laboratory tests including electrocardiogram, complete blood count with differential, urinalysis, SMA 12, serum electrolytes, blood urea nitrogen, creatine phosphokinase, thyroxine, and fasting glucose. Subjects also received a *DSM-III* and SADS-RDC diagnosis.

Ovine CRF Studies

Twenty-one normal controls and twenty-eight depressed (RDC major depressive disorder or bipolar depressed) patients were studied. There was no significant difference in age or sex composition between the control and depressed groups.

At around 7:30 a.m. an indwelling heparin lock catheter (19-gauge "butterfly") was inserted in the subject's forearm; after 30 min of accommodation baseline blood samples (8 cc) were obtained from the catheter at 15-min intervals for 30 min.

At 8:30 a.m. synthetic ovine corticotropin releasing factor (oCRF) was infused into the heparin lock at a dosage of 0.03 µg/kg in 5 cc of normal saline solution over 5 min. Blood samples (8 cc) were then obtained every 15 min for 2 h subsequent to the CRF infusion (i.e., at 8:50, 9:05, 9:20, 9:35, 9:50, 10:05, 10:20, and 10:35 a.m). Vital signs (blood pressure and pulse) were monitored and recorded at each blood withdrawal. Blood samples were collected in polypropylene tubes with EDTA on ice, immediately centrifuged in a refrigerated centrifuge at 15,000 rpm for 20 min, then stored in a $-80°C$ freezer for subsequent ACTH and cortisol measurements.

Ovine CRF was synthesized by Drs. Wylie Vale and Jean Rivier of the Salk Institute and prepared and packaged for human use by Drs. Stan Watson and Huda Akil of the University of Michigan.

hGRF

Fourteen normal controls, three remitted major affective disorder subjects, and four actively ill subjects with major depression were studied. All subjects were male, and there was no significant difference in age composition among the three groups.

At around 07:30 a.m. an indwelling heparin lock catheter (19-gauge "butterfly") was inserted in the subject's forearm; after 30 min of accommodation baseline blood samples (8 cc) were obtained from the catheter at 15-min intervals for 30 min. (hGRF was provided by Dr. Guillemin, Director of the Laboratories for Neuroendocrinology of the Salk Institute, La Jolla, California. The peptide hGRF was synthesized and characterized by Dr. Nicholas Ling of these laboratories.) At 8:30 a.m. synthetic hGRF or placebo was infused into the heparin lock at a dosage of 1 µg/kg in 5 cc of normal saline solution over 5 min. Blood samples (8 cc) were then obtained every 15 min for 2 h subsequent to the hGRF or placebo infusion (i.e., at 8:50, 9:05, 9:20, 9:35, 9:50, 10:05, 10:20, and 10:35 a.m.). Vital signs (blood pressure and pulse) were monitored and recorded at each blood withdrawal. Blood samples were collected in polypropylene tubes with EDTA on ice, immediately centrifuged in a refrigerated centrifuge at 15,000 rpm for 20 min, then stored in a $-80°C$ freezer for subsequent hGH measurements. hGRF and placebo administrations were separated by at least 1 week and were performed in a double-blind randomized, counterbalanced paradigm.

Results

oCRF Studies

Depressed patients had a nonsignificant but strong trend toward a "blunted" or reduced ACTH response compared with the matched normal control group (Fig. 58.1A). (Peak post-CRF ACTH response − minimum pre-CRF ACTH baseline:

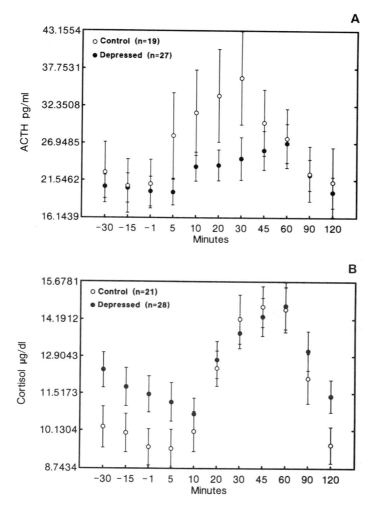

FIGURE 58.1. A: Plasma ACTH before and after intravenous CRF in depressed and control subjects. B: Plasma cortisol before and after intravenous CRF in depressed and control subjects.

$F = 3.324$; DF 1, 46; $p = 0.07$. Peak post-CRF cortisol − minimum pre-CRF cortisol baseline was not significantly different: $F = 1.418$; $DF = 1, 47$; $p = 0.24$) (Fig. 58.1B).

hGRF Studies

There were no significant changes in pulse or blood pressure or behavioral effects of hGRF or placebo administered in the paradigm used. Placebo administration had no significant effects on plasma levels of growth hormone, whereas hGRF administration significantly increased plasma levels of growth hormone in all subjects. Growth hormone levels peaked 15 min after hGRF infusions were still elevated at about 50% of maximal increase (i.e., level at 15 min post-hGRF infusions) at 120 min post-hGRF infusion, the last plasma sampling time-point. It is of interest that, as noted in Figure 58.2, the depressed patient group had significantly diminished or "blunted" plasma growth hormone increases in response to hGRF administration compared to the age- and sex-matched normal control group and remitted affective disorder patients.

Discussion

oCRF Studies

The results of the oCRF studies parallel those in the reports of Gold and colleagues[1] and Holsboer and colleagues,[2] suggesting that depressed patients have a subsensitive, or "blunted," ACTH responsivity to intravenous oCRF. It has been interpreted by Gold (personal communication) as due to classical negative feedback of excess cortisol secretion on the pituitary in depressed patients. In addition, Nemeroff (personal communication) has suggested that this reduced pituitary responsivity to intravenous oCRF in depressed patients could be due to a "down-regulated," or reduced, pituitary CRF receptor number secondary to excessive portal CRF concentrations. The failure to demonstrate a statistically significant reduction in ACTH response in this study could be due to our infusions of CRF being done during the early morning hours when the HPA system is more activated than during the evening hours when Gold and Holsboer and their colleagues performed their studies (Gold, personal communication); alternatively, it could be due to our use of a significantly lower dose of oCRF, i.e., 0.03 μg/kg.

In the studies of Gold and colleagues[1] and Holsboer and colleagues[2] and in our present study, subsequent adrenal cortisol secretion after intravenous administration of oCRF did not differ between depressed patients and cortisol despite reduced pituitary ACTH responsivity. This finding has been interpreted by Gold

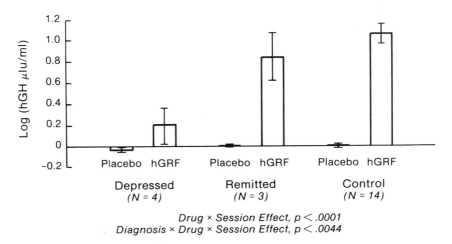

FIGURE 58.2. Mean change (± SEM) in log (hGH μIU/ml) from baseline to 15 min after injection.

and others as possibly due to adrenal cortical hypertrophy secondary to tonically increased plasma ACTH stimulation of the adrenals in depressed patients.

Thus all studies to date suggest that there is reduced pituitary responsivity to intravenous CRF administration in depressed patients but a subsequently normal adrenal cortisol response.

hGRF Studies

To our knowledge, this study is the first demonstration of a diminished pituitary growth hormone response to the hypothalamic releasing factor hGRF in depressed patients. Because remitted patients did not differ from controls in growth hormone responsivity to hGRF, these preliminary data suggest that a reduced growth hormone response to hGRF in depressed patients is a "state" marker.

Although we can only speculate about the mechanism involved in the pathophysiology of this diminished response of the pituitary to administered hGRF in depressed patients, it is known that intravenously administered hGRF does not appear to cross the blood-brain barrier and therefore does not act centrally in this paradigm. Therefore the loci of the action of hGRF must be at the pituitary somatotroph. An elegant study of Mendlewicz and colleagues[3] has demonstrated an elevation in 24-h growth hormone secretion in both bipolar and major depressive disorder patients. It is possible that chronically elevated plasma growth hormone concentrations could "down-regulate" or diminish the pituitary somatotroph GRF receptors and/or provide increased negative feedback when hGRF is intravenously administered.

Conclusions

These data suggest that, in addition to altered CNS regulatory mechanisms in affective illness, there are altered pituitary responses to provocative challenges with these neuropeptides in affective illness. These results offer further insight into the nature of neuroendocrine dysfunction in affective disorders.

References

1. Gold PW, Chrousos G, Kellner C, et al. Psychiatric implications of basic and clinical studies with corticotropin releasing factor. Am J Psychiatry 1984;141:619–627.
2. Holsboer F, Bardeleben U, Gerken A, et al. Blunted corticotropin and normal cortisol response to human corticotropin releasing factor in depression. N Engl J Med 1984;311:1127.
3. Mendlewicz J, Linkowski P, Kerkhofs M, et al. Diurnal hypersecretion of growth hormone in depression. J Clin Endocrinol Metab 1985;60:505–511.

59. TRH Stimulation Test in Psychiatry

PETER HERRIDGE AND MARK S. GOLD

In 1972 the serum thyrotropin (thyroid- stimulating hormone; TSH) response to thyrotropin-releasing hormone (TRH) was reported to be blunted in some euthyroid patients with major depression.[1] Since then approximately 60 studies involving well over 1,000 patients have confirmed that several types of psychiatric illness are associated with a blunted TSH response to TRH. It is now established as one of the most consistent findings in biological psychiatry with profound clinical and theoretical implications. (For reviews see references 2,3.)

A number of factors must be considered when evaluating the results of the TRH test in psychiatric patients, the most obvious one being the presence of thyroid disorder, as even mild hyperthyroidism causes a blunted response. Other factors that may influence the TRH test are age, gender, chronic renal failure, Klinefelter's syndrome, recent weight loss, dementia, repetitive administration of TRH, and recent administration of thyroid hormone, glucocorticoids, somatostatin, neurotensin, or dopamine.

The test is apparently not affected by tricyclic antidepressants or neuroleptics. However, chronic lithium administration can increase the TSH response after TRH most likely by its direct thyroid suppressant effect. Several commonly used drugs can cause blunting of the TSH response, including steroids, aspirin, barbiturates, opiates, cocaine, amphetamines, theophylline, and bromocriptine.

Definition of Blunting

The Δmax TSH is defined as the maximum TSH value occurring after TRH injection minus the baseline TSH value. Most investigators have defined a blunted response as a Δmax TSH of less than 5.0 μIU/ml,[2] whereas other investigators defined it as a Δmax TSH of less than 7.0 μIU/ml.[4]

TRH Test in Depression

In 1972 Prange et al. first reported a blunted TSH response to TRH in euthyroid, depressed women.[1] Since then this finding has been repeatedly confirmed.[2,3] From the studies so far reported, this phenomenon seems to occur in at least 25% of depressed patients.[3]

Some investigators have found no difference in the likelihood of blunting in primary versus secondary depression or unipolar versus bipolar depression. However, others have found increased frequency of blunting in primary versus secondary depression and in unipolar versus bipolar depression.[3,4]

It has been known for some time that elevated cortisol can cause a reduced TSH response in normal subjects and in patients with endocrine disorders.[3,5] Because some depressed patients show activation of the pituitary-adrenal-cortical axis it has been proposed as a cause of blunting in depression. However, several studies have found no association between TSH response and serum cortisol level in depression, and TSH blunting and cortisol nonsuppression after oral dexamethasone appear to be independent phenomenon.[3]

Variations in TRH pharmacokinetics do not appear to account for TSH blunting. In one study patients with blunted responses had postinjection TRH levels significantly higher than those in normal subjects. This finding suggests that thyrotroph cells in patients with TSH blunting are less responsive to TRH and not that less TRH is available to stimulate them.

Although most studies have shown that depressed patients with TSH blunting are euthyroid, some patients, paradoxically, have low serum thyroid hormone levels, suggesting a disturbance in feedback inhibition. One author, however, has reported an increased free thyroxine (T_4) index (FT_4I) in depressed patients. Another study has looked at the TSH response to TRH and serum concentration of free thyroxine (FT_4) and 3,5,3'- and 3,3',5'-triiodothyronine (FT_3 and FrT_3, respectively) in depressed patients before and after clinical recovery induced by electroconvulsive shock therapy (ECT). One group had reduced Δmax TSH and elevated FT_4 levels, which both normalized after ECT. The second group had reduced Δmax TSH and elevated FT_4 levels both before and after ECT. The authors concluded that their data were compatible with the assumption that the decreased TSH response to TRH in patients with endogenous depression is secondary to an increase in circulatory FT_4.[5]

Suicidal Behavior

There is evidence of an association between TSH blunting and suicidal behavior. Two studies have reported a significant negative association between Δmax TSH and a history of violent suicidal behavior.[6] One study has found a strong correlation between violent suicidal behavior and a virtually absent TSH response (Δmax less than 1.0 μIU/ml).

State-Trait Consideration

Most studies have found that a blunted TSH response in depression normalizes in only about one- half of patients after clinical recovery. Thus blunting may be a state marker in some patients and a trait marker in others.[2,6,7]

TRH Test as Predictor of Response and Relapse

A more complex question concerns the value of TSH blunting as a prediction of response to treatment and likelihood of relapse in depression. Several studies have compared the TRH test both in depression and during remission and used the difference in Δmax TSH ($\Delta\Delta$max TSH) as the independent variable. Two studies found that a positive trend in ΔΔmax TSH was correlated with a favorable response to treatment. These studies found that a persistently low TSH response predicted early relapse, i.e., within 6 months.[7]

TRH Test in Other Psychiatric Disorders

In addition to depression, several other psychiatric disorders are associated with a blunted TSH response to TRH in some patients.

Alcoholism

Approximately 50% of patients in acute alcohol withdrawal show blunting of the TSH response. However, in about one-third of alcoholic patients the blunting may persist long after all withdrawal symptoms have remitted. Thus blunting may be a trait marker in alcoholism.

Borderline Personality Disorder

Several investigations have found a blunted TSH response in patients with borderline personality disorder. In at least some of these patients there were no depressive symptoms at the time of testing or in the past and no history of substance abuse.

Mania

Several investigators have studied the TSH response in mania. One study found 18 of 30 mania patients to have a blunted response (Δmax TSH less than 7.0 μIU/ml).[8]

Schizophrenia

Most investigators have found that schizophrenic patients rarely have a blunted TSH response to TRH injection. In one study 31 of 41 unipolar depressed patients (76%) showed a blunted response, but none of 14 schizophrenic patients did.[4]

Causes of TSH Blunting

The TRH stimulation test directly measures the responsiveness of the pituitary thyrotroph cells to stimulation by TRH. The most obvious explanation for a blunted response would be hypersecretion of TRH with subsequent down-regulation of thyrotroph cell TRH receptors. The serum levels of free thyroid hormone have been reported as elevated in patients with blunted response,[5] which is consistent with the TRH hypersecretion hypothesis.

If this report is true, what does it suggest about brain neurotransmitter activity? Norepinephrine and dopamine stimulate TRH production, and serotonin inhibits it. Thus increased norepinephrine or dopamine activity or decreased serotonergic activity might be related to increased TRH secretion. One study has found a significant negative correlation between TSH response in depressed patients and 5-hydroxyindoleacetic acid (5-HIAA) levels in cerebrospinal fluid. Other investigators have looked for associations between urinary 3-methoxy-4-hydroxyphenylglycol (MHPG) and the TRH-induced TSH response with conflicting results.

Another explanation for TSH blunting is that the thyrotroph cells themselves are disordered in some way, or that they receive inhibitory input from some other source. It may be due to increased somatostatin or neurotensin activity or to some as yet unknown agent.

Whatever the cause of a blunted response, there is some evidence of a hereditary component. In one study two of six normal relatives of a depressed patient also showed blunting.

Summary

Although the cause of the blunting of the TRH-induced TSH response in psychiatric illness is not known, the phenomenon itself has emerged as one of the most reproducible findings in biological psychiatry. In the clinical practice of psychiatry the TRH test can be used to great advantage to (a) uncover subtle thyroid disease; (b) aid in diagnosis of depression and bipolar disorder; (c) predict treatment response and risk of relapse; and (d) assess risk of violent suicide attempts.

References

1. Prange AJ Jr, Wilson IC, Lara PO, et al.: Effect of thyrotropin-releasing hormone in depression. Lancet 1972;2:999–1002.
2. Loosen PT: The TRH-induced TSH response in psychiatric patients: a possible neuroendocrine marker. Psychoneuroendocrinology 1985;10:237–260.
3. Loosen PT, Prange AJ Jr: The serum thyrotropin (TSH) response to thyrotropin-releasing hormone (TRH) in depression: a review. Am J Psychiatry 1982;139:405–416.
4. Gold MS, Pottash ALC, Extein I, et al.: The TRH test in the diagnosis of major and minor depression. Psychoneuroendocrinology 1981;6:159–169.
5. Kirkegaard C, Faber J: Influence of free thyroid hormone levels on the TSH response to TRH in endogenous depression. Psychoneuroendocrinology 1986;11:491–497.
6. Kjellman BG: The function of the hypothalamic-pituitary-thyroid axis in affective disorders. Thesis, Karolinska Institute, Department of Psychiatry and Medicine, St. Goran's Hospital, Stockholm, and University of Linkoping, Stockholm, 1983.
7. Targum SD: The application of serial neuroendocrine challenge studies in the management of depressive disorder. Biol Psychiatry 1983;18:3–19.
8. Extein I, Pottash ALC, Gold MS, et al.: Using the protirelin test to distinguish mania from schizophrenia. Arch Gen Psychiatry 1982;39:77–81.

60. Luteinizing Hormone and Prolactin Response to Buprenorphine in Depression and Schizophrenia

C. Schmauss, K.M. Pirke, D.E. Bremer,
M.M. Weber, and H.M. Emrich

An association of hyper- or hypoactivity of endogenous opioids with depressive and schizophrenic psychoses has, to date, not been convincingly demonstrated. Such an assumption could, however, imply an altered sensitivity of structures involved in the mediation of opioid effects. The effects of opioids on pituitary prolactin (PRL)[1,2] and luteinizing hormone (LH) release[3,4] in man are well described, and there is little doubt that these effects are mediated through distinct opioid receptor populations. We have demonstrated that the partial opioid agonist buprenorphine exerts both antidepressive and antischizophrenic effects.[5] We report here on LH and PRL responses of depressed and schizophrenic patients to acute buprenorphine medication in comparison to respective responses of healthy volunteers.

Methods

Subjects

The control segment of the study comprised 53 healthy volunteers aged 20–40 years; 71.7% were men and 28.3% women. The women participated on days 1–5 of their menstrual cycles and were free of contraconceptive medication. The other segment of the study comprised 30 acutely admitted patients (50% men, 50% women; age 18–50 years) suffering from a first manifestation or an acute exacerbation of either schizophrenia ($n = 18$) or major depressive disorder ($n = 12$), diagnosed by *DSM-III* criteria. Patients were drug-free at least 5 weeks before initiation of the study. Informed written consent was obtained from all participants.

Drugs and Blood Sampling

To study the pharmacology of the effect of buprenorphine on pituitary LH and PRL release, subjects of the control group underwent various treatments with naloxone, buprenorphine, and placebo (Fig. 60.1). All patients received buprenorphine 0.2 mg. At 30 min before initiation of the study an intravenous catheter was inserted. Prior to administration of the drugs, a 10-ml baseline blood sample was obtained.

FIGURE 60.1. Effect of naloxone pretreatment on buprenorphine (bup)-induced stimulation of PRL and inhibition of LH release. Data are derived from healthy volunteers, who received one of the following treatments: (a) bup 0.2 or 0.4 mg (*n* = 20; data for 0.4 mg not shown) or placebo (*n* = 8; data not shown); (b) naloxone 0.04–0.4 mg (*n* = 10) or placebo (*n* = 5; data not shown); (c) bup 0.2 mg following a naloxone pretreatment 0.04 and 0.4 mg (*n* = 10). Subjects were blind to the application of either drug or placebo. Buprenorphine and placebo (Reckitt & Colman) were administered as sublingual tablets. Naloxone (Dupont) and placebo (0.9% NaCl) were administered as bolus intravenous injections.

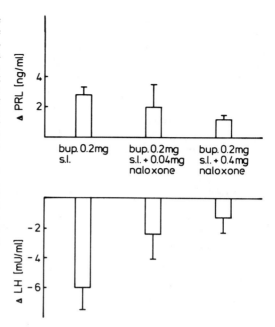

Control subjects remained in a reclining position during the study period and 10-ml blood samples were repeatedly obtained at 30-min intervals following drug administration. Blood samples of patients were obtained twice (baseline and 240 min after buprenorphine administration). So far as possible, the patients were also asked to remain in a reclining position during the study period. No food or drink was allowed.

Determination of LH and PRL Levels and Statistical Analysis

All blood samples were immediately centrifuged, and serum was stored at $-20°C$. LH and PRL levels were determined by radioimmunoassay (Serono-RIA, Diagnostiks, Freiburg). A two-tailed Student's *t*-test was employed to obtain proof of the significance of differences of LH and PRL responses to 0.2 mg buprenorphine between groups.

Results

Healthy Volunteers

Buprenorphine (0.2 and 0.4 mg) dose-dependently increased plasma PRL levels. The peak of effect was obtained 240 min after sublingual (s.l.) application (ΔPRL 2.8 ± 0.9 and 6.65 ± 1.3 following 0.2 and 0.4 mg of buprenorphine, respectively). Interestingly, an inverse dose response was obtained for the inhibition of LH release (ΔLH -6.0 ± 1.5 and -2.0 ± 0.59 for 0.2 and 0.4 mg of buprenorphine, respectively). This finding is compatible with previous reports of bell-shaped dose-response curves for this partial agonist.[6]

Placebo (sublingual and intravenous) treatment did not change plasma LH and PRL levels. Whereas naloxone (0.04–0.40 mg i.v.) had no effect on plasma PRL levels, a dose-dependent stimulation of LH release was found (data not shown). Figure 60.1 shows the effect of naloxone pretreatment on the buprenorphine (0.2 mg s.l.)-induced increased PRL and decreased LH levels. A tenfold higher dose of naloxone was required to sufficiently block the effect of buprenorphine on PRL release than to block the effect on LH release, indicating that the opioid receptor involved in the modulation of LH release is more sensitive to naloxone than the opioid receptor involved in the modulation of PRL release.

Depressed Patients and Schizophrenics

Figure 60.2 demonstrates that the PRL response to 0.2 mg buprenorphine of 18 schizophrenic patients (ΔPRL 3.2 $\pm$ 1.1) and of 12 depressed patients (ΔPRL 2.5 $\pm$ 1.4) did not differ from that of controls. The LH response of depressed patients shows a trend toward blunted responses (ΔLH -3.7 ± 2.0) but does not significantly differ from control responses ($p < 0.1$). In schizophrenics, however, the LH response was significantly blunted when compared to that of controls ($p < 0.02$).

Discussion

Studies on the pharmacology of the effects of naloxone on plasma LH and PRL levels provided evidence that LH release, in particular, is under the control of endogenous opioids, whereas naloxone does not affect PRL levels.[3,4] Using the LH response to an opioid compound with agonist activity as a tool for investigations

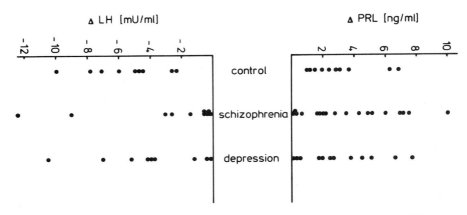

Figure 60.2. Changes in plasma LH (ΔLH) and PRL (ΔPRL) levels 240 min following buprenorphine (0.2 mg s.l.) application. Data were obtained from drug-free patients suffering from either major depression or schizophrenia. Because of the later decision to examine LH responses in these patients as well, the number of reported LH responses is smaller than the number of PRL responses.

of opioid receptor sensitivity in endogenous psychoses seems therefore more plausible than examination of PRL responses in such patients.

The PRL response to opioid agonists in depression has been repeatedly investigated, and results varied from "deficient" PRL responses,[7] to "blunted" PRL responses,[8,9] to normal PRL responses of patients with major depression compared to healthy controls.[10] In agreement with the latter finding, we report no different PRL responses in either depressed or schizophrenic patients compared to controls. The LH response to buprenorphine of depressed patients does not significantly differ from controls but shows a tendency toward lower mean levels. Most striking, however, is the finding of a significantly blunted LH response in schizophrenic patients. The significance of this finding remains to be elucidated.

References

1. Tolis G, Hikey J, Guyda H. Effect of morphine on serum growth hormone, cortisol, prolactin and thyroid stimulating hormone in man. J Clin Endocrinol Metab 1975;41:797–800.
2. Mendelson JH, Ellinboe J, Mello NK, et al. Buprenorphine effects on plasma luteinizing hormone and prolactin in male heroin addicts. J Pharmacol Exp Ther 1982;220:252–255.
3. Delitala G, Devilla L, Arata L. Opiate receptors and anterior pituitary hormone secretion in man: effect of naloxone infusion. Acta Endocrinol (Copenh) 1981;97:150–156.
4. Veldhuis JD, Worgul TJ, Monsaert R, et al. A possible role for endogenous opioids in the control of prolactin and luteinizing hormone secretion in the human. J Endocrinol Invest 1981;4:31–35.
5. Schmauss C, Emrich HM. Narcotic antagonist and opioid treatment in psychiatry. In Rodgers RJ, Cooper SJ (eds): Endorphins, Opiates and behavioral Processes. London: Wiley 1987;327–351.
6. Dum JE, Herz A. In vivo receptor binding of the opiate partial agonist, buprenorphine, correlated with its agonistic and antagonistic actions. Br J Pharmacol 1981;74:627–633.
7. Extein J, Pottash ALC, Gold MS, et al. Deficient prolactin response to morphine in depressed patients. Am J Psychiatry 1980;137:845–846.
8. Judd LL, Risch S, Parker DC, et al. The effect of methadone challenge on the prolactin and growth hormone responses of psychiatric patients and normal controls. Psychopharmacol Bull 1983;18:204–207.
9. Robertson AG, Jackman H, Meltzer HY. Prolactin response to morphine in depression. Psychiatry Res 1984;11:353–364.
10. Zis AP, Haskett RF, Albala AA, et al. Prolactin response to morphine in depression. Biol Psychiatry 1985;20:287–292.

61. Neuroendocrine Factors in Antidepressant Drug Therapy

GERHARD LANGER, GRETA KOINIG,
GEORG SCHOENBECK, AND REINHOLD HATZINGER

The reliable prediction of recovery and relapse and the identification of the therapeutic mechanisms of action of drugs given in the treatment of depressed patients remain unresolved issues in psychiatry and clinical psychopharmacology. Psychoneuroendocrine techniques have been used with some success in the attempt to improve the accuracy of prediction of treatment outcome.[1] Among such techniques the application of the thyrotropin-releasing hormone (TRH) test, i.e., the response of thyrotropin (thyroid-stimulating hormone; TSH) to TRH, has proved of most practical utility.[2]

This chapter is a synopsis of our studies covering 8 years of research in this interdisciplinary field of neuroendocrinology, psychopharmacology, and psychopathology of depression. We have arrived at the conclusions that (a) the combination of two neuroendocrine tests (TRH and insulin tolerance test) may considerably improve the accuracy of recovery-prediction and (b) the TRH test may be helpful in relapse prediction; (c) furthermore, the TRH test may help in elucidating the therapeutic mechanisms involved in symptomatic recovery from depression. Interestingly, our findings point to common mechanisms operative in the pathophysiology and symptomatic recovery[3] of the various functional psychoses (affective and schizophrenic psychoses).

Neuroendocrine Tests and Therapeutic Outcome

Prediction of Recovery

The TRH test was found in several studies to be of predictive value in the treatment of depression (for review see ref. 2). In our own investigation of 83 depressed patients, 90% of those patients on clomipramine who recovered within 9 weeks of treatment had shown at admission a blunted (i.e., abnormally low) TSH response (less than 5 mU/l) to TRH.[2] The respective number for the recovered patients with a normal TSH response was 76%. The difference in outcome between the two groups of patients was even more striking for the opposite prediction, i.e., the proportion of patients remaining nonrecovered for at least 9 weeks of treatment: There were 23% nonrecovered patients with a normal TSH response at admission, in contrast to only 5% nonrecovered with a blunted TSH response.

The insulin tolerance test (ITT) was performed in most of these depressed patients and in patients with functional psychoses other than depression. For statistical purposes data of patients with different diagnosis could be pooled because the findings were similar, analogous to our report with the TRH test.[2] When comparing the possible predictive value of the TRH test and the ITT by applying a statistical model (logistic regression), both tests proved useful: The two tests show interactional rather than additive effects in predicting therapeutic outcome within 4 weeks of clomipramine or haloperidol treatment (Fig. 61.1). For statistical computation, the four variables in the ITT (i.e., the glucose nadir being the necessary stimulus plus the hormonal responses of growth hormone, cortisol, and prolactin)

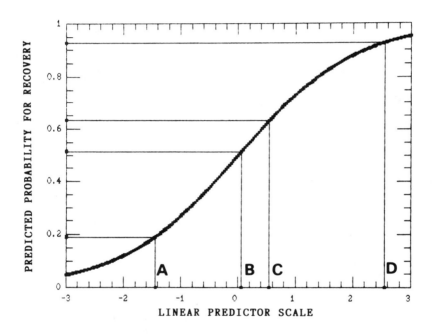

NEUROENDOCRINE VARIABLES		RECOVERED	NONREC.	PREDICTED PROBABILITY FOR RECOVERY	GROUP
TSH < 5	IR < −0.5	6	0	0.928	D
	IR ≥ −0.5	19	11	0.633	C
TSH > 5	IR < −0.5	4	17	0.191	A
	IR ≥ −0.5	18	17	0.514	B

FIGURE 61.1. Prediction of recovery by TRH and insulin tolerance test (ITT). Patients (*n* = 92) with various functional psychoses were treated with clomipramine or haloperidol. The statistical logistic regression model reveals interactional effects between the TSH response to TRH and the ITT (as expressed by the insulin response factor, IR). For further details, see the text.

were expressed by the "insulin response factor" (IR, Fig. 61.1), a factor derived by applying the statistical method of principal component analysis. As shown in the contingency table in Figure 61.1, the predicted probability for recovery of various patients with functional psychoses was 93% if the ITT had been normal and the TSH response had been blunted; in contrast, the predicted probability for recovery was only 19% if both tests had been normal at admission. The dexamethasone suppression test (DST) was of no statistically demonstrable predictive value for treatment outcome using our data.

Prediction of Relapse

Of the 83 depressed patients who entered the inpatient part of the study outlined above, 60 patients were also included in the outpatient part. We found that the blunted (less than 5 mU/l) TSH response at discharge was associated significantly with relapse of depression.[2] In these patients the instantaneous risk (statistical "survival" analysis) of relapse was relatively high during the first 2 months after discharge, i.e., 29% versus 15% in the patients with normal TSH response; throughout the rest of the year the difference in risk of relapse remained constant at 52% versus 36% at 12 months after discharge.

With our data the DST was of no significant value in the prediction of relapse. The data on the ITT for 12 months' follow-up were too few to allow for statistical "survival" analysis.

Therapeutic Mechanisms

The question arose as to whether the TSH response to TRH may change during inpatient treatment; that is, a blunted TSH response may convert to normal and vice versa, and, if so, if such different TSH response patterns during treatment can be statistically associated with therapeutic outcome.

To investigate this possible relation, 98 patients with various functional psychoses (two-thirds of the patients were depressives) were subjected to weekly TRH tests during their 3–9 weeks of treatment with the antidepressant clomipramine or the neuroleptic haloperidol, respectively.[3] The statistical analysis revealed that patients with a "disblunting TSH pattern" (i.e., blunted TSH response at admission that becomes normal during treatment) had a nearly 12-fold higher estimated chance of recovery than the patients with a "normal TSH pattern" (i.e., a normal TSH response on all TRH tests during the treatment period). Neither the diagnostic category of patients nor the kind of drug treatment (antidepressant or neuroleptic) was of noticeable importance in this respect.

Conclusion

The mechanisms of action of psychotherapeutic drugs can be studied at different levels of complexity. On the rather complex level of psychoneuroendocrine research, our strategy was aimed at evaluating possible common mechanisms in the therapeutic effects of "major tranquilizers" (i.e., antidepressants and neuroleptics). For this purpose patients presenting with various psychopathological symptoms of functional psychoses had been studied, most of whom were major depressives.

The blunted TSH response to TRH as a predictor of treatment outcome apparently provides varying information depending on the psychopathological state a patient is in at the time of the TRH test. If a patient is tested during manifest symptoms, the blunted TSH response predicts a more favorable outcome (recovery) of treatment with antidepressants or neuroleptics. However, if tested at recovery, a patient's blunted TSH response points to the risk of early relapse despite antidepressant maintenance medication.

This apparent paradox may be resolved by the following hypothesis: Drugs such as antidepressants and neuroleptics could be particularly effective in the symptomatic improvement of patients whose psychopathological syndromes are associated with a special, as yet uncharacterized, abnormal psychobiological state, one indicator of which is the blunted TSH response to TRH. Normalizing this abnormal psychobiological state with drugs (which goes along with normalization of the abnormal TSH response) would support the process of—but not be identical with—symptomatic recovery.[3] Patients who show a psychopathological syndrome that is not associated with such abnormal psychobiological state (i.e., normal TSH response at admission), however, might benefit less from such drugs.

Our findings for prediction of relapse can be interpreted correspondingly: If a patient recovers "symptomatically" during treatment but continues to show a blunted TSH response at discharge, the persistent psychobiological state could make this patient more vulnerable to symptomatic relapse compared to the patient with a normal TSH response.

This neuroendocrine parameter of blunted TSH respose may indicate a biological state of "malactivation" that is particularly amenable to treatment with tricyclic antidepressant and neuroleptic drugs ("major tranquilizers"). The maintenance of the "malactivation" despite psychopathological recovery predicts an early relapse. We therefore hypothesize that this sequence of TSH patterns may indicate the involvement of common pathophysiological factors in the phenomenology of different psychopathological syndromes and in the recovery. The precise nature of these pathophysiological factors themselves is unknown; the hypothalamic-pituitary-thyroid axis may be involved in a manner yet to be identified.[3]

Acknowledgment. Supported in part by "Fonds zur Foerderung der wissenschaftlichen Forschung", grants 4416, 4565, 5116, and 5260 (Dr. Langer et al.).

References

1. Gold MS, Lydiard RB, Carman JS. Advances in Psychopharmacology: Predicting and Improving Treatment Response. Boca Raton: CRC Press, 1984.
2. Langer G, Koinig G, Hatzinger R, et al.: Response of thyrotropin to thyrotropin-releasing hormone as predictor of treatment outcome: prediction of recovery and relapse in treatment with antidepressants and neuroleptics. Arch Gen Psychiatry 1986;43:861–868.
3. Langer G, Resch F, Aschauer H, et al. TSH-response patterns to TRH stimulation may indicate therapeutic mechanisms of antidepressant and neuroleptic drugs. Neuropsychobiology 1984;11:213–218.

62. Neuroendocrine Studies of the Mechanism of Action of Antidepressant Drugs

S.A. CHECKLEY

A central question in the psychopharmacology of depression is whether tricyclic antidepressants increase or reduce monoaminergic neurotransmission. In the case of norepinephrine uptake inhibitors such as desipramine, the chronic effects of down-regulation at α_2-autoreceptors and up-regulation at postsynaptic α_1-adrenoceptors increase noradrenergic neurotransmission. However, the down-regulation of postsynaptic β_1-adrenoceptors reduce noradrenergic neurotransmission, and it is not known if the net effect of chronic desipramine treatment is to increase noradrenergic neurotransmission in man.[1]

The neuroendocrine control of melatonin secretion is a convenient model for investigating this question in experimental animals[2] and depressed patients. The basis of this model has been reviewed elsewhere[3] and is summarized in this chapter.

Norepinephrine and Melatonin

The addition of norepinephrine (NE) to cultured pineal cells results in the accumulation of cyclic adenosine monophosphate (cAMP), the activation of N-acetyltransferase (NAT), and a consequent increase in the synthesis of melatonin. In man also NE regulates melatonin synthesis, as it is increased following treatment with the selective NE uptake inhibitor $(+)$-oxaprotiline. $(-)$-Oxaprotiline, which does not inhibit NE uptake, does not affect melatonin.[4]

α_2-Adrenoceptors and Melatonin

In rat pineal tissue NE release is inhibited by the α_2-agonist clonidine and is increased by the α_2-antagonist yohimbine. In man melatonin secretion is reduced by clonidine but increased by the α_2-antagonist Org 3770.[5]

β_1-Adrenoceptors and Melatonin

β_1-Adrenoceptors have been demonstrated on pinealocytes, and the stimulation of these cells with isoprenaline results in the accumulation of cAMP, activation of NAT, and increased secretion of melatonin; each of these effects has been blocked by the β-blocking drug propranolol. In man also the activation of β-adrenoceptors is needed for the stimulation of melatonin synthesis, as melatonin secretion in man is abolished by propranolol and by the selective $β_1$-antagonist atenolol.

Adenylate Cyclase and Melatonin

In the rat pineal $β_1$-adrenoceptors are coupled to adenylate cyclase, and dibutyryl cAMP has been shown to increase the activity of NAT and the synthesis of melatonin. In man cAMP also influences the secretion of melatonin, as it is increased by the selective phosphodiesterase inhibitor rolipram.[6]

$α_1$-Adrenoceptors and Melatonin

$α_1$-Adrenoceptors have been demonstrated on rat pinealocytes, and a functional synergism has been demonstrated between $α_1$- and $β_1$-adrenoceptors for their effects on cAMP accumulation and melatonin synthesis. In sheep and man the $α_1$-antagonist prazosin inhibits melatonin secretion.[5]

In summary, the model described above is an appropriate one for asking the question whether chronic antidepressant treatment increases or reduces noradrenergic neurotransmission in animals and man.

Effects of Chronic Imipramine Treatment on Melatonin Synthesis in the Rat

Among the various studies of the effects of antidepressant drugs on melatonin synthesis in animals, the study of Friedman et al.[7] is of particular relevance to clinical practice. Treatment given for 3 weeks resulted in plasma imipramine concentrations that would be considered within the therapeutic range. This treatment resulted in a 31% reduction in pineal β-adrenoceptor binding sites, 36% reduction in NAT activity, 25% reduction in the pineal concentration of its product N-acetylserotonin (NAS), and 23% reduction in pineal melatonin concentrations. In the case of the rat pineal, chronic treatment with imipramine reduced not only the number of pineal β-adrenoceptors but also net noradrenergic signal transmission. Presumably the effect of down-regulation at β-adrenoceptors is greater than the other chronic effects of desipramine on the noradrenergic system in the rat pineal.

Effects of Chronic Desipramine Treatment on Melatonin Secretion in Depressed Patients

In contrast to the animal study of Friedman et al.,[7] no clinical study has yet reported that tricyclic antidepressants reduce noradrenergic neurotransmission. A statistically significant increase in plasma melatonin concentrations was reported by our group[8] following treatment with desipramine for 3 weeks. After 4 weeks of treatment with desipramine there was a nonsignificant trend toward increased plasma concentrations of melatonin in a study of Fraser et al.[9] In four depressed patients Sack and Lewy[10] reported an increase in the urinary excretion of melatonin sulfate following treatment with desipramine for 1 and 3 weeks.

Conclusion

The number of patients studied is still too small to permit a definite conclusion, but the comparisons between animal and clinical studies are striking. Whereas imipramine reduces noradrenergic neurotransmission in the rat pineal, the closely related metabolite of imipramine, desipramine, does not reduce melatonin secretion in depressed patients. Although the pineal is a good model of central neurotransmission, it is not part of the brain and consequently is a model only of central neurotransmission. Within the limits of the model, however, the data reviewed in this chapter seriously question the hypothesis that the mechanism of action of antidepressant drugs involves a reduction in noradrenergic neurotransmission as a result of down-regulation at β-adrenoceptors.

References

1. Checkley SA, Corn TH, Glass IB, et al. Neuroendocrine and other studies of the mechanism of antidepressant action of desipramine. In Murphy DL (ed): Antidepressants and Receptor Function. Ciba Foundation Symposium 123. New York: Wiley, 1986;126–158.
2. Klein DC. Photoneural regulation of the mammalian pineal gland. In Short R (ed): Photoperiodism, Melatonin and the Pineal. Ciba Foundation Symposium 117. New York: Wiley, 1985;51–70.
3. Checkley SA, Park W. The psychopharmacology of the human pineal. J Psychopharmacol 1987;1:109–125.
4. Checkley SA, Thompson C, Burton S, et al. Clinical studies of the effect of (+) and (−) oxaprotiline upon noradrenaline uptake. Psychopharmacology 1985;87:116–118.
5. Palazidou E, Franey C, Arendt J, et al. Use of the pineal neuroendocrine model to investigate the mechanism of action of antidepressant drugs. In: Abstracts of the British Association of Psychopharmacology Meeting, 1987, Cambridge. J Psychopharmacol 1987;1:No. 1:104.
6. Checkley SA, Winton F, Franey C, et al. Effects of a phosphodiesterase inhibitor upon the urinary excretion of 6 sulphatoxy melatonin in man. J Psychopharmacol 1987;1:20–22.
7. Friedman E, Yocca FD, Cooper TB. Antidepressant drugs with varying pharmacological profiles alter pineal beta adrenergic function. J Pharmacol Exp Ther 1984;228:545–549.
8. Thompson C, Mezey G., Corn TH, et al. The effect of desipramine upon melatonin and cortisol secretion in depressed patients and normal subjects. Br J Psychiatry 1985;147:389–393.
9. Fraser A, Brown R, Kocsis J, et al. Patterns of melatonin rhythms in depression. J Neural Transm [Suppl] 1986;21:269–290.
10. Sack RL, Lewy AJ. Desmethylimipramine treatment increases melatonin production in humans. Biol Psychiatry 1986;21:406–409.

63. Growth Hormone Response to Clonidine Stimulation in Affective Disorders: Effects of Lithium Therapy

F. Brambilla, M. Catalano, A. Lucca,
P. Della Maggiora, and E. Smeraldi

Data in the literature suggest that alterations of the noradrenergic (NE) system may exert a pathogenetic influence on affective disorders.[1-3] Impairments of α- and β-NE receptor sensitivity have been reported, and it has been suggested that the efficacy of lithium prophylaxis may be related to its effects on the β-NE receptor.[4]

Because it has also been proposed that the therapeutic effects of antidepressants might be the consequence of α_2-NE receptor desensitization[5] we undertook a study of the effects of lithium administration on the α_2-adrenergic receptors in a group of patients with recurrent depressive illness during a normothymic phase of the disease. The growth hormone (GH) response to acute administration of clonidine, a typical α_2-adrenergic receptor stimulant,[6] was used as an indirect indicator. The implementation of the study during a normothymic phase of depression was intended to avoid any possible interference from depressive or manic symptomatology on the NE-GH-releasing hormone (GRF)-GH axis, which has been demonstrated to be impaired during the active phase of the disease.[3,7-9] We wanted to study the functioning of the α_2-NE receptors in the absence of overt depressive symptomatology and in the meantime observe the direct pharmacological mechanism of action of lithium without regard to clinical evaluations of its effects on the periodicity and course of depressive illness.

Material and Methods

We studied 12 patients (1 male and 11 female) diagnosed as suffering from primary affective disorders (RDC) or major affective disorders (*DSM-III*) and as being in a normothymic phase of the disease. Five subjects had bipolar disorders and seven major depression, recurrent type. The patients' ages ranged from 36 to 62 years; two women were of fertile age, and nine were menopausal. The duration of the disease ranged from 2 to 46 years, with 2 to 18 previous manic or depressive episodes. The group had been in normothymia from 3 weeks to 5 months. All had previously been treated with tricyclic antidepressants, benzodiazepines, neuroleptics, and lithium salts but had had no treatment 2 weeks to 5 months before the study. All subjects were outpatients. Ten healthy volunteers matched for sex and age were used as controls.

Patients and controls underwent the first clonidine stimulation test after an overnight fast and 1 h of bed rest. GH was assayed at 15- to 30-min intervals for 2 h after administration of 150 μg of clonidine as an intravenous bolus at 9:00 a.m. Lithium carbonate was administered orally twice a day (at 9:00 a.m. and 9:00 p.m.) at a dosage of 600 mg/day. After 15 days for patients and 7 days for controls the clonidine test was repeated as described above. At this time, lithium levels were measured in both plasma and red blood cells (RBCs) and were expressed as RBC Li$^+$/plasma Li$^+$ (Lithium ratio). Blood pressure was measured during the clonidine tests. GH concentrations were assayed radioimmunologically using the commercial kits of Sorin (Italy). Lithium levels were measured by atomic absorption spectrophotometry according to the method of Frazer.[10] The data were analyzed statistically by student's t-test for paired samples and by analysis of variance according to Statistical Package for Social Sciences (SPSS) and Biomedical Package for Statistical Software (BMDP).

Results

The results are reported in Figure 63.1. Pretherapy GH basal levels were normal in patients and did not differ from those of controls. There was no change in these levels in either group after lithium administration.

In the controls (Fig. 63.1A), clonidine administration before lithium therapy induced a substantial GH rise, with the mean peak time at 45 min. The mean (±SD) area under the curve (AUC) was 561.4 (± 301.4). The response was reduced after lithium administration, and the AUC was 421.3 ± 240.1, with the mean peak again at 45 min. The difference between the AUC before and after therapy was statistically significant ($p < 0.05$).

In depressives (Fig. 63.1B) the GH response to clonidine administration before lithium therapy was blunted, the mean AUC being 201.3 ± 126 with the mean peak time at 45 min. The difference between the basal response of depressives and controls also was statistically significant ($p < 0.05$). After therapy the GH response to stimulation was slightly increased (AUC 218.8 ± 151.2), with the mean peak time again at 45 min. The difference between the AUC before and after therapy was not statistically significant.

Considering the individual GH responses to stimulation before and after therapy in each subject, we observed that eight of the ten controls had a good pretherapeutic response that decreased afterward; one had no response and no change, and one had a blunted response that increased after therapy. Among the patients, eight had no response, three a blunted response, and one a low-normal GH response to clonidine before therapy. Among the 11 patients with no or blunted responses, seven showed an increased response after lithium therapy that reached normal values in only one. In the other five there was a slight decrease in response. The only patient who had a normal response before therapy had a slight decrease after it. At 15 days of therapy mean lithium blood levels, expressed as the lithium ratio, were not significantly different in depressive and controls (mean ± SD = 0.36 ± 0.12 versus 0.33 ± 0.15). Mean blood pressure (BP) before treatments ranged from 128 ± 9/80 ± 6 at 0 time to 106 ± 10/70 ± 7 at 45 min in controls and from 128 ± 5/81 ± 4 at 0 time to 97 ± 4/65 ± 3 at 45 min in patients. No significant differences

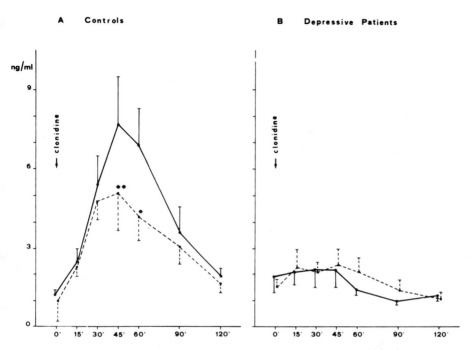

FIGURE 63.1. GH response to clonidine stimulation in 10 controls (A) and 12 patients with depressive disorders (B) before (●————●) and after (■– – –■) lithium therapy. *$p < 0.05$; **$p < 0.02$.

were observed between patients and controls. No significant BP variations were observed after lithium therapy in either group.

Analysis of variance for repeated measures according to BMDP on patient–control differences in GH responses to clonidine stimulation before and after lithium therapy revealed an interaction of diagnosis per time; that is, the pattern of the GH response before and after therapy is exactly opposite in the two groups of subjects examined: negative in controls, and positive in patients. This difference is statistically significant ($p = 0.03$). Analysis of variance according to SPSS also revealed that the difference (Δ) between responses before and after therapy was significantly negatively correlated with the pretherapy response ($p < 0.001$). Thus the different pattern of responses in the two groups seems to depend on the different type of GH response to clonidine before lithium therapy. All the other main effects and covariates (age and sex of the subjects and the lithium ratio) showed no significant interference with the Δ patterns.

Discussion and Conclusions

Our data revealed two phenomena. First, depressed patients in a normothymic phase of the disease, off therapy, showed a blunted GH response to clonidine as it has been reported to occur during the symptomatologically active phases of depression and considered an expression of α_2-NE receptor subsensitivity.[6-8,11-13] The occurrence of this receptor subsensitivity during an asymptomatic phase of the illness has already been observed in small groups of patients.[14] These findings and our results suggest that the α_2-NE receptor subsensitivity may be a trait marker of depression, as it seems to be present during the entire course of the illness. A longitudinal study in a group of patients with and without blunted GH response to clonidine during symptomatic and asymptomatic phases of the disease would be necessary to confirm this hypothesis and to validate the observation that the phenomenon is present only in endogenous and not in neurotic-reactive depressed subjects, as reported by Matussek et al.[7] and Boyer et al.[11]

The second observation stemming from our data is the opposing pattern of the α_2-NE receptor response to lithium administration shown by patients and controls, the first group presenting an increase and the second a decrease of NE receptor sensitivity after lithium therapy. This apparently paradoxical response to the same type of treatment finds its logic in the observation that the response to lithium is based on the state of sensitivity of the α_2-NE receptors before treatment, as revealed by the GH response to clonidine. In other words, lithium would act as a modulator, increasing or decreasing the receptor sensitivity in relation to its initial state of functionality. The significant correlation between the type of α_2-NE receptor response to lithium therapy and depressive illness is a consequence of the initial state of sensitivity of the NE system. In other words, lithium up-regulates α_2-NE receptors in depressed patients because they are initially subsensitive to stimulation. The apparently contradictory effect of lithium in both depressed and manic patients may find its logic in this context; however, a longitudinal study on the effects of long-lasting therapy on the NE system would be necessary to confirm this hypothesis.

References

1. Schilkraut JJ. Current status of the catecholamine hypothesis of affective disorders. In Lipton MA, Di Mascio A, Killam KF (eds): Psychopharmacology: A Generation of Progress. New York: Raven Press, 1978;1223–1234.
2. Charney DS, Menkes DB, Heninger GR. Receptor sensitivity and the mechanism of action of antidepressant treatment: implications for the etiology and therapy of depression. Arch Gen Psychiatry 1981;38:11–60.
3. Siever LJ, Uhde TW, Silberman EK, et al. The growth hormone response to clonidine as a probe of noradrenergic receptor responsiveness in affective disorder patients and controls. Psychiatry Res 1982;6:171–183.
4. Trieser S, Kellar KJ. Lithium effects on adrenergic receptor supersensitivity in rat brain. Eur J Pharmacol 1979;58:85–86.
5. Siever LJ, Insel T, Uhde T. Noradrenergic challenges in the affective disorders. J Clin Psychopharmacol 1981;1:193–206.
6. Erickson E. Experimental Psychoneuroendocrinology: Brain α_2-Adrenoceptor Function and Growth Hormone Release. Goteborg: Universitas Regia & Goteburgensis, 1985.
7. Matussek N, Achenheil M, Hippius H, et al. Effect of clonidine on growth hormone release in psychiatric patients and controls. Psychiatry Res 1980;2:25–36.
8. Charney DS, Heninger GR, Sternberg DE, et al. Adrenergic receptor sensitivity in depression. Arch Gen Psychiatry 1982;39:290–294.
9. Chekley SA, Slade AP, Shur E. Growth hormone and other responses to clonidine in patients with endogenous depression. Br J Psychiatry 1982;138:51–55.
10. Frazer A. Determination of the lithium ratio of human erytrocytes in vivo. In Cooper TB, Gershon S, Kline NS, et al (eds): Lithium: Controversies and Unresolved Issues. Amsterdam: Excerpta Medica, 1979;527–532.

11. Boyer P, Scaub C, Pichot P. Growth hormone response to clonidine test in depressive states. Neuroendocrinol Lett 1982;4:178.
12. Siever LJ, Insel TR, Hamilton JA, et al. A comparison between the growth hormone response to amphetamine and clonidine. Psychiatry Res 1985;16:79–82.
13. Watanabe A, Manome T, Kaneko M, et al. H. Human growth hormone response to clonidine in patients with affective disorders. In: Abstracts, XVI International Congress of Psychoneuroendocrinology, Kyoto, 1985.
14. Siever LJ, Pickar D, Lake CR, et al. Extreme elevations in plasma norepinephrine associated with decreased α-adrenergic responsivity: two case reports. J Clin Psychopharmacol 1983;3:39–41.

64. Endocrinological Diseases Mimicking Affective Disorders

IRL EXTEIN, MARK S. GOLD, AND
WILLIAM A. RAFULS

Neuroendocrinology[1] is becoming increasingly important for both clinicians and researchers in psychiatry. As we learn more about the brain's role as the master of the endocrine system as well as an end-organ for multiple hormonal effects, the line between primary affective disorder and primary endocrine disorders is becoming increasingly blurred. The earliest manisfestation of some endocrine disorders may include disturbances of mood.[2,3] Primary depression is associated with neuroendocrine dysregulation, tests of which have been suggested as diagnostic markers for depressive illness.[4]

The anatomy of neuroendocrine regulation is summarized in Figure 64.1, illustrating the feedback systems involved. Changes in hormone production affect not only peripheral organs and receptors but also central receptors. The same monoamine neurotransmitters implicated in mood disturbances are involved in neuroendocrine regulation.

Endocrinological diseases commonly associated with mood disturbances include thyroid, adrenal, and parathyroid disorders, hypopituitarism, and hyperprolactinemia (Table 64.1).[2,3] Often disturbances of certain physiological parameters (e.g., the levels of calcium, steroid hormones, glucose, and thyroid hormones) account for psychiatric symptoms, reversible by correcting the chemical abnormality. Patients with preexisting psychiatric disorders may be more vulnerable to psychiatric manifestations of endocrinopathies.

Hall et al.[5,6] have studied the role of medical illnesses in psychiatric symptomatology. Up to 46% of patients are reported to have had a previously undiagnosed medical illness causing or exacerbating their psychiatric problems. Endocrine disorders accounted for 29% of the medical illness, with thyroid disorders being most frequent followed by diabetes mellitus, hypoglycemia, Addison's disease, and hyperparathyroidism.

Hyperparathyroidism is of note because of the high incidence of psychiatric symptoms and the rather clear relation to calcium levels.[7] Gross elevations of calcium above 16 mg/dl are associated with organic brain syndromes, whereas elevations below 16 mg/dl are associated mainly with depression and fatigue.

Hypothyroidism is usually considered in the differential diagnosis of depressive and dementing disorders. Hyperthyroidism is part of the differential diagnosis of activated states, such as anxiety and hypomania. Though a transient elevation in thyroxine (T_4) has been noted in 5–10% of acute psychiatric hospital admissions,

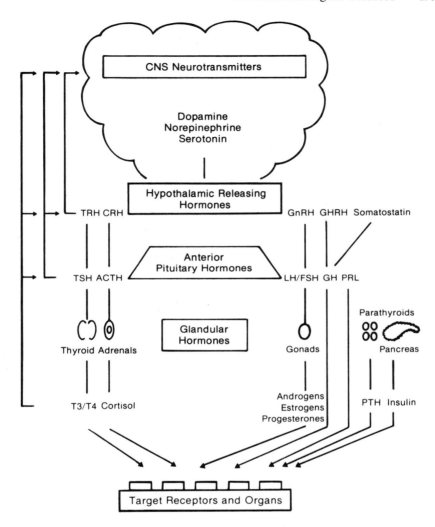

FIGURE 64.1. Neuroendocrine regulation.

hypothyroidism is much more common than hyperthyroidism in psychiatric populations, particularly when considering early stages of hypothyroidism.[8,9] Hypothyroidism is not an all-or-none phenomenon.[9,10] Grade 1 hypothyroidism is clinically overt, with classical physical signs and symptoms and low plasma levels of T_4. Grade 2 is an earlier and milder stage with few clinical symptoms, normal T_4, but elevated plasma levels of thyroid-stimulating hormone (TSH). Grade 3, or subclinical hypothyroidism, an even earlier stage, has none of the classic physical signs or symptoms, normal T_4 and baseline TSH, but elevated TSH response to thyrotropin-releasing hormone (TRH) on the TRH stimulation test. About two-third of the grade 3 patients have autoimmune thyroiditis.[9] About 5–10% of de-

TABLE 64.1. Psychiatric disturbances in neuroendocrine diseases.[a]

Disease	Delirium	Dementia	Anxiety	Apathy	Depression	Irritability	Euphoria	Psychosis	Insomnia	Personality changes
Hypoglycemia	X	X	X		X					X
Hyperglycemia	X	X			X					X
Pancreatic cancer	X				X				X	X
Hypoparathyroidism	X	X	X		X			X		X
Hyperparathyroidism	X	X	X		X	X	X	X		X
Hypocortisolism	X			X	X	X				X
Hypercortisolism		X	X		X	X	X	X	X	X
Hypothyroidism		X			X	X				X
Hyperthyroidism			X	X	X	X	X	X	X	X
Hypopituitarism	X	X	X		X			X		X
Hyperprolactinemia			X		X	X				X

[a]Reprinted from ref. 3, with permission.

pressed patients have subclinical hypothyroidism.[9] Patients with grade 2 and 3 hypothyroidism have been reported to have subtle cardiac and other medical dysfunction.[11]

Depression and fatigue in patients with early grades of hypothyroidism may be an early expression of the endocrine disturbance. A more conservative hypothesis is that the early hypothyroidism colors treatment response. Depressed patients with subclinical hypothyroidism are reported to be more likely to require and respond to thyroid hormone potentiation of tricyclic antidepressants.[12] Bipolar depressed patients with subclinical hypothyroidism are at risk for rapid mood cycling, sometimes tricyclic-induced.[13] Lithium plus thyroid hormone may be the treatment of choice for bipolar patients with laboratory evidence of hypothyroidism.

A large percentage of patients with Cushing's syndrome reportedly have psychiatric disturbances, most commonly depression.[2,3,14] Cushing's syndrome of hypothalamic or pituitary origin is associated more often with mood disturbances than when this disorder originates from an adrenal adenoma or ectopic ACTH-producing neoplasm. Though euphoria has been noted in fewer than 5% of Cushing's syndrome patients, hypomanic-like euphoria and irritability are common side effects of corticosteroid therapy.

The hypercortisolism, elevated ACTH, and dexamethasone nonsuppression of Cushing's syndrome are found commonly in patients with major depression. However, it has been shown that depressed patients have a blunted ACTH/cortisol response to infusion of cortiocotropin-releasing factor (CRF), in contrast to Cushing's disease patients who have an augmented response.[15]

References

1. Martin JB, Reichlin S, Brown GM. Clinical Neuroendocrinology. Philadelphia: Davis, 1977.
2. Leigh H, Kramer SI. The psychiatric manifestations of endocrine disease. Ann Intern Med 1984;29:413–445.
3. Rafuls WA, Extein I, Gold MS, et al. Neuropsychiatric manifestations of endocrine disorders. In Hales RE, Yudofsky SC (eds): Textbook of Neuropsychiatry. Washington, DC: American Psychiatric Press, 1987;307–325.
4. Carroll BJ. Dexamethasone suppression test: a review of contemporary confusion. J Clin Psychiatry 1985;46:13–24.
5. Hall RCW, Gardner ER, Stickney SK, et al. Physical illness presenting as psychiatric disease. Arch Gen Psychiatry 1978;35:1315–1320.
6. Hall RCW, Gardner ER, Popkin ER, et al. Unrecognized physical illness prompting psychiatric admission: a prospective study. Am J Psychiatry 1981;138:629–635.
7. Petersen P. Psychiatric disorders in primary hyperparathyroidism. J Clin Endocrinol Metab 1968;28:1491–1495.
8. Cohn KL, Swigar ME. Thyroid function screening in psychiatric patients. JAMA 1979;242:254–257.
9. Gold MS, Pottash ALC, Extein IL. "Symptomless" autoimmune thyroiditis in depression. Psychiatry Res 1982;6:261–269.
10. Evered DC, Ormston BJ, Smith PA, et al. Grades of hypothyroidism. Br Med J 1973;1:657–662.
11. Cooper DS, Halpern R, Wood LC, et al. L-Thyroxine therapy in subclinical hypothyroidism. Ann Intern Med 1984;101:18–24.
12. Targum SD, Greenberg RD, Harmon RL, et al. Thyroid hormone and the TRH test in refractory depression. J Clin Psychiatry 1984;45:345–346.
13. Cowdry RW, Wehr TA, Zis AP, et al. Thyroid abnormalities associated with rapid cycling bipolar illness. Arch Gen Psychiatry 1983;40:414–420.

14. Reus VI, Berlant JR. Pituitary-adrenal dysfunction in psychiatric illness. In Extein I, Gold MS (eds): Medical Mimics of Psychiatric Disorders. Washington, DC: American Psychiatric Press, 1986;111–130.
15. Gold P, Chrousos G, Kellner C, et al. Psychiatric implications of basic and clinical studies with corticotropin releasing factor. Am J Psychiatry 1984;141:619–627.

III AFFECTIVE DISORDERS IN POPULATIONS AT RISK

III.A. Affective Disorders and Suicide

65. Epidemiology and Psychosocial Risk Factors for Suicide

ROBERT M.A. HIRSCHFELD

This chapter serves as an introduction to the chapters on recent findings on suicide. Space limitation does not allow a comprehensive presentation of the major risk factors for suicide. However, current knowledge on demographic risk factors, including age, sex, marital status, race, and socioeconomic class, are briefly summarized here (Table 65.1). For more detail the reader is referred to relevant reviews.[1-3] Psychiatric risk factors are reviewed.

Rates

Rates of suicide for the major Western and industrialized countries vary sixfold, from less than 6/100,000 per year for Spain, Ireland, Italy, and Israel to more than 20/100,000 for Austria, Switzerland, Denmark, and West Germany.[4] Intermediate rates are reported for the United States, Japan, England, and Canada. The highest rates tend to be found in countries with a high standard of living where the church has relatively little influence. In contrast are more poor countries in which the church, the Catholic church in particular, maintains a strong presence.

Demographic Risk Factors

In the United States the suicide rate for men is more than three times that for women, and this difference has been fairly constant for many years.[5] The rates for both men and women tend to increase in parallel from age 15 to 50. After that point the rates climb sharply for men and decline among women. By age 85 the rate for white women has dropped to about 5/100,000 whereas that for white men has soared to nearly 50/100,000, a tenfold difference

Rates for whites are higher than those for blacks and other noncaucasians of both sexes. In general, ethnic and minority groups have lower suicide rates.

Suicide is most common among single people, followed by the widowed, then the divorced and separated. Married people have the lowest suicide rates.

There is no consistent relation between suicide rates and social class. However, higher social classes tend to have higher suicide rates. The rate of suicide increases in people who have fallen in social status. Some studies have found higher suicide rates among both social class extremes.[6]

Suicide in Psychiatric Patients

Studies of suicide among psychiatric patients have found that risk factors in these subjects differ in several important ways from those in the general population.[7] Rates of suicide in psychiatric patients, particularly inpatients, range from five to six times to nearly 500 times the comparable rate in the general population. Therefore simply being a psychiatric patient puts one at a substantially increased risk of suicide (Table 65.1).

Men are at higher risk for suicide in psychiatric populations, although the sex ratio is substantially lower among psychiatric patients than in the general population. The male/female ratio of suicide in psychiatric patients is below 1.5:1.0.

Among the general population the sex ratio for suicide in the United States was 2.5:1.0 (ranging from approximately 2:1 to 10:1 for various age groups). Therefore being a psychiatric patient tends to increase the risk of suicide in women much more so than it does in men.

In the general population, suicide is very much a phenomenon of older white men. This finding is not nearly as true among psychiatric patients, whose peak suicide rate tends to be during the middle years. Male psychiatric patients tend to commit suicide at a somewhat younger age, perhaps around 25 to 40, whereas the peak in female patients tends to be between 35 and 50.

Caucasian patients kill themselves at a much higher rate than do black and other nonwhite patient groups, as in the general population. Depression, schizophrenia, and substance abuse are also associated with a substantially increased risk of suicide. However, depression, especially psychotic depression or severely incapacitating depression, causes the risk of suicide to soar. Given the high prevalence of depression, its importance as a risk factor puts it at the top of the list.

A psychiatric history increases one's risk of suicide, and a history of prior suicide attempts substantially increases suicide risk. However, the predictive value of suicide attempts does not hold up among psychotic patients, who are much more likely to kill themselves without warning.

Finally, the timing during the course of treatment for the disorder is extremely important. Even though patients are being actively administered to and are being observed for suicidal tendencies while in the hospital, a substantial proportion of them nonetheless do kill themselves while hospitalized. In addition, the 6- to 12-

TABLE 65.1. Summary of risk factors for suicide in psychiatric patients.[a]

Status: psychiatric patient
Gender: male, although the gender distinction is less important than among the general population
Age: middle years, in contrast to the general population
Race: white (at much higher risk than blacks)
Diagnosis: depression and schizophrenia
History
    Suicide attempts, except among psychotic patients
    Undesirable life events, especially humiliating ones or loss of a key person
Timing: during hospitalization and 6–12 months after discharge

[a]From ref. 7, with permission.

month period immediately following discharge is one of very high risk, which is particularly true among women during the first 6 months after hospitalization.

Alcohol is an important consideration in the study of suicide. It may have a disinhibiting effect, breaking down normal constraints on self-destructive behavior. In fact, alcohol is often consumed prior to suicides, and one in five suicide victims are intoxicated at the time of their death.

Risk factors for suicide among alcoholics are similar to those among other psychiatric patients. In contrast to other patients, though, alcoholics are more likely to kill themselves late in the course of their disease. Alcoholics are especially likely to communicate suicidal wishes prior to suicide. The risk substantially increases if there is a concurrent depression.

Certain medical and surgical patients present special suicidal risks and bear more intensive psychiatric attention. Patients with respiratory diseases are three times more likely to suicide than other medical patients. Similarly, patients on hemodialysis are a high risk group. Patients with cancer are slightly more likely to kill themselves than the general population, but if untreated they may be at very high risk. In this group it is unclear how many of the suicides occurred prior to treatment, so generalizations must be tentative.

Conclusion

Suicide continues to be a serious public health problem. We have identified a number of risk factors that help to categorize people according to degree of suicidal risk. However, their value in predicting an individual suicide is unfortunately limited. It is important to remember that being a psychiatric patient substantially increases suicidal risk, and that risk factors that are important in general populations, e.g., a preponderance of men, are not necessarily accurate in psychiatric populations.

References

1. Sainsbury P. The epidemiology of suicide. In Roy A (ed): Suicide. Baltimore: Williams & Wilkins, 1986;17–45.
2. Cross K, Hirschfeld RMA. Epidemiology of disorders in adulthood: suicide. In Cavenar JO, Michels R (eds): Psychiatry, a Multi-volume Textbook. Vol. 6. Philadelphia: Lippincott, 1985.
3. Cross CK, Hirschfeld RMA. Psychosocial factors and suicidal behavior. In Mann J, Stanley J (eds): Psychobiology of Suicidal Behavior. New York: New York Academy of Sciences 1986; in press.
4. Cross K, Hirschfeld RMA. Epidemiology of disorders in adulthood: suicide. In Cavenar JO, Michels R (eds): Psychiatry, a Multi-volume Textbook. Vol. 6. Philadelphia: Lippincott, 1985.
5. Weed JA. Suicide in the United States: 1958–1982. In Taube CA, Barrett SA (eds): Mental Health United States, 1985. Washington, DC: Superintendent of Documents, U.S. Government Printing Office, 1985;135–145.
6. Sainsbury P. The epidemiology of suicide. In Roy A (ed): Suicide. Baltimore: Williams & Wilkins, 1986;17–45.
7. Hirschfeld RMA, Davidson L. Psychiatric risk factors for suicide. In Frances AJ, Hales RE (eds): American Psychiatric Press Review of Psychiatry. Vol. VII. Washington, DC: American Psychiatric Press, 1988;329.

66. Genetics and Suicidal Behavior in the Affective Disorders

ALEC ROY

There are five lines of evidence about genetic factors in suicide in the affective disorders. This chapter reviews data from clinical, twin, Iowa-500, Amish, and Copenhagen adoption studies.

Clinical Studies

Pitts and Winokur[1] found that among 748 consecutively admitted patients 37 reported a possible or definite suicide in a first degree relative (4.9%). In 25 of these 37 cases (68%) the diagnosis was an affective disorder. The statistical probability of this distribution occurring by chance was less than 0.02. When the probable diagnosis in the cases of the first degree relatives who committed suicide were considered, in 24 of the 37 patient-relative pairings both members had affective disorders. Pitts and Winokur[1] estimated that 79% of the suicides of the first degree relatives were associated with probable affective disorder.

Roy[2,3] found that a family history of suicide significantly increased the risk of a suicide attempt in a wide variety of diagnostic groups. Almost half (48.6%) of the 243 patients with a family history of suicide had themselves attempted suicide. More than half (56.4%) of all the patients with a family history of suicide had a primary diagnosis of an affective disorder, and more than one-third (34.6%) had a recurrent unipolar or bipolar affective disorder. Linkowski et al.[4] found that 123 of 713 depressed patients (17%) had a first or second degree relative who had committed suicide. A family history of suicide significantly increased the risk for a violent suicide attempt. Linkowski et al.[4] concluded that "A positive family history for violent suicide should be considered as a strong predictor of active suicidal attempting behavior in major depressive illness."

Murphy and Wetzel[5] found that among suicide attempters with a primary diagnosis of primary affective disorder 17 percent had a family history of suicide and 17 percent a family history of a suicide attempt. As individuals with affective disorders comprise a larger proportion of suicides than individuals with personality disorders, Murphy and Wetzel[5] predicted that more of their patients with affective disorder could be expected to present a significant suicide risk in the future. Therefore they concluded that a "systematic family history of such behavior coupled with modern clinical diagnosis should prove useful in identifying those attempters at increased risk for suicide.''

Twin Studies

Haberlandt[6] pooled the accumulated data from twin studies from various countries. Of the 149 sets of twins where one twin was known to have committed suicide, there were nine sets of twins where both twins had committed suicide. All of these nine twin-pairs were identical twins: No fraternal twins were concordant for suicide ($p<0.0001$). In three of the nine pairs the twins were also concordant for manic-depression.

Iowa 500 Study

In a follow-up study Tsuang[7] found that the first degree relatives of the psychiatric patients in the Iowa 500 study had a risk of suicide almost eight times greater than the risk in the relatives of normal controls. The risk of suicide was significantly greater among the first degree relatives of depressed patients than it was among the relatives of either schizophrenic or manic patients. Among the first degree relatives of the psychiatric patients who had committed suicide, the suicide risk was four times greater than the risk in the relatives of patients who did not commit suicide. The suicide risk was equally high among the relatives of both depressed and manic patients.

Amish Study

In 1985 Egeland and Sussex[8] reported on the suicide data obtained from the study of affective disorders among the Old Order Amish community of Lancaster County in southeast Pennsylvania. Several of the important social risk factors for suicide among individuals in the general population, e.g., unemployment, divorced or separated marital status, social isolation, and alcoholism, are not commonly found among these Amish. Twenty-four of the 26 suicide victims over the 100 years from 1880 to 1980 met RDC criteria for a major affective disorder. Eight of the suicide victims had bipolar I, four bipolar II, and 12 unipolar affective disorder. Another case met diagnostic criteria for a minor depression. Furthermore, most of the suicide victims had a heavy family loading for affective disorders. For example, among the eight bipolar I suicide victims the morbidity risk for affective disorders among their 110 first degree relatives was 29% compared with the 1–4% found among the general population.

Almost three-fourths of the 26 suicide victims were found to cluster in four family pedigrees, each of which contained a heavy loading for affective disorders and suicide. Interestingly, the converse was not true, as there were other family pedigrees with heavy loadings for affective disorder but without suicides. It is also of note that morbidity risk for affective disorders among 170 first degree relatives in other bipolar I pedigrees without suicide was similar to that found in bipolar pedigrees with suicide, also in the 20% range. Thus a familial loading for affective disorders was not in itself a predictor for suicide.

Egeland and Sussex concluded that ''Our study replicates findings that indicate an increased suicidal risk for patients with a diagnosis of major affective disorder and a strong family history of suicide. The number not receiving adequate treatment for manic-depressive illness (among the suicides) suppports the common belief that intervention for these patients at risk is recommended." Also "It appears most warranted in those families in which there is a family history of suicide. The clustering of suicides in Amish pedigrees follows the distribution of affective illness in the kinship and suggests the role of inheritance."

Danish-American Adoption Studies

The strongest evidence for the presence of genetic factors in suicide comes from the adoption studies carried out in Denmark by Kety's group.[9] The Psykologisk Institut has a register of the 5,483 adoptions that occurred in greater Copenhagen between 1924 and 1947. A screening of the registers of causes of death revealed that 57 of these adoptees eventually committed suicide. They were matched with adopted controls for age, sex, social class of the adopting parents, and time spent with their biological relatives and in institutions before being adopted. Searches of the causes of death revealed that 12 of the 269 biological relatives of these 57 adopted suicides had themselves committed suicide compared with only 2 of the 269 biological relatives of the 57 adopted controls ($p < 0.01$). None of the adopting relatives of either the suicide or the control group had committed suicide.

Wender et al.[10] went on to study the 71 adoptees identified by the psychiatric case register as having suffered from an affective disorder. They were matched with 71 control adoptees without affective disorder. Significantly more of the biological relatives of the adoptees with affective disorder, than their controls, had committed suicide. It was particularly adoptee suicide victims with the diagnosis of "affect reaction" who had significantly more biological relatives who had committed suicide than controls. This diagnosis is used in Denmark to describe an individual who has affective symptoms accompanying a situational crisis, often after an impulsive suicide attempt. These findings led Kety[9] to suggest that a genetic factor in suicide may be an inability to control impulsive behavior that has its effect independently of, or additively to, psychiatric disorder. Affective disorder, or environmental stress, may serve "as potentiating mechanisms which foster or trigger the impulsive behavior, directing it toward a suicidal outcome."[9]

Summary

Suicide, like so much else in psychiatry, tends to run in families. The family member who has committed suicide may serve as a role model to identify with when the option of committing suicide becomes a possible "solution" to intolerable psychological pain. However, the family, twin, Amish, and adoption studies reviewed here show that there are genetic factors in suicide. In many suicide victims they are genetic factors involved in the genetic transmission of manic-depression. However, the Copenhagen adoption studies strongly suggest that there may be a genetic factor for suicide independent of, or additive to, the genetic transmission of affective disorder. Support for this possibility comes from the recent Amish studies, which showed that suicide was much more likely to occur when an individual had genetic vulnerabilities to both suicide and to affective illness.

References

1. Pitts F, Winokur G. Affective disorder. P 3. Diagnostic correlates and incidence of suicide. J Nerv Ment Dis 1964;139:176–181.
2. Roy A. Family history of suicide. Arch Gen Psychiatry 1983;40:971–974.
3. Roy A. Genetics of suicide. Ann NY Acad Sci 1987;487:97–105.
4. Linkowski P, Maertelaer de V, Mendlewicz J. Suicidal behavior in major depressive illness. Acta Psychiatr Scand 1985;72:233–238.
5. Murphy G, Wetzel R. Family history of suicidal behavior among suicide attempters. J Nerv Ment Dis 1982;170:86–90.
6. Haberlandt W. Aportacion a al genetica del suicido. Folia Clin Int 1967;17:319–322.
7. Tsuang M. Risk of suicide in the relatives of schizophrenics, manics, depressives, and controls. J Clin Psychiatry 1983;44:396–400.
8. Egeland J, Sussex J. Suicide and family loading for affective disorders. JAMA 1985;254:915–918.
9. Kety S. Genetic factors in suicide. In Roy A (ed): Suicide. Baltimore: Williams & and Wilkins, 1986.
10. Wender P, Kety S, Rosenthal D, et al. Psychiatric disorders in the biological and adoptive families of adopted individuals with affective disorders. Arch Gen Psychiatry 1986;43:923–929.

67. Suicidal Behavior Among Children and Adolescents

CYNTHIA R. PFEFFER

The greatest advances to date in studying suicidal behavior in children and adolescents have been in epidemiological and empirical studies of psychosocial risk factors. Although new developments in understanding biological features of suicidal behavior have been achieved, little information exists about it for youths. Approaches for treatment and prevention also require more concerted efforts in empirically based investigation.

Epidemiology of Suicidal Behavior

Suicide is the second most prevalent cause of death for people aged 15–24 years in the United States. Accidents are the most frequent causes of death, and homicide is the third leading cause of death in this age group. For children less than 15 years old, suicide is the seventh leading cause of death, and the prevalence of suicide in this age group is the lowest for all ages. To illustrate the extent of the problem in recent years, there were in the United States more than 5,000 suicides per year for the 15- to 24-year-old group. Furthermore, it is estimated that there are at least 100 adolescents who attempt suicide for every adolescent who actually commits suicide. These statistical facts reflect a dramatic increase in suicide in the United States over the last several decades. Moreover, it is similar to the rapid rise of youth suicide in other countries in recent years.

Models developed to explain trends for youth suicide have suggested that the proportion of youths in the population at a given time is directly related to youth suicide rates.[1] Holinger and Offer[1] found that between 1933 and 1975 the number of adolescents in the population at a given time is positively correlated with the adolescent suicide rate; i.e., when there are more adolescents in the population at a given time, the adolescent suicide rate increases. There is not a similar relation between the elderly population and elderly suicide rates, which suggests that there is something unique about the incidence of suicide among adolescents and young adults.

Another model suggests that suicide rates are cohort-specific and that in more recently born cohorts the rates are higher than in early cohorts.[2,3]. Furthermore, within a given cohort, as individuals get older their suicide rates increase. This type of model predicts that youth suicide would continue to increase in future years. Another model proposes that there is a period-cohort effect that accounts for the parallel increases of the number of youth psychopathologies.[4] Such a model suggests that both time period and cohort factors interact to cause the youth suicide rates. Specifically, this model suggests something unique about the last several decades that produced a higher suicide rate for adolescents and young adults. These models require additional research validation. Finally, regarding nonfatal suicidal behavior, estimates suggest that there is approximately a 100-fold prevalence of suicide attempts in regard to youth suicide. Accurate epidemiological data on nonfatal suicidal behavior is urgently needed.

Risk Factors for Youth Suicidal Behavior

Youth suicidal behavior is a multidetermined symptom and as a result is in large measure a heterogeneous phenomenon.[5] Among the factors associated with youth suicide are depression and aggression, impulse control, judgment and cognition, quality of interpersonal relations, and early developmental experiences. More research is needed to weigh the relative influence of these factors to produce risk for suicidal behavior.

Other demographic factors are important. For example, suicide is most prevalent in white boys, although nonfatal suicidal behavior occurs more commonly among girls. In the United States, firearms are the leading suicidal methods, although a variety of other techniques are used, including hanging, jumping, and drug overdose.

Symptoms most associated with youth suicidal behavior include affective and antisocial features. Depression, in its mood state and/or as a psychiatric disorder, is a significant feature of youth suicidal behavior. Hopelessness, even more than depression, is related to suicidal impulses. Of course, a history of previous suicidal ideas or acts is a correlate of suicidal tendencies. Insufficient emphasis has been placed on the importance of antisocial symptoms. Although depression seems to be more associated with nonfatal suicidal behavior, especially in preadolescents, and is also important for adolescent suicidal behavior, antisocial symptoms appear to be significant correlates of adolescent suicide. Specifically, drug and alcohol abuse, violence, and impulsivity are notable risk factors for adolescent nonfatal and fatal suicidal behavior.[6]

Family influences have been delineated for youth suicidal behavior.[6] Among them the overriding issue of loss of social supports is evident. Loss of family through death, parental separation or divorce, moves, and illness are significant. Parental psychopathology involving affective and substance abuse disorders and violence is an important element for youth suicidal behavior. These factors may operate through a genetic and/or an experimental component. More research is needed to evaluate the relations between genetic and environmental components of youth suicidal behavior.

An important factor for suicidal risk among youth is the role of imitation. Stimuli that provide models to imitate suicidal tendencies are derived from media presentations of suicide[7,8] and other youths known to have suicidal tendencies. Clusters of suicide in a community may occur after a suicide is publicized. Research is needed to evaluate approaches to decrease imitative suicidal behavior. Furthermore, specific populations of adolescents may be at greater risk for suicide. Such adolescents may encounter certain unique personal and social stresses, such as problems with identity, self-esteem, social isolation, and overwhelming competition. However, there is insufficient research on the factors for such adolescents that involve developmental, biological, sociocultural, and psychological factors in regard to increased suicide risk.

Assessment and Treatment

Early identification of suicidal impulses and their attendent risk factors is essential for prevention of youth suicidal behavior. From a clinical perspective, extensive discussion with a suicidal youngster is necessary to appraise risk. Guides for such an assessment have been offered[5,9] and include focusing on the suicidal episode, current affect states, interpersonal relations, and past developmental experiences. In fact, any talk of suicide should be taken seriously and evaluated carefully. During any clinical assessment of a child or adolescent, the clinician should ask specifically about suicidal ideation and intent: Have you ever felt hopeless? Have you ever felt that life is not worth living? Have you ever wished to die? Have you ever thought about hurting yourself or committing suicide? Have you ever tried to hurt yourself or to attempt suicide? Furthermore, such questions should be asked at various times during the interview process, not just once.[5]

Especially in the assessment and treatment of suicidal youth, involvement of the parents and other family is essential. The quality of supportive resources must be determined. The assessment should include a focus on discovering parental attitudes, family communication pattern, and relationships. A network of other people such as school professionals who are involved with the youngster should be included. Medication is another important aspect of treatment. The type of medication used depends on the symptoms and psychiatric diagnosis of the child or adolescent. Thus an empirical approach to utilization of medications is recommended. As this discussion implies, the treatment must be multifocal, consistent, and of sufficient duration to be effective in minimizing the risk of a future suicidal event.

Other areas of prevention involve decreasing access to lethal suicidal methods, especially guns, medications, and open high places. Screening procedures to appraise early warning signs must be developed. Programs to diminish early precursors of later suicidal tendencies need to be conceptualized. Continued education of professionals working with youthful age groups enhances their capacities to respond effectively so as to lower the suicidal risk among youth. It seems increasingly unlikely that a clinician working alone is able to offer the most effective forms of intervention or prevention of youth suicidal behavior. Instead, newer trends indicate that teams of professionals from different disciplines who collaborate may be most efficacious. Each member of the team may offer a unique input and provide support for the others when caring for suicidal adolescents. Finally, at a more basic level, primary prevention approaches need to be developed to minimize those factors that are early precursors in the etiological processes for the development of youth suicidal behavior.

References

1. Holinger PC, Offer D. Prediction of adolescent suicide: a population model. Am J Psychiatry 1982;139:302–307.
2. Hellon CP, Solomon MI. Suicide and age in Alberta, Canada, 1951 to 1977: the changing profile. Arch Gen Psychiatry 1980;37:505–510.
3. Goldberg RD, Katsikitis M. Cohort analysis of suicide rates in Australia. Arch J Psychiatry 1983;40:71–74.
4. Klerman GL, Lavori PW, Rice J, et al. Birth-cohort trends in rates of major depressive disorder among relatives of patients with affective disorders. Arch Gen Psychiatry 1985;42:689–693.
5. Pfeffer CR. The Suicidal Child. New York: Guilford Press, 1986.
6. Pfeffer CR. Family characteristics and support systems as risk factors for youth suicidal behavior. Presented at the Department of Health and Human Services Secretary's Task Force on Youth Suicide, Bethesda, 1986.
7. Phillips DP, Carstensen LL. Clustering of teenage suicides after television news stories about suicide. N Engl J Med 1986;315:685–689.
8. Shaffer D. Suicide in childhood and early adolescence. J Child Psychol Psychiatry 1974;15:275–291.
9. Maltsberger JT. Suicide Risk: The Formulation of Clinical Judgement. New York: New York University Press, 1986.

68. Death Anxiety in a Psychiatric Population of Suicidal and Nonsuicidal Adolescents

ISRAEL ORBACH, ALAN APTER, ORNA GRUCHOVER, SAM TYANO, AND SHAVI HAR-ZAHAV

Epidemiological studies show that the 15- to 24-year age group is a high risk group for suicide.[1] Various hypotheses regarding suicide in children and adolescents were summarized by Orbach.[2] One of the hypotheses is that youth suicide involves specific processes that lead directly to self-destruction rather than to other forms of maladjustment. In one hypothesis, Orbach et al.[3] suggested that parents' suicidal tendencies can be transferred to their children and that this process may lead specifically to suicide in children. Another hypothesis is that suicide in adolescents is an end result of extreme parental rejection, which is communicated as a *direct message* to commit suicide.[4]

A second hypothesis delineates continuous pressures and an accumulation of negative life events as a causal factor of suicidal behaviors in youngsters. According to this hypothesis, exposure to such pressures exhausts the adolescent's coping abilities so that he is no longer able to confront new pressures.[5] A third hypothesis indicates an interaction between coping abilities, life pressures, and specific familial dynamics as important causal factors in adolescent suicide.

The purpose of the present study was to further investigate a derivative of the "specific factors hypothesis." This hypothesis contends that suicidal behavior is enhanced by a cognitive style that devalues life and idealizes death as a peaceful and rewarding state. Such an attitude is often accompanied by a sharp reduction in death anxiety. When death anxiety is low, suicidal behaviors may ensue.

In other words, death anxiety serves as a buffer against self-destruction. When it is removed, suicide may appear to be the only possible solution for life's problems.[6-10] It has been suggested that this lower death anxiety is a defensive process that enables the troubled child to pursue his or her suicidal wishes. The lack of death anxiety as a defense against self-destruction is one way of minimizing the horror of death and thus suicide.

It is important to emphasize that, contrary to some other arguments,[11] this lack of death fear is not a cognitive deficiency or a temporary cognitive regression due to emotional pressure but, rather, an active mental maneuver to cope with death anxiety in the face of an active suicidal urge. It has been previously demonstrated (in children and to a certain degree in adults) that when death anxiety is stimulated and heightened in suicidal individuals, suicidal behaviors are reduced. Thus studies of death anxiety have far-reaching implications for the prevention and treatment of suicidal behavior.[3,12]

Orbach and co-workers[2,12] have examined death anxiety in the context of a more comprehensive explanatory model of suicidal behavior among children. According to this model, suicidal behaviors are an outcome of a special constellation of attitudes toward life and death: attraction for life, repulsion by life, attraction to death, and repulsion by death. Suicidal children display a unique balance between the four attitudes that facilitates self-destruction. They differ from normal children with respect to the intensity of attraction to and repulsion by death. Thus an important element in the attitudes is the lack of death fear.

The dynamics of death fear were demonstrated in suicidal children and adults. However, thus far there is a conspicuous absence of studies on the fears of death among adolescents. The purpose of this study was to systematically investigate fears of death in this population.

Two groups of adolescents participated in the study: suicidal and nonsuicidal. Both groups came from a hospitalized population. They were evaluated by means of the *DSM-III,* self-report suicidal tendency scale, and a fear of death scale; lethality of previous suicidal attempts was assessed by the staff using an objective and validated scale.

Method

Subjects

The subjects were recruited from the Geha Mental Hospital located in the Tel-Aviv area. Their ages ranged from 15 to 18 years, with a mean of 16.8 years. The suicidal group consisted of 12 girls and 10 boys who attempted suicide prior to the hospitalization. In this group, nine were diagnosed by the *DSM-III* procedure as depressed, four with behavior problems, five borderline, four psychotic, and two manic-depressive. The nonsuicidal subjects were eleven girls and nine boys. Seven subjects were diagnosed as depressed, three anorectic, four borderline, four psychotic, one with behavior problems, and two manic-depressive. The sample came from a mixed population, but most of their families were of middle socioeconomic status. In general, the subjects' intellectual capabilities were normal.

Instruments

Fear of Death Scale.[13] This scale consists of six factors relating to different aspects of death fear: (a) loss of self-actualization (i.e., I am afraid of death because I won't be able to experience new things); (b) deterioration of the body (i.e., I am afraid of death because my body will rot); (c) loss of social identity (i.e., I am afraid of death because nobody will know who I was); (d) loss of family (i.e., I am afraid of death because it will hurt my family); (e) transcendental fears (i.e., I am afraid of the mystery surrounding death); (f) fears of the hereafter (i.e., I am afraid of punishment in the next world). This scale has been previously validated in a series of studies.[13]

Suicidal Tendencies Scale.[14] This is a self-report scale that consists of items on depressive syndromes, suicidal ideation, and suicidal attempts. The standardization, reliability, and validity were successfully established with a sample of more than 400 Israeli adolescents.[14]

Suicidal Lethality Scale.[15] This instrument evaluates the lethality of self-destruction and rank-orders the following: (a) lethality of method; (b) the circumstances; and (c) the manner in which the attempt was discovered. In the present study the scale was slightly modified, and the entire range was divided into four categories of lethality: Category 1 consisted of attempts such as swallowing a few sleeping pills at home with a high chance for discovery; category 2 consisted of attempts such as wrist-cutting while parents were not home; category 3 was jumping from a third floor; the most lethal category consisted of drastic attempts such as hanging. Evaluations on this scale were carried out by the therapist of each subject.

Results

The data were analyzed by means of multivariate analysis of variance (MANOVA) and analysis of variance (ANOVA). In addition, a series of correlations were obtained between the suicidal self-report scale, the lethality of suicidal attempt scale, and the fears of death among the groups of suicidal patients.

Table 68.1 summarizes the means and standard deviations of the six factors of fears of death. The MANOVA indicated an overall significant difference between suicidal and nonsuicidal subjects on all six factors $[F(6,37) = e,6; p < 0.006]$ by the Pillais test, the Hotelling effect, and the Wilks criteria. The ANOVA showed that the suicidal groups exhibited a lower degree of fear of death only with respect to fears concerning self-actualization $[F(1,42) = 17.4; p < 0.001]$, body deterioration $[F(1,42) = 5.5; p < 0.023]$, and transcendental fears $[F(1,42) = 10.4; p < 0.002]$.

One-way analysis employed to evaluate the differences among the six fear factors within each group showed that there was no difference in levels of fears with regard to the six factors in the suicidal group. In nonsuicidals there was significant difference among the six fear factors $[F(5,) = 4.2; p < 0.05]$.

The correlation coefficients between ratings of lethality of the suicide attempt

TABLE 68.1. Six fear factors for suicidal and nonsuicidal groups.

Type of fear	Suicidal group (n = 24)	Nonsuicidal group (n = 20)	p
Body	2.1 ± 1.8	3.6 1.8	0.023
Family	3.1 ± 1.5	3.7 1.7	0.263
Hereafter	2.3 ± 2.3	3.0 2.7	0.392
Self-actualization	2.4 ± 1.6	4.3 1.2	0.000
Social identify	2.3 ± 1.7	2.7 1.8	0.457
Transcendental	2.6 ± 1.8	4.2 1.3	0.002

Results are means ± SD.

and fear of death scale for the suicidal youths indicated a significant negative correlation with regard to three types of fear only: self-actualization ($r = -0.49$; $p < 0.001$), body deterioration ($r = -0.36$; $p < 0.007$), and transcendental fears ($r = -0.37$; $p < 0.006$). These correlations showed that the higher the suicidal lethality the lower the specific fear. The coefficients between self-report suicidal tendency and fears of death in the two groups showed a significant negative correlation for each of the six fear factors: self-actualization ($r = -0.82$; $p < 0.01$), body deterioration ($r = -0.92$; $p < 0.001$), social identity ($r = -0.80$; $p < 0.001$), family concerns $r = -0.49$; $p < 0.005$), transcendental fears ($r = -0.81$; $p < 0.001$), and fear of the hereafter ($r = -0.80$; $p < 0.001$). Again, the correlations indicate that the higher the suicidal tendency the lower the fear.

Discussion

The findings of this study clearly demonstrated that concerns and difficulties in life were reflected in attitudes and fears about death. Suicidal adolescents, like suicidal children and adults, fear death to a far less degree than other suffering adolescents.

Another outstanding finding was the lack of differentiation between the various areas of fear of death in suicidal adolescents. They showed the same low level of death anxiety in regard to all six factors with one possible exception: concerns about the family. On the other hand, the other hospitalized adolescents displayed different levels of death anxiety, with the highest concerns being about self-actualization and transcendental aspects.

The difference in the structure and intensity of fears apparently reflected the experience of total despair about life and an attitude of hopelessness in the suicidal population. The other hospitalized adolescents showed a more differentiated attitude about life, displaying different levels of concern in various areas of life.

There was also a high negative correlation between suicidal tendencies (by both self-report and ratings of lethality) and fear of death. This finding clearly demonstrated the relation between death anxiety and suicidal tendency: the higher the suicidal tendency, the lower the fear of death. It seems that lack of death anxiety is a process related specifically to suicidal tendencies and not to other difficulties in life or to mental problems in general. When a corrosion in fears about death takes place, there is an intensification of the suicidal tendency.

The dynamics of this process may be related to a defense process that takes place when an individual contemplates suicide. The minimization of death fears can be seen as a defense against the horror of death.

Another related hypothesis about this relation has been proposed by Orbach.[2] The lack of fear of death in suicidal adolescents may be one of several dissociative processes that take place in suicidal adolescents. Certain life circumstances coerce the adolescents to form various splits within emotional experiences, his or her social behavior, and within his or her attitudes toward life and death. The only way in which the adolescent can endure some of the pain is by dissociating from certain aspects of his life circumstances and his emotions. The maneuver tends to be generalized to various aspects of functioning including the fears about death.

It is clear that attitudes and fears about death must be a central focus in the therapeutic endeavors with suicidal adolescents. Probing of death anxiety by carefully working through that idiosyncratic perception of death has been proved to be effective with suicidal children.[3] It is most likely that such an approach can be fruitful with adolescents as well.

Finally, the study of death anxieties should be expanded to other groups such as normals. The relations between death anxiety and various clinical syndromes should be studied in detail. Such study can enrich our understanding of the relation between death anxiety, suicidal tendencies, and other pathologies.

References

1. Holinger PC, Luke KW. The epidemiological patterns of self-destructiveness in childhood, adolescence, and young adulthood. In Sudak HS, Ford AB, Rushforth NB (eds): Suicide in the Young. Boston: John Wright, 1984;97–114.
2. Orbach I. Children Who Don't Want to Live. San Francisco: Jossey Bass, 1988.
3. Orbach I, Gross Y, Glaubman H. Some common characteristics of latency age children: a tentative model based on case study analysis. Suicide Life Threat Behav 1981;4:170–180.
4. Sabbath JC. The suicidal adolescent—the expendable child. J Am Acad Child Psychiatry 1985;38:211–220.
5. Cohen-Sondler R, Berman A, King R. Life stress and symptomatology: determinants of suicidal behavior in children. J Am Acad Child Psychiatry 1982;21:178–186.
6. Leviton D. Life and death attitudes of parents of children with problems. Omega 1971;8:333–360.
7. Neuringer C. Changes in attitudes toward life and death during recovery from a serious suicide attempt. Omega 1970;1:201–209.
8. Orbach I, Glaubman H. Children's perception of death as a defensive process. J Abnorm Psychol 1979;88:671–674.
9. Orbach I, Rosenheim E, Hury E. Cognitive functioning in suicidal children. J Am Acad Child Adolescent Psychiatry 1987;26:181–185.
10. Shneidman E. Voices of Death. New York: Harper & Row, 1982.
11. Pfeffer C. The Suicidal Child. New York: Guilford, 1986.
12. Orbach I, Feshbach S, Carlson G, et al. Attraction and repulsion by life and death in suicidal and normal children. J Consult Clin Psychol 1985;51:661–670.
13. Florian V, Kravetz S. Fear of personal death: attribution, structure and religious belief. J Pers Soc Psychol 1983;44:600–607.
14. Bar-Yosef H, Alitzur D. Suicidal Tendencies Scale. Israel: Department of Psychology, Bar-Ilan University, 1985.
15. Smith K, Conroy R, Ehler BD. Lethality of Suicide Attempt Scale. Kansas: Menninger Foundation, 1982.

69. Neurotransmitters and Neurotransmitter Receptors in Depressed Suicide Victims

S.C. Cheetham, J.A. Cross, M.R. Crompton,
C.Z. Czudek, C.L.E. Katona, S.J. Parker,
G.P. Reynolds, and R.W. Horton

Repeated antidepressant drug and electroshock administration to animals alters several classes of cortical neurotransmitter receptors.[1] The role of these adaptive receptor changes in the therapeutic action of antidepressants and the possibility that altered receptors underlie the biological basis of depressive illness can be studied meaningfully only in depressed subjects.

The use of postmortem tissue allows brain receptors to be studied in man. Few postmortem studies of neurotransmitter receptor binding sites have, however, been specifically directed at depressed subjects. Limited studies in elderly depressives dying from natural causes have been reported,[2,3] but more studies have been performed in suicide victims.[4-6] However, suicide victims are a diagnostically heterogeneous group in whom a range of psychiatric illnesses other than depression, e.g., schizophrenia, personality disorder, and alcoholism, may be present.[7] This factor and the possibility of drug treatment prior to death may in part explain the lack of consistency in receptor binding studies in suicide victims.[4-6] Our strategy has been to study only those suicide victims with a definite history of depression (in the absence of symptoms of other psychiatric disorders). These subjects were identified from a large group of confirmed suicide deaths by retrospective psychiatric diagnosis based on hospital and coroner's records and interviews with the subject's medical practitioner, using the classification of Beskow et al.[8] In order to distinguish between receptor alterations that result from treatment with psychoactive drugs (particularly antidepressants) and those related to underlying illness, we have currently restricted our studies to those depressed suicide victims who had not recently been receiving psychoactive drugs and in whom no psychoactive drugs were present in the blood at postmortem examination. Four subjects died by hanging, five by carbon monoxide poisoning, one by drowning, one by stab wound, and two by drug overdose. Control subjects died suddenly from causes not involving the central nervous system (CNS) (mostly cardiovascular disease). The two groups were matched for age, sex, postmortem delay (time from death to storage of tissue at $-80°C$) and duration of tissue storage prior to analysis. Details of the subjects are shown in Table 69.1.

5-Hydroxytryptamine (5-HT, serotonin), 5-hydroxyindoleacetic acid (5-HIAA), dopamine (DA), homovanillic acid (HVA), and norepinephrine (NE) concentrations

TABLE 69.1. Receptor binding sites in the cerebral cortex of depressed suicides and controls.

Receptor binding sites	Frontal cortex		Temporal cortex	
	Depressed suicides	Controls	Depressed suicides	Controls
5-HT$_2$	340 ± 28 (12)	334 ± 16 (12)	397 ± 29 (13)	417 ± 17 (1
Benzodiazepine	1,950 ± 117 (12)	1,688 ± 67 (12)	1,596 ± 160 (8)	1,775 ± 140 (8
GABA$_B$	1,010 ± 80 (11)	1,060 ± 80 (11)	720 ± 70 (11)	610 ± 70 (1

Values are means ± SEM of Bmax (fmol/mg protein). The numbers of subjects are in parenthes Mean ages (± SEM) were 42.5 ± 3.1 years for controls (10M, 3F) and 42.5 ± 3.2 years for depress suicides (10M, 3F). Postmortem delay was 43.0 ± 4.1 h for controls and 32.7 ± 4.4 h for suicides

were determined using high-performance liquid chromatography (HPLC) in frontal and temporal cortex, hippocampus, caudate, and putamen. The concentration of these monoamines and their metabolites did not differ significantly between controls and depressed suicides in the brain regions studied, or between left and right hemispheres within either the control or the suicide group.

The 5-HT$_2$ binding sites were measured by saturation binding of [^{3}H]ketanserin. The equilibrium dissociation constant (Kd) and the number of binding sites (Bmax) (Table 69.1) did not differ between controls and depressed suicides in frontal, temporal, occipital cortex, or amygdala. Depressed suicide victims had lower numbers of 5-HT$_2$ binding sites, but unaltered Kd, in the hippocampus (control 118 ± 9 and depressed 91 ± 7 fmol/mg protein; $n = 13$ for both groups; $p < 0.05$). This effect was more prominent in those suicide victims who died by violent means.

The 5-HT$_2$ binding sites in suicide victims have previously been reported to be increased in number in frontal cortex[4,6] and unchanged in frontal and occipital cortex.[5] Differences between these studies, particularly in terms of the cause of death, the proportion dying by violent means, and the presence and nature of psychiatric illness and drug treatment may contribute to these conflicting results. Our findings in drug-free depressed suicides are supported by a study of elderly subjects with a diagnosis of major depressive disorder who died by natural causes. This study reported no significant difference in frontal cortical 5-HT$_2$ binding compared to control subjects or subjects suffering from dysthymic disorder.[3]

Studies in animals indicate that cortical γ-aminobutyric acid (GABA) receptors are altered by chronic antidepressant drug administration. The number of GABA$_A$ and the functionally linked benzodiazepine (BZ) binding sites are decreased,[9,10] and the number of GABA$_B$ binding sites are increased,[11] We have measured GABA$_A$ site function (the ability of GABA to increase [^{3}H]flunitrazepam binding) and quantitated BZ and GABA$_B$ binding sites in the frontal and temporal cortex of depressed suicides and controls.

The number and affinity of BZ binding sites, the number of GABA$_B$ binding sites (Table 69.1), and GABA$_A$ function did not differ significantly between the two groups. The tendency for a higher number of BZ binding sites in the frontal cortex of the depressed suicide victims compared to controls just failed to reach statistical significance.

Activity of glutamic acid decarboxylase (GAD), an enzyme that has been advocated as a marker of agonal status,[12] did not differ overall between the two groups in frontal or temporal cortex. However, GAD activity was markedly reduced in those suicide victims who died by carbon monoxide poisoning.

In the present study we have investigated neurotransmitters, neurotransmitter metabolites, and receptor binding sites in relation to depressive illness by studying a small but highly selective group of suicide victims with a history of depression who were free from psychoactive drugs during the current episode. These studies are currently being extended to depressed suicides who were receiving antidepressant treatment at the time of death.

Acknowledgment. We thank the Wellcome Trust and Humane Research Trust for financial support. S.C.C. is an MRC Scholar and J.A.C. an SERC Scholar.

References

1. Sugrue MF. Chronic antidepressant therapy and associated changes in central monoaminergic receptor functioning. Pharmacol Ther 1983;21:1–33.
2. Perry EK, Marshall EJ, Blessed G, et al. Decreased imipramine binding in the brains of patients with depressive illness. Br J Psychiatry 1983;142:188–192.
3. McKeith IG, Marshall EF, Ferrier IN, et al. 5-HT receptor binding in post-mortem brain from patients with affective disorder. J Affective Disord 1987;13:67–74.
4. Stanley M, Mann JJ. Increased serotonin-2 binding sites in frontal cortex of suicide victims. Lancet 1984;1:214–216.
5. Owen F, Chambers DR, Cooper SJ, et al. Serotonergic mechanisms in brains of suicide victims. Brain Res 1986;362:185–188.
6. Mann JJ, Stanley M, McBride PA, et al. Increased serotonin-2 and β-adrenergic receptor binding in the frontal cortex of suicide victims. Arch Gen Psychiatry 1986;43:954–959.
7. Barraclough B, Bunch J, Nelson B, et al. A hundred cases of suicide: clinical aspects. Br J Psychiatry 1974;125:355–373.
8. Beskow J, Gottfries CG, Roos BE, et al. Determination of monoamine and monoamine metabolites in the human brain: post mortem studies in a group of suicides and in a control group. Acta Psychiatr Scand 1976;53:7–20.
9. Suzdak PD, Gianutsos G. Parallel changes in the sensitivity of γ-aminobutyric acid and noradrenergic receptors following chronic administration of antidepressants and GABAergic drugs. Neuropharmacology 1985;24:217–222.
10. Suranyi-Cadotte BE, Dam TV, Quirion R. Antidepressant-anxiolytic interaction: decreased density of BZ receptors in rat brain following chronic administration of antidepressants. Eur J Pharmacol 1984;106:673–675.
11. Lloyd KG, Thuret F, Pilc A. Upregulation of γ-aminobutyric acid (GABA) B binding sites in rat frontal cortex: a common action of repeated administration of different classes of antidepressants and electroshock. J Pharmacol Exp Ther 1985;235:191–199.
12. Perry EK, Perry RH, Tomlinson BE. The influence of agonal status on some neurochemical activities of postmortem human brain tissue. Neurosci Lett 1982;29:303–307.

70. Peripheral Serotonin and Catecholamine Levels and Suicidal Behavior

MARIE LUISE RAO AND PETER BRÄUNIG

Reduction in serotonin turnover has been demonstrated in patients with aggressive and autoaggressive, i.e., suicidal, behavior. The concentrations of serotonin (5-hydroxytryptamine, 5-HT) and its metabolite 5-hydroxyindoleacetic acid (5-HIAA) are reduced in the brainstem of suicide victims and in the cerebrospinal fluid of suicidal patients. Violent suicide attempts are associated with low serotonin turnover.[1,2] Mann et al.[3] have shown a correlation between reduced serotonergic activity and suicidal behavior; presynaptic imipramine binding was reduced and 5-HT$_2$ receptors were increased in the frontal cortex of suicide victims. Because serotonin metabolism disturbances seem to be the underlying cause of these psychiatric illnesses, the question is whether they provide a trait, rather than a state, marker; we therefore thought that cross-sectional studies in patients sharing the same symptoms concomitant with a longitudinal study may shed light on some of the pertinent questions in suicide research.

The blood-brain barrier is generally accepted to single out the way bioactive molecules are exchanged between the central nervous system (CNS) and the periphery. These findings do not rule out the possibility that receptor sites for bioactive ligands present in the CNS and the periphery share similar properties. Specific imipramine binding sites have been observed in human platelet membranes; their properties resemble those of central serotonergic receptors.[4] Serotonin accumulated in platelets accounts for more than 98% of whole blood serotonin.[5]

In patients with endogenous depression or schizophrenia, reduced platelet serotonin uptake as well as no changes compared to controls have been found; in the aggregate, information is scarce as regards the relation between peripheral serotonin and mental state. Although blood serotonin may be regarded as a crude indicator of a decrease in serotonin turnover, it allows for the longitudinal assessment of serotonergic activity in that many samples from the same patient may be analyzed. Because aggression and autoaggression may be associated with lowered serotonin turnover and increased catecholaminergic activity as trait markers,[6,7] and because platelet serotonin might reflect serotonin turnover, we investigated the association between suicidality and peripheral serotonin and catecholamines in patients with major psychiatric disorders.

Subjects and Methods

Fifty-nine female inpatients took part in this study; 25 patients showed symptoms meeting ICD 9 criteria for endogenous depression. Thirty-four patients showed Schneiderian first and second rank symptoms for schizophrenia; according to convention the Schneiderian criteria comprise syndromes that may be labeled schizophrenia and schizoaffective disorder. We rated suicidality according to Farberow and MacKinnon.[8] Because depression may be regarded as an integral component of suicidal behavior[9] we rated it by the Hamilton depression score.

Twenty patients took part in a longitudinal study ranging from 3 to 12 months. On account of the Farberow suicide score of more than 130 and a record of previous suicide attempts by violent means we chose four patients and present their clinical status and whole blood serotonin. Blood samples were obtained every fortnight or when the psychopathology of the patient changed.

The patients were treated with neuroleptics and antidepressants as clinically indicated. Patients' age ranged from 18 to 75 years with a mean age of 43 years. For establishment of reference limits we investigated blood serotonin and serum catecholamine concentrations of 26 healthy women with a mean age of 24.5 ± 2.1 years (range 21 to 30 years). We have shown previously that age does not influence the blood serotonin level. We obtained blood samples from patients and subjects by venipuncture between 7:00 and 9:00 a.m. Serotonin was determined in blood by high performance liquid chromatography (HPLC)[10] and the catecholamines in serum by radioenzyme assay.[11]

For technical reasons the Farberow suicide rating scale could be administered to all and the Hamilton depression scale to 16 patients. Blood serotonin was determined in all patients on the second or third day entering the hospital for crisis intervention. Due to failure to stabilize serum adequately, catecholamines could be analyzed in only 11 sera. The significance of difference was established with the Mann-Whitney U-test. Regression analysis was performed to ensure correlation.

Results

We observed a linear relation between blood serotonin levels and the Farberow suicide score in the group of schizophrenic and schizoaffective patients ($r = -0.59$, $p < 0.001$; $n = 34$). It has been stated that a Farberow suicide score of more than 130 represents the breaking point as regards severity of suicidal behavior. Grouping the patients accordingly, schizophrenic women with a Farberow suicide score of less than 130 showed a median serotonin level of 0.74 μmol/l, which corresponded to that of healthy women (0.90 μmol/l); patients with a Farberow score of more than 130 showed a lower serotonin level of 0.28 μmol/l ($p < 0.01$).

Serum norepinephrine ($r = 0.75$, $p < 0.01$; $n = 11$) or dopamine ($r = 0.81$, $p < 0.001$; $n = 11$) levels correlated positively with the Farberow suicide score. Serum dopamine and blood serotonin correlated negatively linearly ($r = -0.72$, $p < 0.01$; $n = 11$). This feature appeared in patients only, as healthy women's serum dopamine and blood serotonin did not correlate ($r = -0.002$). The patient's ratio of serum dopamine to blood serotonin correlated linearly with the Farberow suicide score ($r = 0.50$, $p < 0.05$; $n = 11$).

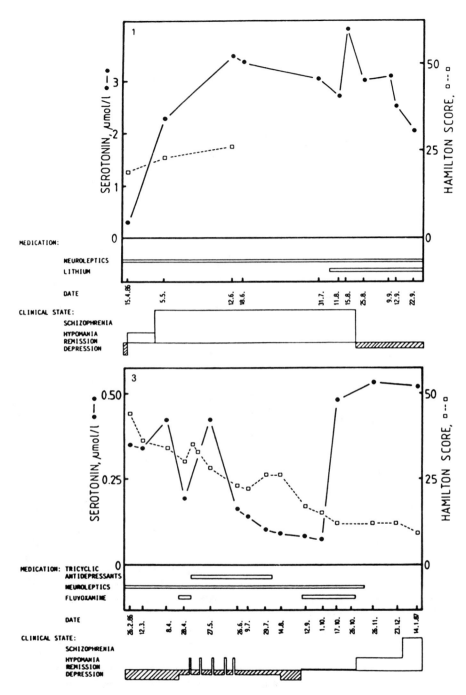

FIGURE 70.1. Longitudinal study of blood serotonin, Hamilton depression score, medication, and clinical state of female patients with schizoaffective disorder. The reference limit (95% confidence limit) of the blood serotonin level in healthy women is 0.5–1.5 μmol/l.

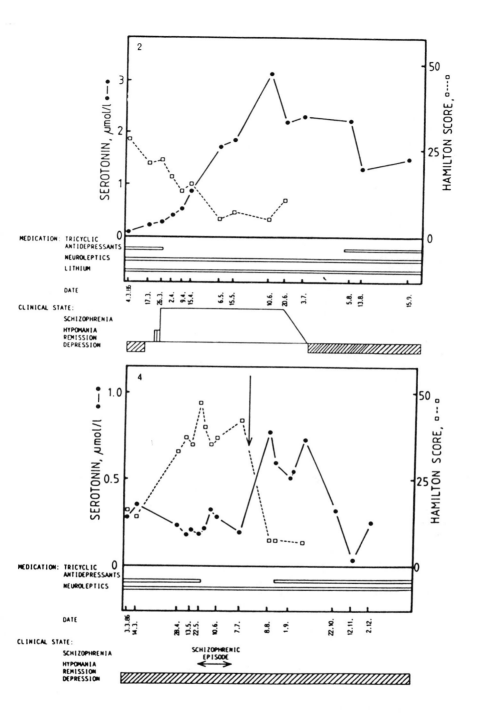

The Farberow suicide score and Hamilton depression score correlated moderately ($r = 0.47$, $p < 0.05$; $n = 16$). Although depression may be regarded as a predictor for suicidality, these results suggested that not all patients were depressed. The Hamilton depression score was not related to blood serotonin or to serum catecholamine levels. We observed no correlation between neuroleptic dose and peripheral serotonin.

In patients with endogenous depression, correlation between any of the parameters mentioned above was low. From a pilot study we observed that intraindividual blood serotonin concentrations varied considerably and that these variations could not be correlated with drug treatment. On account of these observations, we were prompted to investigate longitudinally blood serotonin concomitantly with the clinical state in depressive and schizoaffective patients. From these patients we selected four with a Farberow score of more than 130 and with previous violent suicide attempts. We observed in three patients a switch from a prepsychotic depressive state into a schizophrenic episode (Fig. 70.1). During the time of the study the fourth patient attempted suicide by violent means.

The longitudinal study showed drastic changes in blood serotonin independent of the therapeutic strategy. It may be noted from Figure 70.1 that in three patients blood serotonin levels were low during the depressive phase. During the switch from a prepsychotic depressive to a schizophrenic episode intraindividual whole blood serotonin levels increased by a factor of 7.5–77.0. In the fourth patient the increase in serotonin into the range of the reference limit for healthy women was observed after the violent suicide attempt (Fig. 70.1, lower right diagram, arrow).

Discussion

Our study shows that blood serotonin correlates negatively with suicidality in schizophrenic but not in endogenously depressed patients. No correlation between neuroleptic dose and blood serotonin was observed in our patients, nor was a correlation observed between blood serotonin and suicidality when patients were grouped according to uni- or bipolar disorder. From a pilot study we inferred that a change in the mental state had a far greater influence on blood serotonin than the administration of antidepressants. We argued therefore that if blood platelet function reflects central serotonin turnover and if 98% of the peripheral serotonin circulates bound to blood platelets, the apparent inconsistency as regards serotonin levels and suicidality observed so far might be traced to fluctuations in the 5-HT receptor function as a result of a switch in psychopathology.

Are biological parameters sufficiently stable over time to warrant a one-time measurement? Or are longitudinal studies required to answer this question? The longitudinal approach shows that patients with impulsive and suicidal behavior exhibit a state-dependent[12] lability as regards their peripheral serotonin levels. The decrease in peripheral serotonin was associated with an increase in suicidality; it points to a decreased serotonin bioavailability leading to reduced synaptic serotonergic activity, which may simultaneously provoke an up-regulation in the number of 5-HT$_2$ receptor sites.[3] Previous investigations demonstrated that endogenously depressed patients with low serotonergic activity showed during remission an increase in cerebrospinal fluid 5-HIAA, which points to normalization of the serotonergic activity.[13] Endogenously depressed patients with prolonged low cerebrospinal fluid 5-HIAA levels showed a higher incidence of relapse than those with normal levels.

As shown in the longitudinal study, the most likely explanation of the absence of a correlation between clinical state and blood serotonin in our group of depressed patients may be due to the actual clinical state, which strongly influenced blood serotonin levels. We happened to have a patient who attempted suicide during the time of the study when her peripheral serotonin was low. An increase in peripheral serotonin into the range of the reference limit for healthy women was observed after the suicide attempt (Fig. 70.1, lower right diagram, arrow). This finding may be regarded as a consequence of the cathartic effect observed after the attempt. The observation of low peripheral serotonin levels during the prepsychotic depressive state and the striking increase during the switch into a psychotic episode might provide an explanation for the apparent bimodal cerebrospinal fluid 5-HIAA distribution observed earlier.[13]

Our findings suggest that alterations in serotonin metabolism are expressed as disturbed peripheral transmitter levels on account of the actual mental state.

References

1. Åsberg M, Traskman L, Thoren P. 5-HIAA in the cerebrospinal fluid: a biochemical suicide predictor? Arch Gen Psychiatry 1976;38:1193–1197.
2. Van Praag HM. Biological suicide research: outcome and limitations. Biol Psychiatry 1986;21:1305–1323.
3. Mann JJ, Stanley M, McBride PA, et al. Increased serotonin$_2$ and β-adrenergic receptor binding in the frontal cortices of suicide victims. Arch Gen Psychiatry 1986;43:954–959.
4. Sneddon JM. Blood platelets as a model for monoamine-containing neurones. Progr Neurobiol 1973;1:153–198.
5. Da Prada M, Picotti GB. Content and subcellular localization of catecholamines and 5-hydroxytryptamine in human and animal platelets: monoamine distribution between platelets and plasma. Br J Pharmacol 1979;65:653–662.
6. Linnoila M, Virkunnen M, Scheinin M, et al. Low cerebrospinal fluid 5-HIAA concentration differentiates impulsive from nonimpulsive violent behavior. Life Sci 1983;33:2609–2614.
7. Brown GL, Ebert MH, Goyer PF, et al. Aggression, suicide and serotonin: relationship to CSF amine metabolites. Am J Psychiatry 1982;139:741–746.
8. Farberow NL, MacKinnon D. A suicide prediction schedule for neuropsychiatric hospital patients. J Nerv Ment Dis 1974;158:408–419.
9. Soubrier P. Reconciling the role of central serotonin neurons in human and animal behavior. Behav Brain Sci 1986;9:319–364.
10. Rao ML, Fels K. Beeinflussen Tryptophan und Serotonin beim Menschen die Melatonin-Ausschüttung und damit die Funktion des "Regulators der Regulatoren" (Zirbeldrüse). In Kielholz P, Müller-Oerlinghausen B (eds): Advances in Pharmacotherapy. Basel: Karger, 1987;87–99.
11. Rao ML, Mager T. Influence of the pineal gland on pituitary functions in humans. Psychoneuroendocrinology 1987;12:141–147.
12. Huber G, Penin H. Klinisch-elektroenzephalographische Korrelationsuntersuchungen bei Schizophrenen. Fortschr Neurol Psychiatr 1968;36:641–659.
13. Van Praag HM, de Haan S. Central serotonin metabolism and frequency of depression. Psychiatry Res 1979;1:199–224.

71. Past Suicide Attempt and Monoamine Metabolites: Comparing CSF Concentrations and Angularized Ratios

HANS ÅGREN AND ALEC ROY

Whether depressed suicidal patients have a deranged central serotonin metabolism was questioned by Åsberg et al.[1] They reported low 5-hydroxyindoleacetic acid (5-HIAA) concentrations in patients prone to violent suicide attempts when compared with other depressives and normal controls. From this observation two research paths have emerged: (a) a search for consistent derangements in markers of serotonin turnover and function in depressed suicidal patients, and (b) attempts to link serotonin dysfunction to violent types of behavior. Clearly, results are conflicting. The first contention has found support by at least four groups, whereas three others found no differences between suicidal and nonsuicidal depressed patients (reviewed in ref. 2). The second line has been less equivocal, with fairly consistent findings of an assumedly decreased serotonin turnover, i.e., low cerebrospinal fluid (CSF) 5-HIAA, in brains of patients exhibiting violent behaviors.[3–5]

Also, the question of specificity of abnormality in serotonin mechanisms for these behaviors has been questioned. Three studies have found CSF homovanillic acid (HVA) to be more consistently lower then 5-HIAA in suicidal depression compared with nonsuicidal depression.[2,6,7] This finding raises the problem of interpretability of highly collinear variables (HVA and 5-HIAA typically correlate at the level of $r = 0.8$–0.9); a regulatory serotonin→dopamine causality widely spread in the brain has been suggested based on grounds of clinical and animal data.[8] Lower CSF levels of 3-methoxy-4-hydroxyphenylglycol (MHPG) have also been described in these groups.[9,10]

One obstacle to understanding the meaning of altered CSF concentrations has been different means in various control groups of healthy controls. For example, suicidal depressives were thought to group in the low end of the 5-HIAA distribution whereas controls were higher until a recent National Institute of Mental Health (NIMH) study showed that both old and young controls have *lower* 5-HIAA concentrations than either suicidal or nonsuicidal depressives.[2] In fact, higher 5-HIAA levels in depressed patients than in controls had been reported earlier.[11]

Present Study

Three groups of clinical data are compared here for CSF monoamine metabolite concentrations and certain composite variables designed to elucidate cooperability between monoamine systems. RDC major depressives from (a) Uppsala (64 with and 142 without a history of suicide attempt—an extended series from those previously described[6,9,12]) and (b) intramural NIMH (19 with and 8 without past attempts plus 22 healthy controls[2]), were compared with (c) Åsberg and Träskman-Bendz's published CSF data on 30 patients having attempted suicide[13] and 66 healthy volunteers[14] from Stockholm.

Polar (or "circular") coordinates were used to study cooperability between pairs of monoamine metabolite data. Polar coordinates describe each point in a two-dimensional plot in terms of its distance from origo or the 0:0 point (length of the vector radius) as well as the angle between this vector and the x-axis [arctan (x/y) when expressed in radians, arctan $(x/y) \times 180/\pi$ when expressed in degrees]. Simple ratios between metabolites in fact describe the angle between this vector and the x-axis. Changes in a ratio can be seen as the movement of a data point up to the left or down to the right in a coordinate system. The arctan transform of (x/y) is fully proportional to and contains the same information as arctan (y/x); it is seldom the case with the simple x/y and y/x ratios owing to the easy emergence of outliers.

Results

Comparisons of mean values of CSF 5-HIAA, HVA, and MHPG in the various groups are presented in Table 71.1. In the Uppsala sample, 5-HIAA is significantly *lower* in suicide attempters than in nonattempters, and the Stockholm suicide attempters have significantly *lower* levels than controls. However, the NIMH suicidal patients have nonsignificantly *higher* levels than controls and the nonsuicidal ones are clearly significantly higher. HVA is significantly lower in suicide attempters compared with nonattempters from Uppsala, and the same is found for Stockholm suicidal patients compared with controls. The NIMH suicidal cases have lower HVA levels than controls, but only at trend probability. Finally, MHPG is slightly but significantly *lower* in suicide-attempting patients compared to nonattempters from Uppsala, and NIMH nonsuicidal patients have significantly *higher* levels than controls.

Calculating the polar coordinates for the three pairwise combinations of HVA, 5-HIAA, and MHPG shows significantly *smaller* vector angles from origo to both HVA/5-HIAA points and HVA/MHPG points among the suicide attempters, compared with nonsuicidal patients and controls, but only in the NIMH group.

Plotting the means of the seven groups in three-dimensional space (Fig. 71.1) shows the parallelism between the differences among suicide attempters and nonattempters in the Uppsala and NIMH patient samples. The highest degree of parallelism was found between the HVA/5HIAA differences. The Stockholm controls behave as if they were nonsuicidal depressives.

Nonsuicidal depression is apparently associated with higher concentrations of all three monoamine metabolites in comparison with both depressed patients with past suicide attempts and the American controls; the most distinct similarity in

TABLE 71.1. Measures of CSF monoamine metabolites in three studies.

Variable and study	Depressed suicide attempters (A)	Depressed suicide nonattempters (N)	Controls (C)	Least significant differences[a] [α = 0.95]
5-HIAA (nmol/l)				
Uppsala	87.0 ± 4.6 (65)	99.1 ± 3.1 (142)		A < N
NIMH	83.6 ± 7.6 (19)	107.0 ± 11.5 (8)	72.6 ± 5.8 (22)	C < N
Stockholm	85.2 ± 4.8 (30)		104.1 ± 4.7 (66)	A < C
HVA (nmol/l)				
Uppsala	155.3 ± 8.7 (65)	181.7 ± 6.9 (142)		A < N
NIMH	114.4 ± 16.5 (19)	179.7 ± 25.1 (8)	153.7 ± 12.9 (22)	—
Stockholm	200.8 ± 15.1 (30)		245.9 ± 14.1 (66)	A < C
MHPG (nmol/l)				
Uppsala	39.7 ± 1.3 (65)	43.7 ± 0.8 (142)		A < N
NIMH	43.5 ± 2.8 (19)	47.9 ± 7.0 (8)	37.5 ± 1.3 (22)	C < N
Stockholm	48.3 ± 2.0 (30)		51.2 ± 1.3 (60)	—
Angle HVA/5HIAA (degrees)[b]				
Uppsala	59.9 ± 1.1 (65)	60.0 ± 0.7 (142)		—
NIMH	51.1 ± 2.1 (19)	58.4 ± 2.0 (8)	64.1 ± 0.9 (22)	A < N; A <
Stockholm	65.8 ± 1.2 (30)		65.6 ± 0.9 (66)	—
Angle HVA/MHPG (degrees)[c]				
Uppsala	73.5 ± 1.0 (65)	74.0 ± 0.7 (142)		—
NIMH	65.0 ± 2.6 (19)	73.7 ± 3.2 (8)	74.5 ± 1.4 (22)	A < N; A <
Stockholm	75.0 ± 1.0 (30)		75.5 ± 0.9 (60)	—
Angle 5-HIAA/MHPG (degrees)[d]				
Uppsala	62.9 ± 1.3 (65)	64.0 ± 0.8 (142)		—
NIMH	61.0 ± 1.8 (19)	64.6 ± 4.1 (8)	61.0 ± 1.8 (22)	—
Stockholm	59.4 ± 1.4 (30)		61.6 ± 1.1 (60)	—

Results are means ± SEM.
[a]Fisher's protected t-test on selected contrasts within analysis of variance for each variable.
[b]Arctan (HVA/5-HIAA) × 180/π.
[c]Arctan (HVA/MHPG) × 180/π.
[d]Arctan (MHPG/5HIAA) × 180/π.

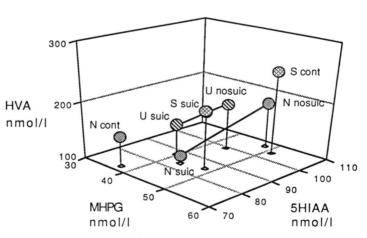

FIGURE 71.1 Three-dimensional representation of means in CSF 5-HIAA (x-axis), MHPG (y-axis), and HVA (z-axis) of all groups analyzed. (U) Uppsala. (N) NIMH (S) Stockholm. (suic) depressed suicide attempters. (nosuic) depressed suicide nonattempters. (cont) healthy volunteers. Pairs of same-center means of the suicide attempter and nonattempter groups are connected in order to demonstrate the parallelism between the Uppsala and NIMH samples. Almost exactly parallel slopes were found in the HVA/5-HIAA projection.

differences is seen in a measure of dopamine/serotonin convariation. Further study must be directed toward understanding the variability of monoamine metabolites in control groups.

Finally, in both the Uppsala and NIMH samples the CSF alterations were unaffected by age or duration of illness (years from first depressive episode). Subdiagnostic comparisons were possible only in the Uppsala sample: the metabolite deviations were found only among unipolar patients.[6,12]

Conclusion

Biochemical covariates to suicidal depression comprise low concentrations of CSF monoamine metabolites and altered interactional measures involving HVA. Prematurely singling out any one amine system as being solely involved appears to be fraught with risks. Clinical interpretations of patient data are complicated by uncertainties of true CSF concentrations in healthy controls, especially as for 5-HIAA. Valid measures more accurately informing about deranged cooperability between different monoamine neurons should be developed.

References

1. Åsberg M, Träskman L, Thorén P. 5-HIAA in the cerebrospinal fluid: a biochemical suicide predictor? Arch Gen Psychiatry 1976;33:1193–1197.
2. Roy A, Ågren H, Pickar D, et al. Reduced CSF concentrations of homovanillic acid and homovanillic acid to 5-hydroxyindoleacetic acid ratios in depressed patients: relationship to suicidal behavior and dexamethasone nonsuppression. Am J Psychiatry 1986;143:1539–1545.
3. Brown GL, Ebert MH, Goyer PF, et al. Aggression, suicide, and serotonin: relationships to CSF amine metabolites. Am J Psychiatry 1982;139:741–746.
4. Lidberg L, Tuck JR, Åsberg M, et al. Homicide, suicide and CSF 5-HIAA. Acta Psychiatr Scand 1985;71:230–236.
5. Virkkunen M, Nuutila A, Goodwin FK, et al. Cerebrospinal fluid monoamine metabolite levels in male arsonists. Arch Gen Psychiatry 1987;44:241–248.
6. Ågren H. Life at risk: markers of suicidality in depression. Psychiatr Dev 1983;1:87–104.
7. Montgomery SA, Montgomery D. Pharmacological prevention of suicidal behaviour. J Affective Disord 1982;4:291–298.
8. Ågren H, Mefford IN, Rudorfer MV, Interacting neurotransmitter systems: a nonexperimental approach to the 5HIAA-HVA correlation in human CSF. J Psychiatr Res 1986;20:175–193.
9. Ågren H. Symptom patterns in unipolar and bipolar depression correlating with monoamine metabolites in the cerebrospinal fluid. II. Suicide. Psychiatry Res 1980;3:225–236.
10. Secunda SK, Cross CK, Koslow S, et al. Biochemistry and suicidal behavior in depressed patients. Biol Psychiatry 1986;21:756–767.
11. Vestergaard P, Sørensen T, Hoppe EJ, et al. Biogenic amine metabolites in cerebrospinal fluid of patients with affective disorders. Acta Psychiatr Scand 1978;58:88–96.
12. Ågren H, Niklasson F. Suicidal potential in depression: focus on CSF monoamine and purine metabolites. Psychopharmacol Bull 1986;22:656–660.
13. Träskman L, Åsberg L, Bertilsson L, et al. Monoamine metabolites in CSF and suicidal behavior. Arch Gen Psychiatry 1981;38:631–636.
14. Åsberg M, Bertilsson L, Mårtensson B, et al. CSF monoamine metabolites in melancholia. Acta Psychiatr Scand 1984;69:201–219.

III.B. Affective Disorders During Childhood and Adolescence

72. Affective Disorders During Childhood and Adolescence: Introduction

MAGDA CAMPBELL

Affective disorders in children and children at risk of affectively ill parents is an area of research that began only a few years ago, and in this short time much knowledge has accumulated. It is important to remember that it was as late as 1973 when Weinberg and his associates[1] published their now classic paper on diagnostic criteria for depression in children. In 1975 the National Institute of Mental Health organized a meeting on depression in childhood,[2] which represented the beginnings of systematic research in the United States.

Affective disorders in this age group is an important area of research. Depressed children and adolescents do exist, and their number is increasing. Suicide in this age group is increasing too, and a subgroup of those children and adolescents suffer from depression that is often unrecognized and untreated. Drug and alcohol abuse in the young is a major problem; and again in a subgroup, drug abuse may be secondary to depression. It is also important to assess the following: First, does affective disorder in parents increase the risk in offspring for psychopathology in general? Second, does it increase the risk specifically for the development of affective disorders? Future prospective studies should tell us if nonspecific behavioral problems seen in offspring during childhood will crystallize into an affective illness during adulthood. The parental contribution may be genetic and/or environmental. The increase of the divorce and separation rates also may contribute to the expression of depression in offspring.

In order to place findings in perspective, controls are required. What constitutes an appropriate control group depends on the type of research questions asked in the future on the basis of current findings. We know that methodology and design influence, or may even determine, the results. Longitudinal studies, twin studies, or adoption studies are needed.

In the meantime, perhaps a different type of research has to focus its efforts on studies of phenomenology and assessment methods. This area has many unanswered questions. Why is it that patients of this age group do not respond to antidepressants as adults do? Why is it that tricyclic antidepressants were not superior to placebo in two major studies involving depressed children[3,4] and in one conducted in adolescents[5]? Unless our diagnostic criteria are valid and unless we are able to diagnose with confidence, we will be unable to develop effective treatments for affective disorders during childhood and adolescence, disorders that can be successfully treated in adult patients. The goals of all research is to treat effectively and ultimately to prevent.

References

1. Weinberg W, Rutman J, Sullivan L, et al. Depression in children referred to an educational center: diagnosis and treatment—preliminary report. J Pediatr 1973;83:1065–1072.
2. Schulterbrandt JG, Raskin A (eds). Depression in Childhood: Diagnosis, Treatment, and Conceptual Models. New York: Raven Press, 1977.
3. Geller B, Cooper TB, McCombes HG, et al. Double-blind placebo-controlled study of nortriptyline in depressed children using "fixed plasma level" design. Psychopharm Bull, 1989; 25 (1).
4. Puig-Antich J, Perel JM, Lupatkin W, et al. Imipramine in prepubertal major depressive disorders. Arch Gen Psychiatry 1987;44:81–89.
5. Ryan ND, Puig-Antich J, Cooper T, et al. Imipramine in adolescent major depression: plasma level and clinical response. Acta Psychiatr Scand 1986;73:275.

73. Study and Treatment of Childhood Depression as a Prototype for the Research and Conceptualization of Other Psychopathologies in Child Psychiatry

Theodore A. Petti

Children with clinically significant dysphoria have been described in the literature for almost a century. Resurgence of interest has centered around theoretical systems developed from work with both children and adults, research demonstrating factors contributing to vulnerability, the availability of effective treatment strategies, and a growing awareness of the similarities between adult and childhood depressives.[1-4]

A similar situation existed in endocrinology between "juvenile onset" and "maturity onset" diabetes. During the past few years, research into the physiology, immunology, and genetics of the disorders have revealed two pathogenetically different disorders: type I (juvenile onset) and type II (maturity onset) diabetes. A triad of markers have been found useful for identifying children at high risk for developing the type I variety. This chapter draws from such analogies to illustrate the thesis that depression in children can serve as a prototype of childhood psychiatric disorders and demonstrate the manner in which such disorders relate to the adult forms of psychiatric disease.

The justification for the depressions of childhood serving as a prototype for study of the other psychopathologies of youth lies in the following areas.

1. *Acceptance of the concept that children do manifest measureable dysphoric symptoms that fit into symptom or disease/disorder categories.*

2. *Availability of instruments to provide surveys of clinical and nonclinical populations, serve diagnostic purposes, and measure changes in symptoms in response to treatment.* A variety of scales for screening, diagnosing, and assessing depression and measuring changes in severity have been developed.[5] Limitations and threats to reliability and validity of such instruments have also been reviewed. The scales developed for childhood depression are based on limited criteria, all of which relate to classifications of adult depressive disorders. As with other childhood diagnoses based on adult models of psychopathology, it may be advisable to maintain a pluralistic perspective and delay premature closure of options by avoiding

the selection of only one set of criteria and discarding the others until methods of validation are available. The continued efforts to develop scales and to test their reliability are critical. The direct interview of the child for data required in diagnosis and efforts to employ a developmental and cognitive approach in the assessment of depressed children can also be expected to generalize across other childhood psychopathologies. The availability of standardized assessment instruments has allowed us to conduct epidemiological investigations.

3. *Development of a body of literature describing the longitudinal course of the disorders.* A limited number of longitudinal studies of childhood depressions have been conducted. Kovacs and associates[6] have provided the most elegant study to date of the natural course of the childhood depressions, including the ages of onset, recovery rates, and risk for new episodes of depressive illness. Separation and divorce, as major stressors on children and adolescents resulting in clinical depression, have been studied and their impact on long-term outcome described. Analogous study is needed for describing the long-term consequences of stressors on affective and other juvenile disorders.

4. *Development of effective treatments for depressed children, the process of which typifies our approach to many other disorders.* Psychodynamic therapy has been the predominant clinical intervention, though a paucity of controlled studies exist. Child psychiatrists are turning with increasing frequency to psychopharmacological agents for treating the more severe depressive disorders of childhood.[2] The methodological problems to be solved for conducting double-blind placebo-controlled studies typify those to be addressed in other disorders. However, our ability to monitor plasma levels of the tricyclics and saliva measures of lithium in children provides tools not previously available. Behavioral or learning theory oriented therapies are being employed to an increasing extent in child psychiatry. The gamut of interventions from social skills, assertion, and conflict resolution training, to social reinforcement schedules, cognitive intervention, and cognitive-behavioral self-control programs are available and can be expected to play an accelerated role in treating depressed and disturbed children. Multimodal therapeutic interventions employing an integrative approach will continue to be of critical importance, particularly for multiproblem children referred for tertiary care. This approach to treating disturbed children may become the expected standard of care in the treatment of psychiatrically and severely disturbed youth.

5. *Beginning development of physiological correlates specific to the disorder.* Many physiological parameters have been identified as potential markers for depressive disorders in children and adolescents. If the more severe psychopathologies of childhood have a physiological dysfunction as a major contributor to etiology, the work with depression assumes even greater importance. Consideration has been given to polysomnographic changes in children serving as state markers for depression, but the results have been inconclusive. Preliminary data demonstrated that major depression, endogenous type, is associated with cortisol hypersecretion in about 50% of affected children and adults.[3] Advances in the use of salivary cortisol levels may facilitate further research into cortisol dynamics and into refining the application of the dexamethasone suppression test (DST). The DST and related physiological measures of the hypothalamic-pituitary-adrenal axis may open up vistas for neuroendocrine study of other childhood disorders and their response to treatment. Preliminary results indicate that hypersecretion of growth hormone may be the first trait, rather state, biochemical marker thus far available in child psychiatry as is insulin-induced hyposecretion of growth

hormone in drug-free children who recovered from a major depression.[3] The results have not been replicated, but this type of association may provide insights into the myriad related neurotransmitters associated with normal and disordered thoughts, emotions, and behavior.

6. *Continuity of the disorders with adult depressive disorders.* As with the diabetes analogy, depression with its onset during childhood and that which develops at a later time may not be identical. The outward clinical manifestations of the disorders may be similar; they may share a number of similar physiological and behavioral patterns and may demonstrate similar responses to treatment. The course of childhood and adolescent depression into adulthood supports the concept of continuity. However, differences related to age in physiological markers, phenomenology, and differences in cognitive capacity to experience depression raise questions concerning the identity of all depressive disorders across the age spectrum, though the diagnoses employing identical criteria may be the same.

7. *Genetic or familial loading of the disorders.* Childhood depression has this characteristic, which is common to many other disorders. The vulnerability of children with parents diagnosed as having a major affective disorder has been documented. Rates of affective diagnoses are high in such children and significantly greater than those found in control groups. Depressive symptoms have also been reported in a high proportion of children of parents with an affective disorder.[4] Delineating the role of parenting styles and behavior on offspring of disturbed parents, particularly depressed mothers, must be a major area of concern for workers in the field. The nurture-versus-nature interaction requires continued research. Issues of competence, personal resources, and social resources are now being studied in the offspring of parents with a bipolar disorder. Some work suggests that disruption of social networks during childhood and the inadequate nurturing of problem-solving skills, feelings of self-worth, control, and competence may be the mechanism through which parental psychopathology is transmitted to these vulnerable youngsters.[7] A limitation of high risk studies based on parental psychiatric disorders is that causality cannot be ascribed. Depression may be based as much on environmental stress as biological vulnerability.

8. *Sharing the complexities of other childhood psychopathologies.* With the positive development of operational criteria for diagnosing childhood and adolescent disorders has come the potential problem of distinguishing the child who "meets criteria" but is not perceived as suffering from a psychiatric disorder. The confounding of diagnostic classifications caused by overlapping psychiatric disorders in children and adolescents is an area best studied with regard to depression. The affect of development on the manifestation of a particular psychiatric disorder, a recurring problem for child psychiatry, is being examined most closely in depressed children. Developmental factors considered important are cognitive, neuroendocrinological, phenomenological, pharmacokinetic, and biopsychosocial. Expected changes in attributional style with puberty and the major contributions of temperament can all be expected to play critical roles in the development of depression in children. These issues also have an impact on and assist in explaining the need for multi-informants in order to obtain data on behavior, thoughts, and internal feeling states and to attain an accurate diagnosis. A body of literature is being developed for childhood depression analogous to that for the physical disorders and diabetes related to adaptation, emotional development, and socialization.

9. *Development and the disorders during early childhood and adolescence, which may portend an especially poor prognosis, as with other childhood disorders.* Youngsters with psychopathology severe enough for referral to a tertiary care center have a particularly guarded prognosis.

10. *Serving as a final common pathway.* Childhood depression as a disorder that results from the interaction of factors related to vulnerability has heuristic appeal. This concept has been described for melancholia.[1] A similar scheme can be applied to children and adolescents wherein physiological stressors, genetic predisposition, psychosocial stressors, and developmental predisposition through early experiences (e.g., early object loss) act to varying degrees to have an impact on postulated neurophysiological functions and mechanisms. These results then influence the diencephalon and perhaps other brain areas, resulting in the development or maintenance of the disorder. The psychoanalytical, behavioral, and biological models provide partial explanations for the development of affective disorders in children and adolescents but can also apply to other disorders in juveniles. Youngsters without threats to their physiological integrity or who are not burdened by a genetic loading for affective disorder may respond to psychosocial stressors by experiencing an adjustment disorder or they may even manage to thrive, whereas others develop a dysthymic disorder and a propensity to major depression. Similar dynamics may be operating in other pediatric disorders. The scientifically based medical model of practice holds clinical diagnoses to represent hypotheses from which the clinician can predict the course of the disorders and effect of treatment. Significant progress had been made in clarifying many critical issues regarding depressed children, though much remains to be understood. The diagnosis of childhood depression must be more than checking off symptoms or assigning a diagnostic label; it must include consideration of the major dimensions discussed when assessing and planning for the care of such children and their families. The diagnosis must also consider the cognitive attributes, social skills, social supports, and other areas of competence available to the child and family. The exquisite studies being conducted with depressed children and adolescents provide models for the study of other major psychiatric disorders as we continue to struggle with the mind-body dichotomy of the twentieth century.

Unlike the physically handicapping disorders of children, which are well diagnosed and treated, childhood affective disorders share a legacy of underdiagnosis, lack of treatment, and inattention. Defining the parameters of childhood affective disorders and their treatment may be the impetus needed for providing the necessary framework to ensure adequate care for all disturbed children.

References

1. Akiskal HS, McKinney WT. Overview of recent research in depression. Arch Gen Psychiatry 1975;32:285–305.
2. Petti TA. Imipramine in the treatment of depressed children. In Cantwell D, Carlson G (eds): Affective Disorders in Childhood and Adolescence. New York: Spectrum, 1983;375–415.
3. Puig-Antich J. Psychobiological markers: effects of age and puberty. In Rutter M, Izard C, Read P (eds): Depression in Young People: Developmental and Clinical Perspectives. New York: Gilford Press, 1986;341–381.
4. Weissman MM, Prusoff BA, Gammon GD, et al. Psychopathology in the children (ages 6–18) of depressed and normal parents. J Am Acad Child Psychiatry 1984;23:78–84.

5. Petti TA. Scales of potential use in the psychopharmacologic treatment of depressed children and adolescents. Psychopharmacol Bull 1985;21:951–977.
6. Kovacs M, Feinberg TL, Crouse-Novak MA, et al. Depressive disorders in childhood. Arch Gen Psychiatry 1984;41:229–237, 643–649.
7. Pellegrini D, Kosisky S, Nackman D, et al. Personal and social resources in children of patients with bipolar affective disorder and children of normal control subjects. Am J Psychiatry 1986;143:856–861.

74. New Hypotheses of the Pharmacotherapy of Childhood and Adolescent Depression

BARBARA GELLER

The differences in future directions of pharmacotherapy research for pediatric compared to adult major depressive disorders (MDDs) stem from the wide gap in reported double-blind placebo-controlled (DBPC) studies to date between the two age groups. Table 74.1 presents the various types of controlled studies reported for adult, prepubertal,[1] and adolescent[2] groups. It does not include several controlled studies of children in which there were fewer than ten subjects. The reason, in part, for the lag in pediatric studies is the more recent consensus on the existence of pediatric MDDs[3] and, concomitantly, the more recent development of pediatric assessment instruments that are comparable to those used in research on adults.[3]

The hypothesis of the two reported pediatric studies was that pediatric and adult MDDs were the same disorder. Therefore children and adolescents with MDDs were expected to have a positive response to tricyclic antidepressants (TCAs). However, neither the Puig-Antich et al. DBPC study of prepubertal children[1] nor the Kramer and Feiguine DBPC study of adolescents[2] found that active drug was significantly better than placebo.

Design problems with these two studies included a small number of subjects in the Kramer and Feiguine work and no placebo washout phase in either study. The importance of the latter was emphasized by the outcome of the Puig-Antich et al. study, i.e., a 56% active response rate but a 68% placebo response rate. Retrospectively, Puig-Antich et al. performed a post hoc analysis that showed an 85% response rate in subjects on active drug who had imipramine (IMI) plasma levels over 150 ng/ml. This finding suggested the possible usefulness of taking plasma levels into account in future IMI DBPC studies of children. An unexpected, and as yet unexplained, finding in the IMI study was a lower response rate (33%) in subjects on active drug with low plasma levels (less than 150 ng/ml) than in the placebo responders (68%).

The initial concerns that TCAs in children would be too cardiotoxic have not been supported.[4] Both children and adolescents have electrocardiographic findings similar to those in adults: a slowing of conduction and an increase in heart rate that are not of known clinical significance.

Clearly, the most crucial future direction is to perform well designed DBPC

TABLE 74.1. Comparison of controlled studies of pharmacotherapy for adult and pediatric depression.

Area	Adult	Adolescent	Child (prepubertal)
No. of DBPC studies[a]	Numerous	One[b]	One[b]
Outcome for episode	Usually significantly better than placebo	Not significantly different	Not significantly different
Drug classes studied	TCA, bicyclic, tetracyclic MAO inhibitors Anxiolytics, anticonvulsants, lithium, amino acid precursors	TCA	TCA
Comparison to nonpharmacotherapy modalities	Several	None	None
Maintenance and prevention	Few	None	None
Effect on future course	Several, controversial	Unknown	Unknown
Atypical or delusional	Few	None	None

DBPC = double-blind placebo-controlled studies.
Studies with more than 10 subjects.

studies that include a placebo washout phase, an adequate number of subjects, and controlled plasma levels.[5]

If studies with these methodological advantages[5] demonstrate a significantly better effect of active compared to placebo drug, the hypothesis that pediatric MDD is the same illness as adult MDD will be supported. If that is the case, future studies could follow the lines of what has already been accomplished in adults, including studies comparing drug to nondrug modalities and maintenance studies.

However, future negative findings will necessitate generating and investigating alternate hypotheses, including the following.

1. That pediatric and adult MDDs are the same illness, but for a subset of children and adolescents early onset signifies greater severity and therefore a different response to interventions. It would be analogous to juvenile- and adult-onset rheumatoid arthritis and diabetes mellitus, where childhood-onset carries a worse course and prognosis and different treatment needs. Thus if a subgroup of early onset MDDs have a more malignant form of the illness, it could explain the poor response to TCAs and perhaps make these subjects analogous to adults with treatment-resistant depressions. If it is the case, the research needs may be similar. That is, treatment resistance at any age may require studies of augmentation of tricylics with lithium, thyroid preparations, or neuroleptics.
2. That a subset of pediatric MDD is an initial episode of a future bipolar course. There are, as yet, no data on predictors of future bipolarity for prepubertal subjects. For adolescents, two groups of investigators have described predictors of a future bipolar course.[6,7] Therefore a research direction would be to design studies in which adolescents with the predictors of future bipolarity are studied separately. It could include a DBPC study of lithium for this group. Using the same reasoning, prepubertal children with first or second degree relatives with bipolar disorders may also be candidates for a DBPC study of lithium.

3. That the "same illness at all ages" hypothesis is not correct for a subset of pediatric MDD, despite a similar clinical presentation. This situation would be analogous to viral or bacterial pneumonia, where treatment is clearly related to the specific pathogen. Testing this hypothesis has similar research requirements at any age. As biological markers became available, they need to be incorporated into treatment study protocols.

4. Another issue is the possibility that a subset of children and adolescents, regardless of family loading for affective disorders, are treatment-resistant because of psychosocial, environmental factors. Thus the expression of a genetic-familial predisposition may be more frequent, of greater severity, and of longer duration in the presence of certain psychosocial factors. Alternately, these environmental factors may be sufficient for the pathogenesis of MDD even without biological vulnerability. Therefore pediatric pharmacotherapy studies need to include psychosocial assessments.

5. Finally, it is possible that a subgroup of prepubertal children who present with MDD have the pathogenetic equivalent of a delusional depression that may not be clinically evident due to their age-appropriate cognitive immaturity.[8] Follow-up studies of treatment-resistant children with MDD may aid in identifying predictors of delusional depression and thus permit incorporating them into future drug study designs.

Summary

The field of pharmacotherapy of pediatric MDD is in its infancy. Future directions, as noted above, depend on whether further studies of TCAs refute or support the hypothesis that MDD is a similar illness with the same treatment needs at all ages.

Acknowledgment. Supported by NIMH grants MH 40273 and MH 40646.

References

1. Puig-Antich J, Perel JM, Lupatkin W, et al. Imipramine in prepubertal major depressive disorders. Arch Gen Psychiatry 1987;44:81–89.
2. Kramer AD, Feiguine RJ. Clinical effects of amitriptyline in adolescent depression. J Am Acad Child Psychiatry 1981;21:636–644.
3. Geller B, Carr LG. Similarities and differences between adult and pediatric major depressive disorder. In Georgotas A, Cancro RM (eds): Depression and Mania: A Comprehensive Textbook. New York: Elsevier Press, 1988;565–580.
4. Geller B, Farooki ZQ, Cooper TB, et al. Serial ECG measurements at controlled plasma levels of nortriptyline in depressed children. Am J Psychiatry 1985;142:1095–1097.
5. Geller B. Components of the design of psychopharmacology studies. Psychopharmacol Bull 1986;22:1077–1080.
6. Strober M, Carlson G. Bipolar illness in adolescents with major depression. Arch Gen Psychiatry 1982;39:549–555.
7. Akiskal HS, Walker P, Puzantian VR, et al. Bipolar outcome in the course of depressive illness. J Affective Disord 1983;5:115–128.
8. Chambers WJ, Puig-Antich J, Tabrizi MA, et al. Psychotic symptoms in prepubertal major depressive disorder. Arch Gen Psychiatry 1982;39:921–927.

75. Depression in Children: Defining the Therapeutic Range for Imipramine

S.H. PRESKORN, E. WELLER, C. HUGHES, AND R. WELLER

The clinical applicability of plasma monitoring of tricyclic antidepressants has been actively studied over the past 15 years. As a result, such monitoring has become a useful tool to guide pharmacotherapy with selected agents. Our studies in children can serve as a model for empirically establishing therapeutic plasma drug monitoring in psychiatry.

This sequential series of studies,[1-4] which was conducted over a 7-year span, was targeted to determine if major depressive disorder (MDD) exists in children. Other questions followed: If it does exist in children, what is the nature of the disorder, and is it responsive to treatment? When these studies began, the prevailing opinion was that MDD could not occur in children, an opinion based on theory alone. Presumably, children did not have sufficient ego development to permit the development of MDD.

Our findings are in significant disagreement with that earlier theoretical supposition. MDD does occur in children aged 6–12 years and is similar to MDD in adults in a variety of ways: (a) phenomenology; (b) familial loading; (c) dexamethasone suppression; and (d) response to antidepressant chemotherapy.[1-4]

Given the potentially life-threatening nature of this disorder, a significant amount of our effort has been directed at treatment, specifically with imipramine (IMI). Our studies with IMI progressed in stages. The first study examined the interindividual variability in drug levels. The second dealt with the relationship between drug plasma levels and both antidepressant response and adverse effects. The third was the classic drug versus placebo double-blind study. The three major studies are summarized below.

Study I: Variability in Plasma Levels

A group of 250 hospitalized patients with MDD ranging in age from 6 to 70 years were studied in terms of the variability in plasma concentrations of IMI and its metabolites. Of these 250 patients, 70 patients were between the ages of 6 and 14 years. The criteria for the study were that (a) all patients had to be hospitalized to ensure compliance; (b) there had to be repeat plasma level determinations; (c) all levels had to be at steady state; and (d) all levels had to be trough levels drawn 10–12 h after the last dose. Plasma levels of IMI (mean 50 ng/ml, range seven-fold), desipramine (101 ng/ml, 11-fold), 2-hydroxyimipramine (77 ng/ml, 33-fold), and 2-hydroxydesipramine (34 ng/ml, two-fold) were quantitated.

Study II: Relation Between Levels and Response

Study II[1,2] was designed to precede a placebo-controlled, double-blind, random assignment study and to test the relationship between plasma levels of IMI and metabolites and antidepressant response. Briefly, patients had to meet the following inclusion criteria: (a) be 6–12 years old and prepubertal; and (b) be hospitalized for MDD, being symptomatically ill for at least 30 days prior to enrollment with a minimum score of 20 on the Children's Depressive Rating Scale (CDRS). Children were excluded if they had organic brain syndrome, attention deficit disorder, an IQ less than 85, and/or psychotic symptoms. Medically unstable children were also excluded.

The design of the study involved three phases: First, the MDD severity was quantitated at baseline using three measures: a clinical global impression (CGI), CDRS, and a self-report scale, the Childhood Depressive Inventory (CDI). For the initial 2 weeks children were treated with daily individual psychotherapy (5 days/week), group psychotherapy (3 days/week), family therapy (2 sessions/week), and milieu therapy including school (4 h/day). They received no drug therapy. Children were reevaluated after these 2 weeks. If unchanged, they were treated with IMI 75 mg at bedtime. Plasma levels of IMI and metabolites were allowed to vary as determined by underlying differences in drug metabolism. The treating team was maintained blind to the plasma drug level achieved. In this sense, the study—although an open, uncontrolled trial—was blind with regard to plasma drug level.

After 3 weeks the treating team could make a single dose change based solely on clinical assessment. This adjustment allowed the study to mimic clinical practice and afforded an additional opportunity to examine the relationship between drug concentration and clinical response. Guidelines were as follows: If the children were improved, the dose was maintained. If not and side effects were present, the dose was reduced to 50 mg at bedtime. If there was no improvement and no side effects appeared, the dose was increased to a maximum of 5 mg/kg/day. Once adjusted, the dose was maintained for an additional 3 weeks.

A more than 70% drug response was observed with IMI plus desipramine plasma drug concentrations between 125 and 250 ng/ml (Fig. 75.1, top). About 50% of the variability in antidepressant response could be attributed to variability in plasma drug level. More than 70% of this variability was accounted for by desipramine plasma levels. Plasma levels of 2-hydroxyimipramine and 2-hydroxydesipramine were not found to correlate with antidepressant response.

Study III. Double-Blind Placebo-Controlled Trial

Inclusion and exclusion criteria were identical to those in the preceding study. Following hospitalization and baseline assessment, children were randomly assigned to receive either placebo or 100 mg of IMI at bedtime. Plasma drug levels were measured at 8 and 12 days. If the plasma level in the IMI-treated children

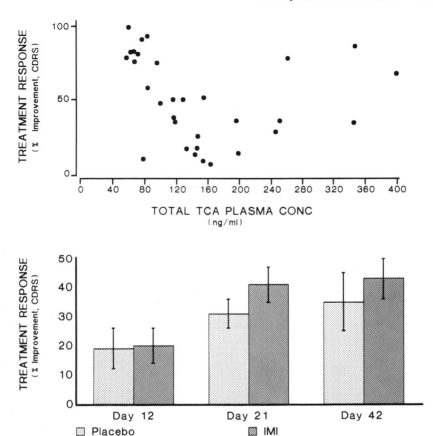

FIGURE 75.1. *Top:* Relation between antidepressant response (as measured by percent reduction in children's depressive rating scale, CDRS, from baseline) versus the total plasma
level of imipramine plus desipramine after 3 weeks of treatment. These data were best fit
by a two-degree polynomial regression equation ($r = 0.68$, $p > 0.001$). *Bottom:* Antidepressant
response (as measured by percent reduction in CDRS from baseline) in patients in placebo
versus imipramine. Imipramine-treated patients had their dosage adjusted by the laboratory
so that optimum plasma drug levels were achieved. Antidepressant response on imipramine
was superior to placebo ($p < 0.05$, ANOVA). This difference was statistically detectable
by 3 weeks.

Results similar to those shown here were obtained for antidepressant response as measured
by a clinican global impression (CGI) scale and a patient self-report scale. The CGI best
demonstrated the overall imipramine versus placebo difference. Results were similar whether
antidepressant response was calculated as percent reduction (as shown), or by raw scores
or residualized scores. The imipramine-placebo difference was most pronounced in DST
nonsuppressors.

was outside the therapeutic range (125–250 ng/ml) determined in study II, the
laboratory could adjust the dose without the treatment team's knowledge by sub-
stituting either active or inactive tablets. Hence the dose could range from 25 to
150 mg/day for the next 4 weeks. This approach eliminated most of the variability
in plasma drug levels. The same severity scales (i.e., CGI, CDRS, CDI) and mea-

surements of adverse events (i.e., side effect scale, blood pressure, other vital signs, electrocardiogram, and mental status examination) were used in this study as in the fixed-dose study (study II).

Imipramine was found to be effective in comparison to placebo.[3] The IMI–placebo difference was apparent within 3 weeks of starting drug therapy (Fig. 75.1, bottom). The placebo-controlled study extended the findings of the fixed-dose study (study II) by being the first study to show that IMI is superior to placebo in the treatment of MDD in children given that therapeutic drug plasma levels (125–250 ng/ml) are achieved. It is of interest that the drug versus placebo difference was more pronounced in DST nonsuppressors in comparison to DST suppressors.

Summary

Based on this work, we have reached the following conclusions. First, IMI is effective in treating MDD in children when compared to placebo. The drug response rate can approach 80% when plasma drug concentration is controlled. In contrast, the placebo response rate is less than 30%. These figures are remarkably similar to those seen in well designed and well executed studies of tricyclic antidepressant response rates in adult MDD. Second, the time course for antidepressant response to IMI is also similar to that observed in adult MDD. Within 3 weeks of initiating IMI, response is observed given that the plasma drug level is within the therapeutic range. Third, the minimum plasma level necessary for antidepressant response in children is remarkably similar to that needed for adult MDD. Fourth, patients who are DST nonsuppressors show the best response to IMI and the poorest response to placebo, similar to reports for adult MDD.

Acknowledgment. Supported by NIMH grants MH 00272 and MH 36739, and by the Psychiatric Research Institute at St. Francis Regional Medical Center, Wichita KS. An earlier version of this chapter appeared in Psychopharmacology Bulletin and is listed as reference 3.

References

1. Preskorn S, Weller E, Weller R. Depression in children: relationship between plasma imipramine levels and response J Clin Psychiatry 1985;43:450–453.
2. Preskorn S, Weller E, Weller R, et al. Plasma levels of imipramine and adverse effect in children. Am J Psychiatry 1983;140:1332–1335.
3. Preskorn S, Weller E, Hughes C, et al. Depression in prepubertal children: DST non-suppression predicts differential response to imipramine versus placebo. Psychopharm Bull 1987;23(1):128–133.
4. Weller E, Weller R, Fristad M, et al. The dexamethasone suppression test in prepubertal depressed children. J Clin Psychiatry 1985;46:511–513.

76. Good Results with the Dexamethasone Suppression Test in Adolescent Inpatients: Implications for Diagnosis in Adolescent Psychiatry

ALAN APTER, ANKE RAM, AND SAM TYANO

There has been a great deal of interest in the association between affective disorders (ADs) and neuroendocrine dysfunction. This interest has greatly increased over the past decade, and it is hoped that such studies will lead to further elucidation of the pathogenesis of these conditions.[1]

Depression is characterized by a number of features reminiscent of hypothalamic disturbance, including mood changes, sleeping problems, and eating and sexual dysfunctions. The hypothalamic pituitary adrenal (HPA) axis has received particular attention in this regard. Work done during the 1970s demonstrated that some affectively ill adults have high basal secretory levels of cortisol and loss of the physiological diurnal variation.[2] These findings have not been reported in children but are present in adolescents, which means that this phenomenon is related to age.[3]

Attempts to suppress cortisol secretion in adult depressives have been made by a number of authors. Many workers, especially the group led by Carroll,[4] have found that more than 50% of endogenously depressed patients failed to suppress cortisol after dexamethasone administration. This nonsuppression occurred in only 5% of patients with other psychiatric illnesses.

The physiological basis of cortisol nonsuppression is unknown. Speculation ranges from diminished tonic inhibition of corticotropin-releasing factor (CRF) to changes in receptor sensitivity along the HPA axis.[5]

The dexamethasone suppression test (DST) could have several clinical applications. It might be useful as an auxiliary diagnostic test for depression,[4] as a guide as to when pharmacotherapy might be discontinued, and perhaps as an indication of the need to initiate tricyclic antidepressant therapy.[6] Initial enthusiam for the DST has waned considerably, however, and there is a great deal of controversy as to the validity of these findings.[7]

The introduction of *DSM-III* criteria for diagnosis has seen a widening of the concept of AD and a narrowing of that of schizophrenia.[8] It has been particularly marked in child and adolescent psychiatry. AD was hardly diagnosed in this age group prior to 1977, but since then the condition has become widely recognized in the United States. Child psychiatrists elsewhere, especially in the United Kingdom,[9] have criticized this swing in the diagnostic pendulum, and there has been much argument about how to differentiate depressive symptoms from depressive syndrome. It is even more problematic during adolescence, where mood swings are common.

One way of improving diagnostic reliability is the use of structured interviews such as the Kiddie-SADS to reduce "information variance." The Kiddie-SADS also yields 11 symptom clusters, four of which are related to depression, (depressed mood, endogenous features of depression, nonendogenous features of depressions, and suicidal tendencies). We have found this instrument to be highly reliable for diagnosis (K = 0.8) and for the symptom clusters (ICC = 0.9).[10]

Systematically investigation of depressive symptomatology among various conditions in psychiatrically ill adolescents has shown the condition to be abundant and widespread (Table 76.1). Thus a biological marker that could separate depressive syndromes would be valuable in adolescent psychiatry. The use of the DST in adolescents has been reviewed by Doherty et al.[11] They reported on seven studies in adolescents (mostly inpatients). Sensitivity ranged from 40 to 64% and the specificity from 88 to 100%.[11]

These findings could be interpreted to mean that many adolescents with depressed symptoms are being diagnosed as having AD. Thus if the diagnosis of major affective disorder (MAD) was restricted to those with definite endogenous (melancholic) symptoms (K-SADS scale score above 23; see Table 76.1) as well

TABLE 76.1. Distribution of 100 plasma cortisol levels after DST.

Cortisol (µg/dl)	Schizoaffective disorder (10%)	Depression (19%)	Other (62%)	Anorexia nervosa (9%)
20				
		x		
15	x	x		
		x		
		x		
		x		x
		x		x
		x	x	x
		x		x
		x		
10	xx			
		xx	x	
	x	x	x	x
	x	xx	x	x
	x	x	x	x
	x	x	x	
5			xxx	
		x		
		xxxxx		
		xxx		
	x	xxxx		x
	x	xxxxx		
	x	x	xxxx	x
	x		xxxxxx	
	x		xxxxxxxxx	

Statistical data were obtained by the Fisher exact test. Frequency of nonsuppressors: depression vs. others, p < 0.0005 (patients with anorexia nervosa were excluded). Sensitivity 84%. Specificity 82% (mainly due to nonsuppression in schizoaffective disorder).

as the other criteria for MAD, sensitivity might be markedly increased. The study described below was designed to test this hypothesis.

Methods

The study population included 100 consecutive admissions to the adolescent inpatient unit at the Geha Hospital. There were 59 girls and 41 boys whose ages ranged from 12 to 18 years (mean 15.5 ± 1.5). Diagnosis was made by:

1. Interviewing with the Kiddie-SADS
2. *DSM-III* criteria with the following modifications:
   a. MAD diagnosed only when the score for mood was more than 15 and that for endogenous symptoms more than 25 on the symptom scale score of the Kiddie SADS
   b. Schizoaffective disorder diagnosed when the mood score was 15 and the endogenous symptoms score was 25 on the Kiddie SADS scale scores, but psychotic symptoms were mood-incongruent and present before or after psychotic symptoms and signs were apparent
3. Observation of the patient over at least 3–4 months.

Cortisol was measured by radioimmunoassay (RIA) at the endocrine laboratory at the Beilinson Medical Center. Dexamethasone 1 mg was given at 11:00 p.m. The following day blood was obtained for cortisol levels 4:00 p.m. and 11:00 p.m. Precautions were taken to ensure the reliability of the RIA in the laboratory especially in the low range of cortisol values.

One serum estimation of less than 5 μg/dl was taken as a positive result. Diagnosticians were completely blind as to the laboratory results.

Results

The result are shown in Table 76.1: 16 of 19 adolescents with MAD showed cortisol nonsuppression. Of the 81 other patients, 20 showed nonsuppression. However, 14 of these patients either had anorexia nervosa or schizoaffective disorder. Thus the sensitivity of DST in our sample is 84%, and the overall sensitivity is 75%. However, when the anorexic patients are excluded, specificity rises to 83%, and when the schizoaffective disorder patients are excluded it increases to 94%.

Forty-three of the adolescents were depressed on admission, and the diagnosis of MAD was considered. Nineteen were later diagnosed as AD on the Kiddie-SADS. Of the 24 who were not, four were nonsuppressors. For these 43 specificity was 83% and sensititivy was 84%.

Discussion

Our results indicate that disillusion with the DST, at least in adolescent patients, is possibly premature. Although the overall findings in this report are similar to those found in the literature,[12] (40–60% sensitivity and 80–100% specificity) the results are greatly improved when conditions known to give false-positive results, e.g., anorexia nervosa, are excluded a priori. In addition to anorexia nervosa, other examples include severe physical illness, trauma, fever, dehydration, temporal lobe epilepsy, pregnancy, Cushing's disease, unstable diabetes, alcoholism, overweight, underweight, and antiepileptic drugs.[4] All these factors are easily recognizable to the clinician.

Two important theoretical considerations with clinical implications are raised by these results: First, some narrowing of the criteria for MAD increases sensitivity but not specificity. The implication is that perhaps MAD is now being overdiagnosed, and that with more detailed quantitative attention to endogenous symptomatology we may be able to delineate a more discrete "melancholic" entity during adolescence. Other adolescents with depressive symptoms may represent a more heterogeneous group of patients. These findings may form some sort of bridge between the broader United States (DSM-III) point of view and the narrower concepts of British child psychiatrists.[9]

The second consideration seems to go against this view, however, in that the DST did not distinguish between MAD and schizoaffective disorder as we defined them. It supports Pope and Lipinski's contention[12] that schizoaffective disorder and good prognosis schizophrenia are really part of the affective disorders.[13] Thus endogenous features of depression may be more related to DST than is depressive syndrome, as defined by DSM-III, which is similar to Van Praag's[13] finding that low cerebrospinal fluid 5-hydroxyindoleacetic acid is more related to dysregulation of aggression than broad syndrome criteria for depression.

The best treatment for psychotic depression and schizoaffective disorder is considered by many clinicians to be similar (combinations of lithium or tricyclics and antipsychotic drugs). These findings do seem to be in line with clinical practice.

Conclusion

By narrowing the diagnosis of AD by emphasizing endogenous features on the one hand and widening the concept of AD by including schizoaffective disorder on the other hand, the DST may be a highly sensitive and specific diagnostic tool. These conclusions are, however, not supported by other workers in the field as yet, and only further validation by genetic treatment and follow-up studies will give a definite answer to the question of how valuable the DST is for adolescent psychiatry.

References

1. Sachar EJ, Asnis G, Halbreich U. Recent studies in the neuroendocrinology of major depressive disorders. Psychiatr Clin North Am 1980;3:315.
2. Sachar EJ, Hellman L, Fukushima DK. Cortisone production in depressive illness: a clinical and biochemical clarification. Arch Gen Psychiatry 1970;23:289.
3. Prug-Antich J, Chambers W, Halpern F. Cortisol hypersecretion in prepubertal depressive illness: a preliminary report. Psychoneuroendocrinology 1979;4:191.
4. Carroll BJ. The dexamethasone suppression test for melancholia. Br J Psychiatry 1982;140:292.
5. Carroll JB, Feinberg M, Green JF. A specific laboratory test for melancholia: standardization, validation and clinical utility. Arch Gen Psychiatry 1981;38:15.
6. Greden JF, Carroll BJ, De Vigne J. Dexamethasone suppression test results and prediction of treatment response. Biol Psychiatry 1981;16:469.
7. Berger M, Pirke KM, Doerr P. The limited utility of the dexamethasone suppression test for the diagnostic process in psychiatry. Br J Psychiatry 1984;14:372.
8. Bleich A, Apter A, Tyano S. Difficulties in the psychiatric diagnosis of adolescents. J Isr Med Assoc 1986⊗4:187.

 9. Shaffer D. Depression, mania and suicidal acts. In Hersov L, Rutter M (eds): Child and
    Adolescent Psychiatry. Oxford: Blackwell, 1985.
10. Laseg M. A Hebrew version of the K-SAD. Doctoral thesis, University of Tel Aviv
    Medical School, 1987.
11. Doherty M, Madansky D, Kraft J, et al. Cortisol dynamics and test performance of the
    dexamethasone suppression test in 97 psychiatrically hospitalized children. J Am Acad
    Child Psychiatry 1986;25(3):100.
12. Pope HG, Lipinski JF. Diagnosis in schizophrenia and manic depressive illness. Arch
    Gen Psychiatry 1978;35:811.
13. Van Praag H. Seminar on Suicide. Jerusalem: Hadassah Hospital, 1986.

77. Social Development of Children at High Risk for Depression: Preadolescence and Early Adolescence

W.R. DAVIS AND L. ERLENMEYER-KIMLING

Many researchers concur that the "diathesis-stress model"[1] by which genetic predispositions become manifest, depending on the presence or absence of unknown environmental factors, is the best model for understanding the etiology of depression. The research presented here is a longitudinal investigation of specific social variables that may be among the unknown factors contributing to the development of depression. Becasue children of depressed parents have a 10–15% risk of developing disorders similar to those of their parents, compared to rates of about 1% in the general population,[2] they are the subjects of choice for this research.

In this report we investigate if having a mentally ill parent predisposes a child toward inadequate social development. Four variables representing specific aspects of social development have been selected for this study. The study children's peer aggression and friendship quality were assessed along with their emotional status in the first testing rounds of two independent samples (A and B). In the second testing rounds, peer network quality and emotional status were measured. The relation of these variables to two important covariates is considered, i.e., socioeconomic status and subjects' full-scale IQ. Many researchers believe that social competence is necessary to establish a social network, and it is included in this study to the extent that it is subsumed by subtests of IQ.

Methods

The New York High-Risk Project, described in detail elsewhere,[3] was concerned with two independent samples of children at risk for schizophrenic or affective disorders. This report focuses on the children at high risk for depression (the AF group), who were defined as having at least one hospitalized parent diagnosed, by the Research Diagnostic Criteria (RDC),[4] to have a major affective disorder or schizoaffective disorder, mainly affective. Each sample also includes a normal control group consisting of children whose parents are not psychiatrically disturbed.

Subsets of questions from the home interview with the "well" parent (the spouse of an AF patient-parent or a randomly selected normal parent) were used to create the parents' versions of the social variables. Children's versions were derived from a child interview. Questions comprising scale variables were selected ac-

cording to face validity, and a psychometric method was used for determining the internal consistency of the questions. Scales developing from the interviews are structured so that high scores indicate problems, and good scores are closer to zero (for details of the scale variables see ref. 5).

Results

Explanatory variables and covariates were tested as discriminators of parental diagnostic groups in both samples using one-way analysis of variance with a fixed-effects model. In sample A the AF children have both lower socioeconomic status and IQ than normal control children ($p<0.001$). As the socioeconomic status was matched in sample B, only IQ replicates the results of sample A, discriminating AF children ($p<0.005$) from normal control children.

Figure 77.1 is a depiction of comparisons between group means of social variables that are either significant or show trends toward significance. Peer aggression is the only explanatory variable that is noteworthy in rounds A1 and B1. In round A1 AF children had a trend toward more peer aggression than normal control children ($p<0.10$), and in round B1 this difference was clearly significant ($p<0.003$). AF children also had significantly less favorable ($p<0.03$) emotional status than normal control children in round B1 and showed a tendency in this direction in round B2 ($p<0.07$). These findings were not obtained in rounds A1 and A2. However, given that the sample B emotional status scales were the most reliable in this study, whereas they were unstable in sample A, the results of rounds B1 and B2 are important.

In round A2, peer network quality shows an unexpected trend ($p<0.14$) toward AF children having more satisfying peer groups than normal control children, but this result is not trustworthy because there was 50% attrition in the AF group between rounds A1 and A2. The expected result occurs in round B2, with normal control children having better peer networks than AF children ($p<0.06$). The round B2 results were more trustworthy, as there was almost no attrition between rounds B1 and B2. Thus by 12.5 years of age, all social variables showed that AF children had trends toward being deficient relative to normal children.

Discussion

The established finding that those with higher rates of impairment have lower IQ and socioeconomic status is also true for children at risk for depression. As social competence is subsumed by IQ, the data suggest that social competence plays an important role in the social development of high risk children. The replication of the result that the AF group had higher peer aggression than normal children in the first rounds of both samples makes this result important. When emotional status scales are reliable, as in rounds B1 and B2, AF children demonstrated lower emotional status than normal children. Thus AF children's high peer aggression scores were associated with low emotional status. The A2 peer network quality results are not reliable because of attrition, but in round B2 the AF children had qualitatively worse network quality scores than the normal children. Taken together these results indicate that by early adolescence AF children are demonstrating social and emotional difficulties similar to those of their parents.

Some theorists[6] have viewed persons prone to depression as highly socialized,

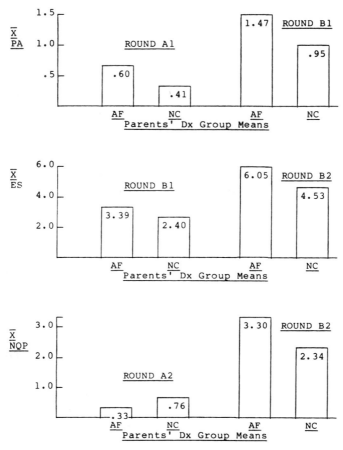

FIGURE 77.1. Histograms of group means for significant social development variables in rounds 1 and 2. (*AF*) high risk for affective disorders. (*NC*) normal control. (*PA*) peer aggression. (*ES*) emotional status. (*NQP*) network quality (peers).

paraphrasing Arieti,[7] who asserted that social overintegration characterizes depression. Watt et al.[8] found that children eventually hospitalized for depression were as socially competent as normal children. Some of the results on children at high risk for depression also indicate that they are as socially friendly as children of normals. In rounds A1 and B1 the peer friendship of the AF group was *not* significantly different from that of the normal group, and the A2 network quality result may be valid even though attrition occurred. Thus although the data seem contradictory, it appears that children of depressed parents are as social as children of normal parents in terms of friendship but have lower IQ scores and demonstrate *less satisfaction* with their social networks, as evidenced by their increased aggression and deficient emotional status relative to the children of normals.

References

1. Rosenthal D, Kety SS (eds). The Transmission of Schizophrenia. Oxford: Pergamon Press, 1968.
2. Depue RA (ed). The Psychobiology of the Depressive Disorders: Implications for the Effects of Stress. New York: Academic Press, 1979.
3. Erlenmeyer-Kimling L, Marcuse Y, Cornblatt B, et al. The New York high-risk project. In Watt N, Anthony EJ, Wynne L, et al (eds): Children at Risk for Schizophrenia: A Longitudinal Perspective. New York: Cambridge University Press, 1984;169–189.
4. Spitzer RL, Endicott J, Robins E. Research Diagnostic Criteria (RDC) for a Selected Group of Functional Disorders. 2nd Ed. New York: New York State Psychiatric Institute, 1975.
5. Davis WR. Coping Resources of Children at Risk for Mental Disorders. Docotoral dissertation. New York: The New School for Social Research, 1986.
6. Phillips L. Human Adaptation and Its Failure. New York: Academic Press, 1968.
7. Arieti S. Manic-depressive psychosis. In Arieti S (ed): American Handbook of Psychiatry. New York: Basic Books, 1959;419–454.
8. Watt NF, Prentky RA, Fryer JH. Childhood social competence in functionally disordered psychiatric patients and in normals. J Abnorm Psychol 1980;89:132–138.

78. Psychiatric Disorders in Children of Depressed Parents

HELEN ORVASCHEL

Children of depressed parents are an important resource for studying risk factors for affective illness. Children's home environments and parental interaction are likely to be affected, as depressed parents have been shown to be more irritable, less involved, and less affectionate with their children.[1,2] Retrospective studies have reported that the childhoods of depressed adults are more likely to include parental rejection, abuse, and family discord. Reviews of first generation research on children at risk for affective illness have been previously published and provide historical perspective and a more detailed summary of the convergence of evidence for risk.[3]

This chapter reports the preliminary findings of a study of the offspring of recurrently depressed parents. Data presented examine the type and magnitude of risk to these children. Parents with recurrent depression (three or more episodes) were selected in an effort to decrease the heterogeneity of affective illness in the patient group and to increase the likelihood of studying familial depression.[4]

Methods

Sample

Sixty-one children from 34 families comprised the high risk group, and 46 children from 29 families comprised the low risk group. All of the children (aged 6–17 years) were identified on the basis of their parents' psychiatric status. In the high risk group, at least one parent in each family was in treatment for recurrent major depression.

Control families were selected for study if neither parent met *DSM-III* criteria for any axis I psychiatric disorder. Most low risk families were obtained from the community of Allegheny County in Pittsburgh. Telephone screens were conducted to determine if the household had children who met our age criteria and were followed with general questions regarding parental psychopathology. This phase was followed by more formal parental assessment. No assessment of children was undertaken until parent assessments were completed and a decision of inclusion was determined.

Assessment Procedures

Demographic information was obtained for all families, and a SADS-L interview provided information about parents' history of psychopathology. Child psychopathology was assessed with the K-SADS-E.[5] A more detailed description of the methodology is reported elsewhere.[6]

Results
Demographic Characteristics

Efforts to match groups for income and social class resulted in no significant differences between groups on these variables. Social class was assigned on the basis on the Hollingshead two-factor index and again differed little between groups. Children ranged in age from 6 to 17 years, with mean ages of 10.7 and 11.1 years for the high and low risk groups, respectively. About 60% of children in both groups were between 6 and 11 years. The low risk group had a somewhat higher proportion of boys than did the high risk group (63% versus 53%). There were no significant differences between groups on verbal IQ (107 versus 109).

Child Psychopathology

Analysis of the psychopathology data was performed using chi-square tests of significance between high and low risk groups. An examination of the diagnostic findings showed consistently higher rates of psychopathology for children of depressed parents than for children whose parents had no psychopathology. Forty-one percent of high risk children met criteria for at least one psychiatric disorder at some time in their lives compared with 15% of low risk children. In addition, the high risk group more frequently met criteria for multiple diagnoses than the low risk group (23% versus 4%, respectively). These group differences were statistically significant.

As another indication of child psychopathology, we looked at the proportion of children in each group who had ever been treated or received medication for emotional or behavioral problems, as well as the percentage of children who had ever made a suicide attempt. About 33% of the high risk group, compared with 9% of the low risk group, have been in outpatient treatment, including long-term care for several, and it was statistically significant. None of the low risk children had ever been hospitalized or received medication for psychopathology, and none had ever attempted suicide, whereas in the high risk group two children had been hospitalized, four had received medication, and three had made suicide attempts. However, these differences were not statistically significant, probably because of the small cell sizes.

Rates of the most frequently occurring psychiatric disorders are presented in Table 78.1. The categories are not mutually exclusive. Significant differences between groups were found for affective disorders and attention deficit disorder (ADD), and a nonsignificant trend was noted for anxiety disorders, all of which were higher for the high risk children. The prevalance rates for ADD in the low risk group were similar to expected population rates for boys and girls, but in the high risk group rates of ADD for boys and girls were almost equal. In the low risk group, one male child had an adjustment disorder with depressed mood and

TABLE 78.1. Prevalence of types of disorders by group.

| | High-risk group | | | Low-risk group | | | |
Type	Male (n = 32)	Female (n = 29)	Total (n = 61)	Male (n = 29)	Female (n = 17)	Total (n = 46)	p
Affective disorder	18.8	24.1	21.3	3.4	5.9	4.3	< 0.008
Anxiety disorder	18.8	20.7	19.7	10.3	5.9	8.7	N.S.
ADD	21.9	17.2	19.7	10.3	0	6.5	< 0.05

one female adolescent had dysthymia, but no low risk child met criteria for major depression (MDD).

Affective Illness

A more detailed examination of affective illness in the high risk group is presented in Table 78.2. Although there were no statistically significant sex differences, girls had somewhat higher rates of MDD and dysthymia, and they were more likely to have both, listed as double depression. Boys and girls were equally likely to be treated for affective illness, but two girls were also hospitalized and three girls had made suicide attempts. All the girls had had a prepubertal onset of affective illness, as had all but one of the boys. The one girl who met the criteria for mania had a postpubertal onset of manic disorder and a prepubertal onset of dysthymia, and her major depression included psychotic symptoms. About 85% of the high risk children who met the criteria for an affective illness had received some form of treatment for their depression.

Discussion

The children in this study were a nonclinically referred sample identified as a function of the presence or absence of parental psychopathology. Prevalence estimates for affective disorders in preadolescent children have been reported to range from 2 to 7%.[7,8] The rate for the low risk children in this study was 5% compared with 21% in high risk children.

Rates of psychopathology in the children of depressed parents were considerably higher when compared with either the low risk group or the estimated rates of disorder for nonreferred children from other studies. In fact, although quantitative differences between the groups were pronounced, qualitative differences (not reflected in the tables) were even stronger. The high risk children had not only

TABLE 78.2. Affective illness in high-risk group.

| | Male (n = 32) | | Female (n = 29) | | Total (n = 61) | |
Illness	No.	%	No.	%	No.	%
Mania	0	0	1	3.4	1	1.6
MDD	4	12.5	5	17.2	9	14.8
Dysthymia	3	9.4	6	20.7	9	14.8
Double depression	1	3.1	4	13.8	5	8.2
Any affective disorder	6	18.8	7	24.1	13	21.3
Treated	5	83.3	6	85.7	11	84.6

higher rates of all types of disorder, but their psychopathology was more severe, as reflected by their impaired functioning and their need for longer-term mental health intervention. Also, the high risk children had a very early age of onset for depression.

We are now examining the psychiatric histories of extended family members of the children in this study, as well as family environment measures, in order to explore possible explanations for the increased prevalence of psychopathology, particularly depression and attention deficit disorder in children of depressed parents. Our findings indicate that these children not only have higher rates of disorder than children of psychiatrically healthy parents, but that they have an early age of onset of psychopathology. We hope to identify specific risk factors associated with the occurrence of these disorders so that we can test their predictive value and examine their potential for primary prevention strategies.

Acknowledgment. This work was supported in part by W.T. Grant Foundation Faculty Scholar Award 8308700.

References

1. Anthony EJ, Ittleson BF. The effects of maternal depression on the infant. Presented at the Symposium on Infant Psychiatry III, San Francisco, 1980.
2. Weissman MM, Paykel ES, Klerman GL. The depressed woman as a mother. Soc. Psychiatry 1972;7:98–108.
3. Orvaschel H. Maternal depression and child dysfunction: children at risk. In Lahey B, Kazdin A (eds): Advances in Clinical Child Psychology. Vol. 6. New York: Academic Press, 1983;169–197.
4. Gershon ES, Weissman MM, Guroff JJ, et al. Validation of criteria for major depression through controlled family study. J Affective Disord 1986;11:125–131.
5. Orvaschel H. Psychiatric interviews suitable for use in research with children and adolescents. Psychopharmacol Bull [Special Issue] 1986;21:737–745.
6. Orvaschel H, Walsh-Allis G, Ye W. Psychopathology in children of parents with recurrent depression. J Abnorm Child Psychol 1988;16:17–28.
7. Kashani JH, Simond JF. The incidence of depression in children. AM J Psychiatry 1979;136:1203–1205.
8. Kashani JH, Barbero GJ, Bolander FD. Depression in hospitalized pediatric patients. J Am Acad Child Psychiatry 1981;20:123–134.

48. High Affinity Imipramine Binding and Serotonin Uptake in Human Platelets as a Peripheral Biological Marker in Neuropsychiatric Disorders

MOSHE REHAVI, RONIT WEIZMAN, AND
ABRAHAM WEIZMAN

High affinity binding sites for [³H]imipramine have been demonstrated and characterized in rat and human brain[1,2] and platelets.[3,4] These binding sites are functionally related to the presynaptic uptake or transport site for serotonin and are probably involved in the well known inhibition effect of tricyclic antidepressants on biogenic amine uptake.[5] A significant decrease in the density of [³H]imipramine binding sites in platelets of severely depressed patients compared to age- and sex-matched controls was reported by Briley et al.[6] and Paul et al.[7] These results were replicated by several investigators (reviewed in refs. 8,9), although other studies have not confirmed this decrease.[10] Chronic imipramine treatment induced parallel decreases in [³H]imipramine binding and serotonin uptake in cat platelets and brain, suggesting that these sites are functionally related.[11] It seems that the decrease in the number of imipramine binding sites in platelets of major depressed patients reflects parallel changes in human brain, as low values of Bmax for [³H]imipramine binding were observed in frontal cortex and hypothalamus of suicides.[12,13] The involvement of the serotonergic system in the pathophysiology of depression is further supported by the low serotonin uptake to platelets of patients with major depression[14] and reduced 5-hydroxyindoleacetic acid (5-HIAA) levels in the cerebrospinal fluid (CSF) of affective patients.[15] It was reported that platelet [³H]imipramine binding might serve as a possible predictor of response to antidepressant treatment[16]; it was also reported to be correlated with the severity of depression[17] and to distinguish among subtypes of depression.[18].

As the manifestations of affective disorder in children and adolescents are not always identical to those of adult affective disorders, we assessed [³H]imipramine binding parameters in platelets of depressed children and adolescents compared to those in normal controls and nonaffective patients.[19] Imipramine binding values did not discriminate between depressed patients and the two control groups. It might be that the young population included in this research has not been exposed to the affective disease for a long enough period or that the symptoms of depression in youngsters do not necessarily imply endogenous depression of the adult type. This possibility is supported by reports suggesting that the dexamethasone suppression test (DST) does not discriminate between major depression and other psychiatric disorders in this age group.[20]

Obsessive compulsive disorder (OCD) is another psychiatric entity associated frequently with depressive symptoms. A serotonergic dysfunction has been suggested to be involved in the pathophysiology of this disorder. This hypothesis is based on the beneficial effect of clomipramine and L-trytophan treatment as well as on the correlation between positive responses to clomipramine treatment and reduced concentration of 5-HIAA in CSF. The maximal binding of [^{3}H]imipramine was significantly lower in both adults and adolescents with OCD compared to matched control subjects. The decreased imipramine binding was not accompanied by a parallel reduction in serotonin uptake.[21] Because a similar lower density was observed in both adolescent and adult OCD patients, it seems that this biochemical correlate is not related to the duration of the disease and may implicate involvement of the serotonergic system in the etiopathology.

A central cholinergic deficit is the most prominent biochemical alteration in dementia of the Alzehiemer's type (DAT). In addition to this impairment there is evidence of hypofunction of the serotonergic system, including reduced serotonergic neurons in the dorsal raphe nucleus, lower serotonin levels in brain, reduced CSF 5-HIAA levels, diminished serotonin turnover, and lower serotonin uptake and imipramine binding to brain tissue.[22] In a study conducted in our laboratory, the [^{3}H]imipramine binding values did not differ between DAT patients and controls.[23] These results are in accordance with a previous study by Suranyi-Cadotte et al.[24] which proposed that imipramine binding to platelets distinguishes depression from DAT. It seems that the decrease in serotonergic activity in DAT is confined to brain tissue and is not extended to the platelets.

Sex steroid hormones as well as the serotonergic system have been suggested to play a role in depression. Affective changes are observed in women during the menstrual cycle, postpartum period, menopause, and oral contraceptive treatment. These observations indicate that alterations in the levels of female gonadal sex hormones can induce affective disorders, hormonal fluctuations that may impact on the regulation of brain biogenic amines. It has been reported that estradiol treatment regulates serotonin turnover and serotonin postsynaptic receptors in rat brain. We investigated the effect of triphasic oral contraceptive (Logynon) treatment in women on the density of [^{3}H]imipramine binding sites in their platelets. Two cycles of Logynon treatment resulted in a significant increase in imipramine binding sites.[25] The pill contains a combination of ethinyl estradiol and levonorgestrel, and it is as yet unclear which of the two hormones is responsible for the up-regulatory effect. It was not clear if this change is accompanied by a similar alteration in the brain. In a comparison study in ovariectomized rats we investigated the effect of chronic estradiol treatment on the serotonin transporter in the brain. Both serotonin uptake and imipramine binding increased by 20–30% in the frontal cortex and hypothalamus after 12 days of 17β-estradiol treatment.[26] The up-regulation of imipramine binding sites observed after estradiol administration may indicate a pharmacological similarity in the activity of estradiol and some of the tricyclic antidepressants at this site. We do not have enough evidence to draw conclusions about the linkage between imipramine binding sites, estradiol level, and depression.

III.C. AFFECTIVE DISORDERS IN THE ELDERLY

79. Diagnostic Criteria for Depression in Alzheimer's Disease

GERALD OPPENHEIM

Depression and Alzheimer's disease (AD) are the two commonest mental disorders in the elderly; coexistence of the two conditions might therefore be expected to be a not infrequent occurrence. Reifler et al.[1] found that 31% of 131 AD patients met *DSM-III* criteria for major affective disorder; and Lazarus et al.[2] scored 20% of 44 AD patients as 17 or above on the Hamilton Scale for Depression.

Symptoms of depression and dementia can be highly similar, a situation that might lead to the depressive syndrome remaining unrecognized and being misperceived as part of the neurodegenerative disease. On the other hand, a significant number of items in commonly used diagnostic criteria for depression (such as *DSM-III* or Hamilton Scale) might fail to distinguish depression from dementia, thus leading to an artificially high rate of diagnosed depression in patients with AD.

As a preliminary investigation aimed at developing diagnostic criteria for depression coexisting with AD, we compared the items of a depressive symptom profile *(DSM-III)* in depressed and nondepressed AD patients.

Methods

Diagnosis of AD

The study subjects were outpatients in our Alzheimer's Disease Treatment and Study Program. Patients are diagnosed as suffering from "probable AD" after psychiatric, neuropsychological, medical, neurological, and clinical laboratory evaluations to exclude other causes of dementia (Work Group on AD[3]).

Diagnosis of Depression

The diagnosis of depression was based on psychiatric evaluation of each patient and an interview of relatives by the author (an experienced geriatric psychiatrist). Clinical depression was diagnosed when a patient was judged to display the definite syndrome of endogenous[4] or vital[5] depression, the primary aim being to distinguish those patients who might respond to antidepressant drug treatment. Sixteen of 58

AD patients (27.6%) were thus diagnosed as suffering from clinical depression. Because of our doubts over the reliability of currently available criteria for diagnosing depression in AD patients, the diagnosis of depression was not based on a score of any standard set of criteria. However, with a view to performing this study, each patient diagnosed as depressed was then screened for "major depressive episode" criteria according to *DSM-III*.[6]

Non-Depressed Group

The control group was 25 AD patients who, at a recent follow-up evaluation, were judged not to be clinically depressed (as described above). Each of these patients was also screened for *DSM-III* criteria for "major depressive episode."

Additional Item ("Recent Rapid Worsening")

In our experience a "recent rapid worsening" in the clinical state of an AD patient may point to a depressive syndrome complicating the dementia; this item was therefore added to the assessment procedure.

Statistics

The two groups were compared on the depression criteria using chi-square with Yates correction (one degree of freedom).

Results

As seen in Table 79.1, 6 of 12 *DSM-III* depression criteria failed to differentiate ($p > 0.05$) between the nondepressed and the depressed group. Stated clinically, six of the depression items are also characteristic features of AD. Four depression items highly significantly differentiated between the two groups: depressed mood ($p = 0.0001$), recent rapid worsening ($p = 0.0001$), loss of appetite ($p = 0.002$),

TABLE 79.1. DSM-III depression criteria in nondepressed and depressed Alzheimer's disease patients.

Criterion	Nondepressed ($n = 25$)		Depressed ($n = 16$)		χ^2	p
Depressed mood	8	(32%)	16	(100%)	15.89	0.0001
Poor appetite	2	(8%)	9	(56%)	9.24	0.002
Weight loss	13	(52%)	10	(63%)	0.11	0.74
Sleep disturbance	6	(24%)	10	(63%)	4.57	0.03
Psychomotor change	9	(36%)	11	(69%)	2.98	0.08
Loss of interest	24	(96%)	16	(100%)	—	—
Loss of energy	4	(16%)	8	(50%)	3.93	0.047
Worthlessness, guilt	8	(32%)	12	(75%)	5.60	0.02
Complaints re thinking	18	(72%)	13	(81%)	0.09	0.76
Evidence re thinking	25	(100%)	16	(100%)	—	—
Death, suicide	5	(20%)	12	(75%)	9.99	0.002
Delusions, hallucinations	13	(52%)	8	(50%)	—	—
Recent rapid worsening[a]	4	(16%)	13	(81%)	14.5	0.0001

[a]Not in *DSM-III* (see "Methods").

and recurrent thoughts of death or suicide ($p = 0.002$). Three additional items were also significant differentiators: worthlessness or guilty ruminations ($p = 0.02$), early wakening or hypersomnia ($p = 0.03$), and loss of energy ($p = 0.047$). These seven items are shown in Table 79.2.

Discussion

This study was based on a valid and well accepted diagnostic instrument for depression, *DSM-III*. The aim was to tease out those items of *DSM-III* that are sensitive and valid indicators of clinical depression coexisting with AD—items capable of pointing to depression despite the coexisting clinical features of the dementing illness.

An in-depth understanding of the clinical phenomenology of AD and of depression is essential for clinical evaluation of such patients, and any set of criteria can act only as an aid to diagnosis. For example, "depressed mood" was found in 32% of the control group but not as the pervasive, continual mood state sometimes with diurnal variation as is seen in clinical depression. AD patients characteristically eat well or excessively but nevertheless lose weight; thus "poor appetite," but not "weight loss," would be expected to be a sensitive depression criterion.

The nature of the sleep disturbance is different in AD and depression: middle of the night awakening with confused disoriented behavior rather than early morning agitated awakening; the only two patients with hypersomnia were in the depressed group. Loss of physical energy in the usually hyperactive AD patient is a significant pointer to depression. Our clinical impression was confirmed that, when asked directly, most AD patients are aware of difficulty with thinking processes and memory, even in quite advanced stages.

Preexisting mood-incongruent delusions or hallucinations were seen equally in both groups, apparently as a clinical feature of AD and unrelated to depression. "Recent rapid worsening" in an AD patient indicated the possibility of depression.

The accuracy of diagnosis of depression in patients with AD has significant implications for epidemiological, clinical, and treatment studies. In addition, drug treatment of such depression may improve the patient's clinical/behavioral state and lessen the burden on the caregiver—important to therapy when dealing with a progressive illness with no known effective treatment.

Our suggested criteria to aid the diagnosis of depression in Alzheimer's disease (DAD) need further evaluation in larger numbers of patients and crosscultural validation.

TABLE 79.2. Suggested criteria for diagnosis of depression in Alzheimer's disease. (DAD)

Continually depressed mood
Recent rapid deterioration
Loss of appetite
Recurrent thoughts of death or suicide
Worthlessness, guilty ruminations
Early awakening or hypersomnia
Loss of energy

References

1. Reifler BV, Larson E, Teri L, et al. Dementia of the Alzheimer's type and depression. J Am Geriatr Soc 1986;34:855–859.
2. Lazarus LW, Newton N, Cohler B, et al. Frequency and presentation of depressive symptoms in patients with primary degenerative dementia. Am J Psychiatry 1987;144:41–45.
3. McKhann GD, Drachman M, Folstein R, et al. Clinical diagnosis of Alzheimer's disease. Neurology 1984;34:939–944.
4. Kiloh LG, Garside RF. The independence of neurotic depression and endogenous depression. Br J Psychiatry 1963;109:451–463.
5. Schneider K. The stratification of emotional life and the structure of the depressive states. Z Ges Neurol Psychiatr 1920;59:281–285.
6. Diagnostic and Statistical Manual of Mental Disorders. 3rd Ed. Washington, DC: American Psychiatric Association, 1980.

80. Association of Somatic Disease with Affective Disorders in Middle and Old Age

MARTIN ROTH

The relation between depression and somatic disease in elderly patients was first submitted to systematic investigation during the 1950s. Patients with depressive illness admitted to psychiatric hospital were found to have a high prevalence of somatic disease.[1,2] This finding could have been due to the higher likelihood of admission in those depressed patients who also suffered from somatic disease. However, epidemiological study of a random community sample of people aged 65 years and over in the same area ruled out this explanation. The prevalence of physical disease among those with psychiatric disorders proved to be significantly greater than that found among mentally healthy controls from the same population.[3,4]

Epidemiological investigation of a sample of individuals on a new housing estate[5] found the same association and showed that the increased prevalence of physical disease among those with psychiatric disorder was to be found in all age groups. Eastwood and Trevelyan[6] recorded similar findings in the course of a study in general practice; they investigated physical and psychiatric status independently using strict and objective criteria for both.

It remained possible that the association was due to the greater propensity of those with depressive illness than mentally healthy subjects to complain of minor physical symptoms. However, those diagnosed as suffering from affective disorder within a random sample of people aged 65 years drawn from the same population as that studied by Kay et al.[3,4] were found to have a significantly shorter life expectation than mentally healthy subjects.[7] This finding tended to invalidate "cry for help" explanations of the connection between affective illness and somatic disease.

Investigations of patients with depression in middle life by Kerr et al.[8] showed the same increased mortality. The authors also reported a significant increase in mortality from carcinoma among their depressed patients. As the neoplastic disease was not discovered until postmortem examination in some patients, the depressive illness could not have been due in all cases to the emotional threat posed by malignant disease. A study by Evans and Whitlock[9] undertaken in a consecutive series of admissions to a Cambridge psychiatric hospital over a 4-year period has confirmed that patients with affective disorder have a mortality rate above normal expectancy. The characteristics of the association (to be described below) were similar to those in the earlier studies cited.

Some Features of the Association Between Affective Disorder and Somatic Disease

In the investigations undertaken in aged subjects in Newcastle cited above the association between physical disease and depression proved to have certain consistent features.

1. Acute physical illness was not found in significant excess among the depressed patients. Only *chronic* physical disease was significantly correlated with depressive illness.

2. The increased prevalence of somatic disease was confined to men; women did not differ significantly in this respect from control subjects.

3. The abridgement of life expectancy was also confined to male subjects. It was not significantly decreased among women.

4. The concomitant somatic disease found in excessive prevalence among the men may have been the entire cause of the increased mortality; this could not be established with certainty. The possibility that the depression had made some independent contribution remained open.

5. The etiological relation between depression and the concomitant somatic disease was complex. The association between psychic and somatic disorder was neither necessary nor sufficient. Even in an advanced stage many patients with physical disease did not suffer from affective disorder. On the other hand, a substantial proportion of patients with severe depressive illness were found to be physically healthy, and the emotional and somatic disease pursued relatively independent courses in some patients. There was a good response to appropriate antidepressant treatment in a proportion of patients in whom somatic disease could only be relieved or in whom it proved untreatable. On the other hand, physical disease might come under control without corresponding change in the depression. The affective disorder would then require treatment in its own right, and it would often prove effective.

6. Whether the course pursued by depression of the aged is similar to that of comparable affective disorders in earlier life is uncertain. The long-term prognosis of depression in the elderly has been found generally poor by some workers. However, any investigation into this question would have to take into account the contribution to prognosis made by chronic and intractable illness, the pain and disablement entailed, and the abridged expectation of life of elderly subjects. No comparative study of prognosis during late and early life that has satisfactorily controlled these variables has been undertaken to date.

7. A wide range of chronic diseases contributes to the association between depressive illness and somatic disease. They include rheumatoid arthritis, diabetes, chronic cardiac disease, myocardial infarction with residual cardiac decompensation, and carcinoma in a variety of sites. Some of the associated conditions, including pulmonary tuberculosis and subacute bacterial endocarditis were, until a few decades ago, diseases mainly confined to earlier life. During old age they present in a relatively "silent" manner, as do pyelonephritis and hyperthyroidism. The latter presents without the characteristic features of this condition in earlier life; exophthalmos, tachycardia, and thyroid enlargement may be absent. A com-

bination of depression, apathy, and atrial fibrillation or other pulse irregularity may be the leading features. Myxedema and hyperparathyroidism may manifest in the first instances in the form of depression of affect, marked fatigue, and suicidal ideation.

Causal Relation Between Somatic Disease and Affective Disorder

It is often assumed that chronic physical disease contributes to the causation of depression by the pain, malaise, and disablement it causes. This is probably the usual direction of causality; the depression is more often than not secondary to the physiological and psychological effects of the organic disease. However, the possibility that depression contributes to the causation of some forms of physical illness through its influence on immunological functions is being investigated to an increasing extent. Moreover, there is a limited body of evidence to *suggest* that complication of a chronic physical illness by a depressive disorder decreases life expectancy.[10]

Among observations that have helped to define the manner in which disorder of affect and chronic disease interact to aggravate the disablement and increase mortality have been those undertaken in the case of cardiac dysrhythmia by Lown and his colleagues.[11] They investigated 117 patients in whom arrhythmias triggered by onerous life events were judged to have developed in 25. This subgroup proved to have less severe cardiac disease but more serious arrhythmias than the remaining patients. In 15 of these 25 patients some threatening life circumstance had been experienced less than 1 h before the onset of arrhythmia; in 17 of the 25 the most common emotional antecedent had been anger.

Personality Variables

Observations have shed light on some of the personality variables underlying these adverse effects of emotional disturbance on cardiovascular disease. There is evidence for a relation between "type A" behavior and ischemic heart disease independent of other risk factors, e.g., smoking, blood pressure, and serum cholesterol level.[12] The concept of type A behavior is controversial. A stricter operational definition of the personality profile to which it refers and more evidence regarding the reliability over time of the measures that are used are needed. Yet the observations placed on record in recent years must be taken into account in clinical practice and also merit other scientific inquiry. A number of laboratory stressors such as mental arithmetic have been found to evoke cardiovascular hyperresponsivity among type A individuals. These stressors also caused increased secretion of cortisol and testosterone in certain situations; a rise in cortisol levels was induced by mental work, and testosterone was increased by tasks that entailed sensory input.

Depression and Arterial Hypertension

The important studies of Sainsbury and his colleagues[13] have established a relation between emotional disorder and essential hypertension. They found a significant correlation in the blood pressure level on the one hand and the duration and number of attacks of illness following recovery from one such attack of depressive illness on the other. Hypertensive and normotensive groups of depressives were significantly differentiated from each other by the number of attacks of depression suffered and their total duration, but not by genetic factors or differing treatments.

Physical Disease and Suicide

Studies of consummated suicides have consistently brought to light an increased prevalence of somatic disease including carcinoma. In a study of suicide in London, Sainsbury[14] found 14 cases of cancer among 390 suicides, an incidence 20 times greater than that found in the general population.

Kreitman[15] compared those suicides who had a history of a previous attempt with those whose first attempt had proved fatal. The age of the former peaked in the 45- to 54-year age bracket distribution and the latter a decade later. The former were characterized by personality disorder or psychopathy often complicated by alcholism or drug dependence, unemployment, and crime. In contrast, those who had made their first attempt proved to be a relatively stable group in whom a recent bereavement or loss ("loss of a significant other") or a physical illness had been a significantly more frequent antecedent to the suicidal act. A family history of suicide was elicited twice as often in those making their first and last attempt.

Barraclough et al.[16] found that most elderly suicides (70–80%) suffered from endogenous depression. The typical subject according to Barraclough et al. is a man whose first attack appears after the age of 40 years, lives alone, has a family history of depression or alcoholism, and has suffered a recent loss. He experiences early morning insomnia, weight loss, reduction in activities, hypochondriasis, guilt, difficulty in concentration, and unobtrusive hypochondriasis.

Role of Personality Factors

Physical illness is not equipotent in producing depression or generating suicidal behavior in all middle-aged and aged persons. It influences certain predisposed individuals, for whom illness and disablement carry a special meaning, with a selective severity. When the first physical illness develops during middle life or later and carries some threat of a chronic aftermath or worse, it tends to overwhelm emotional equilibrium. Yet the coping mechanisms of the individual in question are often found to have been equal in the past for dealing with other forms of stress and challenge. The developmental history and the record of adaptation to a variety of social and personal roles generally provide insight into the menacing significance of physical disablement. A proportion are found to have had a physical deformity of early onset, and in others overinvestment of effort and time in the cultivation of physical fitness will have originated from different causes. A parody of this kind of disorder is provided by the phenonemon of "athlete's neurosis" investigated by Little.[17]

These severe forms of the syndrome may provide some clues to the predominance of men among those in middle and late life whose depressive illness is closely intertwined with the development of physical illness. The threat of disablement that this picture conjures up in men augurs loss of strength and virility, and of prestige and mastery for those in particular in whom self-esteem leans heavily on unfailing physical strength, health, and integrity. Women's experience of physical pain and discomfort is different from that of men. Menstruation, childbirth, and their physical and emotional concomitants familiarize them early in life with the fragility and imperfection of the human physical constitution. Physical strength and endurance, athletic achievement, mastery, and dominance have in the past rarely figured prominently in the self-image of women. Limited impairments that do not disfigure are less of a threat to women's self-esteem.

Summary and Conclusions

The prevalence of somatic disease in depressive illness during the later years of life is significantly in excess of normal expectation. It is with chronic rather than with acute illness that affective disorder of later life is associated. The significant excess is confined to those of the male sex, and it is also only men in whom life expectancy is abridged. Similar associations have come to light in connection with consummated suicide. There are therefore probably genetic and biological dimensions underlying the correlation of somatic and affective disorder during late and middle life. However, there is also evidence to suggest that physical illness and disablement have emotional implications that are particularly threatening for men and that psychodynamic features play some part in the genesis of depressive states in a proportion of patients.

There is a limited body of evidence to suggest that the presence of concomitant depressive disorder is associated with length of survival in patients who suffer from somatic disorder[18] and in those with cancer.[19] The evidence is conflicting, and further studies are needed. Suicide is a relatively rare event in those with chronic disease and even in patients with cancer. However, in the controlled study by Whitlock[20] of 173 suicides and a group of victims of motor accidents matched for age and sex, there were 21 cases of malignant disorder among the suicides compared with two among the victims of motor accidents. There are some difficulties attached to the interpretation of these results, but there is evidence to suggest[21] that it is depressive illness rather than pain and other factors associated with the malignancy, such as its progress, that is associated with the increased prevalence of suicide.

Treatment of the patient with a physical disorder who has a concomitant depression should consist in the first instance of supportives psychotherapy, counseling of the patient and his family, adequate control of pain, and where depression is severe the use of tricyclic compounds or monoamine oxidase inhibitors. However, treatment with drugs should not be undertaken as a matter of routine. In patients with indubitable endogenous features, antidepressive drugs should be administered and their effects carefully monitored and with due caution. Such treatment should also be tried in patients with less specific forms of depression. Clinical observations show that the quality of life is greatly improved in those patients with chronic somatic illness, including malignant disease, in whom depressive illness is diagnosed and treated.

This body of findings should therefore be applied with discrimination and sensitivity in the holistic care of patients in general medicine as well as psychiatry. They define a large new area of scientific investigation for all disciplines within medicine.

References

1. Kay DWK, Roth M. Physical accompaniments of mental disorder in old age. Lancet 1955;2:740–745.
2. Roth M, Kay DWK. Affective disorder arising in the senium. II. Physical disability as an aetiological factor. J Med Sci 1956;102:141–150.
3. Kay DWK, Beamish P, Roth M. Old age mental disorders in Newcastle upon Tyne. I. A study of prevalence. Br J Psychiatry 1964;110:146–158.
4. Kay DWK, Beamish P, Roth M. Old age mental disorders in Newcastle upon Tyne. II. A study of possible social and medical causes. Br J Psychiatry 1964;110:668–687.
5. Hare EH, Shaw GK. Mental Health in a New Housing Estate: a Comparative Study of Health in Two Districts of Croydon. Maudsley Monograph No. 12. Oxford: Oxford University Press, 1965.
6. Eastwood MR, Trevelyan MH. Relationship between physical and psychiatric disorder. Psychol Med 1972;2:363–372.
7. Kay DWK, Bergmann K. Physical disability and mental health in old age: a follow-up of a random sample of elderly people seen at home. J Psychosom Res 1966;10:3.
8. Kerr TA, Schapira K, Roth M. The relationship between premature death and affective disorder. Br J Psychiatry 1969;115:1277.
9. Evans NJ, Whitlock FA. Mortality and late-onset of affective disorder. J Affective Disord 1983;5:297–304.
10. Petty F, Noyes R Jr. Depression secondary to cancer. Biol Psychiatry 1981;16:1203–1220.
11. Lown B, De Silva RA, Reich P, et al: Psychophysiologic factors in sudden cardiac death. Am J Psychiatry 1980;137:1325–1335.
12. Rosenman RH, Brand RJ, Jenkins CD, et al. Coronary heart disease in the Western Collaborative Group Study: final follow-up experience of 8½ years. JAMA 1975;233:862–877.
13. Heine BE, Sainsbury P, Chynoweth TC. Hypertension and emotional disturbance. J Psychiatr Res 1969;7:119–130.
14. Sainsbury P. Suicide in London. Maudsley Monograph No. 1. London: Chapman, 1955.
15. Kreitman N. Parasuicide. Chap. 9. New York: Wiley, 1977.
16. Barraclough B, Bunch J, Nelson B, et al. A hundred cases of suicide: clinical aspects. Br J Psychiatry 1974;125:355–373.
17. Little CJ. The athlete's neurosis—a deprivation crisis. Acta Psychiatr Scand 1969;45:187–193.
18. Stewart MA, Drake I, Winokur G. Depression among medically ill inpatients. Dis Nerv Syst 1965;26:479–485.
19. Achte K, Vonhkonen ML. Cancer and Psyche. Helsinki: Kunnallispaino, 1970.
20. Whitlock FA. Suicide, cancer and depression. Br J Psychiatry 1978;132:269–274.
21. Fox BH, Stanek EJ, Boyd SC, et al. Suicide rates among cancer patients in Connecticut. J Chronic Dis 1982;35:89–99.

81. Excess Mortality in Late Life Depression

E. MURPHY AND J.E.B. LINDESAY

Outcome studies of affective disorders have repeatedly demonstrated a high mortality rate in elderly patients compared with general population groups of the same age. This excess mortality, which is not accounted for by suicides, is particularly marked in men. In one study the mortality during a 1-year follow-up of a group of 124 elderly depressed patients in east London was 19% for men and 11% for women, three times the expected rate for men and double that for women.[1]

The straightforward explanation for this increased mortality is that a proportion of elderly depressed patients have poor physical health. Physical disease and disability are associated with depression in old age and have been demonstrated to adversely affect outcome. The excess mortality associated with depression in this age group may be entirely accounted for by this excess of physical illness. The study reported herein investigated whether physical health problems alone can satisfactorily explain the excess mortality of a group of elderly depressed patients followed up over a 4-year period.

Methods

The study was designed as a comparison between a group of elderly subjects suffering from depression and a psychiatrically fit group of community controls, both groups examined prospectively with regard to their physical health problems and followed up over a 4-year period.

The *depressed group* comprised 124 elderly depressed patients of 65 years and over referred to psychiatric services in east London. Subjects satisfied the Feighner criteria for primary depression.[2] In addition, there were 29 subjects with similarly severe depression found in the community survey who were included with the depressed group.

The *community control group* was a random sample of 266 elderly subjects chosen from the age-sex registers of two general practices in east London, matched by age (60–74 and 75 + years) and by sex with the depressed patient group. Those community subjects with evidence of organic cerebral disorder, anxiety states, and alcohol dependence were excluded. There were a total of 168 community controls who were psychiatrically fit or had minor symptoms only. The transfer of depressed subjects to the depressed group did not affect the comparability of the two groups.

The *interview* of all subjects included demographic data, physical health using a standardized schedule, psychiatric interview using the Present State Examination,[3] the organic questions from the Survey Psychiatric Assessment Schedule,[4] and lastly the Bedford College Life Events and Difficulties Schedule (LEDS).[5] Information about physical health was also collected from medical notes.

On the basis of the medical interviews, the LEDS interview, and information from medical records, for the *physical health rating* each subject was scored on a scale of chronic health difficulties from 1–6. Ratings of 1–3 represented severe health problems, and ratings of 4–6 represented less serious problems. In addition, acute physical illness events that occurred during the year before the interview were also rated on an equivalent 1–6 scale of severity using Brown and Harris's methodology.[5]

Follow-up of patients was done in person, and those alive and agreeable were reinterviewed. The community group was followed up only by inquiry of the general practitioners and by a search in the local death returns of the Environmental Health Department. Causes of death were available for most of the patients who died but not for those in the community group.

Results

Physical Health

A total of 97% (120/124) of patients and 98% (193/197) of community controls were traced 4 years after the initial interview. As expected, there was an excess of poor physical health in the depressed group at initial interview when compared with the nondepressed community group: 53.6% of depressed subjects had experienced a severe health event or had major chronic physical health problems compared with 38.1% of the community group ($p < 0.01$).

Four-Year Mortality

The overall mortality of the depressed group was 34.2% and that of the community group 14%; the difference was more striking in men (Table 81.1). When compared with the expected mortality rate from the local official statistics, the observed mortality rate in the control group was less than expected, especially for men, whereas in the depressed group mortality was significantly greater than expected. The community sample may therefore have been healthier than the overall local

TABLE 81.1. Four-year mortality in depressed and control groups.

Group	Depressed %	No.	Control %	No.	p
Men	41.9	18/43	8.8	5/57	< 0.001
Women	31.0	32/103	16.8	18/107	< 0.05
Total	34.2	50/146	14.0	23/164	< 0.05

population and thus may have contributed to the difference between sexes in the observed excess mortality in the depressed group.

Physical Health and Subsequent Mortality

Table 81.2 shows that physical health problems alone do not explain the increased mortality of the depressed group, which remains excessive when physical health is taken into account. As expected, those in both groups with serious health problems at initial interview were more likely to have died.

Social Factors and Mortality

Socioeconomic group, living alone, marital status, income, and type of housing did not satisfactorily account for the differences in mortality between the two groups.

Discussion

Methodological problems in this study included difficulty assessing the state of the subjects' general physical health by interview and from notes as well as the differences in mortality between the control group and the local population statistics, suggesting that the control group was in relatively better health. However, these results suggest that physical illness is only one factor involved in the increased mortality rates of elderly patients with depression. If this excess mortality is not due to physical illness apparent at the time of initial interview, either there is occult disease present that is specifically associated with depression, the depression itself predisposes to subsequent nonsuicidal mortality, or there are factors that are associated with both depression and an increased risk of death.

Acknowledgment. The authors acknowledge the assistance of Jim Slattery and Rae Smith in completing this study.

TABLE 81.2. Mortality rates in depressed and control groups by physical health problems.

Group	Depressed		Control		
	%	No.	%	No.	p
Severe health event or chronic health difficulty					
Men	50.0	14/28	9.5	2/21	< 0.01
Women	41.2	21/51	24.4	10/41	NS
Total	44.3	35/79	19.4	12/62	< 0.01
Minor health problems only or physically fit					
Men	26.7	4/15	8.3	3/36	NS
Women	21.2	11/52	12.1	8/66	< 0.05
Total	22.4	15/67	10.8	11/102	NS

References

1. Murphy E. The prognosis of depression in old age. Br J Psychiatry 1983;142:111–119.
2. Feighner JP, Robins E, Guze SB, et al. Diagnostic criteria for use in psychiatric research. Arch Gen Psychiatry 1972;26:57–73.
3. Wing JK, Cooper JE, Sartorius N. Measurement and Classification of Psychiatric Symptoms. Cambridge: Cambridge University Press, 1974.
4. Bond J, Brooks P, Carstairs V, et al. Reliability of a survey psychiatric assessment schedule for the elderly. Br J Psychiatry 1980;137:148–162.
5. Brown GW, Harris TO. Social Origins of Depression. London: Tavistock, 1978.

82. Adverse Effects of Antidepressant Drugs in the Elderly

ANASTASIOS GEORGOTAS, ROBERT E. McCUE,
AND NARMADA NAGACHANDRAN

In no other place in psychiatry does the hippocratic caveat "Do no harm" have greater relevance than in treating depressed elderly with antidepressant medications. More so in the elderly than in younger age groups, antidepressant drugs may have a number of undesirable pharmacological properties. Some of them may result from their putative antihistaminic, α-adrenergic, and anticholinergic actions. The greater susceptibility of the elderly to these side effects is usually attributed to the increased prevalence of underlying medical illnesses in the older age group and frequently occurring polypharmacy. In addition, age-related changes in drug metabolism and elimination may play an important role in increasing the susceptibility of the elderly to these undesirable properties. The latter include an appreciable reduction in renal clearance (secondary to decreased cardiac output, decreased total renal tubular mass, renal vasoconstriction, etc.) and hepatic metabolism as well as increased fatty tissue, which results in prolongation of the pharmacological effect of the various antidepressants. Furthermore, decreased levels of circulating proteins may result in higher concentrations of the unbound, pharmacologically active portion of the antidepressant.[1-3] As a result of these changes, plasma levels of antidepressants in the elderly can reach high levels despite modest oral doses. Several studies have already shown it to be true for several tricyclic antidepressants, e.g., amitriptyline, imipramine, and nortriptyline, when plasma levels can be meaningfully measured.[3-5]

At times, the adverse reactions to the various antidepressant drugs cannot be easily distinguished from usual symptoms of depression, such as mild confusion, psychomotor retardation, dry mouth, and constipation. It may frequently result in an over- or underestimation of the true incidence of side effects in the elderly. Therefore carefully noting the existence of symptoms, which may later be confused with side effects, by active questioning prior to treatment is helpful. In most healthy elderly patients, side effects are usually transient, benign, easily managed, and well tolerated. It is often helpful to discuss with patients the likelihood and nature of side effects prior to treatment without exaggerating or taking a defensive attitude. In the authors' experience, an informative discussion with the patient increases compliance and significantly reduces anticipatory anxiety, panicky reactions, and placebo effects.

Frequently Occurring Side Effects

Studies in elderly depressed populations have reported mainly on anticholinergic, central nervous system, and cardiovascular side effects of the various antidepressants.[6]

Anticholinergic Effects

Anticholinergic side effects can range from the more commonly reported ones, such as dry mouth, constipation, and blurred vision, to much more severe but less frequent ones, such as urinary retention, paralytic ileus, confusional states, and delirium. Elderly, debilitated individuals with preexistent physical illnesses are especially prone to these more severe effects. Aside from these problems, anticholinergic side effects are usually easily tolerated by most patients, especially younger ones; tolerance often develops after the first few weeks. On the other hand, older, fragile patients are much more susceptible to confusional states or delirium as signs of central anticholinergic toxicity. Of the tricyclic antidepressants, amitriptyline seems to be the worst offender, with nortriptyline and desipramine having the least anticholinergic toxicity.

Monoamine oxidase inhibitors are less anticholinergic. This finding has been supported by our comparative studies at New York University Medical Center where nortriptyline was compared to phenelzine under double-blind, placebo-controlled conditions in elderly patients suffering from major depressive illness according to Research Diagnostic Criteria (RDC). Our results have shown that nortriptyline has a higher anticholinergic profile than either phenelzine or placebo. The most frequently reported anticholinergic side effects were dry mouth, closely followed by constipation. These problems were present significantly more often in nortriptyline-treated patients. Dry mouth was also reported for a significantly longer period of time (mean 5.6 weeks) by nortriptyline patients than by either phenelzine (mean 3.4 weeks) or placebo (mean 1.4 weeks) patients.[7] No patient in our studies developed delirium or other toxic confusional states.

Of the second generation antidepressants, nomifensine, fluoxetine, and trazodone have been found to be much less anticholingergic in comparison to tricyclics, with trazodone having the fewest adverse effects.[8] Anticholinergic side effects can usually be handled by a proper selection of antidepressant, lowering the dosage, or switching to another family of drugs. Bethanechol, a cholinergic agonist, may be helpful in counteracting peripheral anticholinergic side effects in some patients, but its use should be restricted to cases when all other measures have failed.

Central Nervous System Effects

Of the central nervous system (CNS) side effects, drowsiness and sedation are most frequently reported. Less common but troublesome when they occur are seizures, tremor, impaired balance, and at higher doses speech impairment. Of the tricyclic antidepressants, doxepin and amitriptyline are among the most sedating. In our double-blind studies[7] we found that patients treated with either nortriptyline or phenelzine reported significantly more drowsiness than placebo-treated patients. In addition, phenelzine patients reported drowsiness significantly more frequently than nortriptyline patients.

Of the second generation antidepressants, trazodone appears to be very sedating, which often prevents the dose from being increased to a therapeutic one. A decreased seizure threshold has been reported with maprotiline, especially at higher blood levels and following an abrupt increase in dose.

Cardiovascular Effects

Among the cardiovascular side effects, the most troublesome is orthostatic hypotension, which in the elderly is frequently associated with falls and injuries. Of the tricyclics, nortriptyline seems to be least associated with this side effect, although not totally exempted. Monoamine oxidase inhibitors have been much feared because of their orthostatic effects, although we found them to be comparable to nortriptyline in this respect. In fact, the results of our double-blind studies with elderly patients have shown that orthostatic symptoms such as dizziness were present with approximately equal frequency in both nortriptyline (39 times in 60% of patients) and phenelzine (33 times in 45% of patients) groups and were significantly more frequent in these two groups than in the placebo group (12 times in 21% of patients). There was also a significantly greater mean orthostatic fall in systolic blood pressure in the nortriptyline and phenelzine patients (mean ± SD 9.30 ± 11.38 mm Hg) compared to the placebo group. There was no significant difference between the nortriptyline and phenelzine groups. The orthostatic changes appeared during the first week of treatment and were not correlated with plasma level of nortriptyline, percent platelet monoamine oxidase inhibition, or pretreatment orthostatic changes.

As for electrocardiographic (ECG) changes, we found that after 7 weeks of treatment nortriptyline produced statistically significant increases in both the heart rate and the PR interval, although none of the changes was outside the normal range. Phenelzine produced a significant decrease in the QT interval. None of the patients had pathological ECG changes under the closely monitored treatment conditions of this study. In addition, none of our phenelzine patients experienced a hypertensive crisis.[7,9]

Despite the numerous claims that second generation and antidepressants, such as bupropion, fluoxetine, and mianserin, are superior in terms of cardiovascular safety,[10] there are limited definitive data available on this subject because of the lack of well controlled studies in high risk groups. Substantiation of these claims awaits further investigation.

Epilogue

Treatment of the depressed elderly with antidepressants is by no means devoid of substantial risks from their other pharmacological properties. Yet these risks may have been exaggerated in several studies that compared second generation antidepressants to tricyclics and monoamine oxidase inhibitors. Interestingly enough, in most of these comparative trials, which were mainly supported by major pharmaceutical firms, the newer drugs were compared to tertiary amine tricyclics such as amitriptyline and imipramine, which have a higher anticholinergic, sedative, and perhaps cardiovascular side effects profile, rather than to secondary amines such as nortriptyline and desipramine. Monoamine oxidase inhibitors have not been compared to the newer drugs in elderly depressed patients, although it has been suggested that they produce fewer cardiovascular and anticholinergic side effects. In our experience, both secondary amine tricyclics (nortriptyline, desipramine) and monoamine oxidase inhibitors, if judiciously used, can be safe treatments for the elderly. A meticulous selection of both patients and antidepressants, careful monitoring of dosage and side effects, frequent visits, few dosage readjustments, and the elimination of unnecessary concurrent medication are important factors to be always considered when treating elderly depressed individuals. Properly educating patients and the ones close to them about side effects and reassuring them as to their transient nature, as well as lowering the dose and changing to another antidepressant when side effects are intolerable, are powerful measures to ensure that side effects do not interfere with compliance.

Much more rigorous research is needed in order to develop newer and safer antidepressants. Although several of the second generation agents already on the market appear to be less anticholinergic and potentially less cardiotoxic, they need to be studied in high risk groups before any definite conclusion regarding their safety can be drawn. Another potential drawback to using these newer drugs is the lack of well established therapeutic ranges for plasma levels as are available for older antidepressants such as nortriptyline and imipramine, which may result in diminished efficacy and increased toxicity from their use.

Acknowledgment. Supported by NIMH grant MH35196 (A.M.). (Dr. A. Georgotas).

References

1. Walker JI, Brodie HKH. Neuropharmacology of aging. In Busse EW, Blazwe DG (eds): Handbook of Geriatric Psychiatry. New York: Van Nostrand Reinhold, 1980.
2. Holloway D. Drug problems in the geriatric patient. Drug Intell Clin Pharmacol. 1974;8:632–642.
3. Georgotas A, McCue RE. Affective disorders in the elderly: treatment considerations. In Burrows GD, Norman TR, Dennerstein L (eds): Clinical and Pharmacological Studies in Psychiatric Disorders. London: John Libbey, 1985;326–336.
4. Nies A, Robinson DS, Friedman MJ, et al. Relationship between age and tricyclic antidepressant plasma levels. Am J Psychiatry 1977;134:790–793.
5. Kragh-Sørensen P, Asberg M, Christian EH. Plasma-nortriptyline levels in endogenous depression. Lancet 1973;1:113–115.
6. Georgotas A, Cooper T, Kim M, et al. The treatment of affective disorders in the elderly. Psychopharmacol Bull 1983;19:226–237.
7. Georgotas A, McCue RE, Hapworth W, et al. Comparative efficacy and safety of MAOIs versus TCAs in treating depression in the elderly. Biol Psychiatry 1986;21:1155–1166.
8. Georgotas A, Forsell TL, Mann JJ, et al. Trazodone hydrochloride: a wide spectrum antidepressant with a unique pharmacological profile. Pharmacotherapy 1982;2:255–265.
9. Georgotas A, McCue RE, Friedman E, et al. A placebo-controlled comparison of the effect of nortriptyline and phenelzine on orthostatic hypotension in elderly depressed patients. J Clin Psychopharmacol 1987;7:413–416.
10. McCue RE, Georgotas A. Newer generation antidepressants and lithium. In Georgotas A, Cancro R (eds): Depression and Mania. New York: Elsevier, 1988;372–383.

III.D. AFFECTIVE DISORDERS AND REPRODUCTIVE CYCLICITY IN WOMEN

83. Menarche and Menstrual Symptoms: Psychosocial Perspectives

A large number of physical discomforts and affective changes have been associated with the menstrual cycle. Although there have been numerous attempts to describe the etiology of menstrual symptomatology, such an understanding has remained elusive. Sociocultural as well as physiological and personality factors have been examined. This psychosocial research has shown the importance of beliefs and attitudes as factors influencing women's reports of symptoms.[1]

Our research has extended this sociocultural perspective to the study of the developmental and socialization processes associated with menstruation. We have been concerned with developmental changes in adolescent girls' reported experiences of menstrual symptoms and their acquisition of information about symptoms. Menarche, as the biological symbol of a shift from child to woman, may represent a time of change in self-identity or self-definition. At a minimum, this event signals a need for the girl to determine what it means to be a menstruating woman—how the physical and psychological changes she has heard about may translate into personal experiences. In addition, the definition of the experience established at this time may be difficult to change in that subsequent experiences are perceived in terms of and may be distorted by this definition.[1] Thus perceptions of and information received about the menstrual experience during menarche and shortly after may have a long-lasting effect.

Study 1: Adolescent Girls' Constructions of the Menstrual Experience

In one study we included a combination of longitudinal and cross-sectional designs. The cross-sectional sample consisted of 639 public school girls in grades 5–8, (10–13 years) and 11–12 (16–17 years).[2,3] The longitudinal design employed a matching procedure to control for repeated testing: A premenarcheal girl, matched on age and school, was paired with each girl who reached menarche. Using this procedure, 46 pairs of girls completed both the pre- and postmenarcheal phases of testing. At each testing the girls completed a lengthy questionnaire that included sections on incidence and severity of menstrual and premenstrual symptoms, attitudes about menstruation, and sources of menstruation-related information.

What are girls' beliefs about symptoms as they approach their first experience with menstruation? Our data showed that even the youngest premenarcheal girls we studied expected to experience the same symptoms commonly reported by adult women, and there were few changes right after menarche. Thus a girl enters menarche with a clear set of expectations, many of which are negative. Her experience of menstruation is therefore primed to be a self-fulfilling prophecy. Indeed, additional analyses of our longitudinal data suggest that the prophecy is fulfilled, at least to some extent. Symptom reports of postmenarcheal girls at the second testing were significantly correlated with their premenarcheal expectations at the first testing. There were no significant relations found between expectations at time 1 and time 2 for the girls who remained premenarcheal. Thus the correlations are not simply a response bias. Instead, it is as if expectations present at the time a girl begins to menstruate provide the definition of that experience, whereas expectations of premenarcheal girls continually change, presumably in response to age-related changes in the information available.

Because self-definitions with long-lasting significance may occur at menarche, it is important to examine factors that influence how positive or negative the experience is. Previous literature suggests that two such factors are adequacy of preparation and age of menarche.[4,5] Our analysis of these two variables differed from previous studies in several ways: (a) The girls were younger and thus recollections were based on more recent experiences; (b) the sample was large, and so we could look at more extreme variations; and (c) a longitudinal sample reporting on immediate experiences was included. Effects that did emerge were generally in the predicted direction, though many of the differences failed to reach statistical significance. Girls who were unprepared or early to mature reported more negative reactions and more symptoms, and (in the seventh grade) their self-image ratings were more negative.

A third factor likely to affect positive/negative experiences at menarche is girls' perceptions of the reactions of significant others. That is, we expected that girls who received more information from sources viewed as having positive attitudes would have more positive attitudes themselves. The correlations were generally consistent with these predictions. Perceiving menstruation in positive terms and comfort talking about it were positively correlated with amount learned from positive sources of information (e.g., parents and physician). In addition, premenarcheal girls who reported learning more from male sources (who are generally viewed as negative) reported experiencing greater menstrual and premenstrual distress after menarche. Thus receiving information premenarcheally from sources perceived to be negative appears to be associated with more negative perceptions of symptoms after menarche.

Study 2: Socialization Influences on Girls' Reports of Menstrual Symptoms

More recently we have examined self-definitional processes at menarche in a different way. Because we have argued that girls construct an image of the experience based on prevalent cultural and subcultural beliefs, we studied adolescent girls from two cultures (white and Hispanic of comparable socioeconomic levels).[6] In addition, we examined the influences of two context factors likely to affect the experience of stress at menarche (and, by extension, the experience of negative symptoms). These two factors were the girl's perceptions of her parents' attitudes about her growing up and if the girl had experienced the transition to junior high school (12–13 years of age). Because of the focus of this volume and because the results were complex, we limit our discussion of the results to affective symptoms.

One might predict that more rigid sex role attitudes and greater restrictions accompanying pubertal development in the Hispanic culture[7] would result in more negative symptom reports for Hispanic than for white girls. On the other hand, there are reasons to expect that Hispanic girls might be less influenced by beliefs about the premenstrual syndrome (PMS), as portrayed by the popular media. To highlight this point, the various makers of sanitary napkins began to publicize in the Spanish-speaking media the use of tampons by adolescent girls only during the early 1980s. This delay of exposing the Hispanic subculture to the use of tampons by adolescents was not due to the negative side effects of toxic shock syndrome but, rather, to the long-held belief in the Hispanic culture that virginal girls are not allowed to wear tampons for fear of breaking the hymen.[8] Thus it seems that Hispanic girls may be exposed to the current trends and/or beliefs of some aspects of menstrual cycles at a much slower pace. For this reason, and because affective symptoms are more subjective than physical symptoms, it is perhaps not surprising that we found that white girls were overall more likely to associate negative affect (e.g., depression) with menstruation than were Hispanic girls. In addition, among postmenarcheal girls, white girls were less likely to report positive affect (e.g., feelings of well-being) during menstruation. There were no differences for physical symptoms.

There were also cultural differences in the impact of perceived parental attitudes. The attitude measures consisted of three scales for each parent: positive, negative, and avoidant. We found that girls who perceived that their mothers had negative attitudes about them growing up reported more menstrual-related negative affect, but this finding was significant only for white girls. Perceptions of fathers' negative attitudes were related only to pain and total symptom reports, not to affect per se. However, perceptions that the father was uninterested or *avoidant* about his daughter's growing up was associated with *less* menstrual-related negative affect, perhaps because it is a more normative pattern for fathers. In addition, girls' perception of their father as both positive and avoidant were associated with more menstrual-related positive affect (arousal). Thus expected relations between perceived parental attitudes and menstrual-related affect did emerge, with girls who perceived their parents as more negative or less positive reporting, respectively, more negative or less positive affective symptoms associated with menstruation. The exact nature of the relation varied, however, across father and mother and across cultures.

Finally, girls who experienced a transition to junior high school, an event shown to be stressful for pubertal girls in earlier research,[9] reported more menstrual-related negative affect. Once again, however, this finding was significant only for white girls.

In summary, these data also show the importance of social context factors on reports of menstrual symptoms, particularly affect. We interpret the pattern of results as reflecting two factors: (a) the strength of the association between menstruation and affect (in this case a cultural association); and (b) the existence of stressful events at the time this association is made. That is, white girls were more likely to associate menstruation with negative affect, and the experience of stressful events—negative maternal attitudes and transition to junior high school—

strengthened this association. It may be that the culturally accepted expression of menstrual distress (i.e., PMS) provided an explanation for stress-produced negative affect experienced by some girls. The only exception to this pattern was that the effect of fathers' attitudes did not vary by culture, perhaps because there was less power in these analyses, as about one-half of the sample reported a single-parent household.

Implications for Understanding Menstrual-Related Affective Disorders

We have argued that around the time of menarche girls construct a definition of the menstrual experience from various sources of information, of which direct knowledge of symptoms is only one. Our data suggest that adolescent girls' symptom reports are correlated with their own premenarcheal expectations, suggesting that the direct experience of menstruation is interpreted in terms of expectations previously formed. Moreover, individual differences in symptom reports can be predicted from the context in which self-definitions are initially formed. Current negative reports of symptoms in postmenarcheal girls are related to being unprepared for menarche, being early to mature, receiving information from sources perceived as negative, cultural definitions, and stressful socialization experiences.

Findings that psychosocial factors influence individual differences in girls' perceptions of menstruation have important implications for understanding affective disorders associated with the menstrual cycle, such as PMS. Adolescent experiences may create the foundation for an association between the premenstrual phase and negative affect, particularly if premenarcheal expectations are learned in a culture that emphasizes this association. Thus experiences at menarche may prime some women to be ready to attribute new problems to the menstrual cycle. As PMS receives increasing attention and publicity, therefore, it becomes more likely that PMS will be part of girls' premenarcheal expectations and, presumably, subsequent reported experiences.

Acknowledgment. Preparation of this chapter was supported in part by research grant 37215 and in part by Research Science Development Award 00484, both from the National Institute of Mental Health.

References

1. Ruble DN, Brooks-Gunn J. Menstrual symptoms: a social cognition and analysis. J Behav Med 1979;2:171–194.
2. Brooks-Gunn J, Ruble DN. The development of menstrual-related beliefs and behaviors during early adolescence. Child Dev 1982;53:1567–1577.
3. Ruble DN, Brooks-Gunn J. The experience of menarche. Child Dev 1982;53:1557–1566.
4. Rierdan J. Variations in the experience of menarche as a function of preparedness. In Golub S (ed): Menarche. Lexington, MA: Lexington Books, 1983;119–126.
5. Petersen AC. Pubertal development as a cause of disturbance. Gen Psychol Monogr 1987;111:205–232.
6. Maluf J, Ruble DN. Cultural and family influences on adolescent girls' perceptions of menstrual symptoms. 1988∞ preparation.
7. Canino G. Transactional family patterns. In Zambrana RE (ed): Work, Family, and Health: Latina Women in Transition. New York: Hispanic Research Center, 1982.

8. Zambrana RE. Latina women in transition. In Zambrana RE (ed): Work, Family, and Health: Latina Women in Transition. New York: Hispanic Research Center, 1982.
9. Simmons R, Blyth DA, McKinney KL, et al. The social and psychological effects of puberty on white females. In Brooks-Gunn J, Petersen AC (eds): Girls at Puberty. New York: Plenum, 1982.

84. Affect and Nurturance in First-Time Mothers: Role of Psychobiological Influences

ALISON S. FLEMING, HOWARD KRIEGER, AND P.Y. WONG

Considerable research has been done on the psychobiology of maternal behavior in rats and other small mammals.[1] This chapter attempts to delineate some of the factors regulating maternal behavior in humans, highlighting areas of similarity between humans and these animal models. It is argued that for rat and human mothers the hormones of pregnancy and the parturitional period facilitate the early expression of maternal behavior, but that they do so by altering a number of behavioral propensities simultaneously, including the mother's responsiveness to infant-related cues, the ease with which she learns about these cues, and her overall affective state.[1,2] Once maternal, however, experiences of interacting with the young assume control of the behavior. Extensive discussion and referencing of rodent maternal behavior may be found in Fleming and Orpen[1] and therefore this subject is only briefly discussed below.[2,3]

Rat Model

Primiparous rat mothers show a highly stereotyped and complicated pattern of maternal behavior soon after parturition, without the benefit of prior experience caring for young. The nurturant behavior of the parturient female rat is in marked contrast to the behavior of the inexperienced nulliparous female rat, which initially either neglects or actively rejects neonatal foster pups.

Although primiparous mothers usually do not have the opportunity to exhibit maternal behavior prior to parturition, as schematized in Figure 84.1, responsiveness actually develops during the pregnancy, peaking immediately prepartum,[1] and is sustained for a period after birth. This pattern of changing maternal responsiveness has been shown to be hormonally mediated. In the rat elevated levels of estradiol and possibly prolactin and oxytocin against a background of declining progesterone underlie the periparturitional rise in maternal responsiveness.

Studies indicate that the hormonal induction of maternal behavior is accomplished by acting directly on substrates that underlie the expression of maternal behavior, as well as by increasing the females' attraction to the odor of pups and by reducing the animal's natural timidity and neophobic tendency to avoid the unfamiliar pups. Thus the hormonal profile that facilitates maternal behavior when

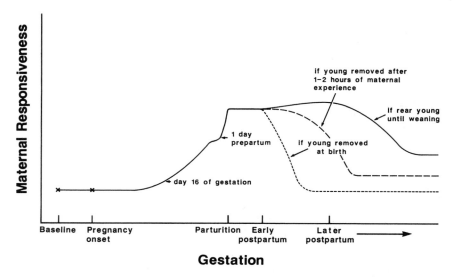

FIGURE 84.1. Changes in maternal responsiveness across gestation and the early postpartum period in rats receiving different amounts of postpartum pup stimulation.

injected into nulliparous female rats also acts to increase the animal's preference for the odor of neonatal pups and decrease the animal's natural timidity and avoidance of novel stimuli.

Once female rats have become maternal under the influence of the periparturitional hormones, the mother's subsequent maternal responsiveness is maintained by experiences interacting with the young. Orpen and Fleming[1] found, for instance, that as little as 30 min of interaction with pups on the day following cesarean delivery resulted in prolongation of the postpartum period of heightened responsiveness. These observations suggest that in rats, as well as other mammalian species,[1] hormones of parturition prime the female rat to respond maternally to young by altering emotional and perceptual components of the response and possibly by facilitating the learning or retention of experiences acquired during the early postpartum period.

Human Studies

Many of the factors shown to influence maternal behavior in the rat have also been shown to play a role in more advanced mammals, including some (although not all) of the primates.[1] These cross-species similarities raised the possibility that similar influences may play a role in the regulation of maternal behavior in first-time human mothers.

Although there are large cross-cultural differences in modes of interaction between human mothers and their offspring,[3] as in other animals, among humans the biological mother is usually the primary caretaker and engages in behaviors that ensure her close contact and proximity to the infant. Because of the relative variability and complexity of human maternal responsiveness, we used multiple measures to assess mothers' attachment to their infants or maternal responsiveness.

Assessments made during pregnancy were based on mothers' self-report responses on clusters of questionnaire items that "tap" women's feelings of warmth toward their fetuses and new babies. We also obtained information on women's feelings about other infants, as well as mothers' feelings about caretaking activities and feelings of their own adequacy in the mothering role. After the birth we obtained not only these self-report measures but also measures of mothers' interactions with their infants. In general, mothers and infants were observed during a feeding session, and behaviors were clustered into approach or affectionate behaviors (including contact behaviors of a noninstrumental nature, e.g., pats, strokes, hugs) as well as caretaking (or instrumental) behaviors.

The first question of interest to us concerned the development of maternal responsiveness across pregnancy. When mothers become pregnant they clearly show changes in a variety of behaviors that may contribute to the development of the fetus or that anticipate the young, but that may not be directly related to conscious feelings of attachment to their infants. Thus pregnant women experience strong aversions to certain foods that may be harmful to the fetus[4]; they also become more home-bound and inner-directed; and toward the end of pregnancy they engage in a form of nesting behavior that involves preparation of the infant's room, etc.[5] They also acquire increasing amounts of information about infants and their care.[6] and show heightened autonomic arousal responses to the cry stimulus of an infant.[7] Although these data suggest that pregnancy does in some sense prepare the mother for impending motherhood, we were interested in whether women experience a change in their conscious feelings of attachment to their infants. A group of first-time mothers filled out questionnaires at six time points: four during the pregnancy and two during the first 6 postpartum weeks. When the scores of all women were analyzed we found a small increase in mothers' positive feelings of attachment to their infants at 20 weeks, after the "quickening," as well as a more precipitous increase between term and 4 days postpartum. However, other maternal attitudes did not change appreciably during pregnancy but did show clear elevations by 2 months postpartum, after some experience with the infant had been acquired. These relations are represented in Figure 84.2.

In our next analyses we were interested in the relative contributions of hormones and psychosocial factors to the variation of maternal responsiveness during the prepartum and early postpartum periods. We measured plasma levels of a variety of hormones during pregnancy and at 6 weeks postpartum and found no relation between any measure of maternal responsiveness and any hormone or combination of hormones at these time points. In contrast, background and social factors clearly account for much of the variance in maternal responsiveness during pregnancy. In one study Fleming et al.[8] assessed women's maternal attitudes during pregnancy and at 1 and 3 months postpartum and found that feelings of maternal adequacy and about caretaking during pregnancy were predicted by such factors as the woman's prior experience of caring for infants and her affective state. Maternal attitudes during pregnancy are also positively associated with the mother's desire to be pregnant.

Although hormones were not found to play a role in maternal attitudes during pregnancy or indeed during the *later* postpartum periods, they may play a role during the earlier postpartum period. Fleming et al.[9] investigated this possibility by assessing women during pregnancy on their maternal attitudes and then observing them with their infants on days 3 and 4 postpartum, when hormonal assays were also done. There were no relations between levels of estradiol or progesterone

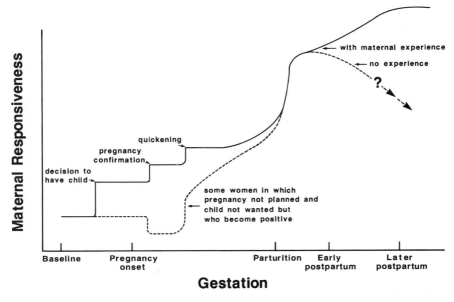

FIGURE 84.2. Changes in maternal responsiveness across gestation and the early postpartum period in human primiparous mothers.

or the ratio of these two hormones and either self-report or behavioral measures of maternal responsiveness, as has been reported in the rat; however, cortisol levels were strongly associated with approach behaviors and showed effects that were additive with prior maternal attitudes. Thus mothers who felt more positively and who had higher cortisol levels showed the highest amount of maternal approach responses. These hormonal effects were no longer present at 2 months postpartum, after considerable experience with the young had been acquired.

How might cortisol be exerting an effect? As indicated by the animal work, hormones could be acting indirectly by influencing mothers' reactions to infant cues as well as the learning of those cues, and/or they could be altering the woman's mood state.

There is, unfortunately, no direct evidence that hormones influence women's response to infant cues, as this particular relation has not been investigated. However, there is some indication that mothers with as little as 1 h of contact with young are able to identify their infants based solely on their odors and, moreover, that they learn these characteristics quickly.[10] Additionally, Schaal[10] reported that mothers show heightened olfactory acuity during the first 3 postpartum days. There is also evidence that the experience of interacting with the infant during the first postpartum hours may facilitate the mother's responsiveness to her infant during the subsequent few days, although the effects of such early contact are apparently short-lived.[11]

Evidence for a relation between puerperal hormones and postpartum mood state is also not strong.[12,13] Steiner et al. found no relation between circulating hormones and any number of measures of mood state at 3–4 days postpartum.[14] However, we did find that mothers with higher cortisol levels after birth felt greater well-being at 2 months postpartum (unpublished observations). Regardless of the role of hormones in mood, Fleming et al.[8] found that mothers who are more dysphoric or depressed at 1 and 3 months postpartum have more negative maternal attitudes and respond less affectionately, and in some analyses less contingently, to their infants than do the happier mothers, although there are no differences in the amount of instrumental caretaking responses shown by the two groups. By 16 months postpartum earlier postpartum depression no longer influenced mothers' interactions with their children.

Although these studies indicate that hormones may facilitate a mother's responsiveness to her infant during the first few postpartum days, hormones are neither necessary nor sufficient for responsiveness to occur. Of greater importance are the attitudes mothers bring to the situation, which in turn may be influenced by women's affective state as well as a variety of psychosocial factors including their concurrent and prior experience with infants.

References

1. Fleming AS, Orpen G. Psychobiology of maternal behavior in rats, selected other species, and humans. In Fogel A, Melson G (eds): Origins of Nurturance. Hillsdale, NJ: Lawrence Erlbaum, 1986.
2. Fleming AS, Anderson V. Affect and nurturance: mechanisms mediating maternal behavior in two female mammals. Prog Neuropsychopharmacol Biol Psychiatry 1987;11:121–127.
3. Fleming AS, Corter C. Factors influencing maternal responsiveness in humans: usefulness of an animal model. Psychoneuroendocrinology 1988;13:189–212.
4. Hook EB. Influence of pregnancy on dietary selection. Int J Obes 1980;4:338–340.
5. Grossman FK, Eichler LS, Winickoff SA, et al. Pregnancy, Birth, and Parenthood. San Francisco: Jossey-Bass, 1980.
6. Deutsch F, Ruble DN, Fleming AS, et al. Becoming a mother: information-seeking and self-definitional processes. Presented at the Annual Meeting of the Eastern Psychological Association, New York, 1986.
7. Bleichfeld B, Moely BE. Psychophysiological responses to an infant cry: comparison of groups of women in different phases of the maternal cycle. Dev Psychiatry 1984;20:1082–1091.
8. Fleming AS, Ruble DN, Flett GL, et al. Postpartum adjustment in first-time mothers: effects of mood on maternal attitudes and behavior. Dev Psychiatry 1988;24:77–81.
9. Fleming AS, Steiner M, Anderson V. Hormonal and attitudinal correlates of maternal behaviour during the early postpartum period in first-time mothers. J Reprod Inf Psychol 1987;5:193–205.
10. Schaal B Contributions olfactives a l'establissement du lien mere-enfant. In Tremblay RA, Provost M, Strayer F (eds): Ethologie et Developpement de l'Enfant. Paris: Stock, 1986:187–211.
11. Goldberg S. Parent-infant bonding: another look. Child Dev 1983;54:1355–1382.
12. Nott PM, Franklin M, Armitage C, et al. Hormonal changes and mood in the puerperium. Br J Psychiatry 1976;128:379–383.
13. Handley SL, Dunn TL, Waldron G, et al. Tryptophan, cortisol and puerperal mood. Br J Psychiatry 1980;136:498–508.
14. Steiner M, Fleming AS, Anderson VN, et al. A psychoneuroendocrine profile for postpartum blues? In Dennerstein L, Fraser I (eds): Hormones and Behaviour. Amsterdam: Elsevier, 1986; 327–335.

85. Myth of Menopausal Depression

MEIR STEINER

Menopause is regarded as the consequence of a chain of events that leads to a change in programming along the hypothalamic-pituitary-gonadal axis. The mechanism of the biological clock that initiates the onset of neuroregulatory changes leading toward menopause is unknown. What is known is that the ensuing steady state of gonadotropin secretion causes ovarian noncyclicity, and with further passage of time ovarian function diminishes and the blood levels of ovarian estrogens decrease to only small, barely detectable amounts. This notion unfortunately led to the development of the concept of menopause as a disease. Adopted primarily by medical practitioners, menopause has become synonymous with a state of estrogen deficiency, which is to be treated with hormone replacement therapy (HRT).

The misconception of menopause as a psychosocial malaise has its deep roots within the traditional psychoanalytical movement. Statements made by leading female psychoanalysts describing the menopausal process as "organic decline," "narcissistic mortification," and "partial death"[1] eventually leading to "desexualization" and "diminished integrative personality strength"[2] are still widely accepted.

A twofold increase in the prevalence of depression among women has been consistently observed[3] and is even more notable during middle life.[4] Because it is widely assumed that the mind–body relation is closer for women than for men, it is expected that the hormonal changes that accompany female reproductive cyclicity are bound to have negative consequences. As stated by Parlee,[5] "It sometimes seems as if the only thing worse than being subjected to the raging hormonal influences of the female cycle is to have those influences subside."

Female vulnerability to depression during the menopause has been attributed to, or attempted to be explained on the basis of, physiological, psychological, or social factors. The evidence (or lack of such) for an association between clinical features of the menopause and these factors is briefly reviewed.

The only specific pathophysiological changes that occur in relation to menopause are the presence of hot flushes, night sweats, and atrophic vaginitis. Climacteric women visiting outpatient clinics complain mostly of these symptoms, although they sometimes also complain of other physical and psychological distress. Some of the behavioral symptoms include irritability, tension, nervousness, fatigue, anxiety, and depression, none of which are age- or sex-specific. Although the hypothesis that hormonal changes at the menopause determine these symptoms is an attractive one, research findings provide only marginal support. Even the vasomotor complaints do not correlate well with hormone levels or cytology and as such are not helpful when planning treatment.[6] Despite the fact that estrogen replacement seems to be effective in alleviating the disability of hot flushes and urogenital atrophy, the medical community seems to be in appreciable disagreement about this treatment regimen.[7,8]

The extent of an association between the menopause and psychiatric disorders is also controversial. It was believed that the preponderance of depression in women can mainly be attributed to an increase in their susceptibility to depression during the menopausal years. Thus a distinct clinical entity, "involutional melancholia," became part of the official nomenclature.[9,10] Further studies failed to support the distinctiveness of postmenopausal depression. The prevalence of depression in women during menopausal years was found to be similar to the risk for depression during other times of the life-span.[11] Women who are depressed during their menopausal years do not have a distinct symptom pattern, do not exhibit an absence of previous episodes, and have life-stress precipitants similar to those in women in other age groups.[12] The age- and sex-specific psychosocial vulnerability to life events during the climacterium hypothesis has also been reevaluated. In one study a simple association between total life stress and the menopausal psychological syndrome (including crying spells, worrying, depressed mood, and panic attacks) seemed to explain only 24% of the variance.[13] Thus it seems that the category of "involutional melancholia," arose from what was essentially a comparison between unipolar and bipolar depression but which ignored the differences in the modal age of onset distribution.[14] Some of the currently used neuroendocrine biological markers for melancholia have also been applied to the menopause. Most of these studies reported that menopausal depressed women have the same degree of "abnormality" on these tests when compared to other groups of melancholic patients (for details see ref. 15). Clinically, it is also important to note that suicide attempts are less common during the menopause[11] and treatment for major psychiatric disorders associated with menopause is the same as for similar disorders occurring in other age groups or in men. Last but not least, menopause is not perceived universally as a loss. To some women, depending on their sociocultural background, menopause is only a relative loss, and to others it is even a gain.[16] Nevertheless, in Western society the menopause coincides with an increased incidence of hospital admissions for depression, an increase in self-reported psychological symptoms, and an increase in illness behavior.[17]

Hypoestrogenism has been linked, on theoretical grounds, to the catecholamine (CA) deficiency hypothesis of depression. Thus although there is no proof as yet for depression during the menopause to be hormone-dependent, several studies claim that this depression is at least somewhat hormone-responsive.[18] In the first study that reported positive results, very large doses of oral conjugated estrogen were administered, but the antidepressant effect was only moderate.[19] When a closer to physiological replacement regimen was applied, the results were tentative,[20] negative,[21,22] or close to a placebo effect.[23] Thus with both HRT and placebo therapy having such a highly significant "mental tonic" effect, the specificity as well as the risk/benefit aspects of long-term HRT for depression are to be seriously questioned. The exception seems to be for younger women with mood changes following surgical menopause. Results indicate that in these women HRT mitigates affective symptoms related to the sudden and drastic postoperative change in endocrine state.[24]

The significance of gonadal hormones for balanced CA processes in the brain is not fully understood. Aging is known to be associated with a decline in CA synthesis and an increase in monoamine oxidase (MAO) activity.[25] It is possible that during menopause this age-related decline in CA, coupled with hypoestrogenism, causes a change in central adrenoceptor sensitivity that in some predisposed women may lead to dysphoric states. It is now known that several of the hormonal states associated with high MAO activity are also associated with depressive states,[19] but MAO inhibitors have not yet been tried in a systematic fashion during the climacterium. It has also been suggested that lower basal luteinizing hormone (LH) levels in some menopausal depressed women represent altered hypothalamic adrenoceptor sensitivity.[26] Nighttime hot flushes, believed to be associated with pulsatile release of LH, are known to chronically disrupt the normal sleep pattern, which may in turn be the cause for daytime irritability, anxiety, and dysphoria. Clonidine, an α-adrenergic agonist, is being used successfully in the treatment of hot flushes. Most placebo-controlled trials show that clonidine is significantly superior to placebo in reducing the number of hot flushes,[27] but surprisingly the behavioral effects of this treatment are not reported.

The theme that emerges is that altered neuroendocrine profiles may not provide mutually independent information. Hot flushes, being one of the specific pathophysiological changes associated with menopause, may be related to dysphoria in more than one way.

It has been suggested that a "menopausal index" be established.[28] With the establishment of this index it is conceivable that future research will be more supportive of the notion that "menopause is part of the normal aging process which in itself does not require therapeutic intervention" and that "the health status of women during this period is not a simple endocrine-deficiency state which could or should be corrected by attempting to recreate for each woman a premenopausal normal environment."[28] It will also help avoid the further medicalization of the menopause[29] and probably identify a much smaller subgroup of dysphoric menopausal women who suffer a minor transient and correctable neuroendocrine dysregulation.

References

1. Deutsch H. The Psychology of Women. New York: Grune & Stratton, 1945;456–487.
2. Benedek T. Climacterium: a developmental phase. Psychoanal Q 1950;19:1–27.
3. Tennant C. Female vulnerability to depression. Psychol Med 1985;15:733–737.
4. Jorm AF. Sex and age differences in depression. Aust NZ J Psychiatry 1987;21:46–53.
5. Parlee MB. Social factors in the psychology of menstruation, birth, and menopause. Primary Care 1976;3:477–490.
6. James CE, Breeson AJ, Kovacs G, et al. The symptomatology of the climacteric in relation to hormonal and cytological factors. Br J Obstet Gynaecol 1984;91:56–62.
7. Padwick ML, Pryse-Davies J, Whitehead MI. A simple method for determining the optimal dosage of progestin in postmenopausal women receiving estrogens. N Engl J Med 1986;315:930–934.
8. MacDonald PC. Estrogen plus progestin in postmenopausal women—act II. N Engl Med 1986;315:959–961.
9. Titley WB. Prepsychotic personality of patients with involutional melancholia. Arch Neurol Psychiatry 1936;36:19–33.
10. Barnett J, Lefford A, Pushman D. Involutional melancholia. Psychiatr Q 1953;27:654–662.

11. Winokur G. Depression in the menopause. Am J Psychiatry 1973;130:92–93.
12. Weissman MM. The myth of involutional melancholia. JAMA 1979;242:742–744.
13. Cooke DJ. Psychosocial vulnerability to life events during the climacteric. Br J Psychiatry 1985;147:71–75.
14. Hamilton M. Depression in the fifties. Gerontology 1986;32(suppl 1):14–16.
15. Steiner M. Psychobiologic aspects of the menopausal syndrome. In Buchsbaum HJ (ed): The Menopause. New York: Springer-Verlag, 1983;151–160.
16. Maoz B, Antonovsky A, Apter A, et al. The perception of menopause in five ethnic groups in Isreal. Acta Obstet Gynaecol Scand 1977;65:69–76.
17. Ballinger SE. Psychosocial stress and symptoms of menopause. Maturitas 1985;7:315–327.
18. Gambrell RD. The menopause: benefits and risks of estrogen-progestogen replacement therapy. Fertil Steril 1982;37:457–474.
19. Klaiber EL, Broverman DM, Vogel W, et al. Estrogen therapy for severe persistent depressions in women. Arch Gen Psychiatry 1979;36:550–554.
20. Holsboer F, Benkert O, Demisch L. Changes in MAO activity during estrogen treatment of females with endogenous depression. Mod Probl Pharmacopsychiatry 1983;19:321–326.
21. Strickler RC, Borth R, Cecutti A, et al. The role of oestrogen replacement in the climacteric syndrome. Psychol Med 1977;7:631–639.
22. Shapira B, Oppenheim G, Zohar J, et al. Lack of efficacy of estrogen supplementation to imipramine in resistant female depressives. Biol Psychiatry 1985;20:570–583.
23. Montgomery JC, Appleby L, Brincat M, et al. Effect of oestrogen and testosterone implants on psychological disorders in the climacteric. Lancet 1987;1:297–299.
24. Sherwin BB, Gelfand MM. Sex steroids and affect in the surgical menopause: a double-blind, cross-over study. Psychoneuroendocrinology 1985;10:325–335.
25. Robinson DS, Nies A, Davis JN, et al. Ageing, monoamines, and monoamine-oxidase levels. Lancet 1972;1:290–291.
26. Amsterdam JD, Winokur A, Lucki I, et al. Neuroendocrine regulation in depressed postmenopausal women and healthy subjects. Acta Psychiatr Scand 1983;67:43–49.
27. Hammar M, Berg G. Clonidine in the treatment of menopausal flushing: a review of clinical studies. Acta Obstet Gynaecol Scand [Suppl] 1985;132:29–31.
28. Report of a WHO Scientific Group. Research on the menopause. WHO Techn Rep Ser 1981;670:3–120.
29. Bell SE. Premenstrual syndrome and the medicalization of menopause. In Ginsburg BE, Carter BF (eds): Premenstrual Syndrome. New York: Plenum Press, 1987;151–173.

IV. RELATED AFFECTIVE SYNDROMES

IV.A. ANXIETY DISORDERS

86. Epinephrine-Induced Anxiety and Regional Cerebral Blood Flow in Anxious Patients

ROY J. MATHEW AND WILLIAM H. WILSON

Little is known about the effect of acute anxiety on cerebral circulation. Kety reported increased cerebral blood flow (CBF) in a patient who had an anxiety attack during CBF measurement with the nitrous oxide inhalation technique.[1] Mathew and associates found an inverse correlation between state anxiety and CBF in a group of patients with generalized anxiety disorder.[2]

We measured CBF before and 2 min after intravenous infusions of epinephrine 0.2 µg/kg or saline given under double-blind conditions over a period of 3 min to two groups of 20 patients with generalized anxiety disorder (*DSM-III*). The epinephrine group (EG) had the following characteristics: age 42 ± 10 years (mean ± SD); trait anxiety, measured by the State Trait Anxiety Inventory,[3] 53 ± 12; Beck Depression Inventory 8 ± 5. The placebo group (PG) had these characteristics: age 46 ± 8 years; trait anxiety 53 ± 11; Beck Depression Inventory 8 ± 6. All participants were right-handed, were physically healthy, and had been drug-free for 2 weeks. There were 12 men and 8 women in each group. The patients were assigned to the epinephrine and placebo groups on a random basis.

The CBF was measured with the xenon-133 inhalation technique[4] using our standard laboratory procedures and usual precautions.[5] During each CBF measurement pulse, respiration, and end-tidal carbon dioxide ($PECO_2$) were measured; and after each measurement venous hematocrit and state anxiety (STAI)[3] were measured.

Epinephrine infusions were followed by significant elevations in state anxiety, respiration, and pulse rate, and nonsignificant decreases in $PECO_2$ (repeated measure analysis of variance). No such changes were seen in the PG subjects. There were no significant differences between the EG and PG subjects on pre- or post-hemispheric or regional CBF, with and without correction for differences in $PECO_2$[6] (Table 86.1) (repeated measure analysis of variance: group × hemisphere × region).

Next we computed Pearson correlations between changes in state anxiety, the physiological indices, and CBF in the two groups. The EG patients showed inverse correlations between state anxiety and CBF (right hemisphere: $r -0.51$, $p < 0.05$; left hemisphere: $r -0.52$, $p < 0.05$), whereas in the PG subjects it correlated positively (right hemisphere: $r +0.50$, $p < 0.05$; left hemisphere: $r +0.44$, $p < 0.05$).

Table 86.1. Changes associated with epinephrine and placebo.

	Epinephrine		Placebo		F (group $\times$ period)	p
Variable	Pre	Post	Pre	Post		
State anxiety	45.8 ± 12	54.9 ± 12	44.1 ± 12	40.4 ± 13	10.5	< 0.003
CBF[a]						
Right hemisphere	75.2 ± 12	74.1 ± 13	69.7 ± 11	66.4 ± 9		NS
Left hemisphere	75.9 ± 11	74.8 ± 13	71.1 ± 12	66.6 ± 9		NS
PECO$_2$ (mm Hg)	37.7 ± 5	35.6 ± 5	37.4 ± 5	36.1 ± 5		NS
Respirations (/min)	10.7 ± 3	15.7 ± 8	11.7 ± 3	11.9 ± 4	7.33	< 0.02
Pulse (/min)	79.2 ± 14	84.4 ± 24	75.9 ± 14	70.1 ± 14	4.2	< 0.05
Hematocrit (%)	40.8 ± 4	40.6 ± 5	39.7 ± 3	39.5 ± 3		NS

Results are means ± SD.
[a]Gray matter flow given as milliliters per 100 g per min uncorrected for PECO$_2$. All comparisons were made with repeated measure analysis of variance.

PECO$_2$ correlated significantly with global CBF in the PG subjects (r +0.42, p <0.05) but not in the EG patients (r +0.14, NS).

At first glance the results seem to indicate that epinephrine-induced anxiety is not associated with any CBF changes. However, on closer inspection the results are complex and difficult to explain.

Acute changes in PECO$_2$ are well known to be accompanied by parallel CBF changes. As a matter of fact, CO$_2$ is believed to be the single most powerful determinant of CBF.[6–8] CBF and PECO$_2$ did not correlate in the EG patients; however, in the PG subjects they correlated significantly. Changes in PECO$_2$ in the EG patients were not associated with CBF changes. Thus the data indicate that the relation between CBF and PECO$_2$ is distorted in acute anxiety. In a previous study conducted in our laboratory[9] subjects who became anxious following CO$_2$ inhalation showed less CBF increase compared to those who did not. In that study correlation between CBF and CO$_2$ was weaker in the subjects who became anxious. Differences between the EG and PG cohorts on the PECO$_2$/CBF relation make comparisons of CBF between the two groups difficult.

At the moment the nature of an anxiety-related factor or factors responsible for the distorted relation between CO$_2$ and CBF is unclear. It may be argued that respiration is disturbed by acute anxiety, making it difficult to record true end-tidal CO$_2$ levels. None of the subjects hyperventilated or showed irregular or shallow breathing patterns. Thus in all probability, the close association between arterial and end-tidal CO$_2$ was preserved in the EG patients.

A number of physiological changes that accompany acute anxiety can influence CBF, including an increase in nonspecific arousal, which is known to increase CBF and two cerebral vasoconstrictive factors, i.e., increased hematocrit (blood viscosity)[10] and sympathetic tone.[11] Vasconstrictive factors seem to be of importance, as the EG patients showed an inverse correlation between CBF and state anxiety. We found a similar inverse correlation between state anxiety and CBF in two separate groups of patients with generalized anxiety disorder.[2,9] Hematocrit is unlikely to be of relevance, as it did not change following anxiety induction. Similar results were obtained in previous experiments in which anxiety was induced with epinephrine infusions (similar to the present study)[12] and CO$_2$ inhalation.[9]

Cerebral blood vessels receive sympathetic innervation from the superior cervical ganglia, stimulation of which reduces CBF.[11] Sympathetic control of CBF compared to several peripheral vascular beds is believed to be weak. However, cerebral vasculature may be oversensitive to sympathetic stimulation in patients with anxiety disorders. It should be noted that symptoms suggestive of transient cerebral ischemia have been reported in patients with panic disorder[13] and generalized anxiety disorder.[14] Additional studies need to be carried out to evaluate the role played by the sympathetic nervous system in the control of CBF during acute anxiety.

Anxiety is generally regarded as a hyperarousal state.[15] Evidence from a variety of sources indicates a close, parallel relation between arousal and CBF.[15] Thus one would expect anxiety to be associated with an increase in CBF. Mild changes in anxiety may indeed be accompanied by an increase in CBF. It should be noted that the PG subjects who showed a modest change in anxiety (3.7 units) showed a positive correlation between state anxiety and CBF. Severe anxiety, on the other hand, might trigger such vasoconstrictive factors as sympathetic tone, which could overshadow the arousal-related CBF increase. EG patients who showed an inverse correlation between state anxiety and CBF had an increase in the former by 9.1 units.

References

1. Kety SS. Consciousness and the metabolism of the brain. In Abramson HA (ed): Conference on Problems of Consciousness. New York: Josiah Macey Jr. Foundation, 1952;11–75.
2. Mathew RJ, Weinman ML, Claghorn JL. Anxiety and cerebral blood flow. In Mathew RJ (ed): The Biology of Anxiety. New York: Brunner/Mazel, 1982;23–33.
3. Spielberger CD, Gorsuch RL, Lushene RD. STAI Manual. Palo Alto, Ca: Consulting Psychologists, Press, 1970.
4. Obrist WD, Thompson HK, Wang HS, et al. Regional cerebral blood flow estimated by[133] xenon inhalation. Stroke 1975;6:245–256.
5. Mathew RJ, Wilson WH, Tant SR. Determinants of resting regional cerebral blood flow in normal subjects. Biol Psychiatry 1986;21:907–914.
6. Maximilian VA, Prohovnik I, Risberg J. Cerebral hemodynamic response to mental activation to normo- and hypercapnia. Stroke 1980;11:342–347.
7. Olesen J. Carbon dioxide. Acta Neurol Scand [Suppl 57] 1974;50:11–18.
8. Purves MJ. Regulation of cerebral vessels by carbon dioxide. In: The Physiology of the Cerebral Circulation. Cambridge: Cambridge University Press, 1972;173–199.
9. Mathew RJ, Wilson WH. Carbon dioxide-induced cerebral blood flow changes in anxiety. Psychiatry Res 1978; in press.
10. Thomas DJ. Whole blood viscosity and cerebral blood flow. Stroke 1982;13:285–287.
11. Edvinsson L. Sympathetic control of cerebral circulation. Trends Neurosci 1983;5:425–429.
12. Mathew RJ, Wilson WH. Anxiety and hematocrit. J Psychosom Res 1986;30:307–311.
13. Coyle PK, Sterman AB. Focal neurologic symptoms in panic attacks. Am J Psychiatry 1986;143:648–649.
14. Mathew RJ, Wilson WH, Nicassio PM. Cerebral ischemic symptoms in anxiety disorders. Am J Psychiatry 1987;144:265.
15. Lader M. Biological differentiation between anxiety, arousal and stress. In Mathew RJ (ed): The Biology of Anxiety. New York: Brunner/Mazel, 1982;11–22.
16. Ingvar DH. Hyperfrontal distribution of the cerebral grey matter flow in resting wakefulness; on the functional anatomy of the conscious state. Acta Neurol Scand 1979;60:12–25.

87. Neurobiological Mechanisms of Panic Anxiety: Review of the Behavioral, Biochemical, and Cardiovascular Effects of Three Panicogenic Stimuli

DENNIS S. CHARNEY, SCOTT W. WOODS, AND GEORGE R. HENINGER

The major results of a series of investigations of experimentally induced anxiety in panic disorder patients are presented here. The data obtained are relevant to the question of which neuronal systems may be involved in the pathophysiology of panic states. The ability of drugs with actions on noradrenergic (yohimbine), serotonergic (*m*-chlorophenylpiperazine), and adenosine (caffeine) function to produce panic anxiety was determined in three independent samples of patients meeting *DSM-III* criteria for agoraphobia with panic attacks or panic disorder and healthy subjects.

Methods

Yohimbine test days: Sixty-eight patients (49 women, mean age 39 ± 2 years; 19 men, mean age 38 ± 2 years) and 20 healthy subjects (11 women, mean age 43 ± 2 years; 9 men, mean age 34 ± 3 years) participated in two test days. Fifty-seven patients and 17 healthy subjects received four placebo-yohimbine capsules on the first test day and four capsules each containing 5 mg of yohimbine on the second test day. The rest of the patients and healthy subjects received the opposite sequence.

Caffeine test day: Twenty-one patients (15 women, mean age 38 ± 3; 6 men, mean age 38 ± 5) and 17 healthy subjects (11 women, mean age 36 ± 3; 6 men, mean age 36 ± 1) participated in two test days. They received oral caffeine-placebo on the first test day and caffeine citrate 10 mg/kg on the second test day.

m-Chlorophenylpiperazine (MCPP) test days: Twenty-four patients (17 women, mean age 36 ± 8; 7 men, mean age 34 ± 7) and 19 healthy subjects (15 women, mean age 37 ± 7; 4 men, mean age 38 ± 8) participated in two test days. They received an intravenous infusion of placebo (e.g., 0.45% saline) over 20 min on one test day and an intravenous infusion of MCPP 0.1 mg/kg on another test day. Twelve patients and 9 healthy subjects received placebo initially.

Complete and more extensive reports of these individual investigations may be found elsewhere.[1-4]

Results

Yohimbine-Induced Panic Attacks

Behavioral Changes. Yohimbine produced panic attacks in 37 of the 68 panic disorder patients and only 1 of the 20 healthy subjects ($p<0.001$, Fisher exact test) (Table 87.1).

Biochemical Changes. The patients who reported that yohimbine induced panic attacks had greater increases in plasma 3-methoxy-4-hydroxyphenylglycol (MHPG) following yohimbine than the healthy subjects or the patients who did not experience panic attacks. Significant yohimbine–placebo differences were identified between the patients who experienced panic attacks and the patients who did not and healthy subjects, respectively, at 120, 180, and 240 min (Fig. 87.1).

Only the patients who experienced panic attacks had significant increases in cortisol from baseline, which occurred at 60 and 90 min following yohimbine administration. These increases were significantly greater than the changes in cortisol after yohimbine administration in the patients who did not report panic attacks and healthy subjects.

In patients who experienced yohimbine-induced panic attacks following yohimbine, growth hormone ($n = 7$) and prolactin ($n = 9$) levels were determined. At no time point was there a significant change in growth hormone or prolactin following yohimbine in comparison to placebo.

Cardiovascular Changes. Yohimbine–placebo differences were significantly greater in the patients for sitting systolic blood pressure at 60 and 90 min. The patients who reported yohimbine-induced panic attacks had slightly greater effects on blood pressure compared to patients who did not (Fig. 87.2). Only the patients experiencing panic attacks had significant yohimbine–placebo increases in heart rate: The increase in sitting heart rate at 180 min was 7 ± 3 mm Hg ($p<0.01$); the

TABLE 87.1. Frequency of panic attacks[a] induced by yohimbine, caffeine, and MCPP in healthy subjects and panic disorder patients.

Test	No. of patients				No. of healthy patients			
	Yes	(%)	No	(%)	Yes	(%)	No	(%)
Yohimbine[b]	37	(54)	31	(46)	1	(5)	19	(95)
Caffeine[b]	15	(71)	6	(29)	2	(12)	15	(88)
MCPP	12	(52)	11	(48)	6	(32)	13	(68)

[a]Two criteria had to be satisfied for the behavioral effect to be designated a panic attack: (a) *DSM-III* criteria requiring a healthy subject or patient to experience a discrete period of severe subjective anxiety accompanied by an increase over baseline on four or more of the 12 *DSM-III* symptoms of a panic attack; and (b) the patient reported that the anxiety state experienced was similar to that of a naturally occurring panic attack.
[b]$p < 0.001$, patients versus healthy subjects, Fisher exact test (two-tailed).

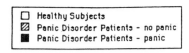

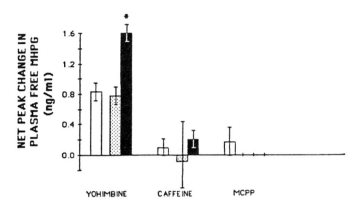

Figure 87.1. Net peak changes (± SEM) in plasma free MHPG in healthy subjects and panic disorder patients who did and did not report panic attacks following yohimbine and caffeine. MHPG data regarding the effects of MCPP was available only in ten healthy subjects. In these subjects the change from baseline following MCPP was not significantly different from the change following placebo at any time point. The net peak change was calculated by subtracting the peak increase from baseline following active drug from the peak increase from baseline following placebo. *$p < 0.001$, net peak change, patients reporting panic attacks versus healthy subjects and patients not reporting panic attacks, Students's t-test (two-tailed).

increase in standing heart rate at 60 min was 6 ± 2 mm Hg (p<0.05), and at 180 min it was (6 ± 2 mm Hg (*p*<0.05).

Caffeine-Induced Panic Attacks

Behavioral Changes. Caffeine produced panic attacks in 15 of the 21 panic disorder patients and in 2 of the 17 healthy subjects (*p*<0.001, Fisher exact test); (Table 87.1).

Biochemical Changes. Caffeine administration did not significantly alter plasma free MHPG levels in either the healthy subjects or the patients who did or did not report caffeine-induced panic attacks (Fig. 87.1).

Caffeine did not significantly increase cortisol levels, but caffeine–placebo differences were significant at 60, 90, and 120 min in both healthy subjects and patients. The effect of caffeine on plasma cortisol levels was not different among the healthy subjects and patients who did and did not experience panic attacks.

Growth hormone and prolactin levels were determined in eight patients who experienced panic attacks following caffeine. At no specific time point was there a significant change in growth hormone or prolactin following caffeine in comparison to placebo.

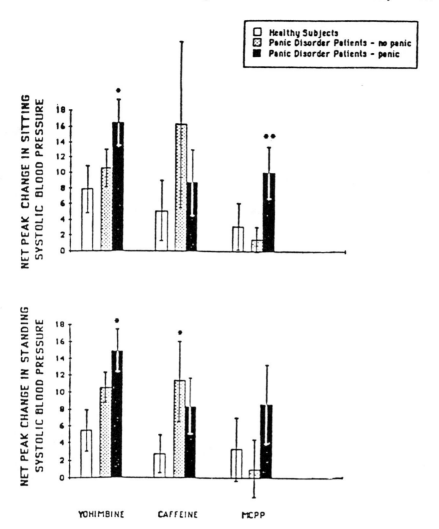

FIGURE 87.2. Net peak change in sitting and standing systolic blood pressures (mm Hg ± SEM) in healthy subjects and patients who did and did not report panic attacks following yohimbine, caffeine, and MCPP. *$d < 0.05$, net peak change, patients versus healthy subjects, Students's t-test (two-tailed). **$p < 0.05$, net peak change, patients reporting panic attacks versus patients not reporting panic attacks, Students's t-test (two-tailed).

Cardiovascular Changes. Caffeine–placebo increases from baseline were significantly greater in the patients for sitting diastolic blood pressure at 60 min and tended to be higher for sitting systolic blood pressure at 30 and 60 min.

Similar caffeine-induced effects on blood pressures were observed when patients who did and did not report panic attacks were compared to the matched healthy subjects (Fig. 87.2). The effects of caffeine on standing heart rate appeared to be more pronounced in the patients experiencing caffeine-induced panic attacks. Caffeine–placebo differences in standing heart rate were significantly greater in these patients at 30 min: $(9 \pm 3$ versus $- 1 \pm 2$ mm Hg $(p<0.01)$.

MCPP-Induced Panic Attacks

Behavioral Changes. The 20-min infusion of MCPP produced panic attacks in 12 of the 23 panic disorder patients and in 6 of the 19 healthy control subjects (NS, Fisher exact test) (Table 87.1).

Biochemical Changes. The comparison of the cortisol, prolactin, and growth hormone increases following MCPP in the healthy subjects and patients revealed that at no time point was there a significant difference in the MCPP–placebo increases in these hormones from baseline between the two groups.

The patients and healthy subjects who reported MCPP-induced panic attacks did not have greater increases in cortisol, prolactin, or growth hormone after MCPP than the healthy subjects or patients who did not have panic attacks.

Preliminary work indicates that MCPP has no significant effect on plasma MHPG levels in ten healthy subjects who did $(n = 3)$ and did not $(n = 7)$ experience panic attacks.

Cardiovascular Changes. The MCPP-induced changes in blood pressure and heart rate were not significantly different in the patients who experienced MCPP-induced panic attacks compared to patients and healthy subjects who did not except for a significantly greater MCPP–placebo increase from baseline in sitting systolic blood pressure at 180 min (Fig. 87.2).

Comment

A major conclusion from this study is that drugs with actions on a variety of neuronal systems, including noradrenergic, adenosine, and serotonergic systems, are capable of producing panic anxiety states defined by standard criteria in susceptible individuals. The observed behavioral, biochemical, and cardiovascular effects of the anxiogenic probes in patients and healthy subjects indicates that drugs that produce similar panic anxiety states can have markedly different actions on neurotransmitter function, hormone secretion, and cardiovascular activity. These data suggest that panic anxiety is unlikely to be uniformly associated with abnormalities in a single neurotransmitter system but, rather, may be produced by dysfunction of a variety of neuronal systems. Although it is possible that panic anxiety may be mediated by a single, as yet undetermined, "final common neuronal pathway" that is regulated by neurotransmitter systems such as those tested in these investigations, a greater degree of redundancy probably exists because of the importance that anxiety and fear play in behaviors essential for species survival.

The increased anxiogenic effects in panic disorder patients of yohimbine, caffeine, and, in previous work, CO_2 and lactate[5-8] suggest that the abnormal responses of panic disorder patients to these drugs may reflect different subtypes of panic disorder. Alternatively, it is possible that abnormal responses to these agents are indicative of a more fundamental molecular dysfunction in the regulation of neuronal excitability than exists within multiple neuronal systems.

Another implication of the demonstration that drugs with pharmacological effects on different neuronal systems produce anxiety states that satisfy *DSM-III* criteria for panic attacks is that current diagnostic criteria for panic attacks define a behavioral state that is neurobiologically heterogeneous. The results emphasize the limitations of the use of descriptive methods for psychiatric classification designed for etiological purposes and the need for clinically applicable biological tests capable of determining specific neurobiological dysfunctions in psychiatric disorders.

References

1. Charney DS, Heninger GR, Breier A. Noradrenergic function in panic anxiety: effects of yohimbine in healthy subjects and patients with agoraphobia and panic disorder. Arch Gen Psychiatry 1984;41:751–763.
2. Charney DS, Heninger GR, Jatlow PI. Increased anxiogenic effects of caffeine in panic disorders. Arch Gen Psychiatry 1985;42:233–243.
3. Charney DS, Woods SW, Goodman WK, et al. Serotonin function in anxiety. II. Effects of the serotonin agonist, MCPP, in panic disorder patients and healthy subjects. Psychopharmacology 1987;92:14–24.
4. Charney DS, Woods SW, Goodman WK, et al. Neurobiological mechanisms of panic anxiety: biochemical and behavioral correlates of yohimbine-induced panic attacks. Am J Psychiatry 1987;144:1030–1036.
5. Woods SW, Charney DS, Loke J, et al. Carbon dioxide sensitivity in panic anxiety: ventilatory and anxiogenic response to CO_2 in healthy subjects and panic anxiety patients before and after alprazolam treatment. Arch Gen Psychiatry 1986;43:900–909.
6. Gorman JM, Askanazi J, Liebowitz MR, et al. Response to hyperventilation in a group of patients with panic disorder. Am J Psychiatry 1984;141:857–861.
7. Liebowitz MR, Fyer AJ, Gorman JM, et al. Lactate provocation of panic attacks. I. Clinical and behavioral findings. Arch Gen Psychiatry 1984;41:764–770.
8. Liebowitz MR, Gorman JM, Fyer AJ, et al. Lactate provocation of panic attacks. II. Biochemical and physiological findings. Arch Gen Psychiatry 1985;42:709–719.

88. Caffeine Model of Panic

THOMAS W. UHDE AND JEAN-PHILIPPE BOULENGER

Much attention has been focused on the neurobiology of panic disorder. According to the *DSM-III-R* classification of panic disorders, panic attacks are given central importance in the genesis and maintenance of secondary complications such as agoraphobia, anticipatory anxiety, and, in a subgroup of patients, major depressive symptomatology. Given this perspective, it is important to understand the pathophysiology and biological correlates of "spontaneous" or "unprovoked" panic attacks.

Unfortunately, the study of "spontaneous" panic attacks in the research setting is made impractical by the infrequent and unpredictable occurrence of natural panic attacks. As a result, laboratories have developed reliable, safe clinical techniques for inducing panic attacks in panic-prone individuals. The most widely studied chemical models of panic are those induced by intravenous sodium lactate, orally administered yohimbine, and inspired carbon dioxide. Our laboratory has developed the caffeine model of panic.

The initial impetus for the development of this model was twofold. First, many anecdotal reports in the literature had suggested that caffeine could induce anxiety and panic attacks if consumed in toxic proportions. Second, extensive observations of patients in our Unit on Anxiety and Affective Disorders at the National Institute of Mental Health indicated that patients with panic disorder were particularly vulnerable to the anxiogenic effects of caffeine. These preliminary observations were later substantiated in more systematic fashion with a retrospective survey. The results of this survey, developed by Boulenger and Uhde,[1] indicated that patients with panic disorder, but not affectively ill patients or normal controls, had levels of self-rated anxiety and depression that correlated with their 24-h caffeine consumption. Moreover, the panic disorder patients reported increased sensitivity to the effects of one cup of coffee.[2] These data suggested that panic disorder patients were more sensitive to the psychoactive effects of caffeine. However, these tentative conclusions were based on self-rated measures and lacked confirmation by a direct test using a caffeine challenge. Therefore our unit developed the caffeine challenge method for investigating the effects of caffeine in humans.[3-6]

Methods

Fourteen normal controls (7 men and 7 women; mean age 31.4 years free from medical or psychiatric illnesses participated in the study. Twenty-four panic disorder patients (9 men and 15 women; mean age 33.6 years) were also studied and remained medication-free during the time of the study. Both controls and patients maintained a caffeine-free diet for at least 10 days prior to and during the study. Twelve controls received placebo and three caffeine doses (240, 480, and 720 mg p.o.), and two controls and eight panic disorder patients received placebo and 480 mg of caffeine. An additional 16 drug-free panic disorder patients received 480 mg of caffeine, but not placebo, as part of a separate study.

The drugs were always administered in the morning after a rest period of at least 30 min. Several behavioral measures, using standardized rating scales, were assessed at baseline and at 60 and 150 min after drug administration. Blood samples for norepinephrine (NE), 3-methoxy-4-hydroxyphenylethylene glycol (MHPG), cortisol, glucose, and lactate were obtained at baseline and at 30, 60, 90, 120, and 150 min after drug administration. In a subgroup of subjects urine samples for MHPG, normetanephrine, and metanephrine were obtained. These urine samples were collected during the 3-h period immediately following drug administration.

Results

Effects of Caffeine in Normal Controls

Caffeine induced a dose-related increase in Zung and Spielberger State anxiety in the normal controls (ANOVA, $p < 0.0001$ and $p < 0.004$, respectively); 2 of 12 normal controls also developed panic attacks after administration of the 720-mg dose. Caffeine induced significant increases by ANOVA in plasma levels of cortisol ($p < 0.0001$), glucose ($p < 0.0004$), and lactate ($p < 0.002$) and an increase in mean arterial blood pressure ($p < 0.007$).

In a subgroup of six normal controls, we evaluated the effects of caffeine on urinary MHPG, normetanephrine, and metanephrine during the 3 h after drug administration. One-way repeated measures ANOVA indicated that there was no difference in any of these catecholamine metabolites across the placebo and three caffeine conditions.

In a subgroup of eight normal controls, we investigated the effects of oral caffeine administration on both plasma caffeine and adenosine levels. As expected, there was a dose-related increase in plasma caffeine ($p < 0.0001$) levels. However, there was no significant change in plasma adenosine. We also examined the relation between plasma caffeine and changes in anxiety (1-h score minus baseline score) by determining the best-fitting lines to the bivariate plot of anxiety versus plasma caffeine level for each individual. Most of the normal controls demonstrated a positive correlation between levels of caffeine in the blood and ratings of anxiety. Thus a significantly greater number of normal controls showed a positive relation between their caffeine levels and changes in Zung (sign test, $p < 0.004$) and state anxiety (sign test, $p < 0.035$) scores than would be expected by chance according to the binomial distribution.

Effects of Caffeine in Patients with Panic Disorder

After administration of 480 mg of caffeine, 9 of 24 panic disorder patients but none of 14 controls experienced panic attacks. This apparent hypersensitivity to caffeine's anxiogenic effects was also reflected in a greater increase in placebo-corrected measures of Zung anxiety found in a smaller subgroup of eight panic patients compared to 14 normal controls (ANOVA, $p<0.01$). Compared to baseline values, caffeine induced significant increases in mean arterial pressure, cortisol, glucose, and lactate in both panic disorder patients and normal controls. Although the caffeine-induced increases in mean arterial pressure were similar, there was a significantly greater main effect increase in cortisol in the panic disorder group compared to controls ($p<0.02$). There was also a significant (group $\times$ time) interaction between the panic patients and normal controls with significantly greater glucose ($p<0.05$) and lactate ($p<0.04$) levels at 90 min following the caffeine administration. Moreover, the "panicking" versus "nonpanicking" panic disorder patients had significantly greater increases in lactate ($p<0.03$).

Discussion

These findings suggest that caffeine has dose-related anxiogenic effects in normal controls; moreover, normal controls may experience panic attacks with caffeine doses above 700 mg. This panicogenic dose of caffeine is roughly equivalent to the amount of caffeine contained in six to ten cups of coffee. It should be emphasized that some normal controls experienced an increased sense of well-being, but not anxiety, following caffeine. In contrast, almost all panic disorder patients reported increased ratings of anxiety after caffeine. In fact, 38% of the patients experienced panic attacks following a 480-mg challenge of caffeine compared to none of the normal controls. Thus our findings with a direct challenge confirmed our initial hypothesis that the panic disorder patients would be more vulnerable to the psychoactive properties of caffeine.

The increased behavioral reactivity to caffeine was also accompanied by a greater increase in blood levels of glucose, cortisol, and lactate in the panic disorder patients compared to normal controls. It is of interest that the panicking patients had significantly greater increases in lactate, but not cortisol or glucose, compared to the nonpanicking panic disorder patients. These data suggest that there may be an important relation between increases in lactate levels and caffeine-induced anxiety. The exact mechanism of caffeine-induced anxiety in humans, however, remains uncertain. Because plasma NE, MHPG, and urinary metabolites of catecholaminergic function did not increase after caffeine, the noradrenergic system appears to be an unlikely candidate for the mediation of the anxiogenic effects of caffeine. Of course, caffeine might stimulate noradrenergic activity in selected brain pathways without increasing levels of NE or its metabolites in peripheral pools. Our data indirectly support a role for adenosine receptor systems in caffeine-induced anxiety states, as caffeine levels reached after administration of 720 mg, the only dose that in the normal controls produced panic attacks, are in a range (44–73 μ M) known to compete with the binding of various ligands to the adenosine receptors in human brain (Ki 35–115 μM).[7] Because the reuptake of adenosine displaced from *brain* receptors is probably rapid, a lack of increase in *plasma* adenosine is not unexpected and not inconsistent with the hypothesis that central adenosinergic function plays a role in caffeine-induced anxiety states.

In summary, the caffeine challenge paradigm provides a new chemical model for investigating the neurobiology of human anxiety. Future studies are required, however, to elucidate the molecular basis of caffeine-induced panic and related caffeine intoxication syndromes.

References

1. Boulenger JP, Uhde TW. Caffeine consumption and anxiety: preliminary results of a survey comparing patients with anxiety disorders and normal controls. Psychopharmacol Bull 1982;18:53–57.
2. Boulenger JP, Uhde TW, Wolff EA, et al. Increased sensitivity to caffeine in patients with panic disorders: preliminary evidence. Arch Gen Psychiatry 1984;41:1067–1071.
3. Uhde TW, Boulenger J-P, Jimerson DC, et al. Caffeine: relationship to human anxiety, plasma MHPG and cortisol. Psychopharmacol Bull 1984;20:426–430.
4. Uhde TW, Boulenger JP, Post RM, et al. Fear and anxiety: relationship to noradrenergic function. Psychopathology 1984;17(3):8–23.
5. Uhde TW, Boulenger J-P, Vittone B, et al. Human anxiety and noradrenergic function: preliminary studies with caffeine, clonidine and yohimbine. In Pichot R, Berner P, Wolf R, et al (eds): Psychiatry: The State of the Art. New York: Plenum Press, 1985;693–698.
6. Boulenger J-P, Bierer LM, Uhde TW. Anxiogenic effects of caffeine in normal controls and patients with panic disorder. In Shagass C, Josiassen RC, Bridger WH, et al (eds): Biological Psychiatry 1985. New York: Elsevier, 1986;454–456.
7. Boulenger J-P, Patel J, Marangos PJ. Effects of caffeine and theophylline on adenosine and benzodiazepine receptors in human brain. Neurosci Lett 1982;30:161–166.

89. Pharmacological Treatment of Panic Disorders

JAMES C. BALLENGER

Effective pharmacotherapy of panic disorder and agoraphobia with panic attacks was introduced during the early 1960s, when almost simultaneously it was reported that both monoamine oxidase inhibitors (MAOIs) and tricyclic antidepressants (TCAs) reduced symptoms of panic and phobic avoidance. This chapter reviews the accumulated evidence regarding the effective pharmacotherapy of these disorders.[1]

Tricyclic Antidepressants

Imipramine

Most of the evidence for tricyclic efficacy in the treatment of agoraphobia with panic attacks has been with imipramine. Five of the six double-blind, placebo-controlled trials of imipramine demonstrate clear superiority of imipramine over placebo, and its effectiveness has been further demonstrated in open trials.[2-13] Results from the four largest research trials report that 70–90% of patients experience moderate or marked improvement in phobic symptoms and secondary disability, but often only after 6–12 weeks of treatment.[4-7,10,11,14]

Other Tricyclic Antidepressants

Clomipramine has been shown to be effective in agoraphobia with panic attacks in open trials and in three placebo-controlled trials.[15-23] Otherwise, there is little evidence of controlled trials with other TCAs. In two open trials, zimelidine, a serotonin reuptake inhibitor, demonstrated significant efficacy. There is also limited and generally anecdotal evidence suggesting that desipramine,[24,25] nortriptyline,[26] maprotiline,[27] doxepin,[13] and amitriptyline[13] are clinically effective and useful. Bupropion is the only TCA shown to be *in*effective in a controlled trial.[28] Although trazodone has been reported to be effective in some patients, evidence suggests that it may be less effective than other TCAs.[27] Anecdotal evidence suggests that amoxapine may also be less effective than the other tricyclics.

Despite the importance of the issue, there are no published comparisons of most of the various TCAs in the treatment of these disorders.

Monoamine Oxidase Inhibitors

There are now six placebo-controlled trials, five with phenelzine[6,7,29–32] (Nardil) and one with iproniazid,[33] that have demonstrated the effectiveness of MAOls. Tyrer and colleagues[29] reported that 65–70% of patients improved and maintained this improvement for 8 months. However, overall these MAOl studies are less convincing than those involving the TCAs because the number of studies is smaller; moreover, they involve smaller sample sizes, have utilized diagnostically mixed patient samples, and have usually involved low doses of the MAOls.

Ballenger et al.[6] and Sheehan et al.[7] reported what is probably the most definitive placebo-controlled trial of an MAOl. Agoraphobics with panic attacks were treated with phenelzine 45 mg/day, imipramine 150 mg/day, or placebo over a 12-week period. All patients received self-exposure instructions and encouragement in every-other-week supportive group therapy sessions. Although there was significant improvement with group therapy alone (plus placebo), both phenelzine and imipramine achieved significantly greater reduction in phobic anxiety and fears, general anxiety, agoraphobic avoidance, and work and social disability. The phenelzine group consistently had greater levels of improvement than the imipramine group, although this difference was generally nonsignificant. However, as assessed on the two physician- and patient-rated behavioral scales measuring severity of phobic and avoidance symptoms and the patients' work and social performance, the phenelzine group showed significantly more improvement than the imipramine group. Approximately 75% of the patients in the phenelzine group had a clinically significant improvement and rated themselves as almost free of symptoms.

In an early open and retrospective study of 246 phobic patients treated with various MAOls, Kelly et al.[34] reported that approximately 75% had responded at 1 month, and this improvement was maintained 1 year later. The panic attacks were blocked in approximately 40% during the first month of treatment, and approximately 90% of patients experienced major improvement of their symptoms.

Benzodiazepines

Although most experienced clinicians and investigators had believed that benzodiazepines were usually only partially effective, preliminary trials suggest that alprazolam, a triazolobenzodiazepine is effective when taken regularly and in sufficiently high doses.

Chouinard and colleagues[35] reported the first double-blind trial of alprazolam versus placebo in patients with both panic disorder and generalized anxiety disorder. Eight of 14 patients had a moderate or excellent response to relatively low doses of alprazolam (mean 2.06 mg/day). Sheehan et al.[36] reported a single-blind, 8-week comparison of alprazolam and ibuprofen. There was little response in patients taking ibuprofen, but there was significant improvement in physican global ratings and in anticipatory anxiety episodes in those receiving alprazolam. Alexander and Alexander[37] reported the treatment of 27 patients with agoraphobia with panic attacks with alprazolam in a private practice setting. Approximately 85% of patients became panic-free on 3–4 mg/day.

Preliminary results from a large, multicenter, double-blind, placebo-controlled trial of alprazolam have been reported.[38] Approximately 560 patients were treated with a flexible-dose schedule using a mean dose of 5.6 mg/day. The investigators reported significantly greater reductions in panic attacks, phobias, anxiety, work and social disability, and overall global ratings in the alprazolam group compared to the placebo group. In this 8-week trial 88% of alprazolam patients and 38% of placebo patients had a moderate or better response. Alprazolam was well tolerated, with a less than 5% dropout rate due to side effects.[39] The principal side effect experienced was sedation, which resolved or improved either over time or with dose reduction.

The only other benzodiazepine study conducted under controlled conditions is a preliminary trial comparing diazepam with propranolol.[40] Noyes and colleagues were able to demonstrate moderate or better improvement in 86% on diazepam but only 33% on propranolol.[40]

Recommended Doses

Mavissakalian and Perel[41] reported that patients treated with imipramine have a significantly higher rate of response on doses of more than 150 mg/day. Zitrin et al.[4,5,14] have consistently recommended that although some patients may respond to low doses of imipramine (e.g., 25 mg/day) most require 150–200 mg/day and some may require 200–300 mg/day.

The optimal serum level of imipramine has been investigated in two published studies. In a 12-week study, Ballenger et al.[11] treated two groups of 18 patients each with doses that maintained their serum level of imipramine plus its principal metabolite desipramine at 100–150 and 200–250 ng/ml, respectively. Approximately 75% achieved an excellent response, with no important differences in response between the two groups. In contrast, Mavissakalian et al.[42] observed a significantly positive correlation between plasma imipramine (not desipramine) and reduction in symptoms in 15 panic disorder patients.

In the largest MAOI trial,[6,7] more than 75% of the patients did well on phenelzine 45 mg/day, although some subsequently improved on doses of 60 mg/day or higher. Patients in preliminary trials with alprazolam have responded to doses as low as 1.0–2.0 mg/day, although most seem to need 3.0–6.0 mg/day, and some 6.0–12.0 mg/day.

Length of Treatment

Systematic data on optimal length of treatment with TCAs, MAOIs, and benzodiazepines are currently unavailable. There is some evidence from controlled trials that patients continue to improve up to 6 months,[4,14] and most clinicians believe that patients continue to improve over most of the first year of treatment.

Relapse

In the three published reports[4,5,14] 15–30% of agoraphobic patients relapsed after discontinuation of antidepressant treatment. There are no published data on relapse rates with the use of alprazolam, but preliminary reports suggest that the relapse rate is comparable to or even higher than that with the antidepressants.

Difference Among the Medications

The three most commonly used drugs at this time–imipramine, phenelzine, and alprazolam–are probably roughly equivalent in terms of efficacy and side effects, although controlled trials comparing them are certainly needed. Clinicians generally choose between them based on differences in their associated side effects.

Termination of Medications

After 6 and often 12 months of successful treatment it is reasonable to consider discontinuation of these medications. The TCAs, MAOls, and alprazolam should all be tapered gradually over a 1- to 3-month period to reduce the patient's anxieties about relapse, allow early detection of a potential relapse, and reduce withdrawal symptoms (with alprazolam). Alprazolam doses should be reduced no more rapidly than 0.5 mg/day once or twice per week. When patients relapse after discontinuing these medications, most if not all respond well to the reinstitution of the medication.

References

1. Ballenger JC. Pharmacotherapy of the panic disorders. J Clin Psychiatry 1987;47(6):27–32.
2. Klein DF. Delineation of two drug-responsive anxiety syndromes. Psychopharmacologia 1964;53:397–408.
3. Klein DF, Fink M. Psychiatric reaction patterns to imipramine. Am J Psychiatry 1962;119:432–438.
4. Zitrin CM, Klein DF, Woerner MG. Treatment of agoraphobia with group exposure in vivo and imipramine. Arch Gen Psychiatry 1980;37:63–72.
5. Zitrin CM, Klein DF, Woerner MG, et al. Treatment of phobias. I. Comparison of imipramine hydrochloride and placebo. Arch Gen Psychiatry 1983;40:125–138.
6. Ballenger JC, Sheehan DV, Jacobsen G. Antidepressant treatment of severe phobic anxiety. In: Abstracts of the Scientific Proceedings of the 130th Annual Meeting of the American Psychiatric Association, Toronto, 1977.
7. Sheehan DV, Ballenger J, Jacobsen G. Treatment of endogenous anxiety with phobic, hysterical and hypochondriacal symptoms. Arch Gen Psychiatry 1980;37:51–59.
8. Marks IM, Gray S, Cohen D, et al. Imipramine and brief therapist-aided exposure in agoraphobics having self-exposure homework. Arch Gen Psychiatry 1983;40:153–162.
9. McNair DM, Kahn RJ. Imipramine compared with a benzodiazepine for agoraphobia. In Klein DF, Rabkin JG (eds): Anxiety: New Research and Changing Concepts. New York: Raven Press, 1981.
10. Mavissakalian M, Michelson L. Agorphobia: behavioral and pharmacological treatments, preliminary outcome, and process findings. Psychopharmacol Bull 1982;18:91–103.
11. Ballenger JC, Peterson GA, Laraia M, et al. A study of plasma catecholamines in agoraphobia and the relationship of serum tricyclic levels to treatment response. In Ballenger JC (ed): Biology of Agoraphobia. Washington, DC: APA Press, 1984.
12. Mavissakalian M, Michelson L, Dealy RS. Pharmacological treatment of agoraphobia: imipramine versus imipramine with programmed practice. Br J Psychiatry 1983;143:348–355.
13. Lydiard RB, Ballenger JC. Antidepressants in panic disorder and agoraphobia. *J Affective Disord* 1987;13:153–168.
14. Zitrin CM, Klein DF, Woerner MG. Behavioral therapy, supportive psychotherapy, imipramine, and phobias. Arch Gen Psychiatry 1978;35:307–316.

15. Colgan A. A pilot study of Anafranil in the treatment of phobic states. Scott Med J 1975;20(Suppl 1):55–60.
16. Waxman D. An investigation into the use of Anafranil in phobic and obsessional disorders. Scott Med J 1975;20(Suppl 1):61–66.
17. Carey MS, Hawkinson R, Kornhaber A, et al. The use of clomipramine in phobic patients: preliminary research report. Curr Ther Res 1975;17:107–110.
18. Beaumont G. A large open multicentre trial of clomipramine (Anafranil) in the management of phobic disorders. J Int Med Res 1977;5:116–123.
19. Gloger S, Grunhaus L, Birmacher B, et al. Treatment of spontaneous panic attacks with chlorimipramine. Am J Psychiatry 1981;138:1215–1217.
20. Grunhaus L, Gloger S, Birmacher B. Chlorimipramine for panic attacks in patients with mitral valve prolapse. J Clin Psychiatry 1984;45:25–27.
21. Escobar JI, Landbloom RP. Treatment of phobic neurosis with chlorimipramine: a controlled clinical trial. Curr Ther Res 1976;20:680–685.
22. Karabanow O. Double-blind controlled study in phobias and obsessions. J Int Med Res 1977;5:42–48.
23. Amin MM, Ban TA, Pecknold JC, et al. Chlorimipramine (Anafranil) and behavior therapy in obsessive-compulsive and phobic disorders. J Int Med Res 1977;5:33–37.
24. Lydiard RB. Desipramine in panic disorder: an open, fixed-dose study. Presented at the Annual Meeting of the American Academy of Clinical Psychiatry, San Francisco, 1985.
25. Rifkin A, Klein DF, Dillon D, et al. Blockade by imipramine or desipramine of panic induced by sodium lactate. Am J Psychiatry 1981;138:676–677.
26. Muskin PR, Fyer AJ. Treatment of panic disorder. J. Clin Psychopharmacol 1981;1:81–90.
27. Sheehan DV. Current views on the treatment of panic and phobic disorders. Drug Ther 1982;12:74–93.
28. Sheehan DV, Davidson J, Manschreck T, et al. Lack of efficacy of a new antidepressant (Bupropion) in the treatment of panic disorder with phobias. J Clin Psychopharmacol 1983;3:28–31.
29. Tyrer P, Candy J, Kelly D. A study of the clinical effects of phenelzine and placebo in the treatment of phobic anxiety. Psychopharmacologia 1973;32:237–254.
30. Solyom L, Heseltine GFD, McClure DJ, et al. Behavior therapy versus drug therapy in the treatment of phobic neuroses. Can Psychiatr Assoc J 1973;18:25–32.
31. Mountjoy CQ, Roth M, Garside RF, et al. A clinical trial of phenelzine in anxiety depressive and phobic neuroses. Br J Psychiatry 1977;131:486–492.
32. Solyom C, Solyom L, LaPierre Y, et al. Phenelzine and exposure in the treatment of phobias. Biol Psychiatry 1981;16:239–247.
33. Lipsedge MS, Hajioff J, Huggins P, et al. The management of severe agoraphobia: a comparison of iproniazid and systematic desensitization. Psychopharmacologia 1973;32:67–80.
34. Kelly D, Guirguis W, Frommer E, et al. Treatment of phobic states with antidepressants: a retrospective study of 246 patients. Br J Psychiatry 1970;116:387–398.
35. Chouinard G, Annable L, Fontaine R, et al. Alprazolam in the treatment of generalized anxiety and panic disorders: a double-blind, placebo-controlled study. Psychopharmacology 1982;77:229–233.
36. Sheehan DV, Coleman JH, Greenblatt DJ, et al. Some biochemical correlates of panic attacks with agoraphobia and their response to a new treatment. J Clin Psychopharmacol 1984;4:66–75.
37. Alexander DE, Alexander DD. Alprazolam treatment for panic disorders. Presented at the 137th Annual Meeting of the American Psychiatric Association, Los Angeles, 1984.
38. Ballenger JC, Burrows G, DuPont RL Jr, Lesser JM, et al. Alprazolam in panic disorder and agoraphobia: results from a multicenter trial. I. Efficacy in short-term treatment. Arch Gen Psychiatry 1988;45(5):413–422.
39. Noyes R Jr, DuPont RL Jr, Pecknold JC, et al. Alprazolam in panic disorder and agoraphobia: Results from a multicenter trial. II. Patient acceptance, side effects, and safety. Arch Gen Psychiatry 1988;45(5):423–428.
40. Noyes R, Anderson D, Clancy J. Diazepam and propranolol in panic disorder and agoraphobia. Arch Gen Psychiatry 1984;41:287–292.

41. Mavissakalian M, Perel J. Imipramine in the treatment of agoraphobia: dose-response relationship. Am J Psychiatry 1985;142:1032–1036.
42. Mavissakalian M, Perel JM, Michelson L. The relationship of plasma imipramine and N-desmethylimipramine to improvement in agoraphobia. J Clin Psychopharmacol 1984;4:36–40.

IV.B. OBSESSIVE COMPULSIVE DISORDER

90. Heterogeneity and Coexistence in *DSM-III-R* Obsessive Compulsive Disorder

STEVEN A. RASMUSSEN AND JANE L. EISEN

Less than a decade ago obsessive compulsive disorder (OCD) was thought of as a rare illness with a poor prognosis. This belief has been challenged by epidemiological and treatment outcome studies that have set the stage for a resurgence of interest in OCD.

The clinical symptoms of OCD have captivated the attention of psychoanalysts, behaviorists, and biologists alike. Despite this interest, relatively little systematic research has been done in OCD in comparison to other anxiety and depressive disorders. Undoubtedly, the single most important factor that has contributed to this situation has been the mistaken belief that OCD is a rare illness, a belief based on a series of follow-up studies initiated during the 1950s and 1960s. These studies consistently reported that the incidence of OCD in psychiatric inpatient and outpatient settings was only 1–2%.[1] Despite its low prevalence in psychiatric populations, most investigators thought that these figures significantly underestimated the illness's prevalence in the general population. In 1953 Rudin estimated the disorder's prevalence in the general population at 0.05%.[2] In 1984 preliminary results from the National Epidemiology Catchment Survey (ECA) were published.[3] The ECA study was a large-scale epidemiological survey that interviewed 15,000 subjects in the general population in order to determine the prevalence rates of psychiatric disorders in the United States. Among the most striking findings were the high lifetime (2.5%) and 6-month (1.6%) prevalence rates of OCD. If these figures are valid, it would make OCD the fourth most common psychiatric disorder in the general population—twice as prevalent as schizophrenia or panic disorder and 50 times more common than Rudin's 1953 estimate.

When we initiated our work, we were surprised to discover that there had been no large-scale phenomenological or epidemiological study of OCD in the last 20 years. We began to study the heterogeneity of OCD and its coexistence with other psychiatric disorders in a subgroup of 44 patients who met *DSM-III-R* criteria for OCD by administering a semistructured interview to each of the probands.[4] The interview covererd demographics; obsessive and compulsive symptoms; course of illness; a checklist of symptoms for depression, psychosis, other anxiety disorders, and personality disorders; and family history. We have subsequently interviewed 50 additional OCD probands using the SADS-LA. We were particularly interested in whether OCD is a heterogeneous diagnosis, and, if so, could it be divided into homogenous subgroups? We were also interested in the question: What other psychiatric disorders were likely to coexist with OCD?

Can OCD be subdivided by symptoms or course of illness into homogeneous subtypes? The most common obsession, found in 55% of the patients, was fear of contamination (Table 90.1). This obsession took many forms, the most common being the fear of unseen dirt, germs, poisons, or toxins. The next most common obsessive thought, present in 42% of the patients, was pathological doubt or the fear that they would be responsible for something terrible happening. Twenty-six percent of the patients complained of sexual obsessions, most commonly fears of sexual impulses that went against their value system or fears of sexual perversions. Twenty-eight percent complained of aggressive obsessions or impulses. As with the patients with sexual obsessions, these patients were often unable to make a clear distinction between having an unacceptable thought and acting on it. Sixty-eight percent of the patients with aggressive obsessions also had fears about their sexual impulses. As a group, the patients with sexual and aggressive obsessions were usually preoccupied with guilt, at times of near delusional proportions. These patients commonly had need to ask or confess compulsions.

Thirty-four percent of the patients had somatic obsessions. Often their lives were dominated by incessant, compulsive checking rituals carried out to reassure them that they did not have a serious illness. Of the 15 patients with somatic obsessions, 73% had checking rituals.

Thirty-four percent of the patients had obsessive thoughts that involved what we have termed the need for symmetry, or exactness. Examples would be the man who felt he had to walk through an office door exactly in the middle and sit at a 90° angle to the therapist, a woman who had to lean objects at just the right angle before she could complete a motor action, and a man with Tourette's syndrome who, if he had a certain number of tics on one side of his body that were involuntary, had to "even them up" with the same number of voluntary movements mimicking the tics on the other side. Patients could usually not express the reason behind these obsessions other than a fear that something bad would happen if they did not "even things up." Most patients with this symptom also had checking and counting rituals. Most were perfectionistic and had had compulsive personalities from an early age. This obsession was significantly more common in men than women ($t = 8.05, f = 1, p < 0.05$) and was associated with a poor prognosis.

The average age of onset was 15.4 ± 0.9 years for men and 24.1 ± 1.7 years for women. Each patient's course of illness was determined as falling in one of three categories: episodic, continuous, or deteriorative (Table 90.1). Only 3% of

TABLE 90.1. Obsessions and compulsions in OCD.

Obsessions ($n = 100$)	%	Compulsions ($n = 100$)	%
Contamination	55	Checking	78
Pathological doubt	42	Washing	47
Somatic	35	Need to ask or confess	25
Aggressive	28	Counting	22
Sexual	26	Symmetry and precision	18
Need for symmetry	24	Hoarding	8
Other	13	Multiple primary compulsions	41
Multiple obsessions	60		

the patients had an episodic course; 84% were classified as having a continuous course and 14% as having a chronic deteriorative course. Twenty-four percent of the patients could identify an environmental precipitant that appeared to trigger their illness, and 68% could not; 8% were unclear on this question. Increases in responsibility such as the birth of a child, promotion to a new job, or significant losses such as the death of a family member or loss of a job were the most common precipitants noted. Almost all of the patients reported an increase in obsessive compulsive symptoms coincident with stressful life events. Most of the women (68%) noted that the severity of obsessive compulsive symptoms increased the week before their menstrual period.

The frequencies of coexisting axis I psychotic disorders in the sample we have interviewed are given in Table 90.2. One-third of the patients had a major depressive disorder on admission. The next most common secondary diagnoses were simple phobia, social phobia, eating disorders, alcohol abuse, panic disorder, and Tourette's syndrome. Lifetime diagnoses of coexisting anxiety disorders suggest that OCD patients have an increased vulnerability to almost all of the other anxiety disorders. Of particular interest is the high lifetime incidence of separation anxiety disorder. The incidence of lifetime major depression was 67%, a figure close to that seen for lifetime major depression in panic disorder. Axis II diagnoses (Table 90.3) included compulsive, passive aggressive, histrionic, schizotypal, schizoid, and dependent personalities.

One can look at the coexistence question from a different angle by asking how many patients with other primary psychiatric diagnoses have significant obsessions or compulsions. Chart review studies of the Chestnut Lodge Follow-up study[5] have shown that about 10% of schizophrenics have obsessions and compulsions. Several authors have found that a high percentage of Tourette syndrome patients have coexisting OCD.[6,7] Breier et al.[8] have reported that 15% of patients with primary panic also have OCD. The incidence of obsessions and compulsions in a clinical sample of major depression is unknown. A controlled interview study that is designed to determine the frequency of obsessions and compulsions in representative clinical samples of depressed and psychotic patients would be useful.

The heterogeneity of the illness, difficulties in establishing valid and reliable exclusion criteria, and the coexistence of OCD with other psychiatric disorders can directly or indirectly influence the results of biological and treatment outcome studies.

At first glance there is a marked dissimilarity between the phenomenological or clinical presentations of the patient with one type of obsession in comparison

TABLE 90.2. Coexisting axis I diagnoses in primary OCD ($n = 100$).

Diagnosis	Current (%)	Lifetime (%)
Major depressive disorder	31	67
Simple phobia	7	22
Separation anxiety disorder		21
Social phobia	11	18
Eating disorder	8	17
Alcohol abuse (dependence)	8	14
Panic disorder	6	12
Tourette's syndrome	5	7

TABLE 90.3. Coexisting
axis II diagnoses in
primary OCD (*n* = 100).

Diagnosis	%
Compulsive	52
Passive aggressive	16
Histrionic	9
Schizotypal	8
Schizoid	7
Borderline	6
Dependent	6
None	36

to another (e.g., need for symmetry versus aggression obsessions). This dissimilarity stimulated our interest in attempting to identify homogeneous diagnostic subtypes. To our surprise, the disorder proved to be much more homogeneous than we expected. The evidence arguing for relative homogeneity of the disorder includes the following: (a) Patients often present with multiple obsessions and compulsions. (b) Patients who are troubled primarily by fears of contamination and washing rituals can subsequently develop pathological doubt with checking and vice versa. (c) There are few significant differences in the course of the illness, prognosis, treatment response to pharmacological agents, sex, and coexisting psychiatric illness between clinical subtypes. As our sample size has increased, the only subtype that has begun to appear to be distinct from the rest of the group has been patients with the need for symmetry or precision.

Classifying patients into groups whose compulsions are driven by the anxiety attached to a particular cognition in contrast to those who have no reason why they repeat the compulsions is more fruitful than subtyping the disorder by the clinical presentation. Other possible subgroups include those whose symptoms are brought on by internal versus external cues and those classified according to whether the proband has insight into the irrationality of the compulsions. Differential response to pharmacological trials have yet to identify homogeneous subgroups, but this approach may be productive in trials with a large sample size currently in progress.

A high percentage of patients with OCD have coexisting anxiety and depressive disorders. A significant number of patients who present with a chief complaint of anxiety or depression have primary OCD. They do not tell anyone about the obsessions or compulsions because they do not want to reveal the more bizarre symptoms. Coupled with the fact that most mental health professionals still do not ask for a history of obsessions and compulsions on routine mental status screening, it can lead to missed diagnosis and an underestimation of the incidence of the disorder. Inclusion and exclusion criteria for neurobiological and treatment studies need to be carefully reviewed in light of the coexistence data. Inclusion of patients with severe depression, psychosis, or severe personality disorders can create significant differences between studies that are otherwise similar in design.

A more careful characterization of the heterogeneity of the illness and its coexistence with other psychiatric disorders in a large OCD sample is needed. It would be equally important to determine the incidence and significance of obsessive compulsive symptoms in panic disorder, schizophrenia, major depression, and

Tourette's syndrome. A comparison of a large clinical population with a cohort of OCD subjects identified in the ECA study using identical structured instruments is necessary to determine the true prevalence rate of the disorder in the general population. A careful controlled family study is needed to help determine the relative contribution of genetic and psychosocial factors to the pathogenesis of the illness. Finally, a prospective follow-up study of the children of adult patients in this sample would help to provide information about the natural history, high risk factors, and pathogenesis of OCD.

References

1. Rasmussen SA, Tsuang MT. Epidemiology of obsessive compulsive disorder: a review. J Clin Psychiatry 1984;45:450–457.
2. Rudin E. Einbeitrag zurfrage der zwengskrunkheit, insobesondere ihrere hereditaren. Arch Psychiatr Nervenkr 1953;191:14–54.
3. Myers JK, Weissman MM, Tischler GL, et al. Six month prevalence of psychiatric disorders in three sites. Arch Gen Psychiatry 1984;41:959–971.
4. Rasmussen SA, Tsuang MT. Clinical characteristics and family history in DSM-III obsessive compulsive disorder. Am J Psychiatry 1986;143:317–322.
5. Fenton WS, McGlashan TH. The prognostic significance of obsessive-compulsive symptoms in schizophrenia. Am J Psychiatry 1986;143:437–441.
6. Nee LE, Caine EO, Polinsky RJ, et al. Gilles de la Tourette syndrome: clinical and family study of 50 cases. Ann Neurol 1982;7:41–49.
7. Pauls DL, Cohen DT, Heimbuch R, et al. Familial pattern and transmission of Gilles de la Tourette syndrome and multiple tics. Arch Gen Psychiatry 1983;38:1091–1093.
8. Breier A, Charney DS, Heninger GR. Agoraphobia with panic attacks. Arch Gen Psychiatry 1986;43:1029–1036.

91. Applicability of Models of Anxiety to Obsessive Compulsive Disorder

ASHOKA JAHNAVI PRASAD

The nosology of obsessive compulsive disorder remains a matter of fierce dispute. It is, for instance, still unclear whether it is a variant of depressive illness or of anxiety disorder, or if it constitutes a nosological entity in its own right.

DSM-III,[1] in a radical departure from its earlier editions, categorized it as an anxiety state along with panic disorder, generalized anxiety disorder, and post-traumatic stress disorder. The final judgment was probably influenced by the very high levels of anxiety obvious in these subjects.

Pharmacological models of anxiety have been proposed. The following are the more popular models that have been subjected to relatively high degree of scientific scrutiny: lactate model; carbon dioxide model; caffeine model; isoproterenol model; and yohimbine model.

Lactate Model

Pitts and McClure[2] demonstrated that an infusion of $105M$ sodium lactate 10 mg/kg produced symptoms of panic anxiety in a high percentage of subjects suffering from anxiety compared to normal controls. Since then, several other trials have replicated this finding.[3-7] The last trial (at this writing) was conducted by Prasad et al,[8] who reported a more than 50% panicking rate of anxious subjects who fulfilled the *DSM-III* criteria for anxiety state as opposed to 19% of the controls with an average panicking time of 15 min. On subdivision of the anxious subjects who panicked, it was found that 86% of them suffered from panic attacks, whereas the remainder fulfilled the criteria for generalized anxiety disorder, thereby suggesting that this model is more applicable to the former rather than latter.

Carbon Dioxide Model

Gorman and his team[9] reported a high rate of panic in subjects suffering from anxiety disorder when they were subjected to 15 min of breathing with 5% CO_2. This finding has since been replicated by Vandenhout et al.[10] Unlike lactate, CO_2

has been known to produce symptoms in both generalized anxiety subjects as well as panickers.[10]

Caffeine Model

Caffeine intake has been associated with high scores of anxiety.[11,12] In doses more than 600 mg, it has been known to precipitate symptoms indistinguishable from those of a generalized anxiety state and panic disorder.[13]

Isoproterenol Model

Isoproterenol is a β-adrenergic agonist and has been known to cause symptoms of panic anxiety in patients fulfilling the *DSM-III* criteria of panic anxiety.[14]

Yohimbine Model

Charney et al.[15] have reported high rates of panic in patients with generalized anxiety as well as panic attacks when infused with yohimbine, and α_2-adrenoceptor antagonist, compared to controls. This finding contrasted with some of the earlier reports indicating that normal subjects were just as susceptible to yohimbine-induced panic.

Specificity of These Models to Anxiety

Anxiety, being a heterogeneous condition, has proved difficult and elusive to researchers endeavoring to construct pharmacological models. Nevertheless these models do provide useful initial leads. Further trials are no doubt necessary to ascertain the validity of these results, but the initial findings hold much promise. It is interesting to note that in all the trials alluded to earlier the definition of subjects excluded obsessive-compulsives. This trial was attempted to test the hypothesis that, should OCD be an anxiety disorder, the subjects should react in a pharmacological manner similar to that of the anxious subjects.

Lactate Provocation in OCD

Sodium DL-lactate (0.5 M) was infused intravenously over 20 min in doses of 10 ml/kg body weight in seven symptom-free OCD patients fulfilling *DSM-III* criteria and eight controls. Two of the controls panicked, and only one of the OCD subjects showed minor signs of panic.

Caffeine Consumption Test in OCD

Three doses of oral caffeine (240, 480, 720 mg) were administered to four symptom-free subjects who fulfilled the *DSM-III* criteria for OCD and seven controls after a 5-day caffeine-free diet. They were then periodically rated on Spielberger's state anxiety scores. The results are illustrated in Figure 91.1, and it is interesting to note a higher anxiety score in the subjects than in the controls.

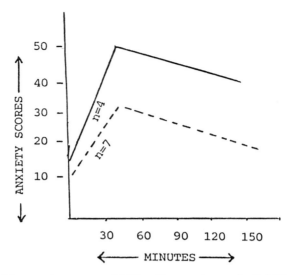

FIGURE 91.1. Mean anxiety scores of OCD subjects and controls. Solid line represents the patients and the broken line the controls.

Isoproterenol Test in OCD

Isoproterenol hydrochloride 5 mg was administered to nine symptom-free subjects fulfilling the *DSM-III* criteria for OCD and eight controls. Only one of the eight controls showed minor signs of panic, whereas seven of nine subjects experienced major panic symptoms.

Discussion

Any biological correlation between OCD and anxiety states is likely to be regarded as premature unless the nosological status of anxiety is clearly defined. However, if the present biochemical status of anxiety is confirmed on the basis of our results, it appears that anxiety and OCD do *not* have identical biochemical profiles. Apart from one other study on OCD patients, where Gorman et al.[16] attempted to ascertain the effect of lactate provocation and came up with broadly similar findings to our group, to the best of my knowledge ours is the first study to attempt a pharmacological provocation of OCD. For obvious ethical reasons, the numbers were small; and for any meaningful conclusions to be drawn, it would have to be replicated and the other remaining models tested. Nevertheless, it does provide a useful base from which to study OCD from a biological perspective and hopefully will help our nosological understanding.

Acknowledgment. The author would like to thank Dr. K. V. Rao and J. Arora for their help, and Susi Schiltz for typing the manuscript.

References

1. Diagnostic & Statistical Manual. 3rd Ed. Washington, DC: American Psychiatric Association, 1980.
2. Pitts F, McClure J. Lactate metabolism in anxiety neurosis. N Engl J Med 1967;277:1329.
3. Fink M, Taylor M, Volavka J. Anxiety precipitated by lactate. N Engl J Med 1969;281:1429.
4. Kelly D, Michell-Heggs N, Sharman D. Anxiety and effects of sodium lactate. Br J Psychiatry 1971;119:129.
5. Appleby I, Liebowitz M, Fyer A, et al. Lactate provocation of anxiety attacks. Arch Gen Psychiatry 1984;41:764.
6. Lappiere Y, Knott V, Gray R. Physiological correlates of sodium lactate. Psychopharmacol Bull 1984;20:50.
7. Pohl R, Raimey J, Ostiz A, et al. Isoproterenol-induced anxiety states. Psychopharmacol Bull 1985;21:424.
8. Prasad AJ, O'Hare A, Kohli D. Lactate provocation in anxiety. 1987; in preparation.
9. Gorman J, Askanazi J, Liebowitz M, et al. Response to hyperventilation. Am J Psychiatry 1984;141:857.
10. Vandenhout M, Grieg E. Panic symptom after inhalation of CO_2. Br J Psychiatry 1984;144:503.
11. Winstead D. Caffeine consumption amongst psychiatric patients. Am J Psychiatry 1978;135:963.
12. Greden J, Fontaine P, Lubetsky M, et al. Anxiety and depression associated with caffeinism. Am J Psychiatry 1978;135:963.
13. Charney D, Heimeger G, Jatlow P. Increased anxiogenic effects of caffeine in panic disorders. Arch Gen Psychiatry 1985;42:233.
14. Raimey J, Effegin E, Pohl R, et al. β-receptor isoprotenol anxiety states. Psychopathology 1984;17(3):40.
15. Charney D, Heimeger G, Brier A. Noradrenergic function in anxiety. Arch Gen Psychiatry 1985;42:450.
16. Gorman J, Lieboritz M, Fryer A, et al. lactate infusions in OCD. Am J Psychiatry 1985;142:864.

92. Frontal Lobe Involvement in Obsessive Compulsive Disorder: Electroencephalographic Evidence

SUMANT KHANNA, C.R. MUKUNDAN, AND S.M. CHANNABASAVANNA

The evidence for biological abnormalities in obsessive compulsive disorder (OCD) has been gradually mounting.[1] Reports on evoked potentials[2,3] have tried to determine the process involved in the pathology of OCD. There have been few studies that have attempted to identify a specific site as being the seat of the psychopathology. Flor Henry[4] used a neuropsychological battery to conclude that there was a frontal lobe dysfunction, but these results were not replicated by Insel et al.,[5] who also found normal computed tomography scans. However, by contrast, children have consistently shown evidence of delayed maturity on neuropsychological and other evaluations.[6,7] With regard to the electroencephalogram (EEG) most studies have shown nonspecific findings.[8] In the only other study where the computerized EEG was analyzed,[4] evidence for a dominant hemisphere dysfunction emerged from the centroparietal leads. In this chapter we highlight findings from two of our studies on the electrophysiology of OCD that have tended to implicate the frontal lobe.

Electroencephalography

We studied 50 subjects with OCD according to *DSM-III* criteria and compared them to an age- and sex-matched normal volunteer control group. Bipolar recordings of the EEG were obtained from two montages with eight channels each. Log power, ratio power, laterality ratio, response to eye opening, and coherence were studied. A statistically significant decrease in log power in the right frontomedial and posterior temporal regions emerged in the OCD sample. This decrease in power was in all bands, and there was a resultant shift in laterality but no difference in the ratio of various bands to the absolute power from these recordings. Findings from coherence analysis suggested more efficient posterior brain functioning due to increased coherence, again more on the nondominant side. Other findings on coherence were too scattered to appear clinically significant.

Bereitschaftspotential

In a paradigm involving the bereitschaftspotential we have reported an investigation with the same sample where there was a decrease in onset latency with a trend toward increased amplitude in the OCD sample.[9] In this context we have tried to apply the model of complex motor programming[10] and to evolve a neurobiological substrate for this circuit. The role of the supplementary motor area has been stressed. We believe that our evidence is the first to support the hypothesis of a deficit in complex motor programming in OCD,[11] possibly of frontal origin.

Discussion

In this study temporal lobe recordings have shown a decrease in power in OCD in the right posterior region, with a suggestion of increased coherence between this area and the centroparietal region. It suggests a hypofunctioning posterior temporal region in the nondominant hemisphere that is working in greater harmony with the posterior part of the cerebral cortex. Whether it is due to increased efficiency of this region or the fact that the working of this region is deficient and its pacemakers inactive, as a result of which the centroparietal region takes over the pacemaker function, is speculative.

The focus of our work has been the frontal region. For purposes of simplicity we have chosen to designate the three leads as frontomedial (FP2-F4 and FP1-F3), frontolateral (FP2-F8 and FP1-F7), and frontoposterior (F4-F8 and F3-F7). The right frontomedial region has shown a decreased power in all the ranges with a subsequent shift in laterality. The bereitschaftspotential, thought to originate at least in part from the supplementary motor area, which overlies the frontomedial region, has similarly been found to show decreased readiness by shortened onset latency. Thus two independent procedures have implicated the frontal lobe as being dysfunctional in OCD.

There are various technical limitations in the study of computerized EEGs. The duration of analysis, the duration of recording for each subject, the parameters taken for analysis, and various other related factors are difficult to control for and account for most variance across centers. Secondly, in interpretation, too little is known about the origin and spread of waves as identified in the computerized EEG to reach definite conclusions. Does decreased power mean hypofunctioning or more efficient basal functioning? How does it correlate with coherence? These areas are some issues that have yet to be adequately settled.

Within these limitations we believe that our studies provide some laboratory evidence for the association of frontal lobe dysfunction with OCD. Earlier we reported a case[12] where OCD developed after head injury. Neuropsychological evaluation was suggestive of predominant bilateral frontal lobe dysfunction. There we had commented on the similarity between obsessions and perseveration. Both could be due to frontal dysfunction, the latter being differentiated by an inability to change set. The importance of stimulus-linked obsessions is being stressed. A further comparison can be drawn with the premotor syndrome described by Luria[13] as an early sign of involvement of the prefrontal cortex, which precedes a later stage of development of obvious perseveration.

Other evidence for frontal lobe involvement in OCD comes from psychosurgery, where sectioning of frontal pathways is consistently associated with a decrease in obsessionality.[14] A dominant frontal lobe dysfunction has been proposed based on a combination of electrophysiological and neuropsychological studies.[4] Isolated case reports of frontal lobe lesions producing obsessive compulsive phenomenon also exist.[8] The evidence implicating the basal ganglia and temporal lobe is, however, meager.[8,11]

Thus our studies and a review of the literature tend to support an association between nondominant frontomedial dysfunction and OCD, with replicable findings across two paradigms. There are three ways of explaining it. First, the association may be coincidental. Second, the association may be the result of the illness. Finally, the dysfunction may be the cause of the illness. It would be premature at this point to reach any definite conclusions, although we have tried herein to argue a case for the last possibility.

References

1. Turner SM, Beidel DC, Nathan RGS. Biological factors in obsessive compulsive disorders. Psychol Bull 1985;97:430–450.
2. Beech HR, Cieselki KT, Gordon PK. Further observations of evoked potentials in obsessional patients. Br J Psychiatry 1983;142:605–609.
3. Shagass C, Roemer RA, Straumanis JJ, et al. Distinctive somatosensory evoked potentials in obsessive compulsive disorder. Biol Psychiatry 1984;19:1507–1524.
4. Flor Henry P, Yeudall LT, Koles ZJ, et al. Neuropsychological and power spectral EEG investigations of the obsessive compulsive syndrome. Biol Psychiatry 1979;14:119–130.
5. Insel TR, Donnelly EF, Lalakea ML, et al. Neurological and neuropsychological studies of patients with obsessive compulsive disorder. Biol Psychiatry 1983;18:741–751.
6. Rapoport J, Elkins R, Langer DH, et al. Childhood obsessive compulsive disorder. Am J Psychiatry 1981;138:1545–1554.
7. Behar D, Rapoport JL, Berg CJ, et al. Computerised tomography and neuropsychological test measures in adolescents with obsessive compulsive disorder. Am J Psychiatry 1984;141:363–369.
8. Jenike MA. Obsessive compulsive disorder: a question of a neurologic lesion. Compr Psychiatry 1984;25:298–304.
9. Khanna S, Mukundan CR, Channabasavanna SM. Obsessive compulsive disorder: is it a problem of complex motor programming? Indian J Psychiatry 1987;29:41–47.
10. Marsden CD. The mysterious motor function of the basal ganglia: the Robert Wartenberg lecture. Neurology 1982;32:514–539.
11. Cummings JL, Frankel M. Gilles de la Tourette syndrome and the neurological basis of obsessions and compulsions. Biol Psychiatry 1985;54:767–775.
12. Khanna S, Narayanan HS, Sharma SD, et al. Post traumatic obsessive compulsive disorder—a single case report. Indian J Psychiatry 1985;27:337–339.
13. Luria AR. The Working Brain. New York: Basic Books, 1973.
14. O'Callaghan MAJ, Carroll D. Psychosurgery: A Scientific Analysis. Lancaster: MTP Press, 1982.

93. Pharmacological Treatment of Obsessive Compulsive Disorder

STUART A. MONTGOMERY, NAOMI FINEBERG, AND DEIRDRE MONTGOMERY

The most widely used drug for the treatment of obsessive compulsive disorder (OCD) is clomipramine. It may therefore be helpful to review the evidence for efficacy for clomipramine alone and in relation to other antidepressants to be found in double-blind controlled studies.

Double-Blind Placebo-Controlled Studies of Clomipramine

There have been six studies comparing clomipramine with placebo, all of which have found clomipramine to be superior to placebo some time between 4 and 6 weeks. This consistency of results is unusual in relatively small studies and argues strongly for the effectiveness of clomipramine in OCD.

The studies of Thoren et al.[1] used a comparison against nortriptyline as well as placebo. There was a significant improvement with clomipramine on a CPRS obsession scale, whereas nortriptyline was no different from placebo.

Insel et al.[2] used clorgyline as an active comparator in a crossover study. Clomipramine was apparently significantly superior to clorgyline and placebo on both a CPRS obsession scale and self-rating scales at 4 and 6 weeks.

Marks et al., in their 1980 study[3] showed significance at 4 weeks on self-rating scales only using patients who were required to be ritualizers. This study was complicated by the use of concomitant exposure behavior therapy after 4 weeks. The absence of a comprehensive scale that registers changes in the range of symptoms complained of by obsessional patients might have compromised this study. A more recent study by the same group largely supports these findings, with clomipramine showing significant superiority over placebo at 8 weeks.[4]

The study of Flament et al.[5] examined the effects of clomipramine in children and found a significant benefit on a CPRS obsessional scale, which was observed at 3 and 5 weeks.

The single study that excluded patients who were concomitantly depressed using both the criteria of absence of primary depression and absence of secondary depression was a small crossover study by Montgomery,[6] which also found a significant advantage for clomipramine over placebo at 4 weeks on a CPRS obsessional scale.

Preliminary results from a study of more than 500 patients treated with clomipramine or placebo appear to confirm the findings of the smaller studies.[7]

Double-Blind Comparisons of Clomipramine with Reference Antidepressants

Many of the studies of clomipramine compared with other drugs are too small to make a direct comparison of efficacy. It is surprising therefore that despite the small size of the studies clomipramine was superior to clorgyline,[2] amitriptyline,[8] and desipramine.[9,10] In a study by Volavka et al.[11] clomipramine was superior to imipramine in self-rating scales only, but this finding is weakened by the fact that the pretreatment baseline was higher for those patients treated with imipramine. The superiority of clomipramine over imipramine is supported by the findings of Foa et al.,[12] where imipramine was no different from placebo on obsessional measures but was superior on measures of depression. The superiority of clomipramine over nortriptyline is supported by the study by Thoren et al. where clomipramine was not significantly superior to nortriptyline on a direct comparison, but clomipramine was superior to placebo and nortriptyline was not. Clomipramine was found to be superior to zimelidine by Zohar and Insel,[8] but there were only five patients treated with zimelidine in this study, which is too small a sample on which to base conclusions.

These studies indicate that clomipramine is the most effective drug for the treatment of OCD. The superiority of clomipramine over other tricyclic antidepressants suggests that there is something about clomipramine that is specifically useful. The findings also suggest that the effect of clomipramine is not mediated simply by its antidepressant action. Clomipramine is a powerful serotonin uptake inhibitor, although its active metabolite is not. These findings therefore provide some support for the serotonin hypothesis of obsessional behavior. Studies on the newer serotonin uptake inhibitors fluoxetine and fluvoxamine also tend to support the serotonin hypothesis.

Effect of Clomipramine on Obsessional Thoughts

An analysis of the response to treatment with clomipramine compared with placebo in the study by Montgomery[6] throws some interesting light on the question of the selective effect of clomipramine. In this study (Table 93.1) there was significant improvement in compulsive thoughts and inner tension on clomipramine. There was a trend in favor of clomipramine on the two other obsessional thinking items: indecision and worrying over trifles. It indicates that a specific effect of clomi-

TABLE 93.1. Amelioration of obsessional symptoms with clomipramine using CPRS obsession scale ($n = 14$).[a]

CPRS item	CMI vs. PLAC (parallel design at 4 weeks)	CMI vs. PLAC (crossover design at 8 weeks[b])
Compulsive thoughts	$p < 0.01$	$p < 0.02$
Phobias	NS	NS
Inner tension	$p < 0.05$	NS
Rituals	NS	NS
Indecision	$p < 0.1$	NS
Worrying over trifles	$p < 0.1$	NS
Six-item obsessional scale	$p < 0.01$	$p < 0.01$
MADRS depression scale	NS	NS

[a]Reprinted from ref. 6, with permission.
[b]Each patient acts as his own control.

pramine was seen on the pattern of symptoms associated with ruminations. Interestingly, in this study there was no change in the item of rituals, providing further support for the separation in treatment terms of rituals from ruminations. Clomipramine appears to have a specific advantage in reducing the ruminations associated with obsessional compulsive disorder. These findings raise the interesting possibility that clomipramine is exercising a primary effect on obsessions in contrast to behavior therapy, which is primarily concerned with rituals.

Conclusion

Pharmacotherapy of obsessive compulsive disorder appears to have established its effectiveness in a large number of studies. The most widely studied drug, clomipramine, is better than placebo in the presence or the absence of coexisting depressive illness. This effect appears to be independent of its action as an antidepressant. Clomipramine is reported to be more effective than a range of other antidepressants. However, there is some evidence of potential efficacy for some of the other antidepressants, although they are not as effective as clomipramine. The selective effect of clomipramine in nondepressed patients with OCD on obsessional thoughts, but not on rituals, suggests that the primary effect of clomipramine on OCD might be on the ruminations with secondary effects on rituals. The primary effect of behavior therapy on OCD seems to be on rituals. There is no evidence of a negative interaction between pharmacotherapy and exposure therapy, and there should be no reason why they may not be used concomitantly. The primary indication for behavior therapy seems to be in ritualizers, where it is the treatment of choice. The primary indication for clomipramine seems to be in ruminators, where it should be the treatment of choice.

References

1. Thoren P, Asberg M, Cronholm B, et al. Clomipramine treatment of obsessive compulsive disorder. Arch Gen Psychiatry 1980;37:1281–1285.
2. Insel TR, Murphy DL, Cohen RM, et al. Clomipramine and clorgyline in OCD. Arch Gen Psychiatry 1983;40:605–612.
3. Marks IM, Stern RS, Mawson D, et al. Clomipramine and exposure for obsessive compulsive rituals. Br J Psychiatry 1980;136:1–25.
4. Marks IM, Lelliott P, Basoglu M, et al. Clomipramine, self-exposure and therapist-aided exposure. Br J Psychiatry 1988;152:522–535.
5. Flament MF, Rapoport JL, Berg CJ, et al. Clomipramine treatment of childhood obsessive-compulsive disorder. Arch Gen Psychiatry 1985;42:977–983.
6. Montgomery SA. Clomipramine in obsessional neurosis: a placebo controlled trial. Pharm Med 1980;1:189–192.
7. DeVeaugh-Geiss J, Katz R, Landau P. A multi-centre trial of Anafranil in obsessive compulsive disorder. Psychopharm 1988; 96 Suppl.: 80.
8. Ananth J, Pecknold JC, Van den Steen N, et al. Double blind study of clomipramine and amitriptyline in obsessive neurosis. Prog Neuropsychopharmacol 1981;5:257–262.
9. Zohar J, Insel TR. Drug treatment of obsessive-compulsive disorder. J Affect Disorders 1987;13:193–202.
10. Leonard H, Swedo S, Rapoport JL, Coffey M, Cheslow D. Treatment of childhood obsessive compulsive disorder with clomipramine and desmethylimipramine: a double-blind crossover comparison. Psychopharmacology Bulletin. 1987;2493–95.
11. Volavka J, Neziroglu F, Yaryura-Tobias JA. Clomipramine and imipramine in obsessive-compulsive disorder. Psychiatr Res 1985;14:83–91.
12. Foa EB, Steketee G, Kozak MJ, et al. Effects of imipramine on depression and on obsessive-compulsive symptoms. In: Abstracts, Annual Meeting, American College of Neuropsychopharmacology, 1985;38.

94. Use of Antiandrogens in the Treatment of Obsessive Compulsive Disorders: Theoretical Considerations

M. CASAS, E. ALVAREZ, P. DURO, M.C. PINET,
A. TEJERO, C. UDINA, J. RODRIGUEZ-ESPINOSA,
J. TOMAS-VILALTELLA, AND J. MASANA

The treatment of obsessive compulsive disorder (OCD) is one of the most difficult problems facing psychiatry today. Despite many attempts at treatment, the only therapies that have been effective to date are some antidepressants, such as clomipramine, monoamine oxidase inhibitors (MAOIs) and some behavior therapy techniques. The results, however, are not completely satisfactory.[1]

Based on casual observations concerning the beneficial effects of treatment with cyproterone acetate (CA) in obsessive compulsive patients[2] we carried out two pilot studies,[2,3] one with women and the second with men.

In the first we studied six female outpatients, four with severe OCD, one with a schizophrenia-like psychosis with marked obsessive symptoms, and one with a phobic disorder including complex ritual-like behavior. The results obtained were as follows: The patients tolerated the treatment well with no undesirable side effects. There was a notable improvement in the obsessive symptoms associated with a decrease in compulsive rituals while under treatment (50–75 mg CA). General mood improved, and the level of anxiety dropped. Although after some months in treatment a certain degree of tolerance seemed to appear, the patients did not relapse to the state experienced before treatment.

The second pilot study is being done with three male outpatients with OCD. To date, all patients have shown both clinical and behavioral improvements as well as better social adjustment. Before the onset of treatment (on the fourth day of the menstrual cycle in women) patients underwent a plasma hormonal study that included prolactin, follicle-stimulating hormone, luteinizing hormone, testosterone, sex hormone-binding globulin, free testosterone index, 17β-estradiol, progesterone, Δ4-androstenedione, and dehydroepiandrosterone sulfate. Pretreatment results were within the usual range; while on CA, changes in testosterone, sex hormone-binding globulin, and free testosterone index were found in the three men but they became normal during the first month after CA withdrawal.

The positive results from these initial studies led us to design two double-blind crossover studies in patients with OCD using CA 75 mg/day versus placebo in one, and clomipramine 200 mg/day and CA 75 mg/day versus clomipramine and placebo in the other. These studies are at present under way.

We have found no clear explanation for the improvement of obsessive patients treated with antiandrogens. However, after reviewing the literature we are able to expose some theoretical links between OCD and aggressive behavior, their biological correlates, and the possible action of CA as an antidepressant, which might account for its positive effect in OCD.

Antiandrogens are substances that are able to block or reduce the physiological effects of androgens on target tissues. CA is among the most potent. It also possesses progestational activity, suppresses the secretion of gonadotropins, and, as a result, suppresses the production of testosterone by the testes. CA reduces most biological and behavioral parameters related to male sexuality. Inhibition of the male sexual response, a decrease in aggressive impulses, apathy, and a decrease in energy level and general drive have been observed with the use of this drug.

In studies of patients under treatment with CA, Itil and Itil[4] have shown several aspects of this drug that could open a new field in its clinical use. These authors, using computerized electroencephalogram analysis (CEEG), which provides a profile of the pharmacological effects of various substances on the central nervous system, found that at low doses (50–100 mg) the CEEG profile of CA was similar to that of the "sedative" antidepressants. It is interesting at this point to emphasize that such doses were used in our studies.

In some clinical studies a high incidence of extrapunitive aggressive impulses has been observed in OCD patients.[5] The use of projective tests in these patients elicits impulsive responses, which often adopt the form of obsessive thoughts. It also seems clear that hostility is an important component of ritualistic behavior, and violence is the major content of obsessive thinking. On the other hand, irritability seems closely linked to the degree of severity and interference of the symptoms. It therefore seems that in addition to anxiety and depression, hostility and irritability are common mood states among OCD patients.[6] These findings agree with the observation of some psychoanalysts that hostile and sadistic impulses are the main component of OCD. Eysenck and Eysenck[7] found that aggressiveness or lack of impulse control (psychoticism) was a common personality trait in these patients. Furthermore, in one study impulsivity correlated positively with the severity of the obsessive compulsive symptoms and the level of anxiety.[8]

Animal studies support the theory that the neurobiological substrate for aggressive behavior is influenced by hormonal variables,[9] and many data suggest a relation between testosterone and aggressive behavior. Although no clear relation regarding levels of testosterone and human behavior has yet been demonstrated, response to threat has been directly related to testosterone in healthy individuals.[10] Furthermore, data from studies with openly violent criminals and individuals who present pathological alterations of testosterone levels show a clear correlation between testosterone and aggressive behavior.[11]

If OCD is related to aggressiveness, and aggressiveness is influenced by testosterone, we could suggest that a decrease in testosterone effect, by means of antiandrogenic treatment, could be responsible for the improvement of the obsessive compulsive patients we are studying.

Conclusions

Although the data thus far are not conclusive, it has been shown that: (a) Male and female patients with OCD improve under antiandrogenic therapy in two pilot studies. (b) CA has a CEEG profile similar to that of sedative tricyclic antidepressants and therefore perhaps a similar clinical action. The antidepressant action of CA could also account for its beneficial effect in obsessive compulsive patients. (c) Aggressiveness and OCD have been clinically related. As CA may reduce aggressive impulses in OCD, an improvement in general clinical symptoms can be expected.

References

1. Insel TR. New Findings in Obsessive-Compulsive Disorder. Washington, DC: American Psychiatric Press, 1984.
2. Casas M, Alvarez E, Duro P, et al. Antiandrogenic treatment of obsessive-compulsive neurosis. Acta Psychiatr Scand 1986;73:221–222.
3. Casas M, Alvarez E, Duro P, et al. The use of CA in the treatment of OCD: clinical findings. In: Abstracts of the International Conference on New Directions in Affective Disorders, Jerusalem, 1987.
4. Itil TM, Itil KZ. Computer-EEG of second and third generation of psychotropic drugs. In: Proceedings of the 14th Collegium Internationale Neuro-Psychopharmacologicum Congress. Vol. 7. Suppl. 1. New York: Raven Press, 1984.
5. Millar DG. Hostile emotion and obsessional neurosis. Psychol Med 1983;13:813–819.
6. Farid BT. Obsessional symptomatology and adverse mood. Br J Psychiatry 1986;149:108–112.
7. Eysenck HJ, Eysenck SBG. Psychoticism as a Dimension of Personality. London: Hoder & Stonghton, 1976.
8. Hoehn-Saric R, Banksdale VC. Impulsiveness in obsessive-compulsive patients. Br J Psychiatry 1983;143:177–182.
9. Valzelli L. Psychobiology of Aggression and Violence. New York: Raven Press, 1981.
10. Olweus D, Mattsson A, Schalling D, et al. Testosterone, aggression, physical and personality dimensions in normal adolescent males. Psychosom Med 1980;2:253–269.
11. Schalling D. Personality correlates of plasma testosterone levels in young delinquents—an example of person-situation interaction? In Mednick S, Moffitt T, Stack SA (eds): The Course of Crime: New Biological Approaches. Cambridge: Cambridge University Press, 1987;283–291.

IV.C. POSTTRAUMATIC STRESS DISORDER

95. Psychobiology of the Trauma Response

BESSEL A. VAN DER KOLK

When Kardiner first described the full syndrome of what is now called posttraumatic stress disorder (PTSD)[1] in 1941 he called it a "physioneurosis," a mental disorder with both psychological and physiological components. People with PTSD continue to suffer from "enduring vigilance for and sensitivity to environmental threat." The response to trauma is consistent across traumatic stimuli: The central nervous system has a limited and rather consistent response to terrifying experiences. After a traumatic event most victims go through a period of phasic reliving, with intrusive reexperiences, such as visual images and physiological arousal, alternating with denial and numbing of responsiveness to the environment. In many people the condition becomes chronic, with various degrees of residual symptoms, for example physiological hyperreactivity, a subjective sense of loss of control, chronic passivity alternating with uncontrolled violence against the self or others, sleep disturbances, and reenactments of traumatic events.[2] Often symptoms become evident only during later periods of life stress, when current stressful events can be experienced as a partial reliving of earlier trauma. The degree to which traumatic experiences become interwoven in the totality of a person's characterological responses depends on (a) the psychobiological maturation of the victim, (b) the severity of the stressor, (c) the presence of prior traumatizing experiences, and (d) the quality of social support.[3] We hypothesize that the emotional and behavioral responses to trauma are driven by neurobiological alterations and propose the following specific postulates.

Thesis 1: The severity of physiological arousal during the trauma determines the severity of posttraumatic symptomatology. The degree of physiological disorganization as well as the cognitive capacities during the experience determine the subjective interpretation of the event. What makes an experience traumatic is the lack of capacity to fit the event into existing conceptual schemata: It overwhelms both conceptually and physiologically, leaving people in a state of "unspeakable terror," with an inability to process physiological arousal with words and symbols. Social support and prior exposure to stresses that have been mastered mitigate against overwhelming physiological disorganization, which may result in a conditioned response that leads to poor tolerance for subsequent arousal. Increased autonomic arousal interferes with the capacity to make an appropriate psychological assessment of the stimulus and thus leads to an emergency response to relatively minor stimuli. This condition inhibits symbolic and linguistic processing and promotes physical responses, including acts of aggression against the self or others, or social and emotional withdrawal—the all-or-nothing responses.[3] The resulting lack of affect tolerance interferes with the ability to grieve and to work through ordinary conflicts, thus limiting the capacity to accumulate restitutive and gratifying experiences. Because they respond with hyperarousal to emotional or sensory stimuli, traumatized individuals have difficulty modulating their anxiety, aggression, and the extent of their intimate involvement with others. This persistent difficulty in modulating the intensity of affect seems to be an important causative factor in the self-medication with alcohol and drugs in many traumatized individuals.

Thesis 2: The animal model of inescapable shock elucidates the biology of the trauma response in humans. It is surprising that the animal model of inescapable shock has principally been applied as a model for affective illness in which traumatic antecedents have not been clearly identified as etiological factors, rather than to understanding the physiological response in PTSD and the biological substrate of its psychological effects.[4] Inescapable stress results in norepinephrine (NE), serotonin, and dopamine depletion (presumably due to the fact that utilization exceeds synthesis). The helplessness syndrome seen after exposure to inescapable shock is due to the lack of control of the animal to terminate shock: The behavioral and biochemical sequelae of escapable shock tend to be in the direction opposite to those of inescapable shock. When shock is escapable, NE levels are not lowered and may even increase. Neurotransmitter depletion may become a conditioned response to further aversive stimuli, giving rise to receptor supersensitivity.[3]

The behavioral sequelae of catecholamine depletion following inescapable shock in animals closely parallel the negative symptoms of PTSD in people. We have proposed that the diminished motivation, decline in occupational functioning, and global constriction seen in PTSD are correlates of a relative NE depletion. The clinical symptomalogy of hyperreactivity coincides with the establishment of chronic receptor supersensitivity following repeated, transient catecholamine and serotonin depletion.[3]

Thesis 3: Opioid-mediated stress-induced analgesia may account for compulsive reexposure to trauma. Animals exposed to inescapable shock develop stress-induced analgesia upon reexposure to another stressor within a brief period of time. This analgesic response to prolonged or repeated stress is mediated by endogenous opioids and is readily reversible by naloxone. Christie and Chester[5] have demonstrated that prolonged stress in animals activates brain opiate receptors in a manner analogous to repeated application of exogenous opiates. Both naloxone injections and termination of the stressful stimuli produced opiate withdrawal symptoms. These results indicate that severe, chronic stress may result in a physiological state resembling dependence on high levels of endogenous opioids.

In humans, elevations of endogenous opioids have been reported following a variety of stressors, such as surgery, marathon running, thermal stress, and habitual self-mutilation. In a recent study we found that reexposure to a traumatic stimulus evoked an endogenous opioid response equivalent to 8 mg of morphine in Vietnam veterans with PTSD, but not in combat in animals after mild stressors veterans without PTSD. Thus reexposure to stress can have the same effect as the temporary application of exogenous opioids. This effect may account for the compulsive reexposure to traumatic stimuli reported by many traumatized individuals.[3]

Thesis 4: Memory disturbances following traumatization are produced by long-term potentiation and are related to increased opioid and cortisol secretion. The ubiquitous disturbance of memory for the trauma may take the form of both hypermnesia and amnesia. Hypermnesia seems to occur after a single traumatic event, whereas amnesias dominate after prolonged or multiple trauma. The locus ceruleus, the primary source of NE innervation of the limbic system, also plays a role in memory retrieval facilitation by means of the noradrenergic tracts emanating from the locus ceruleus to the hippocampus and amygdala.[6] We have hypothesized that NE-mediated long-term augmentation of these pathways following trauma underlies the repetitive intrusive reliving of the trauma under conditions of subsequent stress.[3] After repeated or prolonged traumatization, relative increases in both endogenous opioid and cortisol release, both of which interfere with memory storage through direct action on the hippocampus, could account for dissociative and amnestic phenomena. The storage of traumatic memories recapitulates the modes of memory consolidation in early life: enactive, iconic, and symbolic/linguistic. Amnesia can occur when traumatic experiences are encoded in sensorimotor or visual form and therefore cannot be easily translated into symbolic language necessary for linguistic retrieval.[3]

Thesis 5: There is a correlation between childhood trauma, the capacity to dissociate, and the infliction of deliberate self-harm. In a recent double blind study we found a very significant relationship between a childhood history of physical and sexual trauma, and self-mutilation and self-starvation in adulthood. Self-mutilation is reported as a response to abandonment and is accompanied by analgesia and an altered state of consciousness. Self-harm provides relief and return to normalcy. Endogenous opiates seem to play a role in chronic self-injurious acts. This hypothesis is supported by direct measurements of endogenous opioids in self-mutilators and by the effect of naloxone or naltrexone on this behavior.[3] The relation between dissociation, childhood trauma, and self-mutilating behavior is a subject of further investigation.

Thesis 6: Traumatization of children affects maturation of the central nervous system. Abused children frequently have been noted to have soft neurological signs and nonspecific electroencephalographic abnormalities. There are intriguing similarities between patients with multiple personality disorder, a dissociative disorder caused by severe childhood abuse, and some of the symptomatology of temporal lobe epilepsy. It is possible that kindling phenomena leading to lasting neurobiological and behavioral (characterological) changes are produced by repeated traumatization, as with child abuse, or by one trauma followed by intrusive reexperiences. The limbic system matures primarily after birth; and, at least in lower primates, this maturation is strongly influenced by the quality of the social attachment systems. Disruption of attachment systems during critical periods appears to have a lasting adverse effect on the capacity to form secure and satisfying attachment bonds later in life.[7]

Conclusion

The symptoms of posttraumatic stress disorder are caused by neurobiological alterations, the severity of which depend on the maturational state of the organism and the severity and duration of the stress. Conditioning of these neurobiological responses results in partial reliving experiences in response to subsequent stressors, which may take the form of somatic sensations, visual images, or physical reen-actments. Particularly in children, the traumatic origin of the resulting symptoms may not be readily evident and may take the form of anxiety and dissociative and conduct disorders.

References

1. Kardiner A. The Traumatic Neuroses of War. New York: Hoeber, 1941.
2. Horowitz MJ. Stress Response Syndromes. 2nd Ed. New York: Jason Aronson, 1985.
3. Van der Kolk BA.: Psychological Trauma. Washington, DC: APA Press, 1987.
4. Maier SF, Seligman MEP.: Learned helplessness: theory and evidence J Exp Psychiatry Gen 1976;105:3–46.
5. Christie MJ, Chester GB. Physical dependence on physiologically released endogenous opiates. Life Sci 1982;30:1173–1177.
6. Delaney R, Tussi D, Gold PE. Long-term potentiation as a neurophysiological analog of memory. Pharmacol Biochem Behav 1983;18:137–139.
7. Reite M, Field T. The Psychobiology of Attachment and Separation. Orlando: Academic Press, 1985.

96. Psychophysiology of Posttraumatic Stress Disorder

ROGER K. PITMAN AND SCOTT P. ORR

Posttraumatic stress disorder (PTSD) is characterized by a constellation of symptoms falling into three major categories[1]: (a) intrusion symptoms, involving recurrent, distressful recollections of the event in various forms, including nightmares and flashbacks; (b) avoidance symptoms, involving numbing of responsiveness and avoidance of stimuli associated with the distressing event; and (c) arousal symptoms, including insomnia, irritability, difficulty concentrating, hypervigilance, exaggerated startle, and (last but not least) "physiological reactivity to events that symbolize or resemble an aspect of the (traumatic) event." It will be seen that the diagnosis of PTSD is primarily based on data obtained through patient self-report and, as such, is vulnerable to any factors that might consciously or unconsciously distort verbal report. This consideration, along with the fact that claims of PTSD are often complicated by important compensation and other secondary gain considerations, has led to the expression of skepticism about the validity of PTSD as a mental disorder[2] and (even if its validity is granted) its true incidence in various stressed populations, such as veterans of the Vietnam conflict.[3]

An important task for research is to establish objective means for assessing PTSD. Validation by objective methods would support the credibility of the PTSD concept and could be useful for identifying false positives, discovering undetected cases, separating PTSD from other mental disorders, and gauging treatment response. In this regard, psychophysiology may be of value. As used here, psychophysiology refers to the measurement of inferred mental processes or disorders through their bodily (usually autonomic) manifestations.

There have been four previously published major psychophysiological studies of PTSD, all involving veterans of military combat. These studies (and an additional one of our group) are summarized in Table 96.1. All four studies attempted to document physiological reactivity to events related to the trauma by exposing PTSD and various control subjects to recorded combat sights and sounds in the laboratory while various physiological responses were measured.

Dobbs and Wilson[4] studied eight "decompensated" World War II veterans with combat neuroses (most or all of whom would likely receive a PTSD diagnosis by today's criteria), 13 "compensated" combat veterans without psychiatric symptoms, and 10 noncombat student controls. All were exposed to an 8-min tape of

TABLE 96.1. Psychophysiological studies of posttraumatic stress disorder.

Study	Subject groups	Experimental stimuli	Control stimuli	Significant variables	PTSD response	Discriminant analysis (%)
Dobbs & Wilson (1960)[4]	8 PTSD 13 Combat C 10 Noncombat C	Combat sounds, flashes	None	HR		100 Spec 91 Sens 96 Disc
Blanchard et al. (1982)[5]	11 PTSD 11 Noncombat C	Combat sounds	Music, arithmetic	HR SBP EMG	9 BPM 8 mm Hg	
Malloy et al (1983)[6]	10 PTSD 10 Combat C 10 Noncombat psych. C	Combat slides	Shopping slides	HR SR	11 BPM 3 SRRs	80 Disc
Blanchard et al. (1986)[7]	57 PTSD 34 Combat C	Combat sounds	Music, arithmetic	HR	11 BPM	90 Spec 70 Sens 77 Disc
Pitman et al. (1987)[9]	18 PTSD 15 Combat C	Combat imagery	Neutral, other imagery	SC EMG	0.62 µmhos 1.90 µV	100 Spec 61 Sens 79 Disc

(PTSD) posttraumatic stress disorder. (C) control. (HR) heart rate. (SBP) systolic blood pressure. (EMG) electromyogram. (SR) skin resistance. (BPM) beats per minute. (SRR) skin resistance response. (SC) skin conductance. (Spec) specificity. (Sens) sensitivity. (Disc) overall discrimination. See also Blanchard et al.[7]

artillery barrage, small arms fire, and aerial bombardment sounds accompanied by flashes from a photic stimulator. Eight of the 13 "compensated" veterans showed a moderate or marked increase in pulse rate compared to one of ten controls. The behavioral responses of the "decompensated" veterans were so marked as to prevent measurement of their physiological responses; five of eight requested that the tape be turned off.

A study conducted by Blanchard et al.[5] compared 11 Vietnam veterans with PTSD with a matched group of noncombat controls on their physiological responses to mental arithmetic and to an audiotape of combat sounds played at gradually increasing volume levels. Whereas both groups showed physiological arousal to the mental arithmetic, only the PTSD patients were aroused by the combat sounds, where increases in heart rate, blood pressure, and electromyogram (EMG) significantly distinguished the groups. The PTSD patients also chose to terminate the combat stimuli at a significantly lower decibel level than the controls.

Malloy et al.[6] studied three matched groups of ten subjects each, including Vietnam combat veterans with PTSD, Vietnam combat veterans without PTSD, and non-PTSD psychiatric inpatient controls. All were exposed to audiovisually presented scenes of combat in Vietnam. Scenes of a shopping trip served as control scenes. The results showed significantly greater increases in heart rate and skin resistance responses in the PTSD group compared to the two control groups during the combat scenes. These physiological changes paralleled self-reported anxiety and a behavioral measure (latency to termination of the tape by button press). Finally, in a second study expanding their earlier work, Blanchard et al.[7] found higher heart rate responses to combat sounds in a large group of PTSD subjects in comparison to a combat control group.

The above studies were not without flaws, which included group discrepancies in age, educational level, and extent of combat experience; the use of medicated subjects or failure to specify subjects' medication status and higher baseline physiological arousal in the PTSD subjects. However, considered together, these studies lend considerable credence to PTSD's validity. A limitation common to all four of the reviewed studies, however, is the use of standard combat stimuli; that is, the same stimuli were presented to each subject. Standard stimuli may not fully capture the unique traumatic experience of the individual subject. Attempts to establish physiological correlates of PTSD symptomatology should optimally take into account the individual specificity of the underlying traumatic experiences.

We have been attempting to meet this desideratum, utilizing Lang's bioinformational theory of emotion[8] as the conceptual basis for our own psychophysiological investigation of PTSD. Lang has proposed that emotion is defined by a specific information structure in memory, consisting of stimulus, meaning, and response propositions (including autonomic changes), organized into an associative network. When a critical number of propositions are accessed, the network is processed as a unit. We have hypothesized that PTSD consists of pathological emotional networks that can be instigated through various means, including mental imagery. Following Lang's methodology, we have exposed medication-free PTSD patients and combat controls matched for age, educational level, combat exposure, and event severity to self-generated mental imagery of their own specific traumatic events while recording physiological measures. The method and results of our work to date, which appear in detail elsewhere,[9] are outlined in Table 96.1. Compared to combat controls, we have found dramatically higher physiological responses to traumatic imagery stimuli in PTSD subjects, indicating that traumatic emotion in PTSD is not recalled in tranquility.

An additional advantage of the individualized imagery method is that it lends itself to the study of treatment interventions, as treatment is concerned with helping persons adjust to the specific past experiences that trouble them. The psychophysiological study of PTSD treatment poses a challenge to future PTSD research, as does the extension of this research to the many kinds of PTSD unrelated to military combat.

References

1. American Psychiatric Association. Diagnostic and Statistical Manual of Mental Disorders. 3rd Ed., revised. Washington, DC: American Psychiatric Association, 1987.
2. Silsby HD, Jones FD. The etiologies of Vietnam post-traumatic stress syndrome. Milit Med 1985;150:6–7.
3. Fleming RH. Post Vietnam syndrome: neurosis or sociosis? Psychiatry 1985;48:122–139.
4. Dobbs D, Wilson WP. Observations on the persistence of war neurosis. Dis Nerv Syst 1960;21:40–46.
5. Blanchard EB, Kolb LC, Pallmeyer TP, et al. A psychophysiological study of post traumatic stress disorder in Vietnam veterans. Psychiatr Q 1982;54:220–229.
6. Malloy PF, Fairbank JA, Keane TM. Validation of a multimethod assessment of posttraumatic stress disorders in Vietnam veterans. J Consult Clin Psychol 1983;51:488–494.
7. Blanchard EB, Kolb LC, Gerardi RJ, et al. Cardiac response to relevant stimuli as an adjunctive tool for diagnosing posttraumatic stress disorder in Vietnam veterans. Behav Ther 1986;17:592–606.
8. Lang PJ. The cognitive psychophysiology of emotion: fear and anxiety. In Tuma AH, Maser J (eds): Anxiety and the Anxiety Disorders. Hillsdale, NJ: Lawrence Erlbaum Associates, 1985;131–170.
9. Pitman RK, Orr SP, Forgue DF, et al. Psychophysiologic assessment of post-traumatic stress disorder imagery in Vietnam combat veterans. Arch Gen Psychiatry 1987;44:970–975.

97. From CSR to PTSD

ZAHAVA SOLOMON

Combat stress has often been implicated in the genesis of psychiatric disturbances.[1,2] Combat-related trauma may be conceived of as a multistaged process.[3,4] During a war or shortly therafter the most common pathological manifestation is combat stress reaction (CSR). After the actual threat of war is lifted, the most common and conspicuous variety of combat pathology is posttraumatic stress disorder (PTSD). CSR is characterized by labile polymorphic manifestations ranging from overwhelming anxiety through total withdrawal and resulting in extreme behavior and seriously impaired functioning.[3] PTSD is characterized by reexperiencing the traumatic event, numbing of responsiveness to or reduced involvement with the external world, and a variety of autonomic, dysphoric, or cognitive symptoms.

The long-lasting effects of combat have received considerable attention. At the same time only a few studies have investigated the long-term consequences of combat stress reaction, and their findings were inconsistent. Kettner,[5] in a study of the long-term adjustment and mental health of 35 Swedish United Nations soldiers serving in the Congo (Zaire) in 1961 who had been diagnosed as CSR casualties, found that in the long run these men did not significantly differ from controls in either adjustment or mental health.

An earlier study of our group,[6] however, which assessed the military adjustment of CSR casualties following the 1973 Yom Kippur War found a marked decline in the military fitness ratings of CSR casualties. Similarly, several studies of Lebanon War veterans have found that 1 and 2 years after the war Israeli CSR casualties showed more PTSD,[7,8] more psychiatric symptomatology,[9] and more impaired social functioning[10] than comparable controls without CSR.

During and immediately after the Lebanon War, the Israel Defense Forces (IDF) had several hundred CSR casualties. Concerned with their well-being, the IDF initiated an extensive multicohort longitudinal research project on many aspects of the disorder ranging from its causes through its diagnosis, course, and treatment. In this chapter we aim to (a) asses the prevalence, intensity, and type of PTSD in CSR casualties 1, 2, and 3 years after the 1982 Lebanon War; and (b) delineate the unique profile of PTSD among Israeli soldiers with and without antecedent CSR.

Method

Two groups of subjects participated in this study. The *CSR group* included soldiers who fought on the front line during the Lebanon War and had been identified by IDF mental health personnel as CSR casualties. The *control group* consisted of soldiers who fought in the same combat units as the CSR group but did not show symptoms of CSR. The controls were pairwise matched for age, education, military rank, and assignment. Detailed descriptions of procedures, inclusion criteria, sampling procedure, and response rates can be found in our earlier publications.[7,8]

Measures and Procedure

The PTSD Inventory consists of 13 statements describing the *DSM-III* symptoms of PTSD as adapted for war trauma. The respondent was asked to indicate if he had experienced each of the described disturbances within the past month. Validity and reliability of this measure were assessed with good results.[7,8] Subjects were then interviewed and asked to complete a battery of questionnaires 1, 2, and 3 years following their participation in the 1982 Lebanon War.

Results and Discussion

Prevalence

Assessments demonstrated that in all three study years PTSD was overwhelmingly more prevalent among CSR casualties (62%, 56%, 43%, respectively) than among their matched controls (14%, 17%, 9%). These results clearly point to the long-term sequelae of CSR. However, PTSD was also found to be prevalent in the control group, which was an untreated group.

Although it is well recognized that many psychiatric disorders, including PTSD, go untreated, the high rate of cases in the control group was surprising in the current Israeli context, as veterans who sought help in an IDF clinic would have averted the very real risk of being sent back to the front. Their reluctance to seek treatment may have derived from their continuing high motivation to serve in the army, as in Israel masculine identity and status are strongly associated with army service.

Change in Prevalence

Results also show that PTSD rates in both groups changed over time. The literature on psychic trauma suggests two somewhat contradicting theories for predicting psychological recovery: residual stress perspective and stress evaporation perspective.[11] The *residual stress perspective* holds that traumatic events leave emotional scars in most people for an extended period of time. The *stress evaporation perspective* holds that although some individuals react to stress maladaptively time is a healer, and so the detrimental effects are transient and short-lived. Our results show that rates of PTSD were stable in both groups during the first 2 years after the war but significantly dropped during the third year. In other words, both theories hold. The drop coincides with Israel's finally withdrawing most of its forces from Lebanese soil. Although the heavy fighting lasted only several weeks of the summer of 1982, Israeli soldiers remained in Lebanon, where periodic flare-ups continued to occur. Our subjects, like other Israeli men in their age group, still served in the reserves and could have been sent back to Lebanon at any time. The continuing threat may have impeded their recovery. When the third year measurements were taken, both the lifting of the actual threat and the decreased dwelling on the war in the media and national consciousness may have reduced the stress the veterans were under and contributed to their recovery.

Clinical Type: Symptoms and Severity

Close scrutiny of the PTSD symptom profile in the two study groups revealed several patterns. First, the symptom profiles of all four study groups (CSR/PTSD, CSR/no-PTSD, no-CSR/PTSD, no-CSR/no-PTSD) during the first study year were almost parallel. Neither the presence or absence of PTSD nor group affiliation led to a differently shaped curve. Whether symptoms were highly endorsed or less so, they received relatively proportional endorsement in all four groups. This parallelism means that we are dealing with the same clinical entity in all four groups and that the crucial difference is one of degree. Second, although the parallelism indicates the general validity of the *DSM-III* criteria for PTSD, it also shows that not all symptoms are equally endorsed and that some are more prevalent than others. For example, whereas recurrent recollections of the war are endorsed by almost all PTSD casualties, survivor guilt and reduced expression of anger are endorsed by few. Third, subjects with current PTSD who had prior CSR tended to report more of each of the 13 *DSM-III* symptoms than PTSD subjects in the control group. Fourth, time had a differential effect on the symptom profile in the two study groups. In the CSR group the composition of the disorder remained intact, and the change was one only of degree, with the rate endorsement of PTSD symptoms decreasing proportionally with time. In the control group the passage of time changed not only the severity of the PTSD syndrome but also its composition.

One of the facts that became clear from the symptom profile is that neither guilt feelings nor reduced anger were highly endorsed by our subjects. This finding is a departure not only from the *DSM-III* symptomatology but also from ample evidence of a wide range of other studies of PTSD. Guilt feelings, especially survivor guilt, have been found to be a key variable in psychiatric morbidity induced by traumatic experiences in such widely differing groups as survivors of concentration camps, Japenese who survived the atomic bomb, survivors of the Buffalo Creek flood, veterans of World War II, and Vietnam veterans.[12]

The low endorsement of guilt and reduced expression of anger in our group may be explained by "the unique but commonly recognized features of the specific war."[13] In the Lebanon War, the absence of atrocities, the positive attitude of the Israeli population toward returning soldiers as protectors of their country, and the widespread public criticism of the war may all have had a salutary effect. Survivor guilt has been found to be mitigated when it can be channeled into an open expression of anger.[14] In Israel the open anger of much of the public about the Lebanon War may have supported precisely such an externalization.

Conclusion

The results suggest that the detrimental effects of combat are deep and enduring, and are especially so for CSR casualties. Close scrutiny of the clinical data suggests that PTSD is a complex entity encompassing a large variety of manifestations that differ in quality and quantity from one group to another. More studies are needed to refine diagnostic criteria, which have considerable bearing on treatment.

References

1. Grinker RR, Spiegel JP. Men Under Stress. Philadelphia: Blakiston, 1945.
2. Stauffer SA, Lumsdaine AA, Lumsdaine MH, et al. The American Soldier, Vol III: Combat and Its Aftermath. Princeton, NJ: Princeton University Press, 1949.
3. Kardiner A. War Stress and Neurotic Illness. New York: Hoeber, 1947.
4. Titchner JL, Ross WO. Acute or chronic stress as determinants of behavior, character and neuroses. In Arieti S, Brody EB (eds): Adult Clinical Psychiatry: American Handbook of Psychiatry. New York: Basic Books, 1974.
5. Kettner B. Combat stress and subsequent mental health—a follow-up of Swedish soldiers serving in the United Nations Forces 1961–62. Acta Psychiatr Scand [Suppl] 1972;230:5–112.
6. Solomon Z, Oppenheimer B, Noy S. Subsequent military adjustment of combat stress reaction casualties—a 9 year follow-up study. Milit Med 1986;151:8–11.
7. Solomon Z, Weisenberg M, Schwarzwald J, et al. Post-traumatic stress disorder among frontline soldiers with combat stress reaction: the 1982 Israeli experience. Am J Psychiatry 1987;144:448–454.
8. Solomon Z. Combat-related posttraumatic stress disorder among Israeli soldiers—a two year follow-up. Bull Menninger Clin 1987;51:80–95.
9. Solomon Z, Mikulincer M, Bleich A. Characteristic expressions of combat-related post-traumatic stress disorder among Israeli soldiers in the 1982 Lebanon War. Behav Med 1988;14(4):171–178.
10. Solomon Z, Mikulincer M. Combat stress reaction, PTSD and social adjustment—a study of Israeli veterans. J Nerv Ment Dis 1987;175(5):277–285.
11. Figley CR. Psychological adjustment among Vietnam veterans: an overview of the research. In Figley CR (ed): Stress Disorders Among Vietnam Veterans—Theory, Research and Treatment. New York: Brunner/Mazel, 1978.
12. Hendin H, Haas AP. Wounds of War: The Psychological Aftermath of Combat in Vietnam. New York: Basic Books, 1984.
13. Laufer RS, Gallops MS, Frey-Wouters E. War stress and post-war trauma. J Health Soc Behav 1984;25:65–85.
14. Lifton RJ. Death in Life: Survivors of Hiroshima. New York: Random House, 1986.

98. Social Support Versus Self-Sufficiency in Traumatic and Posttraumatic Stress Reactions

NORMAN A. MILGRAM

Some of the assumptions underlying current conceptualizations of social support are challenged in this chapter. A rationale is offered for several propositions discussed below, and partial evidence is offered in their support.

Historical Background

Considerable research has shown that social support mitigates or buffers the adverse psychological impacts of exposure to stressful life events and thereby reduces the probability of psychiatric disorders in general and of posttraumatic stress disorders in particular.[1,2] Social support has been defined as assistance in coping[3] and refers to emotional, informational, instrumental, and companionate functions performed for a distressed individual by significant others such as family members, friends, co-workers, relatives, and neighbors. These functions may also be performed by professionals—physicians, clergy, psychiatrists, psychologists, and social workers.

The early research in this field was marked by adherence to the *availability imperative,* the notion that availability of social support is a guarantee of its utilization and beneficial effect. The availability imperative has since been replaced by the *time lock-and-key imperative.* For every lock, there is a key that opens it at an appropriate time. For every individual in stress there is a social support system optimally effective at a particular point in the coping process. This statement implies that social support becomes available to a given individual or group as a function of the efforts of others. It is proposed here that people exposed to stressful situations engage spontaneously in sequential search and selection of social supports. They actively recruit social support and weigh the various kinds of social support available to them before selecting one to match their personal resources and current level of symptomatology.

The notion of sequential search and selection does not necessarily assume that that all people in stressful situations need support systems to mitigate adverse stress reactions and lower the probability of chronic sequelae. On the contrary, some people who reject available social support are self-sufficient and have the personal resources to cope with some stressful situations on their own, without jeopardy.

Research Findings

My colleagues and I examined these issues in a preliminary manner in two studies. The first was a long-term follow-up of the grief and stress reactions of 415 seventh grade children following the death of 19 classmates and the serious injuries of the 14 survivors in a schoolbus accident.[4-6] During the week after the disaster children attended the mass funeral, engaged in commemorative ceremonies and activities to honor the dead, and were offered group and individual sessions with professional personnel—the guidance teacher, school psychologist, and other volunteer mental health workers on the scene.

They were asked in a self-report questionnaire 1 week after the accident which of the following individuals helped them to cope with their distress—themselves, parents, siblings, relatives, neighborhood friends, schoolmates, classroom teachers, guidance teachers, or psychologists. Self was checked off by 86% of the children followed by parents 65%, teachers 44%, and so on down to psychologists 18%. The children checked off an average of 3.14 sources of social support. When asked which of these sources helped the most, nearly 50% again said themselves, 31% their parents, etc.

These reports on social support were correlated with kind and frequency of professional sessions received, interest in future sessions, and frequency of stress reactions. Data were consistent with a sequential search and selection model: The children who reported relatively few stress reactions depended on themselves, received few sessions with a professional worker, and were not interested in professional treatment. Children with greater distress turned to others for social support—family members and age peers at school—and when their symptomatology was not relived they turned to professional adults and showed interest in further treatment of this nature. Children with highly atypical, extreme stress reactions turned to professional workers from the start because they believed their friends and family could not help them with problems of this magnitude.

A follow-up self-report questionnaire after 1 year and behavioral follow-up by teachers and the school psychologist over the next 2 years gave no credence to the argument that self-sufficient children were denying an urgent unmet need for help. We concluded that many children prefer to cope on their own with the grief and stress reactions that follow the death of schoolmates and appear to be symptom-free thereafter. Self-sufficiency may have been effective in this instance because coping was emotion-focused rather than problem-focused and took place in the absence of life-threatening stressors. We predict, however, that few if any people insist on going it alone when exposed to life-threatening situations, as in combat stress.

Musketeer Syndrome (or There Are Times when You Need All the Friends You Can Get)

In the well known novel *The Three Musketeers* by Alexander Dumas, the motto of the heroes is "One for all and all for one." A modern psychological term that represents this kind of contract is *group cohesiveness,* defined as a mutual support system in which members provide all forms of social support to one another.

Field research studies[7,8] on posttraumatic reactions in combat soldiers have demonstrated the buffering effect of serving in units characterized by high group cohesiveness as contrasted with units characterized by low cohesiveness. Not infrequently the incidence of psychiatric casualties was lower in a cohesive unit exposed to combat of greater intensity and duration than in a less cohesive one exposed to lower levels of combat stress. Evidence cited for the remarkable stress-buffering efficacy of group cohesiveness is based on group comparisons, i.e., the incidence of psychiatric casualties in combat of military units with high versus low group cohesiveness. Few if any studies have investigated these relations within individual soldiers, each from a different military unit.

The Israeli involvement in Lebanon between 1982 and 1985 provided an opportunity to assess the relation between group cohesiveness, combat intensity, and stress reactions in two distinct time periods.

The first was the initial invasion (June 6–30, 1982). This period was characterized on the *negative* side by high military and civilian casualties and on the *positive* side by the high consensus within Israeli society about goals and achievements of the war. The second was the subsequent holding operation until withdrawal 2 years later. This period was a mirror image of the earlier one and was characterized on the *positive* side by few casualties, military or civilian, and on the *negative* side by increasing dissatisfaction within the army and the society about the war.

In this study[9] retrospective self-report data by 48 Israeli soldiers were obtained in April 1984 as withdrawal from Lebanon was under way. We found a marked decline in level of combat-related stressors, bodily stress reactions, and belief in the war's goals, and a moderate decline in emotional stress reactions, group morale, and primary loyalty to the group over one's family. There was, however, no corresponding decline in the motivation to serve to the best of one's ability, group cohesiveness, or military performance. Group cohesiveness was the major factor affecting military performance during both time periods; group loyalty was second. The other variables, including one's ideological orientation (left versus right), had no effect. Level of combat stressors was related to emotional and bodily stress reactions but not to military performance. We concluded that the major factor in sustaining military performance under stressful conditions is the mutual social support of comrades-in-arms.

References

1. Cobb S. Social support as a moderator to life stress. Psychosom Med 1976;38:300–314.
2. Kessler RC, McLeod JD. Social support and mental health in community samples. In: Cohen S, Syme SL (eds): Social Support and Health. New York: Academic Press, 1985;219–240.
3. Thoits PA. Social support as coping assistance. J Consult Clin Psychol 1986;54:416–423.
4. Toubiana YH, Milgram NA, Strich Y, et al. Crisis intervention in a school community disaster: principles and practices. J Community Psychol 1988;16:228–239.
5. Milgram NA, Toubiana YH, Klingman A, et al. Situational exposure and personal loss in children's acute and chronic stress reactions to a school disaster. J Traumatic Stress 1988;1:339–352.
6. Milgram NA, Toubiana YH. Confronting vs avoidant behavior and support systems in children's coping with a school bus disaster. Unpublished paper. Tel Aviv: Tel-Aviv University, 1987.

7. Milgram NA, Hobfoll S. Generalizations from theory and practice in war-related stress. In Milgram NA (ed): Stress and Coping in Time of War: Generalizations from the Israeli Experience. New York: Brunner/Mazel, 1986;316–352.
8. Noy S, Nardi C, Solomon Z. Battle and military unit characteristics and the prevalence of psychiatric casualties. In Milgram NA (ed): Stress and Coping in Time of War: Generalization from the Israeli Experience. New York: Brunner/Mazel, 1986;73–77.
9. Milgram NA, Orenstein R, Zafrir E. Stressors, interpersonal resources and interpersonal supports in wartime military performance. J Milit Psych, in press.

99. Pharmacotherapy Trials in Posttraumatic Stress Disorder: Prospects and Problems

BERNARD LERER, PETER BRAUN, AVRAHAM BLEICH, HAIM DASBERG, AND DAVID GREENBERG

Although a clinical symptom picture resembling the currently accepted *DSM-III* diagnosis of posttraumatic stress disorder (PTSD) has been recognized for decades, focused trials of psychopharmacological agents are a relatively recent development. The initial report by Hogben and Cornfield[1] of a dramatic effect of treatment with the monoamine oxidase inhibitor phenelzine in patients with "traumatic war neurosis" has been followed by a spate of positive reports. These reports have attributed beneficial effects to a variety of drugs including tricyclic antidepressants,[2,3] the limbic anticonvulsant carbamazepine,[4] and the β-receptor blocker propranolol.[5] Contrary to these generally optimistic reports, our experience with psychotropic agents in Israeli samples of PTSD patients has been less encouraging. This experience has been for the most part prospective and, in two studies, double-blind in nature using a drug/placebo crossover design.

To date, no published studies, including our own, have employed the classic, two-group random-assignment methodology which is a prerequisite for definitive trials of psychopharmacological agents. Notwithstanding this limitation, our findings have led us to seriously question if further drug trials in PTSD may not be rendered counterproductive by the considerable overlap between diagnostic criteria for PTSD and those for major depressive and anxiety disorders. As a result of this overlap, "beneficial effects in PTSD" may be attributed to agents that ameliorate nonspecific symptoms suffered by an essentially heterogeneous population of patients who have in common prior exposure to psychologically traumatic circumstances or events. Briefly summarized, the findings on which these concerns are based were as follows.

Phenelzine

Twenty-five veterans of the 1982–1984 Lebanon conflict who fulfilled *DSM-III* criteria for PTSD were prospectively assigned to treatment with phenelzine (median dose 60 mg/day for 4–22 weeks). Only four had a greater than 30% improvement in posttraumatic symptoms, and none exceeded a 50% change over baseline levels.[6] Posttraumatic symptoms were rated using a scale derived from the *DSM-III* criteria for PTSD. Improvements on the Hamilton Anxiety and Hamilton Depression Scales were of a similar order of magnitude. All four best responders had concurrent *DSM-III* diagnoses in addition to PTSD: panic disorder in two cases and dysthymic disorder in the two others. Sleep disturbance was the only individual symptom that showed clinically impressive improvement in the whole subject group (mean 36%).

A random-assignment, double-blind crossover trial with phenelzine in a different sample of PTSD patients yielded even less encouraging results.[7] Ten patients completed at least 4 weeks of treatment on phenelzine (45–75 mg/day) or placebo, a 2-week placebo period, and then a further 4 weeks on the alternate treatment. This group of subjects did not consist exclusively of military veterans (four subjects) but included civilian victims of terrorist attacks (two subjects) and of traffic and industrial accidents (four subjects) that resulted in the death or injury of others. The rating instruments used included the PTSD, Impact of Events, Hamilton Anxiety, and Hamilton Depression Scales.

Only three subjects responded better to phenelzine than to placebo. One received phenelzine in the second leg of the trial; he had reported no improvement during the prior placebo phase. The two others received phenelzine during the first leg and did not relapse after withdrawal of the active drug. However, three other subjects showed a pattern of response similar to placebo during the first leg, which carried over into their active drug phase. Two of the three phenelzine responders had concomitant *DSM-III* diagnoses of generalized anxiety disorder. The two other patients with concomitant *DSM-III* diagnoses (major depression in both cases) did not respond during either phase of the trial. In the group as a whole there was, as might be expected from the individual outcomes, no significant advantage for phenelzine over placebo on any of the rating scales. Outcome data for the full trial period showed consistent improvement irrespective of treatment and suggested a strong influence of nonspecific factors and/or a prominent placebo effect.

Alprazolam

Alprazolam, a triazolabenzodiazepine, has well documented anxiolytic, antidepressant, and antipanic properties.[8] Because the *DSM-III* criteria for PTSD encompass symptoms of this type, alprazolam appeared to be a logical candidate for a trial in this syndrome. We recently completed a random-assignment, double-blind, crossover trial of alprazolam in PTSD.[9] The protocol for this study employed the same methodology and rating scales used in the phenelzine trial[7] and included a similar patient population. Ten subjects completed both legs of the alprazolam–placebo crossover, undergoing 5 weeks of treatment in each phase (alprazolam dose 2.5–6.0 mg/day) separated by a 2-week placebo period. Hamilton Anxiety Scale ratings revealed a small but significant advantage for alprazolam ($p < 0.02$). There was a similar but nonsignificant trend favoring alprazolam on a self-rated Visual Analog Scale reflecting overall well-being. However, the PTSD, Impact of Events, and Hamilton Depression Scale showed little change on either treatment and no advantage for the active drug. In contrast to the phenelzine crossover trial,[7] improvement irrespective of treatment was not a prominent feature, suggesting that positive effects could be more confidently attributed to the active drug. The best responder to alprazolam in this trial had a concomitant *DSM-II* diagnosis of panic disorder, and another good responder fulfilled criteria for generalized anxiety disorder. Two subjects with concomitant diagnoses of major depression had no discernible benefit from the treatment.

An ongoing, open, prospective trial of alprazolam in a population made up exclusively of military veterans has yielded similar results. Reduction in anxiety symptoms has been the most prominent feature. Patients with the greatest improvement in Hamilton Anxiety Scale (HAM-A) ratings have also reported some reduction in "core" PTSD symptoms (discussed below), but it has been of marginal clinical significance. The most striking response was observed in a patient with a concurrent full-blown syndrome of panic attacks and agoraphobia.

Tricyclic Antidepressants

Retrospective evaluation of 25 veterans with PTSD exposed to a number of psychopharmacological agents indicated "good to moderate" effects in 19 of 28 trials with tricyclic antidepressants.[10] Sleep difficulty was the most consistently improved symptom. The relation of therapeutic response to the severity of anxiety and depressive symptoms was difficult to define because of the retrospective nature of the study. Our subsequent clinical experience has focused on amitriptyline, which appears to be considerably more efficacious than either phenelzine or alprazolam. This experience has yet to be systematically analyzed. An association between severity of depressive symptomatology and therapeutic response has been frequently noted, however, and an improvement in sleep disturbance has been consistently observed.

Conclusions

Our experience with psychotropic agents in the treatment of PTSD has been only minimally encouraging. It has also raised pertinent questions regarding the role of pharmacotherapy in treating this complex disorder. The prospects for further research in this area must be regarded with some reservation until the issues raised have been adequately addressed.

It is our impression that improvements noted with the agents we have studied cannot be regarded as a specific effect on core posttraumatic symptoms. Under this category we include daytime flashbacks, traumatic dreams, preoccupation with the traumatic event and persistent recollections of it, reintensification of symptoms by exposure to related cues, and survivor guilt. The initial report of Hogben and Cornfield[1] attributed specific effects of this type to phenelzine, as did, although less extensively, the prospective study of Davidson et al.[11] in 11 veterans with PTSD. A specific effect of imipramine on night terrors associated with PTSD has been reported by Marshall[12] in three subjects. It has been our experience, however, that even in subjects reporting major clinical improvement the core PTSD symptoms tend to remain relatively unchanged. The most dramatic improvements have, in fact, been noted in subjects in whom symptoms of this type were not initially prominent. This finding suggests that positive effects of antidepressant agents in PTSD may represent a symptomatic improvement in affective and anxiety elements of the clinical syndrome that are not specific to PTSD. Amelioration of sleep disturbance is an important example.

These comments do not imply that antidepressants agents should not be tried in PTSD patients in whom a trial of pharmacotherapy is deemed appropriate. Patients with prominent affective symptoms and sleep disturbance could well benefit from such interventions. On the research level, however, the rigorous definition of a core PTSD syndrome that can be convincingly separated from concomitant affective and anxiety symptoms appears to be strongly indicated. Further drug trials, even if better controlled and encompassing a larger number of subjects than those reported to date, could continue to generate confusing results if they are based on the criteria presently in use.

References

1. Hogben GL, Cornfield RB. Treatment of traumatic war neurosis with phenelzine. Arch Gen Psychiatry 1981;38:440–445.
2. Falcon S, Ryan C, Chamberlain K, et al. Tricyclics: possible treatment for posttraumatic stress disorder. J Clin Psychiatry 1985;46:385–389.
3. Burstein A. The treatment of post-traumatic stress disorder with imipramine. Psychosomatics 1983;25:683–687.
4. Wolf ME, Alavi A, Mosanaim AD. Post traumatic stress disorder in Vietnam veterans—clinical and EEG findings: possible therapeutic effects of carbamazepine. Biol Psychiatry 1987∞ press.
5. Kolb LC, Burris BC, Griffiths S. Propanolol and clonidine in treatment of the chronic post traumatic stress disorders of war. In van der Kolk B (ed): Post Traumatic Stress Disorder: Psychological and Biological Sequelae. Washington, DC: American Psychiatric Press, 1984;97–105.
6. Lerer B, Bleich A, Garb R, et al. Post traumatic stress disorder in Israeli combat veterans: effect of phenelzine treatment. Arch Gen Psychiatry 1987;44:976–981.
7. Shestatzky M, Greenberg D, Lerer B. A controlled trial of phenelzine in post traumatic stress disorder. Psychiatry Res 1987;24:149–155.
8. Fawcett JA, Kravitz HM. Alprazolam: pharmacokinetics, clinical efficacy, and mechanism of action. Pharmacotherapy 1982;2:243–254.
9. Braun P, Greenberg D, Lerer B. Modest effects of alprazolam on anxiety symptoms in post traumatic stress disorder. Submitted for publication.
10. Bleich A, Siegel R, Garb R, et al. Post-traumatic stress disorder following combat exposure: clinical features and psychopharmacological treatment. Br J Psychiatry 1986;149:365–369.
11. Davidson J, Walker JI, Kilts C. A pilot study of phenelzine in post-traumatic stress disorder. Br J Psychiatry 1987;150:252–255.
12. Marshall JR: The treatment of night terrors associated with the posttraumatic syndrome. Am J Psychiatry 1975;132:293–295.

100. Psychobiology of Dissociation

FRANK W. PUTNAM

Dissociation is a psychophysiological process that is best understood by careful investigation of its clinical phenomenology and experimental psychophysiology. It was among the first mental processes to be systematically studied and attracted the interest of such notables as Benjemin Rush, William James, Morton Prince, Alfred Binet, and others associated with the early development of modern psychiatry.[1] Pierre Janet made many important contributions to our current understanding of dissociation, and his doctoral dissertation *L'Automatisme Psycholgique* was hailed from the first as a classic of the psychological sciences; it remains an important clinical document today.

There has been a recognition that dissociation plays an important role in the psychopathology of posttraumatic stress disorder and other traumatically induced psychological reactions.[2] In particular, dissociation is thought to be the primary psychobiological mechanism responsible for such symptoms as amnesias, flashbacks, intrusive images and affects, and abreactions, commonly noted in victims of physical and psychological trauma. Acute dissociative reactions such as psychogenic amnesia and psychogenic fugue states are often noted immediately after a traumatic precipitant.[2] Chronic dissociative disorders, such as depersonalization syndrome and multiple personality disorder, typically follow a history of sustained or repetitive trauma.[2] Dissociation is also thought to make secondary contribution to the depression and disturbances in sense of self commonly found in victims of trauma.

Principles of Dissociation

A number of general principles have been observed to operate across different forms of dissociation.[2] It has long been recognized that dissociation exists on a continuum.[3] Micro- and minidissociative episodes occur in normal individuals daily. More significant dissociative episodes, such as "highway hypnosis" or "breakaway" can occur in normal individuals operating in sensory-deprived or monotonous environments. Transient depersonalization, a mild form of dissociative reaction, frequently occurs in normal adolescents, and its incidence declines with age.[2] Survey data from the Dissociative Experiences Scale (DES) on the frequency of dissociation in various psychiatric populations demonstrates a clear continuum ranging from normal adult subjects on the low end to multiple personality disorder patients at the high end.[3]

Although dissociation serves as an initially adaptive response to acute trauma it frequently becomes maladaptive when it recurs in situations outside of the immediate trauma context. Pathological dissociation, as categorized in the *DSM-III*, is characterized by three general principles. The first is that there is a disturbance in the individual's memory. Generally it takes the form of amnesias such as those seen in psychogenic amnesia or psychogenic fugue states. In depersonalization syndrome and many posttraumatic reactions, the disturbance in memory may be manifest as dream-like recall of the events, often with a detached quality. The patient may report details as if he or she was watching from a distant perspective rather than directly experiencing the event.

The second general principle is that in pathological dissociation there is a marked disturbance in the individual's sense of self. For example, in psychogenic amnesia the patient loses memory for self-referential information although the general fund of knowledge remains intact. In psychogenic fugue states and multiple personality disorder there are secondary identities that control the individual's behavior; and in depersonalization syndrome the individual feels as if he or she were dead, a machine, or unreal. The third principle is that pathological dissociation is almost inevitability associated with acute or chronic traumatic precipitants.[2]

Pathological dissociation is probably best conceptualized as a traumatically induced altered state of consciousness. It shares many of the properties of a discrete state of consciousness, including state-dependent learning (SDL), state-dependent memory retrieval, and a state-dependent biology. Although most traumatically induced dissociative reactions are too short-lived to be adequately investigated in the laboratory, we believe that multiple personality disorder, a chronic dissociative reaction, provides a unique model for studying the psychophysiology of dissociation.[4]

Multiple Personality Disorder as a Model of Dissociation

Multiple personality disorder (MPD), a major form of dissociative disorder, is characterized by the existence of two or more separate and distinct personalities within an individual. These alter-personalities may each have their own complex social patterns and behaviors; when a given personality is dominant, it controls the individual's behavior. Whereas the single most common symptom in MPD is amnesia for life experiences, most of these patients first present with complaints and symptoms suggestive of depression.[5] Typically, these patients are polysymptomatic, with the most common presenting symptoms being depression, "mood swings," suicidality, sleep disturbances, sexual dysfunction, conversion symptoms, fugue episodes, panic attacks, and substance abuse.[5] Most of these patients spend 5 years or more in and out of psychiatric treatment and typically receive numerous diagnoses before being identified as having MPD.[5] They are usually refractory to most standard treatments and typically exhibit a pattern of alternating between relatively high social functioning and apparent brief psychotic decompensations.

A history of significant childhood trauma has been repeatedly noted by all modern clinical investigators, and it is generally accepted that severe or repetitive trauma, typically sexual abuse, occurring before midadolescence is necessary to produce MPD. The alter-personalities, which are dissociative states of consciousness elaborated over time and organized around a specific body image and strong affect, arise as a child's defense against the terror and anger engendered by the trauma. There is a significant correlation between the amount of trauma and the number of alter-personalities.[5]

The alter-personalities can be conceptualized as discrete altered states of consciousness, first initially evoked by the trauma and later reactivated by similar environmental cues. With repeated activation, an alter-personality accumulates a unique history of its own together with a set of behaviors that give it the individuality found so striking by clinicians. Investigations indicate that many of the alter-personalities exhibit state-dependent properties of learning, memory, and psychophysiology. Silberman et al.[6] found evidence of state-dependent learning and memory between alter-personalities using word list tasks and measuring the leakage of information across personalities. Physiological measures including galvanic skin response, electroencephalography (EEG), and evoked potentials have been utilized to study the state-dependent biology of the alter-personalities.[7] Currently investigations are under way with regard to alter-personality-specific changes in cerebral blood flow, EEG, and immune function. Multiple personality disorder may prove to be an important model of how psychological state interacts with bodily physiology.

The treatment is essentially the psychotherapy of a traumatic neurosis and can be significantly facilitated by use of hypnosis to uncover amnesic material. The impression of most experienced clinicians is that the disorder has a good prognosis, though no controlled studies of outcome exist to date.[8]

References

1. Ellenberger HF. The Discovery of the Unconscious: The History and Evolution of Dynamic Psychiatry. New York: Basic Books, 1970.
2. Putnam FW. Dissociation as a response to extreme trauma. In Kluft RP (ed): Childhood Antecedents of Multiple Personality. Washington, DC: American Psychiatric Press, 1985;65–97.
3. Bernstein E, Putnam FW. The development, reliability and validity of a dissociation scale. J Nerv Ment Dis 1986;174:727–735.
4. Putnam FW. The study of multiple personality disorder: general strategies and practical considerations. Psychiatry Annu 1984;14:58–61.
5. Putnam FW, Guroff JJ, Silberman EK, et al. The clinical phenomenology of multiple personality disorder: review of 100 recent cases. J Clin Psychiatry 1986;47:285–293.
6. Silberman EK, Putnam FW, Weingartner H, et al. Dissociative states in multiple personality disorder: a quantitive study. Psychiatry Res 1985;15:253–260.
7. Putnam FW. The psychophysiologic investigation of multiple personality disorder: a review. Psychiatr Clin North Am 1984;7:31–40.
8. Putnam FW. The treatment of multiple personality: state of the art. In Braun BG (ed): The Treatment of Multiple Personality Disorder. Washington, DC: American Psychiatric Press, 1986;177–198.

IV.D. ANOREXIA AND BULIMIA

101. Eating Disorder and Affective Disorder: How Real Is the Relation?

JACK L. KATZ

The traditional view of anorexia nervosa and bulimia has held that they are psychosomatic eating disorder (ED) syndromes that occur primarily in adolescent girls or young women. Attempts to refine our understanding of their development have brought attention to possible specific developmental phenomena or personality characteristics, family styles or patterns, and sociocultural trends or influences that may serve as risk factors for these disorders.[1] Precipitating and perpetuating variables have also been examined.

However, another explanation for the basic pathology of the eating disorders has been proposed. Pope and Hudson,[2] as well as others, have hypothesized that eating disorders are essentially variants of depressive disorder. Thus anorexia nervosa and bulimia are postulated to be manifestations of an underlying affective disorder (AD) that has taken a particular form of expression, perhaps by virtue of sociocultural influences or individual psychobiological vulnerabilities.

In this chapter we examine the evidence for and against this proposal and offer a synthesis that seems to provide the most reasonable and parsimonious explanation for the conflicting data.

Evidence for a Relation

Clinical Data

A number of studies have now documented that the cross-sectional application of reliable diagnostic criteria, such as *DSM-III* or Research Diagnostic Criteria (RDC), to persons diagnosed as having either anorexia nervosa or bulimia yields a concomitant diagnosis of major depression in 23–80% of patients.[3] Most reported figures cluster about an AD rate of 40–50% in both eating disorders, which would mean a frequency of depression of perhaps fivefold that in the general population.

Moreover, the application of these clinical diagnostic criteria in a longitudinal fashion, i.e., in follow-up studies, has generally yielded data indicating that about 30–45% of patients with an index episode of anorexia nervosa or bulimia will at some time develop symptoms that meet criteria for a diagnosis of major depression.[3]

Retrospective studies also indicate that some ED patients clearly meet criteria for major depression prior to their initial episode of eating disorder.[4]

Family Data

The importance of family pathology in supporting a clinical diagnosis has grown substantially in recent decades. Regardless of the mode of transmission, we have come to recognize that similar pathology tends to cluster in families. Hence it is not surprising that several investigators have looked at the incidence of AD in the relatives of ED patients. Almost all have reported a significantly elevated incidence of AD in these relatives when compared to AD incidence figures for the general population.[3]

Response to Pharmacotherapy

Although a condition's response to a specific pharmacological agent does not necessarily tell us about the underlying etiology of that condition—as many drugs have general palliative effects without necessarily attacking the specific cause of a disorder—empirical studies of response to classes of medication can often provide important leads about pathogenesis and sometimes even about etiology. That bulimia has now been reported in several well controlled double-blind studies to respond significantly to antidepressants,[5] whether monoamine oxidase inhibitors or tricyclics, and that lithium has been reported to be helpful in some anorectic and bulimic patients[6] suggest that AD and ED could share underlying pathogeneses or etiologies.

Endocrine Markers

The wide attention to the hypothalamic-pituitary-adrenal (HPA) axis in the affective disorders has now spilled over into the eating disorders. Not only has there been clear-cut evidence of similar activation of this axis in anorexia nervosa and AD patients but actually a higher percentage of anorectics (about 70%) than is typically reported for depressed patients (about 40%) shows aberrant HPA functioning.[7] (The findings with normal-weight bulimics are inconsistent but still more frequently abnormal than in the general population.)

Arguments Against a Relation
Clinical Data

Although an incidence of about 50% of diagnosable major depression in patients with an ED is certainly striking when compared to an incidence of perhaps 10% for the general population, it does not address the possibility that perhaps the appropriate control group should not be the general population but, rather, other psychiatric cohorts. As Strober and Katz have observed,[8] rates of diagnosable concomitant depression comparable to those found in ED patients emerge in studies of both schizophrenic and alcoholic subjects. Thus it is conceivable that there is a limited repertoire of human behaviors and emotions, and chronic psychiatric disorder (and probably chronic physical disorder) simply puts one at risk for what has been termed "secondary" depression.

Indeed, if one looks more closely at the actual depressive symptoms among patients with eating disorders, one finds that, although the features often do qualify for an overall *DSM-III* or RDC diagnosis of major depression, they are anything but melancholic in nature.[8] Thus anhedonia, motor retardation, lack of reactivity to the environment, diminished energy, diurnal variation, etc. are all typically absent.

Moreover, with regard to the longitudinal findings, Keller et al.[9] have demonstrated during careful 1-year follow-up studies with bulimic patients that improved mood did not correlate with decreased binging. This finding suggests underlying pathogenetic mechanisms in eating disturbance and affective disturbance that are not necessarily concordant.

Finally, and perhaps most tellingly, is the argument advanced by Altshuler and Wiener.[10] They have pointed out that symptoms that provide the basis for a diagnosis of major depression have been shown to occur frequently in states of starvation. Thus the studies of Keys et al.[11] with voluntarily starved normal adults revealed the widespread presence of depressed mood, irritability, decreased concentration, constipation, decreased libido, fatigability, obsessional preoccupations, etc. Thus starvation itself can apparently elicit an affective-behavioral-physiological-cognitive state strikingly similar to that seen in ED patients. Even the objection that this argument would not hold for bulimic patients of normal weight may not be valid: We know that most bulimics simply do not eat normally. Thus their nutritional state, as contrasted with their weight, can hardly be termed optimal.

Family Data

Aside from the occasional glaring exceptions to the studies reporting a significantly increased incidence of AD in the relatives of patients with eating disorders,[12] there is other evidence to suggest that these conditions do not share a common familial transmission. First, Strober and colleagues[13] have shown that, although there is indeed an elevated incidence of affective disorders in first degree relatives of hospitalized patients with anorexia nervosa, the incidence of eating disorders among relatives of AD probands, as well as of schizophrenic patients, is no greater than that in the general population. Moreover, when their anorectic subjects were divided into depressed and nondepressed cohorts, it was found that the rate of AD in the relatives of the depressed anorectics was 3.5 times greater (17.3% versus 5.1%) than that among the nondepressed anorectics. Thus affective illness clusters significantly only in the families of *depressed* ED patients, and ED does not cluster at all in the families of noneating-disordered, depressed patients, thereby strongly suggesting that these disorders are transmitted independently.

Response to Pharmacotherapy

Several aspects of the studies on response to medication are disconcerting. That response to antidepressant treatment for bulimia occasionally takes place prior to the usual 10- to 14-day lag time characteristic of response in depression and that improvement in bulimia with antidepressant treatment is commonly independent of the presence or absence of affective features[14] raise the possibility that the effectiveness of the antidepressants in bulimia might have a central biological basis different from that in AD. Moreover, the well known association of both antidepressants and lithium with weight gain suggests that these agents may be acting on appetitive or metabolic pathways in anorectic subjects, rather than on an underlying depression.

Endocrine Markers

Not only is the evidence for overlap between ED and AD far less noteworthy for thyroid and growth hormone indices, as well as for neurotransmitter metabolite excretion,[15] but even the HPA findings must now be considered suspect. The sensitivity and specificity of HPA alterations in depression are not only becoming increasingly controversial, but these precise HPA findings have now been elicited by caloric restriction to between 1,000 and 1,200 kcal/day over 18 days in normal female volunteers; it occurred, it should be noted, in the absence of any sign of depression.[16] Hence the use of endocrine markers to establish a relation between ED and AD must be regarded as of dubious reliability at this time.

Evidence for a Restricted Relation

Biochemical Studies

Given the complexities and ambiguities in the clinical, follow-up, family, pharmacotherapy, and psychoendocrine studies, other possible markers of depression have been examined in ED patients. Biederman and colleagues, in a series of studies,[17-19] have reported significant abnormalities in platelet monoamine oxidase activity, human leukocyte antigen-BW 16 (a genetic marker) frequency, and plasma cyclic adenosine monophosphate (CAMP) concentration in about 30–45% of patients with anorexia nervosa. What makes their findings important is that the subgroup of anorectic subjects characterized by these biological abnormalities was also the same subgroup characterized by symptoms of major depression. These findings thus suggest that a subgroup, but only a subgroup, of ED patients actually have concurrent or underlying AD.

Sleep Studies

Consistent with these studies, the report of Katz and co-workers[20] on sleep variables in ED patients indicates the existence of a subgroup—but again only a subgroup of about 30%—that is characterized by another biological marker of depression, i.e., a substantially shortened latency in the onset of rapid-eye-movement (REM) sleep. Here too it was precisely this subgroup who were most likely to show clinical stigmata and family histories consistent with a diagnosis of AD. Age, percent ideal body weight, duration of illness, and level of activity showed no correlation with duration of REM latency.

Integrating and Interpreting the Data

Two inferences from these data appear reasonable. On the one hand, it seems evident from a wide array of studies that there exists a bonafide *subgroup* of patients with ED, probably in the range of 25–50% of all ED patients (both anorectic and bulimic) who are also characterized by another axis I diagnosis, i.e., major depressive disorder. On the other hand, it seems equally evident that most ED patients are not. Whether clinical, follow-up, family, response to medication, or biological findings are examined, the latter group simply fails to give evidence of also being afflicted by an AD. Thus to equate these two conditions—i.e., to view anorexia nervosa and bulimia as variants or masked equivalents of depression—and to suggest that they share the same etiology is to ignore the substantial data now available in this regard.

However, as some relation other than a shared etiology does appear to exist, given the sizable subgroup characterized by both AD and ED, we propose the following explanatory models.

1. On one side of the pathogenetic sequence exists the likelihood that depression is a risk factor, although only one among several risk factors, for the development of an ED among young women in industrialized cultures. Thus anorexia nervosa with its implicit emphasis on achieving control and identity, and bulimia with its excessive self-feeding, might be culturally induced defenses against the painful and empty feelings of a depression. Indeed, the fact that two of the cardinal features of anorexia nervosa, i.e., starvation and exercise, are known to elicit increments in endorphin levels also suggests a possible biological basis for the utility of anorexia nervosa as a defense against an underlying depression.

2. On the other side, the malnutrition characteristic of the EDs (including bulimia, where normal weight should not be equated with healthy nutrition) presumably can elicit a depressive state in certain individuals. The pioneering work of Keys et al.[11] clearly indicated the feasibility of this sequence. Conceivably, dietary deficiencies in certain neurotransmitter precursors or metabolic cofactors can lead to affective, cognitive, physiological, and behavioral disturbances that overlap those seen in depression.

3. Finally, not only might depression be a risk factor preceding ED in some patients while being a consequence in others, but in still others it might represent a phase in the chronic affective lability of an underlying borderline personality disorder or grief over the social losses and disruptions commonly elicited by EDs.

Summary

The data suggest that there is *not* an etiological relation between affective disorder and eating disorder. Rather, each, in a sense, can be viewed most meaningfully as a risk factor for the development of the other. Different pathogenetic pathways can thus eventually lead to overlapping clinical presentations, and these pathways should not be interpreted to mean that there exists a common underlying etiology.

References

1. Garfinkel PE, Garner DM. Anorexia Nervosa—A Multidimensional Perspective. New York: Brunner/Mazel, 1982.
2. Pope HG, Hudson JI. New Hope for Binge Eaters. New York: Harper & Row, 1984.
3. Katz JL. Eating disorder and affective disorder: relatives or merely chance acquaintances? Compr Psychiatry 1987;28:220–228.
4. Piran N, Kennedy S, Garfinkel PE, et al. Affective disturbance in eating disorders. J Nerv Ment Dis 1985;173:395–399.
5. Herzog DB. Antidepressant use in eating disorders. Psychosomatics 1986;27(suppl):17–23.
6. Gross HA, Ebert MH, Faden VB, et al. A double-blind controlled trial of lithium carbonate in primary anorexia nervosa. J Clin Psychopharmacol 1981;1:376–381.
7. Walsh BT. Endocrine disturbances in anorexia nervosa and depression. Psychosom Med 1982;44:85–91.

8. Strober M, Katz JL. Depression in the eating disorders: a review and analysis of descriptive, family and biological findings. In Garner DM, Garfinkel PE (eds): Diagnostic Issues in Anorexia Nervosa and Bulimia Nervosa. New York: Brunner/Mazel, 1988;80–111.

9. Keller MB, Herzog DB, Lavori PW, et al. One year course of bulimia and affective disorders. Presented at the Annual Meeting of the American Psychiatric Association, Washington, DC, 1986.

10. Altshuler KZ, Weiner MF. Anorexia nervosa and depression: a dissenting view. Am J Psychiatry 1985;142:328–332.

11. Keys A, Brozek J, Henschel A, et al. The Biology of Human Starvation. Vol. 1. Minneapolis: University of Minnesota Press, 1950.

12. Stern SL, Dixon KN, Nemzer E, et al. Affective disorder in the families of women with normal weight bulimia. Am J Psychiatry 1984;141:1224–1227.

13. Strober M, Salkin B, Burroughs J, et al. A family study of anorexia and depression. Presented at the Annual Meeting of the American Psychiatric Association, Washington, DC, 1986.

14. Agras WS, Dorian B, Kirkley BG, et al. Imipramine in the treatment of bulimia: a double-blind controlled study. Int J Eating Disord 1987;6(1):29–38.

15. Halmi K. Relationship of the eating disorders to depression: biological similarities and differences. Int J Eating Disord 1985;4(4A):667–680.

16. Mullen PE, Linsell CR, Parker D. Influence of sleep disruption and calorie restriction on biological markers for depression. Lancet 1986;2:1051–1055.

17. Biederman, J, Rivinus TM, Herzog DB, et al. Platelet MAO activity in anorexia nervosa patients with and without a major depressive disorder. Am J Psychiatry 1984;141:1244–1247.

18. Biederman J, Rivinus TM, Herzog DB, et al. High frequency of HLA-Bw 16 in patients with anorexia nervosa. Am J Psychiatry 1984;141:1109–1110.

19. Biederman J, Baldessarini RJ, Harmatz JS, et al. Heterogeneity in anorexia nervosa. Biol Psychiatry 1986;21:213–216.

20. Katz JL, Kuperberg A, Pollack CP, et al. Is there a relationship between eating disorder and affective disorder? New evidence from sleep recordings. Am J Psychiatry 1984;141:753–759.

102. Neuroendocrine Findings in Depression, Anorexia Nervosa, and Bulimia

GREGORY M. BROWN, ALLAN S. KAPLAN,
AND SIDNEY H. KENNEDY

Numerous endocrine abnormalities have been reported in depression, anorexia nervosa, and bulimia. Similarities in the abnormalities that have been reported may suggest that underlying mechanisms are interrelated. Moreover, anorexia nervosa and bulimia share a number of clinical features and family history. In this chapter, endocrine changes in depression, anorexia nervosa, and bulimia are discussed and the interrelation of these abnormalities between the illnesses is evaluated.

Hypothalamic-Pituitary-Adrenal Axis

Abnormalities in the hypothalamic-pituitary-adrenal (HPA) axis show the most similarity among depression, anorexia nervosa, and bulimia. It is well established that there is an abnormal 24-h pattern of serum cortisol in depression. Overall secretion of cortisol is increased, and the circadian increase may begin earlier.[1] The half-life and clearance of cortisol are normal in affective disorder; hence the increase in cortisol level is due to hypersecretion from the pituitary. In melancholia, nonsuppression is commonly seen on the dexamethasone suppression test. Although there is variability from center to center, the abnormality persists in about 65% of patients studied.[2] Studies employing corticotropin-releasing factor (CRF) demonstrate that the release of ACTH from the pituitary in response to CRF is blunted in depressed patients.[3] It is of considerable interest that infusions of CRF in normal subjects give rise to a similar constellation of changes, suggesting that the abnormalities in the HPA axis in depressed patients are caused by hypersecretion of CRF. These findings in patients with depression contrast with findings in patients with Cushing's disease. Such patients show augmented ACTH secretion following CRF, indicating that the abnormality in Cushing's disease is localized to the pituitary corticotropin cell.

In anorexia nervosa, findings similar to those in melancholia are reported. On the dexamethasone suppression test a marked resistance to dexamethasone is seen, which occurs in 100% of patients with severe weight loss. These abnormalities recover to a certain extent in patients following weight gain. In response to CRF, underweight patients with anorexia nervosa demonstrate a subnormal adreno-corticotropin hormone (ACTH) response similar to that seen in depressed patients.[3] Hence, as in depressive illness, these endocrine changes in anorexia nervosa appear to be secondary to hypersecretion of CRF.

There is much less literature on bulimia and its endocrine manifestations. One published study has reported a normal 24-h pattern of cortisol in such patients[4]; however, we have found that the overnight secretion of cortisol in both underweight and normal-weight bulimic patients is significantly increased with the extent of abnormality being similar whether the patient is underweight or normal weight.[5] In nine studies in the literature examining dexamethasone suppression in bulimic patients, an abnormal response has been reported in 93 of 206 patients studied for a 45% abnormality. In one study[6] we found that suppressors and nonsuppressors were equally likely to be depressed, and so the abnormality appeared not to be related to depressive features. Walsh and co-workers (unpublished data) have described lower levels of dexamethasone in bulimics than in controls, suggesting that peripheral factors may be implicated in the nonresponsiveness. Gold and co-workers reported a normal ACTH response to CRF stimulation in bulimic patients of normal weight who had shown nonsuppression on the dexamethasone suppression test.[3]

Melancholic depressives, underweight anorexic patients, and bulimic patients all show abnormality of the 24-h secretion of cortisol and in dexamethasone suppression. Studies employing CRF, however, differentiate these groups. Both melancholic depressives and underweight anorexic patients show a subnormal ACTH response to CRF, which suggests that the abnormality is secondary to hypersecretion of CRF from the hypothalamus in these patients. In contrast, bulimic patients show a normal ACTH response to the CRF.

There are three major problems with existing studies on HPA function. One issue is the effects of drugs. Withdrawal from antidepressant drugs can cause nonsuppression following dexamethasone for up to 3 weeks.[7] Many studies of the dexamethasone suppression test employ drug withdrawal periods of less than 3 weeks. A second issue is that of weight change, which itself causes changes. The third issue is that of caloric intake; fasting can produce changes in DST without a change in weight. Fichter et al.[8] found increased 24-h plasma cortisol levels, increased cortisol half-life, and abnormal dexamethasone suppression test in normal subjects after a few days of fasting. This change was found with decreases in body weight from 102% to 96% of ideal. Thus both fasting and weight loss may be accompanied by changes in pituitary-adrenal regulation. These effects have obvious significance for anorexia nervosa, although depression is also frequently accompanied by poor appetite and significant weight loss. Hence some of the changes in adrenal regulation in depressed patients may be related to altered nutritional status. Even in bulimics this factor cannot be excluded.

Hypothalamic-Pituitary-Thyroid Axis

Numerous studies have documented a decrease in the thyroid-stimulating hormone (thyrotropin; TSH) response to TRH in 25–30% of depressed patients.[9] A similar finding has been reported in alcoholic patients and in those with borderline states. This change occurs without any alteration in resting triiodothyronine or thyroxine levels. In contrast, in patients with anorexia nervosa, resting levels of triiodo-thyronine are decreased whereas there is an increase in the inactive reverse form of triiodothyronine. Most studies of anorexia report that the TSH response to TRH is of normal magnitude but may show a delay.[10] Studies of bulimic subjects are contradictory. However, in one study the TSH response to TRH was found to be normal in all subjects.[6] Thus there appear to be differences in these three conditions with blunting of the TSH response in some depressed patients; alterations of triiodothyronine, reverse triiodothyronine, and a delay in the TSH response in anorexic patients; and a low incidence of any abnormality in bulimic patients. Once again it is necessary to introduce a cautionary note. Healthy, fasting, female subjects also display a blunting of the TSH response to TRH.[8] Thus acute changes in nutritional status may influence this test.

Growth Hormone Regulation

Numerous studies have shown abnormalities of growth hormone regulation in patients with affective disorder. The test procedure that has become most widely used for study of growth hormone is the clonidine stimulation test. Blunting of this response is widely reported in depressed patients.[11] As this test is believed to depend on stimulation of the postsynaptic α_2-adrenergic receptor, these test results may indicate abnormalities in these receptors in depressed patients. In one study, Brambilla et al.[12] examined the response in patients with anorexia nervosa. In these patients the response to clonidine was normal. In a second study no difference was found between bulimic patients and control subjects.[6] Again, it is of interest that Fichter and co-workers[8] found in normal subjects during fasting no abnormality in growth hormone responses to clonidine until normal body weight was again obtained.

Hypothalamic-Pituitary-Gonadal Axis

A number of studies show little change in gonadal regulation in depressed patients. A normal response is found of both luteinizing hormone (LH) and follicle-stimulating hormone (FSH) to LH-releasing hormone (LHRH) stimulation in primary unipolar depressed patients,[13] whereas the LH response to LHRH is increased in secondary depressed patients.[13] In patients with anorexia nervosa widespread abnormalities are found with amenorrhea, decreased levels of LH and FSH, and impaired response to clonidine and to LHRH with an increased FSH/LH ratio. No data appear to be available for bulimia.

Pineal Gland

In depressed patients a variety of studies have recorded a decreased nocturnal rise in the pineal hormone melatonin.[14] Studies of melatonin in anorexic patients have reported normal[15] or reduced[16] nocturnal melatonin. In other studies of bulimia we have found no alteration in melatonin.[5]

Conclusion

Because many patients with anorexia nervosa display depressive features, it is instructive to compare the endocrine abnormalities in depression and anorexia nervosa. The marked similarity of the changes in adrenal regulation in these two disorders is noteworthy. Studies in fasting normal subjects demonstrate that weight loss itself can reproduce these changes.[16] Hence the abnormality in some depressives and in most anorexic patients may be related to weight loss. However, it is unlikely that the high incidence of abnormality in depression is solely attributable to weight loss.

It is also noteworthy that bulimic patients appear to differ from either anorexic patients or depressed ones; these subjects have a normal response to CRF despite an abnormality on the dexamethasone suppression test (DST). Furthermore, most studies show no relation between depressive features in bulimics and abnormal dexamethasone suppression. Hence DST nonsuppression in bulimic patients may have a different underlying cause, possibly related to purging of the dexamethasone tablets.

With respect to thyroid, growth hormone, pituitary, gonadal, and pineal regulation, there appear to be clear differences between these three conditions, indicating that effects of depression, anorexia, and bulimia are distinct. Moreover, in each instance where the appropriate studies have been done, fasting mimics the effects of anorexia nervosa. Hence endocrine abnormalities occurring in anorexia nervosa for the most part appear to be related either to the alteration of body weight or to lack of some dietary component. One fact that stands out in this literature is that effects of underfeeding are prominent, so much so that endocrine changes that might be specific to anorexia nervosa are certainly obscured by underfeeding. In both depression and bulimia altered feeding patterns are a confounding factor that requires careful control in any future studies.

References

1. Rubin RT, Poland RE. Pituitary-adrenocortical and pituitary-gonadal function in affective disorder. In Brown GM, Koslow SH, Reichlin S (eds): Neuroendocrinology and Psychiatric Disorder. New York: Raven Press, 1984;151–164.
2. Carroll BJ, Feinberg M, Greden JF, et al. A specific laboratory test for the diagnosis of melancholia. Arch Gen Psychiatry 1981;38:15–22.
3. Gold PW, Loriaux L, Roy A. Response to corticotropin-releasing hormone in the hypercortisolemia of depression and Cushing's disease. N Engl J Med 1986;314:1329–1335.
4. Walsh BT, Roose SP, Katz JL, et al. Hypothalamic-pituitary-adrenal-cortical activity in anorexia nervosa and bulimia. Psychoneuroendocrinology 1987;12:131–140.
5. Kennedy S, Costa D, Parienti V, Brown GM. Melatonin regulation in bulimia. In Hudson JI, Pope HG Jr (eds): Psychobiology of Bulimia. Washington, DC: APA Press, 1987;73–97.
6. Kaplan AS, Garfinkel PE, Warsh JJ, et al. Neuroendocrine responses in bulimia. Adv Biosci 1986;60:241–245.
7. Kraus RP, Hux M, Grof P. Psychotrophic drug withdrawal and the dexamethasone suppression test. Am J Psychiatry 1987;144:82–85.
8. Fichter MM, Pirke KM, Holsboer F. Weight loss causes neuroendocrine disturbances: experimental study in healthy starving subjects. Psychiatry Res 1986;17:61–72.
9. Loosen PT, Prange AJ Jr. Serum thyrotropin response to thyrotropin-releasing hormone in psychiatric patients: a review. Am J Psychiatry 1982;139:405–416.
10. Hudson JI, Hudson MS. Endocrine dysfunction in anorexia nervosa and bulimia: comparison with abnormalities in other psychiatric disorders and disturbances due to metabolic factors. Psychiatr Dev 1984;4:237–272.
11. Siever LJ, Uhde TW, Silberman EK. Growth hormone response to clonidine as a probe of noradrenergic receptor responsiveness in affective disorder patients and controls. Psychiatry Res 1982;6:171.
12. Brambilla F, Lampertica M, Sali M, et al. Clonidine stimulation in anorexia nervosa: growth hormone, cortisol, and beta-endorphin responses. Psychiatry Res 1987;20:19–31.

13. Ettigi PG, Brown GM, Seggie JA. TSH and LH responses in subtypes of depression. Psychosom Med 1979;41:203–208.
14. Beck-Friis J, von Rosen D, Kjellman BF, et al. Melatonin, cortisol and ACTH in patients with major depressive disorder and healthy humans with special reference to the outcome of the dexamethasone suppression test. Psychoneuroendocrinology 1985;10:173–186.
15. Dalery J, Claustrat B, Brun J, et al. Plasma melatonin and cortisol levels in eight patients with anorexia nervosa. Neuroendocr Lett 1985;7:159–164.
16. Birau N, Alexander D, Bertholdt S, et al. Low nocturnal melatonin serum concentration in anorexia nervosa—further evidence for body weight influence. ICRS Med Sci 1984;12:477.

103. Antidepressant Therapies for Treatment of Anorexia Nervosa and Bulimia Nervosa

SIDNEY H. KENNEDY

Several authors have enthusiastically argued that a decrease in binge activity after antidepressants supports claims for a common origin to bulimia and affective disorder. The perils of such an argument are well illustrated in the model of diuretic treatment for congestive heart failure (CHF). Using the above logic, CHF would then be a disorder of renal origin.

Genetic and Family Studies

In addition to common symptoms (see Ch. 101) and some neuroendocrine similarities (see Ch. 102), genetic and family studies have provided what seems to be strong evidence of a link between the two groups of disorders. Findings in family studies can be summarized as follows: (a) In most cases about 50% of bulimic patients have family members with an affective disorder.[1,2] (b) Depression is equally common in relatives of anorexic patients with or without bulimia.[3,4] (c) Families of bulimic patients also have a higher rate of alcoholism.[5] However, (d) relatives of affective disorder patients do not show an increase in eating disorders.[6]

There have been few reported genetic studies in eating disorder patients. Monozygotic twins have a 56% concordance rate for anorexia nervosa compared to 7% for dizygotic twins.[7] Biederman and colleagues[8] have also reported a higher incidence of HLA Bw16 among anorexic patients, a finding previously reported for depression. These data suggest genetic overlap between eating and mood disturbances and raise the question of similar neurobiological mechanisms being involved in the regulation of mood and eating behaviors.

Drug Response

The main purpose of this chapter is to outline current research into the treatment of eating disorders with antidepressant drugs and to examine the rationale for such treatment.

Anorexia Nervosa

Initially open studies of tricyclic antidepressants, e.g., amitriptyline, suggested that superior weight gain and attitude to food could be obtained.[9] However, two subsequent controlled double-blind trials involving clomipramine and amitriptyline showed no advantage during active drug treatment.[10,11] These studies also highlighted the extreme reluctance of many patients with anorexia nervosa to take psychotropic medication.

Bulimia Nervosa

So far, studies involving the use of antidepressants in bulimia nervosa have yielded more encouraging results. Pope and colleagues[12] conducted a 6-week study using 200 mg of imipramine. Eight of the nine patients on active drug had a response, based on binge reduction, compared to none of the ten on placebo. Hughes and associates[13] reported on a 6-week study they did with 22 nondepressed bulimics using variable doses of desipramine. Again the group on active drug had a striking response compared to the placebo group. In two other studies[14,15] neither amitriptyline nor mianserin produced significant benefit.

Walsh and colleagues[16] demonstrated a significant response to phenelzine during a 10-week study of this monoamine oxidase inhibitor. Using isocarboxazid, Kennedy and associates[17] used a 13-week crossover design to treat 22 women with bulimia. A significant reduction in binge eating and vomiting occurred during treatment with isocarboxazid compared to placebo.

Differences in outcome among the various studies may relate to the different methods of patient recruitment, choice and dosage of drug used, the presence or absence of concurrent therapies, or duration of the trials.

Rationale for Drug Response

Animal studies have shown that hunger and satiety mechanisms can be altered by manipulating central monoamines, particularly norepinephrine (NE) and serotonin (5-hydroxytryptamine, 5-HT).[18] Because research into the mechanism of action of antidepressants has mainly involved the NE and 5-HT systems it is not surprising that antidepressants have been tried in patients with eating disorders. As was discussed in Chapter 102, noradrenergic (NE) activity may be altered in patients with affective disorders, eating disorders, and panic disorder, although no predominantly noradrenergic antidepressant has been studied under double-blind conditions in anorexia nervosa. Because 5-HT has an inhibitory effect on eating in animals, cyproheptadine, a 5-HT antagonist, was proposed as a useful agent in promoting eating and weight gain among patients with anorexia nervosa. However, under double-blind conditions, no significant clinical benefit was found.[19]

Disturbances of impulse, affect, and eating in bulimia have been associated with altered 5-HT transmission, as have affective disorder, suicide, and alcoholism. In fact, Wurtman and Wurtman[20] proposed that carbohydrate ingestion after a period of carbohydrate abstinence increases brain uptake of tryptophan, the precursor of 5-HT. Thus binges for the bulimic may represent an attempt to regulate affect through the 5-HT system. Preliminary trials of selective 5-HT uptake inhibitors appear to support this hypothesis. Robinson and associates[21] reported a temporary cessation of binge eating following a single oral dose of fenfluramine. This drug appears to advance satiety and slow the rate of food consumption. Fluoxetine, a similar agent, appears in preliminary studies to have a similar effect in reducing both alcohol consumption and food intake. It is currently being investigated for the treatment of bulimia.

Summary

Overlap between the two groups of disorders occurs at several levels. (a) Genetic and family studies support an association. However, because genetic factors in affective disorder continue to be elusive, caution must be exercised in the interpretation of genetic findings among eating disorder patients. (b) Clinical disturbances of affect, eating, and impulse occur in both groups of disorders and may reflect disturbances in NE and 5-HT mechanisms. However, these findings should not be used to link the two groups of disorders etiologically. (c) At a more empirical level, antidepressant drugs have not been shown to have any specific "antianorexia nervosa" effect, although some patients with bulimia nervosa, even in the absence of current depression, may be helped by antidepressants.

Acknowledgment. Support was provided by Physicians Services Incorporated, Toronto, Canada, and Mr. E. Yakovitch, Upjohn Canada. Chris Garner and Carrol Whynot provided technical assistance.

References

1. Pyle RL, Mitchell JE, Eckert ED. Bulimia: a report of 34 cases. J Clin Psychiatry 1981;42:60–64.
2. Piran N, Kennedy S, Garfinkel PE, et al. Affective disturbances in eating disorders. J Nerv Ment Dis 1985;173:395–400.
3. Hudson JI, Pope HG Jr, Jonas JM, et al. Phenomenological relationship of eating disorders to major affective disorder. Psychiatry Res 1983;9:345–354.
4. Gershon ES, Schreiber JL, Hamovit JR, et al. Clinical findings in patients with anorexia nervosa and affective illness in their relatives. Am J Psychiatry 1984;141:1419–1422.
5. Strober M, Salkin B, Burroughs J, et al. Validity of the bulimia-restricter distinction in anorexia nervosa: parental personality characteristics and family psychiatric morbidity. J Nerv Ment Dis 1982;170:345–351.
6. Strober M, Morrell W, Burroughs J, et al. A controlled family study of anorexia nervosa. J Psychiatr Res 1985;19:239–246.
7. Holland AJ, Hall A, Murray R, et al. Anorexia nervosa: a study of 34 twin pairs and one set of triplets. Br J Psychiatry 1984;145:414–419.
8. Biederman J, Rivinus TM, Herzog DB, et al. High frequency of HLA Bw16 in patients with anorexia nervosa. Am J Psychiatry 1984;141:1109–1110.
9. Needleman HL, Waber D. Amitriptyline therapy in patients with anorexia nervosa. Lancet 1976;134:1303–1304.
10. Lacey JH, Crisp AH. Hunger, food intake and weight: the impact of clomipramine on a refeeding anorexia nervosa population. Postgrad Med J 1980;56:79–85.
11. Biederman J, Herzog DB, Rivinus TM, et al. Amitriptyline in the treatment of anorexia nervosa: a double-blind, placebo-controlled study. J Clin Psychopharmacol 1985;5:10–16.
12. Pope HG Jr, Hudson JI, Jonas JM, et al. Bulimia treated with imipramine: a placebo controlled double blind study. Am J Psychiatry 1983;140:555–558.
13. Hughes PL, Wells LA, Cunningham CJ, et al. Treating bulimia with desipramine. Arch Gen Psychiatry 1986;43:182–186.

14. Mitchell JE, Groat R. A placebo-controlled double-blind trial of amitriptyline and bulimia. J Clin Psychopharmacol 1984;4:186–193.
15. Sabine EJ, Yonace A, Farrington AJ, et al. Bulimia nervosa: a placebo-controlled double-blind therapeutic trial of mianserin. Br J Pharmacol 1983;15:195–202.
16. Walsh BT, Stewart JW, Roose SP, et al. A double-blind trial of phenelzine in bulimia. J Psychiatr Res 1985;19:485–489.
17. Kennedy SH, Piran N, Warsh JJ, et al. A trial of isocarboxazid in the treatment of bulimia. J Clin Psychopharmacol 1988;8:391–396.
18. Coscina DV. Brain amines in hypothalamic obesity. In Vigersky RA (ed): Anorexia Nervosa. New York: Raven Press, 1977;97–107.
19. Goldberg SC, Halmi KA, Eckert ED, et al. Cyproheptadine in anorexia nervosa. Br J Psychiatry 1979;134:67–70.
20. Wurtman RJ, Wurtman JJ. Nutrients, neurotransmitter synthesis, and the control of food intake. Psychiatr Annu 1983:13:854–857.
21. Robinson PH, Checkley SA, Russell GFM. Suppression of eating by fenfluramine in patients with bulimia nervosa. Br J Psychiatry 1985;146:169–176.

104. Psychodynamic Reflections on Anorexia Nervosa

EDITH MITRANY

The purpose of this chapter is to describe the author's clinical experience with 30 cases of anorexia nervosa (AN) treated or supervised over the last 15 years. Table 104.1 indicates the gender distribution of this study, which is consistent with the data provided by other authors, i.e., a strong female dominance (90%). Although the average age of onset of the anorexia nervosa is 14.2 years, some patients presented for treatment years later. In some of the cases, ours was a second or third treatment attempt. Of the 30 patients, one was psychoanalyzed and the others were treated by individual psychotherapy, often coupled with family therapy.

Table 104.2 lists the additional psychiatric diagnoses. It is of interest to determine whether we are confronted in these patients with a coexistent emotional disorder or the additional psychiatric disorder is an interrelated, intertwined, or even causative condition. If the latter is true, we might be moving toward the demystification of anorexia nervosa as a unique, exclusive, independent disorder.

Clinical Vignettes

Clinical vignettes are useful for outlining the psychodynamic features of the anorectic patient.

Case 1. An 18-year-old girl came to therapy after having gone through a 2-year period of unstable weight. At first she had put on 20 kg; then she had lost this weight plus 20 kg more. When first seen by me, she was a tense, anxious, emaciated girl recently drafted into the army. She was obsessed with the need to continue dieting, oblivious of her extreme thinness and rather pleased with her appearance weightwise. Because of severe constipation, or what she described as such, she used large amounts of laxatives. Her regression to early object relation patterns was expressed in her panic at having to leave home, even for a day's work and more so whenever on duty overnight. In order to alleviate this intolerable separation anxiety, she permanently carried with her a large bag filled with a variety of home items, such as food she never ate, books she was not going to read, clothes, etc.

The patient underwent psychoanalysis for 6 years. During this period many

TABLE 104.1. Analysis of data from 30 cases with AN.

Parameter	No. of patients	%
Gender		
Male	3	10
Female	27	90
Hospitalization required	18	60
Pediatric patients	15	50
Psychiatric patients	6	20
Pediatric/psychiatric patients	3	10
Anorexia nervosa + bulimia	4	13

Mean age of onset: 14.2 years
Mean duration of psychotherapy: 1.9 years

changes took place in her life, but the difficulty to separate, to part with her primary objects—those in reality as well as those internalized and fantasized—remained largely unchanged despite her increasing insight with regard to this problem. These introjected objects were often hated and repudiated, which might have been the reason for her almost untreatable self-induced vomiting. Over the years she left her parents' house and built a life of her own on the surface. Underneath, however, she kept closing ranks with the parental objects, both consciously and unconsciously. Repeated suicide attempts, alcohol abuse, occasional shoplifting, and vagrancy were meant to convey the message "I cannot or will not look after myself in a responsible, adult way." On the other hand, a superior academic performance, brilliant achievements in her career, the ability to fall in love and be loved in return, to initiate and maintain friendships, and to feel empathy and concern reflected some of her many strengths. Analysis enabled her to gain insight into her refusal to grow up. This refusal was overdetermined: Growing up meant renouncing early dependency gratification, assuming adult responsibilities for her own person and her own life, and being like mother or even outdoing mother (with all the guilt entailed) or failing to measure up to mother (with all the resentment entailed). Father remained the ideal love object of the early oedipal years. No man in her adult life matched up to this idealized, sexually forbidden object.

TABLE 104.2. Psychiatric diagnoses (DSM-III-R) additional to AN.

Diagnosis	No.	%
Axis I		
Major depressive episode	8	27
Identity disorder	3	10
Oppositional defiant disorder	4	13
Separation anxiety	2	7
No additional diagnosis	2	7
Axis II		
Personality disorder	12	40
Borderline	6	20
Narcissistic	1	3
Compulsive	3	10
Schizotypal	2	7

This patient presented fixations at all levels of psychosexual development. Her narcissistic personality disorder encouraged a need to aggrandize and idealize paralleled by an equally great fear of devaluation by herself and others. Her self-concept was either precariously glorified or diminished, self-abused by her hectic behavior and binging. Basically, she was an addict—at times to alcohol, at times to habits or ideas. The preoccupation with eating and weight was, in a way, an expression of this addiction.

Cases 2–4. Three boys were remarkably similar to each other in terms of their psychodynamic makeup. They were 13–14 years of age at the onset of anorexia. All three exhibited cardinal signs of a major depressive episode: dysphoric mood, loss of interest, loss of pleasure, hypoactivity, loss of energy, guilt or self-reproach, and impaired concentration, which negatively affected a previously high level of scholastic achievment. All three had moderate to severe anxiety related to their short stature and to the way their maleness could become affected by their weight loss. This anxiety made its appearance somewhere along the line after some months in therapy, at a point where the obsession with dieting and losing weight changed from ego-syntonic to ego-alien. This change appeared to be momentous in terms of heralding the improvement in both anorectic symptoms and the underlying depression. Only after becoming conscious of and being able to verbalize the fear of smallness, helplessness, and effemination could they discard the anorectic behavior, which so far had been used for externalizing and masking their fears.

Because of their illness, all three boys lost their libido. Already pubertal before the onset of anorexia, they now stopped masturbating and sexually fantasizing. At the turning point described above, they began expressing fears about whether they would ever regain sexual function.

All three boys also dealt with feelings of guilt with regard to predicaments in their families. They felt as if they carried the family's fate on their shoulders, which in essence is a rather grandiose or righteous feeling and a notion not too far remote from the unconscious wish to displace an ineffectual father who also happened to be an oedipal rival.

Case 5. A young woman in her mid-twenties came to therapy because of a consistent reluctance to commit herself to a stable, permanent relationship with a man. Six years prior to the present treatment this patient went through a period of severe anorexia lasting more than 2 years. Psychoanalytical psychotherapy at that time led to a symptomatic cure. This treatment case provided an opportunity to closely examine the aftermath of "cured" anorexia nervosa. The weight had been satisfactory and stable for some years. The menses were regular. However, certain attitudes disclosed her anorectic past. The patient had no tendency to gain weight, although she rigorously watched her diet. Any indulgence was followed by feelings of guilt. Even the fantasy of eating forbidden foods induced a feeling of "sin." She developed a "gastronomic" morality. At the same time, her sexual behavior was rather loose, but here there were no second thoughts; no feelings of discomfort or guilt were ever evoked. The patient reminisced about her years of starvation with tenderness and intense longing. She seemed to imply that by resuming the eating she had renounced her purity, lost her true virginity—the real promiscuity lay in the eating.

Case 6. An 18-year-old girl came to therapy because of a severe obsessive compulsive disorder. Four years previously, at the age of 14, she had gone through a severe anorectic episode that had lasted in its severe form for about a year. At one time she fasted for 20 successive days and lost more than 50% of her body weight. At present, her weight has been normal for years. Her eating habits were affected mostly by her many and bizarre obsessive rituals that invaded her entire life. As in the previous case, here too one had the opportunity to observe the sequelae of anorexia that had been symptomatically cured. Once again, she could identify the retrospective idealization, the yearning for this "superior" ability, this "strength of character" to starve herself, to renounce bodily pleasure.

Mogul[1] regarded this asceticism, which occasionally reaches grotesque proportions, as an "exaggeration of the creative self-discipline" of the healthy adolescent. Through the active phase of the anorexia, this asceticism is consistently overvalued; and after the symptoms have disappeared the memory of this asceticism vividly persists, a lost gift that one wishes retrieved.

Psychodynamic Considerations

The phenomenology of all 30 patients was strikingly uniform and consistent with the description given by most authors. If there were variations, they were mainly quantitative, such as the presence, absence, or frequency of vomiting, the use of laxatives, the overtness and intensity of aggression and resistance to renounce the anorectic position, the shrewdness of manipulations, etc.

The real differences between these patients lay in the fact that in all of them the anorexia was superimposed on different personality structures, or different psychopathologies. Riesen[2] wrote that "we are confronted with a syndrome which can be embedded in various personality structures with varying psychiatric diagnoses." Sours[3] also mentioned the connection to a variety of psychopathologies.

Many of the patients in this sample showed evidence of fixations to pregenital levels of development as well as ego and drive regressions. Their object relations were often characterized by difficulty in separating from the primary objects. Whenever therapy continued long enough to allow deeper insights, some patients expressed fears of merging with or devouring/being devoured by the object. Consequently, a "safe" distance was being maintained in their present interpersonal involvements, a distance that contrasted and came into blatant conflict with otherwise strong dependency needs. The more precarious the sense of mastery, the more controlling these patients became—unrealistically so with regard to their own body, intolerably so in relation to significant others. Many of them, but particularly those who suffered from depression, conveyed a conscious and identifiable feeling of loss, disenchantment, disappointment in others.

Conclusion

Anorexia nervosa is a syndrome whose most consistent characteristic is the uniformity of its phenomenology and the diversity of its psychodynamics. The severity of the condition, the choice of treatment, its course and eventual outcome, and finally the later sequelae are to a great extent determined by the underlying, intertwined psychopathology of which the anorectic episode is an intrinsic, inseparable aspect.

References

1. Mogul SL. Asceticism in adolescence and anorexia nervosa. Psychoanal Study Child 1980;35:155–175.
2. Riesen S. The psychoanalytic treatment of an adolescent with anorexia nervosa. Psychoanal Study Child 1982;37:433–459.
3. Sours J. The primary anorexia nervosa syndrome. In Noshpitz J (ed): Basic Handbook of Child Psychiatry. Vol. 2. New York: Basic Books, 1979;568–580.

IV.E. SCHIZOAFFECTIVE DISORDER

105. Schizoaffective Psychoses: Six Hypotheses

IAN BROCKINGTON

Psychiatry suffers from a scarcity of classificatory ideas. A small number of portmanteau terms, e.g., "schizophrenia," are used to describe a kaleidoscope of clinical pictures. The term "schizoaffective" has come to prominence and has also fallen prey to semantic confusion. Kasanin introduced the term, although few of his patients would meet modern criteria: He described transient delusional illnesses in susceptible persons reacting to an event, similar to the Scandinavian "reactive psychosis" or the French "bouffée delirante."[1] The modern idea of concurrent schizoaffective psychosis was introduced during the 1970s as part of the drive to bring psychiatric diagnosis under definitional control, the Research Diagnostic Criteria (RDC) definition being particularly useful, especially because of its distinction between manic and depressed schizoaffective patients. Concurrent schizoaffective disorder must be distinguished from sequential schizoaffective disorder, i.e., from a mixture of diagnoses in a series of episodes—a small group studied by Sheldrick and Mendlewicz.[1] This chapter deals mainly with concurrent schizoaffective disorder, considering six hypotheses.

Hypothesis 1: Coincidence of Two Diseases

To say that two diseases are present implies the simultaneous presence of two faults distinct at some fundamental level (e.g., genetic level). The explanation of schizoaffective disorders in terms of a "coincidence" of schizophrenia and affective disorders is contradicted by its observed incidence of 0.3–6.0/100,000 per year, depending on definition. This figure is several orders of magnitude higher than the expected coincidence of the two major psychoses. These calculations assume that the two diseases operate independently. It is possible, however, that they interact, aggravate another, or are mutually precipitating—an idea developed further when considering hypothesis 6 (see below).

Hypothesis 2: All Variants of Schizophrenia

The second hypothesis assumes two diseases, only one of which is present, and proposes that it is always schizophrenia; i.e., schizophrenia can excite "nonspecific" emotional symptoms, but affective disorders cannot provoke schizophrenic symptoms. Evidence showing that schizoaffective psychoses behave like schizo-phrenia on discriminating tests favor this hypothesis, but there is little such evidence. An outcome study carried out by Welner showed that most of his patients ran a chronic course, but the definition admitted a group already chronically ill and was weighted in favor of patients with few affective symptoms.[1] There is also evidence from treatment response, in that schizoaffective disorders respond to neuroleptics; but neuroleptic response is obviously a weak discriminator between schizophrenia and the affective psychoses.

Hypothesis 3: All Variants of Affective Psychosis

Without altering the premise that only one disease is present, it can be argued that all schizoaffective patients are suffering from an affective psychosis; that is, schizophrenic and paranoid symptoms are nonspecific, and dementia praecox is excluded by the presence of an affective syndrome. The case for this hypothesis is strong in schizoaffective mania. There is abundant evidence that this disorder responds to lithium, runs a benign course, and is associated with familial affective disorder. For schizoaffective depression the answer is less clear. Such patients respond to electroconvulsive therapy and lithium prophylaxis,[2] but the outcome is less benign: In our follow-up study of 75 schizoaffective depressed patients, we found them to be heterogeneous in terms of history, clinical picture, and outcome; a large minority followed a malignant course, and only a few ran a bipolar course.

Hypothesis 4: Either Schizophrenia or Affective Psychosis

The next hypothesis also assumes two distinct disease entities but holds that schizoaffective disorder may be an expression of either; i.e., it is a provisional symptomatic diagnosis awaiting an etiological diagnosis. This hypothesis would be supported by finding that schizoaffective patients could be split into two groups, each with the markers of one major psychosis. The best evidence comes from genetic studies, which have shown that both diseases are present in the families of schizoaffective patients, e.g., the study of Baron, who distinguished between "mainly affective" and "mainly schizophrenic" schizoaffectives and found that the former had high family rates for unipolar illness and no schizophrenia, and the latter had some unipolar illness and some schizophrenia, thus splitting the schizoaffective patients into two groups with different patterns of heredity.[1]

Hypothesis 5: A Third Psychosis

The next explanation abandons the "two-entities principle" and postulates a third major psychosis. Much has been written about this idea, especially under the name of "cycloid psychosis." The hypothesis would be supported by the absence of sensitive pathognomonic signs of schizophrenia and affective psychoses in schizoaffective patients, as well as the identification of one or more characteristics (symptoms, therapeutic response, aspects of the course, biological associations, mode of inheritance) that are special to the third disease. Because outcome studies of cycloid psychosis distinguish it from schizophrenia but not from affective psychosis, the best evidence comes from genetic studies, which have found a few families with a strong tendency to schizoaffective illness. In Angst's family study, families were grouped according to the disease pictures present (family pedigrees). There were ten families with schizoaffective psychosis breeding true.[1]

Hypothesis 6: Not Discrete Diseases but Interacting Processes

The hypotheses so far considered have assumed that the diseases were distinct and were not present in the same patient at the same time. This assumption seems improbable when one considers how closely pathological processes are interlocked in somatic disease. Somatic disease finds symptomatic expression through disordered physiology with inevitable overlap of clinical manifestations. In the same way, brain disorders produce disorders of experience and behavior through disruptions of normal psychological processes. The sixth hypothesis abandons the premise of "one disease only" and holds that psychotic disease pictures result from the interaction of an array of morbid processes, some of which are discrete inborn deviations and some deviations from the normal limits of safety on psychological parameters. How many processes are required? At least five are needed: (a) manic depression (a group of biogenic disorders including catatonia, cycloid psychosis, and the puerperal psychoses); (b) reactive emotional states of various kinds; (c) delusion formation (which has many determinants and can be subclassified; (d) verbal hallucinosis and other disturbances of psychic unity; and (e) social defects and handicaps, which are also complex. Such an interaction naturally leads to a continuum or spectrum of clinical pictures in which no natural boundaries or zones of rarity are perceivable, the midzone being occupied by the schizoaffective psychoses.

How can such a hypothesis be investigated and compared with its rivals? It is necessary to direct attention to individual patients and investigate them by methods capable of demonstrating the presence of each disease or process independently. In medicine these complex interactions have gradually been unraveled against a background of clearly understood normal structure and function. In psychiatry we require an understanding of normal psychological functioning and its biological substrate. We also require measurable markers of disease processes. If we can find just one sensitive and specific indicator of the presence of each disease, we can look at its presence in schizoaffective patients and see what disease or diseases these patients have. The discriminating variables—pattern of inheritance, treatment response, course and outcome, and some tentative biological associations—are few and unsatisfactory, and they do not have the specificity and sensitivity required.

Conclusion

We have discussed six hypotheses. Perhaps the balance of the evidence is in favor of two or three distinct diseases causing a similar "mixed" clinical picture through the activation of shared pathways of psychological dysfunction. A rather more complex model has also been offered, involving a skein of pathological processes that are simultaneously activated or mutually aggravating. The riddle of the schizoaffective disorders is derived from the unresolvable problems of the "two-entities principle," which is a gross oversimplification. The affective disorders belong to two main groups, and "schizophrenia" never was, never will be, a unitary disease.

References

The studies referred to in this chapter are listed in ref. 1.
1. Brockington IF, Meltzer HY. The nosology of schizoaffective psychosis. Psychiatric Dev 1983;1:317–338.
2. Maj M. Effectiveness of lithium prophylaxis in schizoaffective psychoses: application of a polydiagnostic approach. Acta Psychiatr Scand 1984;70:228–234.

106. Psychopharmacology of Schizoaffective Mania

TREVOR SILVERSTONE

There is considerable evidence from genetic, clinical, and follow-up studies that many, if not most, of the patients exhibiting the features of the manic or excited form of schizoaffective disorder are probably suffering from a variant of bipolar illness.[1-3] One way of testing this theory is to examine the response of patients with the manic type of schizoaffective disorder (hereafter referred to as schizomania) to a range of drugs that have been found to benefit patients with more typical manic illness and to compare this response to that seen in mania as well as to that seen in patients with an unequivocal diagnosis of schizophrenia. Three classes of drugs are considered here in this context: neuroleptics, lithium, and anticonvulsants.

Neuroleptics

Mania

Although chlorpromazine, with its wide range of pharmacological actions, effectively reduces manic hyperactivity and excitement,[4] its pronounced sedative effect makes patients feel sluggish and lethargic. So, except in the early stages of treatment where such an overall sedative effect may be desirable, haloperidol, a neuroleptic that is less sedating, is preferable.[5] The more selective dopamine (DA) receptor-blocking drug pimozide has been shown to be equally effective.[6]

Schizophrenia

There is no need to reemphasize the value of neuroleptic drugs in the management of acute schizophrenia. No other class of drugs comes even close in terms of efficacy. Although all the available antipsychotic drugs block DA receptors or reduce presynaptic DA control,[7] the relation between their pharmacological actions and clinical response in schizophrenia may be less close than has previously been supposed. The time course of response in relation to the rise in prolactin is much closer in mania[8] than in schizophrenia.[9]

Schizomania

Thus the question to be asked is: How closely does the time course of clinical response match that of the rise in the plasma levels of prolactin? There has been no study that addressed this question directly, although antipsychotic drugs are clearly effective in schizomania.[10] A potentially promising approach would be to evaluate in schizomania some of the new specific D_2 receptor-blocking drugs such as remoxipride or raclopride, which have been shown to be effective in schizophrenia but which may be less so in mania.

Lithium

Mania

Following the seminal observation by Cade in 1949 that lithium alleviated states of manic excitement, lithium came to be widely regarded as the treatment of choice for mania, with some workers going to far as to suggest that lithium is specific for mania.[11] Lithium is superior to placebo[12] and has proved equal to chlorpromazine for the treatment of mildly to moderately manic patients, although the more highly active patients do better on chlorpromazine.[13]

Schizophrenia

With schizophrenia the picture becomes less clear. The difficulty arises when deciding which patients described as "excited" and "highly active" are primarily suffering from schizophrenia and which from an affective disorder with schizophreniform features (see below). In patients who appear to fall into the first category, lithium is less effective than chlorpromazine.[14] However, among patients described as having a "schizophreniform" illness (some of whom might well have been classified by others as schizomanics), lithium did lead to improvement.[15] Although one-third to one-half of patients with schizophrenia benefit from lithium, virtually none makes a full recovery.[16] It looks as if the more typical the schizophrenic illness, the less likely is the response to lithium; the more it resembles affective disorder, the greater is the likelihood of response.

Schizomania

Many patients included in the studies purporting to examine the efficacy of lithium in schizophrenia were in all probability suffering from schizomania. Such patients did reasonably well. In addition, there have been three clinical trials confined to patients fulfilling predetermined diagnostic criteria for schizomania. In the largest trial, among 42 patients categorized as being highly active, chlorpromazine was superior to lithium; for mildly active patients both treatments successfully reduced schizophrenic as well as affective symptoms.[17] This finding is similar to what is seen in mania and supports the view that schizomania is best included in the spectrum of affective disorders.

In a small study involving 19 patients with schizomania, of whom 14 completed at least 7 days of treatment, three of the six treated with lithium improved. In the third study patients were categorized as either "primary affective" or "primary schizophrenic."[18] The addition of lithium to haloperidol conferred a "modest but consistent'' benefit over placebo, with no difference between the two diagnostic groups.

Comment

Lithium is clearly not specific for affective *symptoms;* if it is selective for affective *disorder* remains uncertain. The centrally acting anticholinesterase inhibitor physostigmine temporarily reverses manic symptoms. It is therefore interesting to note that among a group of 11 patients with schizophrenia-related illnesses the four who showed a temporary improvement with physostigmine also showed a good clinical response after 2 weeks of treatment with lithium; two of these patients were labeled schizoaffective.[19] By contrast, none of those who failed to respond to physostigmine improved with lithium.

Carbamazepine

Mania

Following encouraging clinical reports of the efficacy of carbamazepine in the treatment of mania,[20] in a double-blind trial some 70% of the patients receiving carbamazepine improved as did 60% of those receiving chlorpromazine.[21] In another study of 19 manic patients, 12 showed improvement with carbamazepine, with six relapsing when placebo was substituted.[22] The patients responding best to carbamazepine were more manic, had a more rapid frequency of recurrence, had not responded well to lithium, and were less likely to have a positive family history. It was concluded that there may be two populations of manic patients—carbamazepine responders and lithium responders—which possibly reflects two stages of the illness. In a direct comparison lithium was found to be effective in a greater proportion of patients than was carbamazepine.[23] As before, there was a suggestion that there may have been two subgroups: carbamazepine responders were rapid cyclers with marked psychotic features who had previously proved lithium-resistant.

Carbamazepine was found to be equal to chlorpromazine in 15 patients.[24] In a double-blind study we compared carbamazepine to haloperidol.[25] Improvement was seen within a week of starting treatment with either drug, with the haloperidol group improving faster. However, by the end of 4 weeks almost all of the nine patients in the haloperidol group had dropped out largely because of extrapyramidal side effects. By comparison, six of the eight patients on carbamazepine stayed the course and achieved a good clinical response.

Schizophrenia

Uncontrolled reports indicate that carbamazepine is a useful adjunct to antipsychotic drugs in the management of violent behavior in disturbed schizophrenics,[26] and the combination of carbamazepine and haloperidol was found to be slightly superior to a placebo–haloperidol combination in patients categorized as exhibiting features of an "excited psychosis."[27] A direct comparison of carbamazepine and lithium added to chlorpromazine revealed no difference in 30 female patients with bipolar illness, schizoaffective disorder, schizophreniform psychosis, or schizophrenia.[28]

Schizomania

A proportion of the patients included in the category of excited psychosis could probably be classified as schizomanic. On the whole, these patients responded well to the addition of carbamazepine to their antipsychotic medication.

Up to now there have been no reports of controlled clinical trials of carbamazepine in selected groups of patients fulfilling diagnostic criteria for schizomania. In the few uncontrolled studies that have been carried out in "selected affective disorders," one patient improved on carbamazepine alone, whereas in another carbamazepine was thought to have augmented the effect of lithium.[29] Carbamazepine also helped in a case of schizoaffective psychosis with lithium-induced nephrogenic diabetes insipidus[30] and in another patient with a 14-year history of "schizoaffective psychosis."[31] Finally, in 11 lithium-resistant patients, seven of whom fulfilled Research Diagnostic Criteria for bipolar illness and four for schizoaffective disorder (three of whom were considered to be of the mainly schizophrenic type[32]), carbamazepine led to improvement in most of the bipolar patients, whereas only one of the schizoaffective patients showed even a "slight" response.

It is impossible to draw any firm conclusions from such a limited series of uncontrolled observations involving an extremely small number of patients with a variety of conditions. Carefully controlled trials involving patients conforming to strict diagnostic criteria are needed.

Conclusion

To repeat the question set at the beginning: "Can differential response to drugs help us characterize schizomania as either a varient of mania, a varient of schizophrenia, a distinct diagnostic grouping separate from mania and schizophrenia, or an interaction between the two?" The answer must be tentative. Those cases that clinicians have classified as primarily affective, albeit with superadded schizophreniform features, respond to lithium and carbamazepine similarly to typically manic patients. Lithium is less effective in nuclear schizophrenia, suggesting that schizomania that responds to lithium is an illness more toward the manic end of the spectrum. The evidence with regard to carbamazepine is as yet too sparse to provide any telling arguments one way or the other.

Of potential promise in helping to resolve the issue are the noradrenergic α_2-blocking drug clonidine,[33] the calcium channel blocker verapamil,[34] and the benzodiazepine clonazepam,[35] each of which has been found to reduce manic symptoms in bipolar patients. The results of studies of these drugs in schizomania are awaited with interest.

References

1. Procci WR. Schizoaffective psychosis: fact or fiction? Arch Gen Psychiatry 1976;33:1167–1178.
2. Clayton PJ. Schizoaffective disorders. J Nerv Ment Dis 1982;170:646–650.
3. Brockington IF, Meltzer HY. The nosology of schizoaffective psychosis. Psychiatr Dev 1983;4:317–338.
4. Prien RF, Caffey EM, Klett CJ. Comparison of lithium carbonate and chlorpromazine in the treatment of mania. Arch Gen Psychiatry 1973;29:420–425.

5. Rees L, Davies B. A study of the value of haloperidol in the management and treatment of schizophrenic and manic patients. Int J Neuropsychiatry 1965;1:263–265.
6. Cookson J, Silverstone T, Wells B. A double blind comparative trial of pimozide and chlorpromazine in mania: a test of the dopamine hypothesis. Acta Psychiatr Scand 1981;64:381–397.
7. Creese I, Burt DR, Snyder SH. Dopamine receptor binding predicts clinical and pharmacological potencies of antischizophrenic drugs. Science 1976;192:481–483.
8. Cookson JC, Silverstone T, Rees L. Plasma prolactin and growth hormone levels in manic patients treated with pimozide. Br J Psychiatry 1982;140:274–279.
9. Silverstone T, Cookson J, Ball R, et al. The relationship of dopamine receptor blockade to clinical response in schizophrenic patients treated with pimozide or haloperidol. J Psychiatr Res 1984;18:255–268.
10. Brockington IF, Kendell RE, Kellett JM, et al. Trials of lithium, chlorpromazine and amitriptyline in schizoaffective patients. Br J Psychiatry 1978;133:162–168.
11. Gershon S, Yuwiler A. Lithium ion: a specific psychopharmacological approach to the treatment of mania. J Neuropsychiatry 1960;1:229–241.
12. Goodwin FK, Zis AP. Lithium in the treatment of mania: comparisons with neuroleptics. Arch Gen Psychiatry 1979;36:840–844.
13. Prien RF, Caffey EM, Klett CH. Comparison of lithium carbonate and chlorpromazine in the treatment of mania. Arch Gen Psychiatry 1973;26:146–153.
14. Shopsin B, Kim S, Gershon S. A controlled study of lithium -v- chlorpromazine in acute schizophrenics. Br J Psychiatry 1971;119:435–440.
15. Hirschowitz J, Casper R, Garver DL, et al. Lithium response in good prognosis schizophrenia. Am J Psychiatry 1980;137:916–920.
16. Delva NJ, Letemendia FJJ. Lithium treatment in schizophrenia and schizoaffective disorders. Br J Psychiatry 1982;141:387–400.
17. Prien RF, Caffey EM, Klett CJ. A comparison of lithium carbonate and chlorpromazine in the treatment of excited schizoaffectives. Arch Gen Psychiatry 1972;27:182–189.
18. Biederman J, Lerner Y, Belmaker RH. Combination of lithium carbonate and haloperidol in schizoaffective disorder. Arch Gen Psychiatry 1979;36:327–333.
19. Edelstein P, Schulz JR, Hirshowitz J, et al. Physostigmine response and lithium in schizophrenia. Am J Psychiatry 1981;138:1078–1081.
20. Okuma T, Inanaga K, Otsuki S, et al. Comparison of antimanic efficacy of carbamazepine and chlorpromazine: a double blind controlled study. Psychopharmacology 1979;66:211–217.
21. Ballenger JC, Post RM. Carbamazepine in manic depressive illness: a new treatment. Am J Psychiatry 1980;137:782–790.
22. Post RM, Uhde TW, Roy-Byrne PP, et al. Correlates of antimanic response to carbamazepine. Psychiatr Res 1987;21:71–83.
23. Lerer B, Moore N, Meyendorf E, et al. Carbamazepine versus lithium in mania—a double blind study. J Clin Psychiatry 1987;48:89–93.
24. Grossi E, Sacchetti E, Vita A, et al. Carbamazepine -vs- chlorpromazine in mania; a double blind trial. In Emrich HM, Okuma T, Muller AA (eds): Anticonvulsants in Affective Disorders. Amsterdam: Excerpta Medica, 1984.
25. Brown D, Silverstone T, Cookson J. Carbamazepine compared to haloperidol in mania. In preparation.
26. Hakola MPA, Laulumaa VA. Carbamazepine in the treatment of violent schizophrenics. Lancet 1982;1:1358.
27. Klein E, Bental E, Lerer B, et al. Carbamazepine and haloperidol -v- placebo and halperidol in excited psychosis. Arch Gen Psychiatry 1984;41:165–172.
28. Lenzi A, Lazzerini F, Grossi E, et al. Use of carbamazepine in acute psychosis: a controlled study. J Int Med Res 1986;14:78–84.
29. Folks DA, King DL, Dowdy SB, et al. Carbamazepine treatment of selectively affected disordered patients. Am J Psychiatry 1982;139:115–119.
30. Brooks SC, Lessin BE. Treatment of resistant lithium-induced nephrogenic diabetes insipidus in schizoaffective psychosis with carbamazepine. Am J Psychiatry 1983;140:1077–1078.
31. Cegalis JA, Possick SG. Carbamazepine and psychotherapy in the treatment of schizoaffective psychosis. Yale J Biol Med 1985;58:327–336.

32. Elphick M. An open trial of carbamazepine in treatment resistant bipolar and schizoaffective psychosis. Br J Psychiatry 1985;147:198–200.
33. Hardy MC, Legrubier Y, Widlocher D. Efficacy of clonidine in 24 patients with acute mania. Am J Psychiatry 1986;143:1450–1453.
34. Giannini AJ, Houser WL, Loiselle RH, et al. Antimanic effects of verapamil. Am J Psychiatry 1984;141:1602–1603.
35. Victor BS, Link NA, Binder RL, et al. Use of clonazepam in mania and schizoaffective disorders. Am J Psychiatry 1984;141:1111–1112.

107. Neuroendocrinology of Schizoaffective Disorders

J.C. COOKSON

Neuroendocrinology may be used to test hypotheses about the relation of schizoaffective disorder to schizophrenia and to affective illness. This chapter reviews the available evidence. The neuroendocrinology of mania has been reviewed previously.[1]

Cortisol Levels

Basal levels of cortisol are raised throughout the day and night in patients with severe depression and severe mania. In less severe cases of mania only the nocturnal levels are raised.[2] Daytime levels may be less than normal in some milder rapid-cycling cases of mania.[3] One of the factors affecting the increase in cortisol levels in mania is severity, as measured by a clinical rating scale.[2] Acute schizomania diagnosed using Research Diagnostic Criteria (RDC) in acute psychotic patients under relatively drug-free conditions is associated with elevated cortisol levels compared to normal controls and to acute schizophrenics.[4] Thus acute schizomania resembles severe mania rather than schizophrenia; findings in chronic schizomania are not reported.

Dexamethasone Suppression Test

The overnight dexamethasone (1 mg) suppression test (DST) has been used extensively in psychiatric patients in recent years. It is now recognized that manic patients show nonsuppression at least as frequently as any other diagnostic group.[5,6] Psychotic manics are as likely as nonpsychotic manics to show nonsuppression.[7] A review of the world literature concluded that acute or atypical psychoses (which would include schizoaffective disorders) were not clearly distinguished from psychotic affective patients by their rate of nonsuppression in the DST.[8] On the other hand, the DST was relatively effective in distinguishing psychotic affective patients from schizophrenics. By contrast, patients with schizodepression (RDC, mainly schizophrenic type) are less likely to show nonsuppression, and in this regard they resemble nondepressed psychotics.[9,33,34]

Prolactin

Basal levels of prolactin are normal or slightly elevated in mania; during treatment with pimozide or haloperidol, prolactin levels rise in parallel with the improvement in clinical state from the 2nd to the 14th day of treatment.[10,11] A similar time course of prolactin change occurs in schizophrenia, but the clinical improvement is markedly slower.[12] The extent and time course of clinical improvement may be an important distinguishing feature of schizoaffective disorders. Some cases of schizomania appear to improve like typical mania, but others seem to show only partial improvement with haloperidol alone.[13] The time course of change of cortisol levels in such patients would also be worthy of study, as has been done in manics with haloperidol and pimozide.[2,14]

Pituitary–Thyroid Axis

Affectively ill patients are more likely than other diagnostic groups to show blunting of the thyroid-stimulating hormone (TSH) response to the thyrotropin-releasing hormone (TRH).[15] Despite early promise that the TRH test might be useful for distinguishing mania from schizophrenia, there is considerable overlap.[16] A review[17] found that among 50 reports of 1,000 depressed patients 25% showed blunting, and there are four reports all agreeing that blunting occurs in mania; however, there are three reports of normal TSH responses in 41 schizophrenic patients and four reports of blunted responses in 20 of 83. Many factors (other than psychiatric diagnosis), including cortisol level, weight loss, and insomnia, may affect the TRH test. Perhaps because of this nonspecificity, the TRH test has not been reported specifically for schizoaffective disorders.

Growth Hormone

Intravenous injection of the α_2-norepinephrine receptor agonist clonidine tends to produce a release of growth hormone. This response is reportedly blunted in major depression.[18] There are two reports that the response may also be blunted in the manic phase,[19,20] raising the possibility that this test could identify a trait marker for affective illness. The original report described blunting in schizoaffective disorders (ICD-9) as well.[18] Unfortunately, other work has not always replicated the original finding of increased blunting in major depression compared to normal controls.[21] A correlation is found between urinary free cortisol and blunting of the clonidine response in depression.[22]

Growth hormone response to the dopamine receptor agonist apomorphine in mania is either no different from that in other diagnostic groups,[23] or it is lower than in normals and depressives[24,25] or in schizophrenics.[26]

There is a developing consensus that the apomorphine response may be increased in association with nonspecific psychotic symptoms. Thus there is an increase in association with first-rank symptoms of Schneider, irrespective of diagnosis,[27] in association with psychosis ratings across all diagnoses,[23] and with total psychosis score and thought disorder score.[28] Using RDC criteria, schizoaffectives (both mainly affective and mainly schizophrenic) had larger responses than manic patients.[26]

Melatonin

Sensitivity to suppression of nocturnal melatonin levels by bright light is increased in bipolar affective disorder compared to normal controls, and it applies even in the euthymic phase.[29] There are as yet no reports of this possible "trait marker" of bipolar disorder in patients with schizoaffective disorder.

Postpartum Psychosis

The presentation of psychosis during the period shortly after childbirth is dominated by schizomania.[30] It may be of relevance that estrogens—hormones whose levels fall at this time—interact with dopamine receptors so that dopamine systems may be supersensitive during the period after childbirth.[31,32] The interaction of estrogens with separate dopamine pathways that may underlie the symptoms of mania and schizophrenia might explain the occurrence of the mixed schizomanic state at this time.

Conclusions

Basal cortisol levels and responses to dexamethasone tend to identify (a) acute schizomania with severe mania and (b) acute and atypical psychosis with psychotic depression and mania. Schizodepression (RDC, mainly schizophrenic-type) resembles nondepressed psychosis in response to dexamethasone. At present, growth hormone responses to clonidine identify schizoaffectives with manics and major depressives. Growth hormone responses to apomorphine identify schizoaffectives with schizophrenics rather than manics or depressives, apparently reflecting the shared nonspecific psychotic features.

References

1. Cookson JC. The neuroendocrinology of mania. J Affective Disord 1985;8:233–241.
2. Cookson JC, Silverstone T, William S, et al. Plasma cortisol levels in mania; associated clinical ratings and changes during treatment with haloperidol. Br J Psychiatry 1985;146:498–502.
3. Joyce PR, Donald RA, Elder PA. Individual differences in plasma cortisol changes during mania and depression. J Affective Disord, 1987;12:1–5.
4. Christie JE, Whalley LJ, Blackwood DHR, et al. Raised plasma cortisol concentrations a feature of drug-free psychotics and not specific for depression. Br J Psychiatry 1986;148:58–65.
5. Stokes PE, Stoll PM, Koslow SH, et al. Pretreatment DST and hypothalamic-pituitary-adrenocortical findings in depressed patients and comparison groups. Arch Gen Psychiatry 1984;41:257–267.
6. Arana GW, Barreira PJ, Cohen BM, et al. The dexamethasone suppression test in psychotic disorders. Am J Psychiatry 1983;140:1521–1523.
7. Godwin CD. The demaxethasone suppression test in acute mania. J Affective Disord 1984;7:281–286.
8. Arana GW, Baldessarini RJ, Ornsteen M. The dexamethasone suppression test for diagnosis and prognosis in psychiatry. Arch Gen Psychiatry 1985;42:1193–1204.
9. Coccaro EF, Prudic J, Rothpearl A, et al. The dexamethasone suppression test in depressive, non-depressive and schizoaffective psychosis. J Affective Disord 1985;9:107–113.
10. Cookson JC, Silverstone T, Rees LH. Plasma prolactin and growth hormone levels in manic patients treated with pimozide. Br J Psychiatry 1982;140:274–279.

11. Cookson JC, Moult PJA, Wiles D, et al. The relationship between prolactin levels and clinical ratings in manic patients treated with oral and intravenous test doses of haloperidol. Psychol Med 1983;13:279–285.
12. Silverstone T, Cookson JC. Examining the dopamine hypothesis of schizophrenia and of mania using the prolactin response to antipsychotic drugs. Neuropharmacology 1983;22:539–541.
13. Klein E, Bental E, Lerer B, et al. Carbamazepine and haloperidol v. placebo and haloperidol in excited psychoses. Arch Gen Psychiatry 1984;41:165–170.
14. Cookson JC, Silverstone T, Besser GM, et al. Plasma corticosteroids in mania—the effects of pimozide. Neuropharmacology 1980;19:1243–1244.
15. Kirkegaard C, Bjørum N, Cohn D, et al. Thyrotropin-releasing-hormone (TRH) stimulation test in manic-depressive illness. Arch Gen Psychiatry 1978;35:1017–1021.
16. Extein I, Pottash AL, Gold MS, et al. Using the protirelin test to distinguish mania from schizophrenia. Arch Gen Psychiatry 1982;39:77–81.
17. Loosen PT. The TRH-induced TSH response in psychiatric patients: a possible neuroendrocrine marker. Psychoneuroendocrinology 1985;10:237–260.
18. Matussek N, Ackenheil M, Hippius H, et al. Effect of clonidine on growth hormone release in psychiatric patients and controls. Psychiatr Res 1980;2:25–36.
19. Watanabe A, Manone T, Kaneko M, et al. Presented at the 16th International Congress of the International Society of Psychoneuroendocrinology, 1985.
20. Ansseau M, Von Frenckell R, Cerfontaine JL, et al. Neuroendocrine evaluation of catecholaminergic neurotransmission in mania. Psychiatr Res 1987;22:193–206.
21. Horton R, Katona C, Paykel E, et al. Unpublished data.
22. Dolan RJ, Calloway SP. The human growth hormone response to clonidine: relationship to clinical and neuroendocrine profile in depression. Am J Psychiatry 1986;143:772–774.
23. Meltzer HY, Kolakowska T, Fang VS, et al. Growth hormone and prolactin response to apomorphine in schizophrenia and the major affective disorders. Arch Gen Psychiatry 1984;41:512–519.
24. Casper RC, Davis JM, Pandey GN, et al. Neuroendocrine and amine studies in affective illness. Psychoneuroendocrinology 1977;2:105–113.
25. Garver DL, Pandey GN, Dekirmejan H, et al. Growth hormone and catecholamines in affective diseases. Am J Psychiatry 1975;132:1149–1154.
26. Hirschowitz J, Zemlan FP, Hitzemann RJ, et al. Growth hormone response to apomorphine and diagnosis: a comparison of three diagnostic systems. Biol Psychiatry 1986;21:445–454.
27. Whalley LJ, Christie JE, Brown S, et al. Schneider's first-rank symptoms of schizophrenia: an association with increased growth hormone response to apomorphine. Arch Gen Psychiatry 1984;41:1040–1043.
28. Zemlan FP, Hirschowitz J, Garver JL. Relation of clinical symptoms to apomorphine-stimulated growth hormone release in mood-incongruent psychotic patients. Arch Gen Psychiatry 1986;43:1162–1167.
29. Lewy AJ, Nurnberger JI, Wehr TA, et al. Supersensitivity to light: possible trait marker for manic-depressive illness. Am J Psychiatry 1985;142:725–727.
30. Dean C, Kendell RE. The symptomatology of puerperal illness. Br J Psychiatry 1981;139:128–133.
31. Cookson JC. Oestrogens, dopamine and mood. Br J Psychiatry 1981;139:365–366 (letter).
32. Cookson JC. Post-partum mania, dopamine and oestrogens. Lancet 1982;2:672.
33. Maj M. Response to the dexamethasone suppression test in schizoaffective disorder, depressed type. J Affective Disord 1986;11:63–67.
34. Katona CLE, Roth M. The dexamethasone suppression test in schizo-affective depression. J Affective Disord 1985;8:107–112.

108. Prophylaxis of Schizoaffective Disorders

MARIO MAJ

The only drug whose efficacy in preventing recurrences of schizoaffective disorders has been tested in a sufficiently large number of controlled trials is lithium. Only a few studies, in fact, have been carried out with carbamazepine, dipropylacetamide, and fluphenazine. Even for lithium, however, the evidence provided by the available literature is far from conclusive; different authors have found that lithium is as effective in schizoaffective disorders as in bipolar affective disorder,[1,2] or that it is effective but less so than in major affective disorders,[3,4] or that it is scarcely useful.[5] These conflicting results reflect, on the one hand, the intrinsic heterogeneity of schizoaffective disorders and, on the other, the discrepancy among the diagnostic criteria used by the various researchers for the selection of schizoaffective patients. For instance, patients selected by Rosenthal et al.[2] on the basis of Research Diagnostic Criteria (RDC[6]), which require the presence of a "full" manic or depressive syndrome, were surely different from those collected by Perris and Smigan,[5] in whom mood-incongruent delusions were prominent and recovery after the first episode was not complete: it is not surprising therefore that their response to lithium was not the same.

Another approach has been proposed for analyzing conflicting results obtained by researchers using different diagnostic formulations. Labeled "polydiagnostic," it is based on the simultaneous application of different sets of diagnostic criteria to the same research population. The approach has been applied by our group to the question of the efficacy of lithium prophylaxis in schizoaffective patients.[7] At the same time, we have tried to extend to schizoaffective patients the study of clinical, historical, and biological factors associated with response or nonresponse to lithium prophylaxis previously carried out in patients with bipolar and unipolar affective disorders,[8] as well as the search for the minimum plasma lithium levels required for effective prophylaxis already performed in bipolar patients.[9] The results of these studies are summarized in this chapter. More precisely, we try to give an at least provisional answer to the following questions: (a) Is lithium effective as a prophylactic agent in broadly defined schizoaffective disorders? (b) Taking for granted that schizoaffective disorders represent a heterogeneous group of conditions, in *which* schizoaffective patients is lithium effective? (c) Are there any clinical, historical, or biological predictors of response to lithium prophylaxis in schizoaffective patients? (d) What are the minimum plasma lithium levels required for effective prophylaxis in schizoaffective disorders?

Methods and Results

Our starting research population included the 62 patients fulfilling ICD-9 criteria[10] for schizophrenic psychosis, schizoaffective type (the broadest diagnostic criteria for schizoaffective disorders that we could find in the literature) who undertook lithium prophylactic treatment between January 1, 1978 and December 31, 1984 at our Center for Prevention and Treatment of Affective Disorders. All these patients were prescribed lithium carbonate, conventional form. Dosage was adjusted in order to obtain 12-h plasma lithium levels in the range 0.6–1.0 mEq/l. The determination of plasma lithium levels and the assessment of patients' psychopathological state was performed monthly or bimonthly. Forty-eight patients completed a 2-year follow-up period with plasma lithium levels that in not more than one occasion were below the expected range; six patients dropped out (three of them after a relapse), and eight were excluded from the study because their plasma lithium levels were constantly below those expected.

The overall effectiveness of lithium prophylaxis was tested (a) by comparing, in the 48 patients who completed the follow-up, the mean number of morbid episodes and the mean total morbidity (expressed in months) during the lithium treatment period with those during the 2-year period preceding the index episode and the start of lithium prophylaxis; (b) by comparing, in the extended sample of 54 patients (the 48 individuals who completed the follow-up plus the 6 dropouts), the mean number of morbid episodes and the mean total morbidity during the lithium treatment period with those during a period of the same length preceding the index episode and the start of lithium prophylaxis. This second comparison was made in order to avoid getting spurious results as a consequence of the exclusion of dropouts. The mean number of morbid episodes and the mean total morbidity were significantly decreased during lithium treatment, which supports the idea that lithium is effective as a prophylactic agent in broadly defined schizoaffective disorders.

The effectiveness of lithium prophylaxis in the various subgroups of schizoaffective patients was tested (a) by applying the above mentioned "polydiagnostic" approach, i.e., by examining the response to lithium prophylaxis in patients fulfilling different sets of diagnostic criteria for schizoaffective disorders, such as RDC, Kendell's criteria,[11] Welner's criteria,[12] Perris and Smigan's criteria,[5] and the original Kasanin's description of acute schizoaffective psychoses as operationalized by Brockington and Leff[11]; (b) by exploring the response to lithium prophylaxis in patients fulfilling RDC for the various subtypes of schizoaffective disorders, i.e., "mainly affective" versus "mainly schizophrenic" and schizomanic versus schizodepressive.

Within the group of 48 patients meeting ICD-9 criteria and completing the 2-year follow-up, RDC were fulfilled by 33 individuals, Kendell's criteria by 39, Kasanin's criteria by 19, Welner's criteria by 18, and Perris and Smigan's criteria by 14. A significant reduction of the mean number of morbid episodes and mean total morbidity during the lithium treatment period, compared with the 2-year period preceding the index episode and the start of lithium prophylaxis, was observed in the first three subgroups but not in the last two. Because Welner's and

Perris and Smigan's criteria emphasize the "schizophrenic" component of schizoaffective pathology, these results suggest that lithium prophylaxis is relatively ineffective in schizoaffective patients showing prominent "schizophrenic" features. On the other hand, the results confirm that the diagnostic criteria used for patient selection play a crucial role in conditioning the research findings concerning schizoaffective disorders, and that this factor can explain a large part of the disagreement existing in the literature about the response to lithium prophylaxis in these conditions.

Only 24 of the 33 patients fulfilling RDC for schizoaffective disorder could be assigned either to the "mainly affective" or the "mainly schizophrenic" subtype, which confirms that a subpopulation of patients escapes such dichotomy and does not fit a neo-Kraepelinian model of schizoaffective disorders as subtypes of either schizophrenia or major affective disorders. A significant reduction of the mean number of morbid episodes and the mean total morbidity during the lithium treatment period was observed in the 14 "mainly affective" but not in the 10 "mainly schizophrenic" patients, thus confirming the relative inactivity of lithium prophylaxis in schizoaffectives with a strong "schizophrenic" component in their pathology. On the other hand, the mean number of morbid episodes and the mean total morbidity during lithium treatment were found to be significantly decreased in the 14 patients defined cross-sectionally as schizomanic but not in the 19 patients diagnosed as schizodepressive. These findings are in line with the previous[8,13] showing the similarity of schizomanic patients to "pure" bipolars with respect to both outcome and response to drug treatments, in contrast to the clear difference, with respect to the above variables, between schizodepressives and "pure" unipolar depressives.

The possible value of different clinical, historical, and biological variables in predicting response to lithium prophylaxis in schizoaffective patients was explored by classifying the 48 patients fulfilling ICD-9 criteria and completing the 2-year follow-up period as responders ($n = 24$) and nonresponders ($n = 24$) to prophylaxis according to the criteria reported elsewhere.[8] The only historical variable that was significantly associated with a favorable response to lithium prophylaxis was a previous bipolar course of the illness. There was also a nonsignificant trend of patients with a family history of affective disorders to be responders and of patients with a previous evidence of a residual "schizophrenic" symptomatology between the morbid episodes to be nonresponders. Clinical variables (including scores on individual CPRS items during the index episode) and biological indices (including mean plasma lithium levels, mean lithium ratio values, frequency of individual HLA antigens, and in schizodepressive patients response to dexamethasone suppression test) did not discriminate between responders and nonresponders. It seems therefore that the most important information concerning the likelihood of a favorable response to lithium prophylaxis is that provided by the assessment of patients' personal and family psychiatric history.

In order to identify the minimum plasma lithium levels required for effective prophylaxis in schizoaffective disorders, 15 patients fulfilling ICD-9 criteria who had completed the 2-year follow-up were randomly recruited for a further trial. In these patients lithium dosage was adjusted in order to obtain plasma lithium levels in the range 0.45–0.60 mEq/l for 1 year. Then the mean number of morbid episodes and the mean total morbidity during this year were compared with those during the second year during which plasma lithium levels had been maintained in the range 0.60–1.00 mEq/l and with those during the year preceding the index episode and the start of lithium prophylaxis. A significant decrease of both the number of episodes and the total morbidity with respect to the prelithium period was observed during the period of treatment with lithium levels in the range 0.60–1.00 mEq/l but not during that of treatment with levels in the range 0.45–0.60 mEq/l. It may be tentatively concluded therefore that prophylactic treatment with low plasma lithium levels (0.45–0.60 mEq/l), which has been found to be effective in bipolar patients,[9] is not useful in schizoaffectives.

Conclusion

On the basis of the above data, an at least provisional answer can be given to the questions put at the beginning of the chapter. Lithium appears to be effective as a prophylactic agent in broadly defined schizoaffective disorders. However, it seems to be scarcely useful in schizoaffective patients with prominent "schizophrenic" features and to be less effective in patients diagnosed cross-sectionally as schizodepressive than in those defined as schizomanic. Consistently, a previous bipolar course of the illness appears to be the most reliable predictor of a favorable response to prophylaxis, whereas the various aspects of the clinical picture during the index episode do not have any predictive value. Finally, it seems that plasma lithium levels required for effective prophylaxis are those included in the range 0.60–1.00 mEq/l, whereas, contrary to what is observed in bipolar patients, lithium levels in the range 0.45–0.60 mEq/l do not appear to be effective.

References

1. Smulevitch AB, Zavidovskaia GI, Igonin AL, et al. The effectiveness of lithium in affective and schizo-affective psychoses. Br J Psychiatry 1974;125:65–72.
2. Rosenthal NE, Rosenthal LN, Stallone F, et al. Toward the validation of RDC schizoaffective disorder. Arch Gen Psychiatry 1980;37:804–810.
3. Angst, J, Weis P, Grof P, et al. Lithium prophylaxis in recurrent affective disorders. Br J Psychiatry 1970;116:604–613.
4. Prien RF, Caffey EM, Klett CJ. Prophylactic efficacy of lithium carbonate in manic-depressive illness. Arch Gen Psychiatry 1973;28:337–341.
5. Perris C, Smigan L. The use of lithium in the long term morbidity suppressive treatment of cycloid and schizoaffective psychoses. Lecture given at the VII World Congress of Psychiatry, Vienna, 1983.
6. Spitzer RL, Endicott J, Robins E. Research Diagnostic Criteria (RDC) for a Selected Group of Functional Disorders. 2nd Ed. New York: Biometrics Research, 1975.
7. Maj M. Effectiveness of lithium prophylaxis in schizoaffective psychoses: application of a polydiagnostic approach. Acta Psychiatr Scand 1984;70:228–234.
8. Maj M, Arena F, Lovero N, et al. Factors associated with response to lithium prophylaxis in DSM III major depression and bipolar disorder. Pharmacopsychiatry 1985;18:309–313.
9. Maj M, Starace F, Nolfe G, et al. Minimum plasma lithium levels required for effective prophylaxis in DSM III bipolar disorder: a prospective study. Pharmacopsychiatry 1986;19:420–423.
10. World Health Organization. Glossary and Guide to the Classification of Mental Disorders in Accordance with the Ninth Revision of the ICD. Geneva: WHO, 1978.
11. Brockington IF, Leff JP. Schizoaffective psychosis: definitions and incidence. Psychol Med 1979;9:91–99.
12. Welner A, Croughan JL, Robins E. The group of schizoaffective and related psychoses. Arch Gen Psychiatry 1974;31:628–631.
13. Maj M. Clinical course and outcome of schizoaffective disorders: a three-year follow-up study. Acta Psychiatr Scand 1985;72:542–550.

109. Treatment of Depression in Schizophrenia

D.A.W. JOHNSON

A review of the literature[1] concluded that depression in schizophrenia is much more frequent than commonly thought (15–50% over 9–24 months). One study found that patients on maintenance therapy were more than twice as likely to experience depression as an acute schizophrenic relapse,[2] and another showed that the risk of hospital admission from depression equaled that due to an acute psychotic relapse.[3] A survey of stable patients maintained in the community reported that affective symptoms were those most frequently complained of by the patients.[4] Other studies suggested a particularly high risk during the postpsychotic[5,6] period.

It is most unlikely that a single etiology explains all depression, and even individual patients may have different causes on different occasions. It is suggested that this complex problem should be considered under a number of headings.

Personality

The relevance of personality development, life events, preillness behavior patterns, and previous depression needs to be explored. Only Roy et al.[7,8] have explored this problem, and they concluded that depressed schizophrenic patients had a more vulnerable personality and experienced more stress than nondepressed patients: The depressed schizophrenic patients were more likely to be living alone, have suffered an early parental loss, been treated for a previous depression, had previous attempts at self-harm, had more undesirable life events during the previous 6 months, and had more hospital admissions.

Genetic Predisposition

A number of authors have suggested that schizophenic patients with relatives suffering from depressive disorders have an increased risk of depression, but no satisfactory controlled trial has evaluated the hypothesis. Galdi et al.[9] supported a concept of "pharmacogenic depression" that occurs in genetically predisposed patients as one type.

Postpsychotic Depression

There is a consensus that 25–50% of patients experience depression during the 6 months following recovery from an acute episode.[5,8,10] The theories of etiology fall into two principal categories: theories of psychological development and the suggestion that depression occurring at this time is only an apparent phenomenon due to the differential response of symptoms. It is important to note that both theories suggest that the appearance of depression at this time is an index of progress. The issues have been debated extensively.[11,12]

Depression as a Symptom of Schizophrenia

Depressive symptoms may be an integral part of schizophrenia. Research results suggest that their presence may be an early warning of relapse or, alternatively, that an acute episode is responding to treatment. The very frequency of depressive symptoms at all stages of both treated and untreated schizophrenia must also suggest a relation with the illness process. More recent research suggests that depression developing after an interval of more than 12 months following recovery from an acute relapse indicates an illness with a relapsing course and a higher risk of acute relapse within the next 2 years.[13]

Relation with Neuroleptic Drugs

It is possible for drugs to be associated with depressive symptoms is one of two ways.

1. Neuroleptic drugs produce a true depression. There are many reasons for believing that even if neuroleptic drugs can cause depression on occasion it must be a minor cause. Historically, depression was recorded before the use of neuroleptic drugs. Depression has been identified as a prodrome to first schizophrenic illness, before the patient has been introduced to drugs. In drug trials the control group on placebo has experienced an equal amount of depression. However, a number of reports claim an association between neuroleptic drugs and depression, and indicate some dose association. Thus the possibility that occasional depression may be a true pharmacological depression cannot be excluded.

2. A number of authors have identified akinetic depression, which is a drug-induced neurological or psychological syndrome of extrapyramidal origin that is so similar to true depression that either the patient or the therapist can confuse the diagnosis. It responds rapidly to anticholingeric drugs.

Schizoaffective Illness

The possibility of a separate diagnostic category has been suggested. At the present time there is no general agreement on the definition of schizoaffective disorder, nor is there prospective evidence that any one of these definitions has a different natural history or outcome. No specific response has been identified.

Treatment

Because there is no single agreed-on etiology—and certainly no single cause for all depression, even in the same patient—there can be no single treatment. However, guidelines can be given for a practical approach.

1. Overall, about one-third of depressions resolve within a 2-month interval without any change of treatment. The proportion is even higher during the postpsychotic period.
2. The emergence of new depressive symptoms during a period of remission, particularly after an interval of 12 months, must raise the question of a possible relapse.
3. Approximately 10–15% of apparently depressed patients on maintenance neuroleptic medication are suffering from the "akinetic" syndrome, which responds rapidly to anticholinergic medication.
4. Recent life events or stress must be evaluated. It must be remembered that stress can cause depression as a prodrome of acute schizophrenic relapse.
5. Pharmacogenic depression must be considered. Dose reduction or even a change of neuroleptic drug may bring relief.
6. Despite the frequent use of tricyclic antidepressants, there is little research evidence supporting their prescription. These drugs may cause schizophrenic deterioration and should be used cautiously.
7. The value of lithium usage remains unclear, with conflicting trial results,[14] but a therapeutic trial in patients with recurrent depressions is a worthwhile strategy.
8. Electroconvulsive therapy may bring short-term benefit in selected patients but has no proved longer-term benefits.
9. It is important to note that the lowest prevalence of depression in schizophrenic patients is in patients maintained on modest doses of neuroleptic medication. The risks are identical for oral or depot injection administration.

References

1. Johnson DAW. Depressive symptoms in schizophrenia. In Kerr A, Snaith P (eds): Contemporary Issues in Schizophrenia. London: Gaskell, 1986;451–459.
2. Johnson DAW. Studies of depressive symptoms in schizophrenia. Br J Psychiatry 1981;139:89–101.
3. Falloon I, Watt DC, Shepherd M. A comparative controlled trial of pimozide and fluphenazine decanoate in the continuation therapy of schizophrenia. Psychol Med 1978;8:59–70.
4. Cheadle AJ, Freeman HL, Korer J. Chronic schizophrenic patients in the community. Br J Psychiatry 1978;133:211–227.
5. McGlashan TH, Carpenter WT. Postpsychotic depression in schizophrenia. Arch Gen Psychiatry 1976;33:231–239.
6. Knights A, Hirsch SR. Revealed depression and drug treatment for schizophrenia. Arch Gen Psychiatry 1981;38:806–811.
7. Roy A, Thompson R, Kennedy S. Depression in schizophrenia. Br J Psychiatry 1983;142:465–470.
8. Roy A. Suicide in chronic schizophrenia. Br J Psychiatry 1982;141:171–177.
9. Galdi J, Rieder RD, Silber D, et al. Genetic factors in the response to neuroleptics in schizophrenia: a psychopharmacogenetic study. Psychol Med 1981;11:713–728.
10. Mandel MR, Severe JB, Schooler NR, et al. M. Development and production of postpsychotic depression in neuroleptic treated schizophrenics. Arch Gen Psychiatry 1982;39:197–203.
11. Galdi J. Depression "revealed" in schizophrenia. In Kerr A, Snaith P (eds): Contemporary Issues in Schizophrenia. London: Gaskell, 1986;462–267.

12. Hirsch SR. Depression "revealed" in schizophrenia. In Kerr A, Snaith P (eds): Contemporary Issues in Schizophrenia. London: Gaskell, 1986;467–469.
13. Johnson DAW. The significance of depression in the production of relapse in chronic schizophrenia. Br J Psychiatry 1988;152:320–323.
14. Delva NJ, Letemendia FJ. Lithium treatment in schizophrenia and schizoaffective disorder. In Kerr A, Snaith P (eds): Contemporary Issues in Schizophrenia. London: Gaskell, 1986;381–396.

V NEW DIRECTIONS
IN TREATMENT

V.A CLASSIFICATION AND PHARMACOTHERAPY

110. Pharmacotherapy and the Overlap Between Affective and Other Psychiatric Disorders

T.A. BAN, M. JAREMA, F. FERRERO, AND B. PETHO

By the late 1960s it had become evident that "the findings which have accumulated during the new psychopharmacological era strongly suggest that the classical nosological groups are only in part homogenous entities."[1] It was also recognized that replacement of artificial diagnostic concepts by concepts that correspond more closely to naturally occurring mental illness is one of the essential prerequisites of psychiatric progress.

However disappointing it might be, one has to accept that empirically derived diagnoses based on therapeutic responsiveness to antidepressants or lithium salts did not prove of value beyond specific experimental situations. In this respect they are less useful to the clinician than the *DSM-III*, which at least can distinguish a therapeutically more responsive patient population with a major depressive disorder from a therapeutically less responsive patient population with a dysthymic disorder and a therapeutically more responsive patient population with bipolar disorder from a therapeutically less responsive patient population with atypical bipolar disorder.[2] The *DSM-III* can provide sufficiently homogeneous patient populations for establishing the therapeutic efficacy of antidepressants and lithium salts. It falls short, however, in the identification of treatment-responsive diagnostic subforms. The same applies to the ICD-9.

Research Diagnostic Criteria Employed at Vanderbilt University

There are indications that the research diagnostic criteria employed at Vanderbilt University (VRDC) can distinguish between lithium and/or antidepressant responsive and refractory forms (and subforms) of psychiatric illness. With the VRDC the diagnostic concepts that evolved from Falret's[3] "folie circulaire" correspond to Leonhard's[4] diagnostic concepts of "phasic psychoses," "cycloid psychoses," and "nonsystematic schizophrenias." They refer to three distinct groups of mental illness, subsumed by Kraepelin[5] under the unitary concept of manic-depressive insanity, each of which is the result of a different psychopathological process. On the basis of the relative frequency of abnormal forms of experience (during episodes), the VRDC distinguishes between seven bipolar (one within the phasic psychoses, three within the cycloid psychoses, and three within the nonsystematic schizophrenias) and 12 unipolar (within the phasic psychoses) clinical syndromes, as well as between "complete" (pure mania and pure melancholia) and "incomplete" (pure euphorias and pure depressions) forms of illnesses within the phasic-unipolar psychoses. Furthermore, and in keeping with the KDK Budapest,[6] the VRDC distinguishes between reactive[7] and endogenous psychoses within the functional (affective) psychoses.

VRDC and Diagnoses Relevant to Affective Disorders

To obtain an estimate on the relative frequency of occurrence of VRDC diagnoses, a clinical study with 200 patients was designed. In the course of this study each consecutively admitted consenting patient was interviewed one to three times within a 2-week period. All VRDC diagnoses were based on the consensus of two to four psychiatrists; and all VRDC diagnoses were compared to *DSM-III* diagnoses based on the patient's clinical record.

Of the 200 consecutively admitted patients, 98 were men and 102 were women, ranging in age from 15 to 83 years (with a mean of 35 and a median of 33) and in number of previous hospitalizations from 0 to 31. It was noted that 30% of the patients had had no previous hospitalization, whereas 44% had had more than one prior admission.

Of the 200 patients, nine refused to give consent for the interview necessary to derive a VRDC diagnosis, and seven were discharged before a VRDC diagnosis could be made. Therefore analyses of data were based on 184 patients. There were 39 different *DSM-III* diagnoses (including nine affective disorders and four other disorders with an affective syndrome) encountered in the study population of 184 patients. Of the 58 patients with the *DSM-III* diagnosis of affective disorder, 47 were diagnosed as major affective disorders, 6 as atypical affective disorder, and 5 as other specific affective disorders. Within the major and atypical affective disorders, bipolar disorders (26 patients) outnumbered unipolar disorder (24 patients), whereas within the other specific affective disorders (4 patients) dysthymic disorders outnumbered cyclothymic disorders (1 patient).

There were 30 different VRDC diagnoses (including ten affective disorders and four disorders related to affective disorders) encountered in the VRDC population of 184 patients. Of the 55 patients with a VRDC diagnosis of affective disorders, 10 were diagnosed as reactive affective psychoses and 45 as endogenous affective psychoses; and of the 45 endogenous patients, 16 were diagnosed as manic-depressive psychosis, 11 as pure melancholia (9 patients) or mania (2 patients), 14 as pure depressions (self-torturing 9, harried 2, hypochondriacal 1, nonparticipatory 1, and suspicious 1), 1 as enthusiastic euphoria, and 3 as affective psychosis undifferentiated. It was noted that self-torturing depression (9 patients) outnumbered all other subforms of pure depression and was encountered as frequently as pure melancholia (9 patients).

There was an overlap between *DSM-III* and VRDC diagnoses of affective disorders in 37 patients. It was noted, however, that the *DSM-III* concept of affective disorder included patients with VRDC diagnoses of both reactive (3 patients) and endogenous (34 patients) affective disorders. Furthermore, the *DSM-III* diagnostic concept of major depression (17 patients) included patients with VRDC diagnoses of pure melancholia (6 patients), pure depression (7 patients), reactive affective psychosis (3 patients), and affective psychosis undifferentiated (1 patient). Similarly, the *DSM-III* diagnostic concept of dysthymic disorder (3 patients) included patients with pure melancholia (1 patient), harried depression (1 patient), and manic-depressive psychosis (1 patient). On the other hand, the *DSM-III* diagnostic concept of bipolar disorder (13 patients) was restricted to VRDC diagnoses of manic-depressive disorder (10 patients), pure mania (2 patients), and affective psychosis undifferentiated (1 patient).

In 21 (36.2%) of the 58 patients with a *DSM-III* diagnosis of affective disorder, VRDC diagnoses were outside of affective disorders. In approximately 25% of these patients, however, the VRDC diagnoses were bipolar disorders and as such were compatible to some extent with a *DSM-III* diagnosis of affective disorder, e.g., anxiety-happiness psychosis (1 patient), periodic catatonia (1 patient), affect-laden paraphrenia (4 patients).

In 18 (32.7%) of the 55 patients with VRDC diagnosis of affective psychosis, *DSM-III* diagnoses were outside of affective disorders. In all these patients, however, *DSM-III* diagnoses were compatible with VRDC diagnoses of affective disorder, e.g., schizoaffective disorder (2 patients), adjustment disorder with depressed mood (9 patients), adjustment disorder with mixed disturbance of emotions and conduct (4 patients), and bulimia (3 patients).

Conclusions

It remains to be seen if the VRDC could provide a valid nosology. However, because its diagnostic concepts are derived from an analysis of all the developmental stages of psychiatric disease, it is reasonable to assume that these concepts are more likely to correspond with naturally occurring mental illness than the diagnostic concepts of some of the other current widely used classifications. In contradistinction to the *DSM-III*, which is based on the consensus of experts, the VRDC is based on the historical development of diagnostic concepts. Whereas the *DSM-III* dismisses it, the VRDC stresses the distinctiveness of personality development and disease process. Probably the most important difference between the two classifications, however, is that in the *DSM-III* the empirical syndromes are primarily based on the content of abnormal experiences, whereas in the VRDC they are based on the relative frequency of abnormal forms. Because it is on the relative frequency of various abnormal forms of experience that our traditional syndromic classification is based, it is not likely that the clinical syndromes of *DSM-III* represent proper diagnostic categorization.[8] Content, with our present state of knowledge, has its roots in the unique life of the individual and as such never lends itself to nosology, because nosology as a rule represents generalization.[9]

At present, it is only a clinical impression that the VRDC can distinguish between lithium and/or antidepressant responsive and refractory populations within affective disorders. On the other hand, it is an established fact that in our survey the total number of patients in the pooled bipolar population of cycloid psychoses (4 patients) and nonsystematic schizophrenias (14 patients) outnumbered the total number of patients with a VRDC diagnosis of manic-depressive psychosis (16 patients). Because it remains questionable whether patients with cycloid psychoses and especially with nonsystematic schizophrenias respond to lithium salts, whereas there is substantial evidence that they respond to neuroleptics, it is reasonable to assume that in our sample of bipolar patients the therapeutic effects of neuroleptics would be superior to those of lithium salts. It is also reasonable to assume that demonstration of the therapeutic efficacy of lithium salts in our bipolar population would have encountered great difficulties, if it would have been possible at all.

Similarly, it is an established fact that in our survey the total number of patients in the pooled unipolar population of reactive affective psychoses (9 patients) and pure depressions (12 patients) outnumbered the total number of patients with a VRDC diagnosis of pure melancholia (12 patients). Because it remains questionable whether patients with reactive affective psychoses and especially with some of the psychotic forms of pure depression respond to cyclic antidepressants, whereas there is some evidence that they respond to neuroleptics, it is reasonable to assume that in our sample of unipolar patients the therapeutic effects of neuroleptics would be at least equal to those of cyclic antidepressants. It is also reasonable to assume that demonstration of the therapeutic efficacy of cyclic antidepressants in our unipolar population would have encountered great difficulties, if it would have been possible at all.

References

1. Ban TA. Psychopharmacology. Baltimore: Williams & Wilkins, 1969.
2. Stewart JW, McGrath PJ, Liebowitz R, et al. Treatment outcome validation of DSM-III depressive subtypes. Arch Gen Psychiatry 1985;42:1148–1153.
3. Falret JP. De la Folie Circulaire. Paris: Thesis, 1854.
4. Leonhard K. Aufteilung der endogenen Psychosen. Berlin: Akademie-Verlag, 1957.
5. Kraepelin E. Psychiatrie. 5th Ed. Leipzig: Barth, 1896.
6. Petho B, Ban TA, Kelemen A, et al. KDK Budapest: Kutatasi Diagnosztikai Kriteriumok funkcionalis psychosiok korismezesehez. Ideggyogyaszati Szemle 1984;37:102–131.
7. Wimmer A. Psychogene Sindssygdomsformer. Copenhagen: Lunds, 1916.
8. Ban TA. Prolegomenon to the clinical prerequisite: psychopharmacology and the classification of mental disorders. Prog Neuropharmacol Biol Psychiatry 1987;11:527–580.
9. Hoenig J. Jaspers view on schizophrenia. In Howell J (ed): Concepts of Schizophrenia. New York: International Universities Press, 1985.

111. Classification of Affective Disorders and Psychopharmacology: Rosetta Stone or Hypothetical Construct?

HEINZ E. LEHMANN

Depression is perhaps the oldest, and certainly the best described, of all mental disorders. Epidemiologists are convinced that it is an illness that has become more prevalent in recent years.[1] Because it is a severely disabling and often life-threatening disorder, the treatment of depression is a pressing issue for clinical psychiatry today.

The first effective antidepressant therapy, electroconvulsive treatment (ECT), introduced during the late 1930s, made an important impact through the reduction of depression-related suicides and the shortening of depressive and manic episodes. Twenty years later the tricyclic and monoamine oxidase inhibitor (MAOI) antidepressants, as well as lithium, established pharmacotherapy as the first-line treatment of affective disorders. These drugs, associated with less severe side effects than ECT and capable of providing long-term maintenance treatment, brought further improvement to the treatment of affective disorders but were far short of being curative. One of their most important contributions to progress was the fact that their action mechanisms presented challenges and clues that led to the opening of many new doors in the neurosciences and to dramatic developments in our understanding of affective disorders. Indeed, the action mechanisms of the modern antidepressants drugs in some way played the role of a rosetta stone to the deciphering of neurotransmitter and receptor dynamics in neuropsychiatry, although the neuroscientists so far have not been able to discover more than some important pathophysiological pathways of depression, leaving its cause still unknown.

However, little progress has been made during the last three decades in the development of new antidepressant drugs that would meet our clinical expectations of shorter therapeutic time lag, greater specificity, and higher predictability of action, or increased safety and freedom from side effects.[2] The "second generation" of antidepressants has been somewhat of a disappointment.

In the very early days, i.e., toward the end of the 1950, it was thought that there might be external criteria for psychopharmacological categories hidden in the responses of nonhuman biological systems, e.g., plants or animals, to drugs. These earliest searches for an external type of biological marker were unsuccessful.

Nosological differences, however, were reflected to some extent in differential indications for antidepressant therapy: ECT was less effective in depressions associated with much anxiety, and pharmacotherapy had subtly different effects in endogenous and psychogenic (neurotic) depressions. For instance, in an early study trimipramine (Surmontil) produced almost equal ratios of improvement in endogenous and neurotic depressions—even a slightly higher proportion in the neurotic—but more "excellent" results in endogenous and more "good" improvement in neurotic depressive states.[3]

During the 1960s intensive epidemiological, phenomenological, and statistical work on the classification of depressions yielded only modest results. Several independent studies established the existence of a category of depressive disorder that resembled Kraepelin's clinical category of endogenous depression, but no clear grouping of neurotic or psychogenic depression emerged.[4] In this case the relative superiority of ECT and antidepressant drugs in the endogenous depressions confirmed nosological distinction, just as the differential efficacy of tricyclics and phenothiazines had confirmed the distinction between affective and psychotic disorders.

It is possible to construct a table of those depressive disorders that should or should not undergo antidepressant physical or pharmacological treatment (Table 111.1).[5] It is also possible to give reasons why certain depressed patients are refractory to antidepressant treatments that are effective for most other patients.[6]

Controlled studies have shown that an impression on which clinicians had acted for many years, i.e., that operationally defined atypical depressions respond better to MAOIs than to tricyclics, has been justified.[7] Beyond the old clinical classifications of endogenous, neurotic, and atypical depressive or manic episodes, however, neither new nosological distinctions nor biological markers have yet produced solidly relevant connections between the classification of affective disorders and psychopharmacology.

A much promoted search for the hypothetical construct of ideally homogeneous groupings of affective disorders has been going on for years. Whether such groupings—homogeneous by whatever criteria—will prove to be valid is by no means certain. Eventually, the postulated association of specific therapeutic responses associated with such homogeneous groupings of depressed patients may well turn out to have been a false hope, a will-o'-the wisp.

TABLE 111.1. Various depressive states: their diagnosis and indications for antidepressant therapy.[a]

State	Diagnosed as depressive	Requiring antidepressant treatment
Grief reaction	+	−
Masked depression	−	+
Psychiatric misdiagnosis	−	+
Acute depressive crisis	+	−
Stress dysphoria (coping distress)	?	−
Existential malcontent	?	−
Endogenous (biological) depression	+	+
Neurotic/reactive depression		
Acute	+	+
Chronic	+	?
Depressive personality	+	?

[a]Reprinted from ref. 5, with permission.

The status of psychopharmacology in the affective disorders today resembles that of general pharmacology in hypertension and arthritis. Although there are many types of hypertension (e.g., primary and secondary, essential, renovascular, renin-angiotensin, aldosterone) and many antihypertensive drugs (e.g., thiazides, β-blockers, enzyme inhibitors, calcium antagonists), these drugs are rarely chosen because of the differential diagnosis of hypertension; they are chosen most frequently because of the number, intensity, and type of their side effects. A similar situation exists in the treatment of arthritis. Regardless of whether a patient suffers from rheumatoid arthritis, osteoarthritis, or even the gouty form of arthritis, most patients are treated with nonsteroidal antiinflammatory drugs. Again the choice of a particular drug depends mostly on its side effects or pharmacokinetics, e.g., how often it must be taken during the day.

Does it mean that we have already reached the final stage of development in the psychopharmacological treatment of affective disorders and that no further refinement may be expected? Such a question should be formulated differently. For instance: Given the fact that several decades of intensive search for clues to better antidepressant and antimanic treatment by means of changed classification or biological markers have not yielded significant results, considering further that the pharmacological industry has not made any breakthroughs for some time and that the neurosciences have failed to discover the causes of affective disorders, where should we look for future improvements in treatment? Personally, I think it should be in clinical fine-tuning.

Mood disorders are natural human conditions that either have become excessive or have persisted too long; they are not essentially new, ego-alien phenomena such as hallucinations, delusions, or other psychotic manifestations. Because of this difference in the nature of these conditions, it may be assumed that affective disorders originate mainly through a disturbance of centrally existing on–off controls. It means that any search for specific physical factors—including the search for specific drugs—for the treatment of affective disorders might be doomed to failure and that an integrated system of conscious and unconscious, emotional and cognitive, and neuropsychological as well as neurophysiological and metabolic factors might have to be considered in the successful management of any but the simplest depressive or manic state.

Instead of hoping forever for new specific drugs to fit hypothetically homogeneous types of depression, we might do better if we aimed at a match between existing individual depressive and manic conditions and carefully chosen antidepressant and antimanic agents that are already available. Here are some examples: a depressed, professional proofreader who could not afford to suffer blurred vision, treated with desipramine to minimize anticholinergic side effects; a depressed woman with chronic irritable bowel syndrome treated with amitriptyline to maximize anticholinergic side effects; a manic-depressive ballet dancer treated with carbamazepine rather than lithium to avoid excessive weight gain; a patient with neurotic depression treated with trimipramine to permit him to have dreams to be analyzed, as trimipramine is almost unique among antidepressants in not suppressing rapid-eye-movement (REM) sleep; a psychiatrist suffering from "double depression", given methylphenidate twice a day in addition to a tricyclic in order to prevent him from falling asleep during psychotherapeutic sessions with his patients; finally, a married couple, suffering from recurrent depressions who faced marital problems and whose marriage was strengthened by what they considered to be a shared danger of hypertensive crisis, from which they had to protect each other by watching their diets when they both received maintenance treatment with MAOIs.

Psychiatry, by its nature, deals with more idiosyncratic human conditions than other branches of medicine, which are faced with more general and operationalized phenomena. Is it not possible that we have already reached the limits of a match between diagnostic classification and further specification in the psychopharmacology of affective disorders? Should we not perhaps learn to refocus the treatment of these illnesses from the generality of classification to the individuality of personal life situations?

References

1. Robins LN, Helzer JE, Weissman MM et al. Lifetime prevalence of specific psychiatric disorders in three sites. Arch Gen Psychiatry 1984;41:949–958.
2. Lehmann HE. Drugs of the future. In Usdin E, Forrest JS (eds): Psychotherapeutic Drugs. New York: Marcel Dekker, 1976;1469–1487.
3. Scarlatesco A, Jacob W, Kelen L. Trimipramine in general practice. In Lehmann HE, Berthiaume M, Ban TA (eds): Trimipramine, A New Anti-depressant. Montreal: Phoenix Printing, 1964;77–86.
4. Lehmann HE. Classifications of depressive states. J Can Psychiatr Assoc 1977;22(7):381–390.
5. Lehmann HE. The clinician's view of anxiety and depression. J Clin Psychiatry 1983;44(8):3–7.
6. Lehmann HE. Therapy-resistant depressions—a clinical classification. Pharmakopsychiatrie 1974;7(3):156–163.
7. Leibowitz MR, Quitkin, FM; Stewart, JW Phenelzine or imipramine in atypical depression: a preliminary report. Arch Gen Psychiatry 1984;41:669–777.

112. Diagnostic Dimensions of the Newcastle Scales and the Response to Antidepressant Treatments

L. CLEMMESEN, P. ALLERUP, P. BECH, AND THE
DANISH UNIVERSITY ANTIDEPRESSANT GROUP
[DUAG]*

During the last decades when many new antidepressants have been evaluated against such reference drugs as imipramine and amitriptyline, rating scales measuring the severity of depressive states have had much more scientific interest than diagnostic depression scales. Using the psychometric methods of Likert, Guttman, and Rasch, it has previously been found that the Melancholia Scale for Severity of Depression (MES) is a valid outcome rating scale for antidepressants.[1-3] Taking the social tradition in clinical psychopharmacology into account, we have recommended use of the Hamilton Depression Scale with the Melancholic Scale (HDMS), which in combination defines a universe of 23 items for the severity of depression, including the *DSM-III* concept of major depression.[4]

Dimension of the Newcastle Diagnostic Scale for Depression

The two Newcastle scales[5] have been developed by use of discriminant function analysis. Each scale consists of ten items which by the multivariate analysis has obtained differential weights (positive and negative). The sum of the weighted items gives the diagnostic rating score, which theoretically ranges on a bipolar dimension of endogenous versus reactive depression. In the literature there have been many studies examining the score distribution on the bipolar dimension. The original study[6] found a bimodal distribution, but more studies have since found a unimodal distribution.[1]

Although the construct validity of the Newcastle scales has been questioned,[7] few have evaluated this aspect of validity. The predictive validity of the Newcastle scales has been found high in some studies[1,8] but low in others.[9]

*Steering Committee: P. Bech, L.F. Gram (Chairman), P. Kragh-Sørensen, Ole J. Rafaelsen, N. Reisby, and P. Vestergaard.

Diagnostic Melancholia Scale

In a previous study[10] we selected ten items from the universe of diagnostic items defined by the two Newcastle scales (Table 112.1). The theory behind the item selection was that the construct of diagnosis should be independent of the construct of severity.[1] Endogenous depression should not be synonymous with psychotic depression. As can be seen in Table 112.1, five of the items are indicative for endogenous depression and five items are indicative for reactive depression.

The first step in our analysis was to test by Rasch models if the two groups of items were each one-dimensional measures of endogenous and reactive depression, respectively. In the study was included 95 patients rated by the Newcastle Scales before treatment with antidepressants (clomipramine or citalopram) in a controlled trial.[11] The results showed that the five endogenous items constituted one dimension and the five reactive items another.

The next step in our analyses was to evaluate if there was a simple mathematical relation between the two dimensions. The results showed that no such relation exists. Of the 95 patients, 31 scored above the cutoff score of 5 on both dimensions (mixed endogenous and reactive depression); 47 patients scored above 5 on the endogenous dimension but below 5 on the reactive dimension (pure endogenous depression); 13 patients scored above 5 on the reactive dimension but below 5 on the endogenous dimension (pure reactive depression); and 4 patients scored below 5 on both dimensions (uncertain diagnosis).

On both Newcastle scales we found a unimodal distribution. The Diagnostic Melancholia Scale (DMS) results showed that around 30% of the patients had a mixed endogenous and reactive depression. The predictive validity of the DMS was evaluated by measuring outcome to treatment. We have argued[12] that for endogenous depression there should be a clear time-dependent improvement curve when using the HDMS as the outcome measurement. The results showed that monotonously ascending improvement curves were found in 76.6% of the patients with pure endogenous depression, whereas it was the case in only 58.1% with mixed endogenous and reactive depression and in 53.8% of patients with pure reactive depression. This difference was statistically significant. When using the Newcastle scales classification no difference between endogenous and reactive depression was obtained.

TABLE 112.1. Diagnostic melancholia scale.

Dimension	Score
Endogenous	
Quality of depression	0–2
Early awakening	0–2
Weight loss	0–2
Diurnal variation, morning worst	0–2
Persistence of clinical picture	0–2
Reactive	
Psychosocial stressors	0–2
Reactivity of symptoms	0–2
Somatic anxiety	0–2
Duration of current episode	0–2
Character neurosis	0–2

Finally, we demonstrated that there was no covariance between the severity score (HDMS) and the diagnostic score (DMS), whereas a slight positive correlation was found between the severity scores and the Newcastle scores for endogenous depression.

Perspectives

The Newcastle scales should be considered as the most frequently used diagnostic scales for depression. The DMS should be considered a two-dimensional classification system by which it is possible to evaluate psychoprovoked endogenous depression and to make assessments in general practice because the psychotic symptoms have been excluded. Whereas the construct validity of DMS is thus superior to the Newcastle scales, further studies are needed for the evaluation of the predictive validity.

References

1. Bech P. Rating scales for affective disorders: their validity and consistency. Acta Psychiatr Scand [Suppl 295] 1981;64:1–101.
2. Bech P, Haaber A, Joyce CRB. Experiments of clinical observation and judgment in the assessment of depression. Psychol Med 1986;16:873–883.
3. Maier W, Philipp M. Comparative analysis of observer depression scales. Acta Psychiatr Scand 1985;72:239–245.
4. Bech P, Kastrup M, Rafaelsen OJ. Mini-compendium of rating scales for states of anxiety, depression, mania and schizophrenia with corresponding DSM-III syndromes. Acta Psychiatr Scand [Suppl 326] 1986;73:737.
5. Roth M, Gurney C, Mountjoy CQ. The Newcastle rating scales. Acta Psychiatr Scand [Suppl 310] 1983;68:42–54.
6. Carney MWP, Roth M, Garside RF. The diagnosis of depressive syndromes and prediction of ECT response. Br J Psychiatry 1965;111:659–674.
7. Eysenck HJ. The classification of depressive illness. Br J Psychiatry 1970;117:249–250.
8. Zimmerman M, Coryell W, Pjohl B, et al. An American validation study of the Newcastle Diagnostic Scale. Br J Psychiatry 1987;150:526–532.
9. Katschnig H, Nutzinger D, Schanda H. Validating depressive subtypes. In Hippius H (ed): New Results in Depression. Berlin: Springer, 1986.
10. Bech P, Gjerris A, Andersen J, et al. World Health Organization Schedule for Standardized Assessment of Depressive Disorders (WHO/SADD-5). Psychopathology 1984;17:244–252.
11. Danish University Antidepressant Group (DUAG). Citalopram: clinical effect profile in comparison with clomipramine. Psychopharmacology 1986;90:131–138.
12. Bech P, Allerup P, Reisby N, et al. Assessment of symptom change from improvement curves on the Hamilton Depression Scale in trials with antidepressants. Psychopharmacology 1984;84:276–281.

V.B. ANTICONVULSANTS IN AFFECTIVE DISORDER

113. Mode of Action of Anticonvulsants in Affective Illness

ROBERT M. POST AND S.R.B. WEISS

A series of anticonvulsant compounds have emerged with interesting and important profiles of clinical efficacy for the treatment of affective illness. As reviewed elsewhere[1] and in this volume, a substantial body of evidence suggests that carbamazepine, in addition to its anticonvulsive and antinociceptive actions, exerts acute and prophylactic effects in the treatment of bipolar manic-depressive patients. Moreover, efficacy has been reported in many of the patients who are relatively poor responders to lithium carbonate, i.e., those with greater manic severity, dysphoria, rapid cycling, and a negative family history of affective disorders in first-degree relatives.[2] The anticonvulsant valproate, when used in combination with lithium, shows rather greater efficacy in mania than in depression, with useful long-term prophylaxis in previously lithium-nonresponsive patients. We may classify electroconvulsive therapy (ECT) as an anticonvulsant, as it is potent in inhibiting the development and completed kindled seizures in the amygdala-kindling model in animals. ECT is effective for the acute treatment of manic and depressive episodes, although its efficacy in prophylaxis remains to be systematically explored. Clonazepam has acute antimanic effectiveness[3]; its antidepressant and prophylactic effects require further study. Conversely, the anticonvulsant alprazolam, which is primarily used for the treatment of panic anxiety syndromes, appears to exert some antidepressant effects in patients with less severe depressions, although its use in bipolar illness may be relatively contravened because of reports of its inducing manic episodes similar to those seen with more traditional antidepressant modalities such as tricyclic antidepressant and monoamine oxidase inhibitors. Although early reports suggested the antimanic efficacy of phenytoin, systematic controlled clinical trials remain to be conducted.

Comparison with Lithium

In contrast to these agents, lithium carbonate is not a potent anticonvulsant and is ineffective in blocking amygdala and hippocampal seizures. Nonetheless, it may be valuable to consider actions of the anticonvulsants (e.g., carbamazepine) that are shared with lithium when considering possible mechanisms for their efficacy in the treatment of affective illness. These might include an ability to decrease γ-aminobutyric acid (GABA) turnover[4] and inhibit norepinephrine-stimulated adenylate cyclase activity. Conversely, because preliminary data suggest that there may be differential clinical response characteristics among lithium and carbamazepine responders (see above), one might look for differential properties of lithium and carbamazepine, which are apparent in most neurotransmitter and peptide systems studied, that could account for their distinct clinical profiles.

Comparisons Among Anticonvulsants

Another strategy for potentially elucidating important mechanisms of carbamazepine and related anticonvulsants in affective illness would be systematic comparisons of common mechanisms of action of anticonvulsants that are effective in affective illness compared to those without demonstrated efficacy. However, there is a lack of studies involving agents with particular efficacy in petit mal epilepsy such as ethosuximide, which may help delineate whether specific classes of anticonvulsants effective in the treatment of complex partial and generalized seizures are selectively effective in bipolar illness. Moreover, the relative efficacy of carbamazepine, especially in comparison to phenytoin, remains to be adequately delineated. Because both carbamazepine and phenytoin bind at and stabilize type 2 sodium channels labeled by [^{3}H]batrachotoxin-A20-α-benzoate,[5] this common mechanism would remain a candidate for carbamazepine's antimanic as well as anticonvulsant efficacy should the two drugs show profiles of equal clinical efficacy.

Selective case studies suggest that some patients may be preferentially responsive to single agents within the anticonvulsant class. For example, we have observed excellent responses to carbamazepine but not phenytoin or valproic acid in a double-blind, crossover comparison in the same patient. Conversely, we have observed good responses to valproate (in combination with lithium), where carbamazepine was ineffective. Thus the differential ability of antimanic agents to exert clinically useful effects in the treatment of affective illness complicates the search for common mechanisms among the anticonvulsants that might account for this aspect of their clinical profile.

In this regard, different mechanisms appear to be involved in the efficacy of these anticonvulsant drugs. Whereas stabilization of the type 2 sodium channels appears important to the anticonvulsant effects of carbamazepine and phenytoin, this ability is not shared by other anticonvulsants. In addition, clonazepam and diazepam exert their anticonvulsant effects through the classical central-type benzodiazepine receptor. In contrast, carbamazepine appears to be active at the "peripheral-type" (P-type) benzodiazepine receptor, as evidenced by greater binding at the site marked by Ro5-4864 and reversal by Ro5-4864 of the anticonvulsant effects of carbamazepine, but not diazepam, on amygdala-kindled seizures.[6] Carbamazepine also appears to be unique among the anticonvulsants in increasing firing of the noradrenergic locus ceruleus. Noradrenergic mechanisms (α_2-related) appear important to carbamazepine's anticonvulsant efficacy, as yohimbine (an α_2-antagonist) blocks effects of carbamazepine on amygdala kindled seizures (Weiss et al., 1986, unpublished observation).

Time of Onset of Efficacy: Relation to Biochemical Mechanisms

A final comparative analysis of time frames of clinical response may be employed in attempts to distinguish mechanisms related to efficacy in affective illness from those related to anticonvulsant or antinociceptive effects of an agent such as carbamazepine. The anticonvulsant and antinociceptive effects appear to be of rapid onset, often coincident with achieving clinically relevant plasma levels. However, the antimanic effect of carbamazepine, although relatively rapid in onset and comparable to those achieved with neuroleptics, nonetheless appear to require 1–2 weeks before they become maximal. The antidepressant effects of carbamazepine show a greater lag, often requiring 3–4 weeks before improvement is maximal.

According to this analysis as well as previous discussions, the most likely candidates for the acute (immediate-onset) anticonvulsant effects of carbamazepine are those involving type 2 sodium channels, P-type benzodiazepine receptors, noradrenergic α_2 mechanisms, and, potentially, alterations in glutamate efficacy. $GABA_B$-like mechanisms of carbamazepine may be involved in its antinociceptive, but not its anticonvulsant, effects. The relatively acute time course of antimanic efficacy could be related to the mechanisms mentioned above or to effects postulated to be altered in the manic syndrome, which include carbamazepine's ability to: increase acetylcholine in the striatum; decrease cerebrospinal fluid (CSF) homovanillic acid (HVA) clinically and dopamine turnover in animals; decrease CSF norepinephrine in manic patients; inhibit adenylate cyclase activity in response to norepinephrine, dopamine, adenosine, or oubain; decrease GABA turnover; or act as a vasopressin agonist. Effects of carbamazepine that require chronic administration to develop may be better candidates for the antidepressant effect of this drug. These include increased substance P sensitivity, increased adenosine receptor binding, greater effects on GABA turnover, ability to decrease the response to apomorphine, increased plasma tryptophan and urinary free cortisol excretion, and decreases in CSF somatostatin. (See the review by Post[7] for complete references.)

Elucidation of which of these potential mechanisms or others is related to carbamazepine's delayed effects in the treatment of acute depression requires a series of convergent clinical and preclinical investigations. The task is further complicated by the lack of adequate animal models of depression and mania. We had initially hoped that elucidation of the possible anticonvulsant effects of carbamazepine might lead to a systematic exploration of whether these same mechanisms could mediate the therapeutic effects of carbamazepine in affective illness, even though affectively ill patients do not exhibit overt or covert evidence of seizure disorder. However, the time frame analysis suggests that these anticonvulsant mechanisms may actually be less likely to be involved in the clinical efficacy of carbamazepine in affective illness and that one should look for effects that develop only with chronic administration.

In this regard, we have elucidated a seizure model that requires chronic administration of carbamazepine to exhibit efficacy. Chronic, but not acute, administration of carbamazepine is able to block the development of pharmacologically kindled seizures induced by cocaine or lidocaine. Hence this atypical seizure model, which requires chronic carbamazepine administration to show efficacy, may be

534 ROBERT M. POST AND S.R.B. WEISS

more relevant to biochemical and physiological mechanisms involved in carbamazepine's efficacy in affective disorders, which also require time to develop and are not exhibited after acute administration.

Summary

It is clear that, in addition to providing a series of new treatment options for the refractory manic-depressive patient, clinical and experimental use of the anticonvulsants may offer new conceptual leverage in exploring mechanisms that are critical to their clinical efficacy in the affective disorders and, ultimately, in elucidating the possible basic mechanisms that are dysregulated in the affective disorders themselves.

References

1. Post RM, Uhde TW. Clinical approaches to treatment-resistant bipolar illness. In Hales RE, Frances AJ (eds): APA Annual Review. Vol. 6. Washington, DC: APA Press, 1987;121–146.
2. Post RM, Uhde TW, Roy-Byrne PP, et al. Correlates of antimanic response to carbamazepine. Psychiatry Res 1987;21:71–83.
3. Chouinard G. Antimanic effects of clonazepam. Psychosomatics 1985;26:7–12.
4. Bernasconi R. The GABA hypothesis of affective illness: influence of clinically effective antimanic drugs on GABA turnover. In Basic Mechanisms in the Action of Lithium. Amsterdam: Excerpta Medica, 1982;183–192.
5. Willow M, Gonoi T, Catterall WA. Voltage clamp analysis of the inhibitory actions of diphenylhydantoin and carbamazepine on voltage-sensitive sodium channels in neuroblastoma cells. Mol Pharmacol 1985;27:549–558.
6. Weiss SRB, Post RM, Patel J, et al. Differential mediation of the anticonvulsant effects of carbamazepine and diazepam. Life Sci 1985;36:2413–2419.
7. Post RM. Mechanisms of action of carbamazepine and related anticonvulsants in affective illness. In Meltzer H (ed): Psychopharmacology: A Third Generation of Progress. New York: Raven Press, 1987;567–576.

114. Acute and Prophylactic Properties of Carbamazepine in Bipolar Affective Disorders

TERUO OKUMA

Several drugs have been investigated as alternatives to lithium for acute and prophylactic treatment of bipolar disorders. They include anticonvulsants such as carbamazepine, valproate, and acetazolamide, antipsychotics such as zotepine, and benzodiazepines such as clonazepam.

Carbamazepine

In many countries, including Japan, affective disorders are not yet included among the indications for carbamazepine (CBZ). The author therefore planned to perform systematic open and double-blind studies on the therapeutic effect of CBZ on affective, schizoaffective, and schizophrenic disorders in order to establish evidence that will enable these disorders to be included among the indications for this anticonvulsant. The double-blind study is not yet complete, and the results of a multi-institutional open trial is therefore presented here.

Subjects of the study were selected from outpatients and inpatients of 55 psychiatric institutions in Japan. The diagnoses of the patients according to the *DMS-III* criteria were as follows: affective disorders 103, schizophrenic disorders 54, schizoaffective disorders 26. Global improvement rates at the conclusion of CBZ therapy in patients with affective, schizoaffective, and schizophrenic disorders are shown in Table 114.1. The highest proportion of markedly improved cases (40.8%; 42/103) appeared in the affective disorders group. The sum of markedly improved and moderately improved affective disorder cases was 72.8% (75/103). The improvement rates were similar to those of our previous open and double-blind studies performed in Japan[1] and those reported in various countries. For schizoaffective disorder the rate of markedly improved case was lower, but the sum of the markedly improved and moderately improved cases was close to that of the affective disorders. In patients with schizophrenic disorders markedly improved cases comprised only 11.1%, but about one-half of the patients showed a moderate improvement.

Improvement of symptoms during CBZ therapy was evaluated by the Clinical Psychopharmacology Research Group in Japan (CPRG) Rating Scale for Mania

TABLE 114.1. Efficacy of carbamazepine classified by maximum daily dose.

Maximum daily dose (mg)	Affective disorders		Schizoaffective disorder		Schizophrenic disorders	
	Marked improvement	Marked + moderate improvement	Marked improvement	Marked + moderate improvement	Marked improvement	Marked + moderate improvement
100–200	0/2	0/2	0/1	1/1	0/0	0/0
300–400	12/20 (60.0)	18/20 (90.0)	2/9 (22.2)	6/9 (66.7)	2/14 (14.3)	11/14 (78.6)
500–600	22/56 (39.3)	42/56 (75.0)	3/7 (42.9)	4/7 (57.1)	4/28 (14.3)	14/28 (50.0)
800–1800	8/25 (32.0)	15/25 (60.0)	1/9 (11.1)	5/9 (55.6)	0/12 (0)	5/12 (41.7)
Total	42/103 (40.8)	75/103 (72.8)	6/26 (23.1)	16/26 (61.5)	6/54 (11.1)	30/54 (55.6)

Percents are given in parentheses.

and the Brief Psychiatric Rating Scale (BPRS). In manic patients symptom items that were significantly improved were basic mood, psychomotor activity, speech, voice, and sleep; the improved symptom items were common among affective, schizoaffective, and schizophrenic groups.

The mean daily CBZ dose in affective disorders was 594 mg in good responders and 677 mg in poor responders; serum concentrations were 7.0 and 7.1 μg/ml, respectively. These findings support the results of previous studies that good or poor responses to CBZ are not directly related to the dose or serum concentration of CBZ.

Carbamazepine and Lithium

It has been reported in several studies that CBZ may have an antimanic effect in lithium nonresponders. In the present open trial, 35 of 103 patients with affective disorders had been treated with lithium with poor response before the CBZ therapy. The present CBZ therapy was effective in all of the 35 lithium poor responders.

There have been several reports that showed in open trials that antimanic and prophylactic effects of lithium and CBZ are almost equal. Kishimoto and Okuma[2] compared the prophylactic efficacy of the two therapies in 30 bipolar patients who had undergone both CBZ and lithium therapy (separately). The number of manic episodes during the CBZ therapy was 0.8 per year, which was a significantly lower figure than that for the control period (1.7/year); the same figure during lithium therapy was 1.1 per year, which was not sigificantly different from that of the control period. A similar result was obtained in terms of the effect on depressive episodes.

The data from 17 patients with bipolar affective disorders who had received all three therapies—prophylactic lithium, prophylactic CBZ, combined lithium and CBZ—have been collected. Prophylactic efficacies of the three therapies were compared using as an indicator the number of manic or depressive episodes during the control period and the three therapy periods. These 17 patients showed no response or only partial improvement on either lithium or CBZ therapy previously, so combined lithium and CBZ therapy was therefore necessary. With regard to the prophylactic effect on manic episodes, the number of episodes was significantly lower than during the control period for all three therapy periods. Among the three therapies, CBZ therapy was superior to lithium therapy, and the combined therapy was superior to CBZ alone or lithium alone. The effect of the three therapies on depressive episodes was similar to that on manic episodes, but a significant decrease in the number of episodes was found only during the combined therapy.

Shortening of the circadian rhythm has been proposed as one of the pathogenetic factors in affective disorders, and the mechanism of action of lithium has been related to its effect of prolonging the shortened circadian rhythm. Mitsushio et al.[3] studied the effect of chronic administration of CBZ on the free-running circadian rhythm of 12 rats. After the stable free-running rhythm was observed, CBZ was administered through the rat meals for 33 or 52 days. The serum CBZ concentration was about 5 μg/ml. It was found that, althouth CBZ did not alter the free-running circadian rhythm during the administration, withdrawal of CBZ shortened the circadian period by 10–20 min in one-half of the rats, and the readministration of CBZ restored and prolonged the period again in these rats. In the other one-half of the rats, however, the free-running circadian rhythm did not change throughout the time recorded.

Zotepine

As for the alternatives to lithium other than CBZ, a new antipsychotic drug, zotepine, has been reported to have a rapid, potent antimanic effect. Zotepine belongs to the thiepines and has been synthesized in Japan for the treatment of schizoprenia. Among several reports on its antimanic efficacy, Harada and Otsuki[4] investigated the antimanic effect on 16 patients diagnosed as having manic-depressive psychosis or shizoaffective psychosis according to ICD-9 and found that marked improvement was attained in 75%; the sum of marked and moderate responses was 94%. The antimanic effect was higher when zotepine was used in combination with lithium. The onset of the antimanic effect was rapid, and some improvement was observed on the first day of administration in 5 of 16 patients. In 9 of the 16 patients, however, a transient depressive state occurred during the zotepine treatment. To elucidate the mechanism of action of zotepine, its potency in terms of competing for binding sites in the brain associated with dopamine, serotonin, norepinephrine, etc. was measured. Zotepine was found to have the most potent activity to $5HT_1$ (serotonin; 5-hydroxytryptamine) receptor among the test drugs. This finding suggested that the activity of the drug at the $5\text{-}HT_1$ receptor might be associated with its antimanic effect.

Clonazepam

As another alternative to lithium, clonazepam, a benzodiazepine anticonvulsant, has been reported to have antimanic effects. Kishimoto et al.[5] reported a significant antidepressant effect of clonazepam in 40 depressed patients. They reported that the sum of markedly improved and moderately improved cases was 72% in major depression, 70% in bipolar disorder, and 75% in other types of depression following clonazepam 1.0–8.0 mg/day (mean 3.4 mg/day). The onset of the antidepressive effect was rapid, and 86% of the cases with favorable response showed improvement within a week. Kishimoto et al.[5] speculated that the antidepressive efficacy of clonazepam may be related to the suppression of serotonergic function through the γ-aminobutyric acid (GABA) system.

Komada et al.[6] studied the therapeutic and prophylactic effects of clonazepam 1.6–10.0mg/day in ten patients with bipolar disorder and nine with major depression. Though the study is still in a preliminary stage, the sum of markedly improved and moderately improved cases was 37.5% (3/8) for manic episodes and 50% (8/16) for depressive episodes.

References

1. Okuma T, Inanaga K, Otsuki S, et al. Comparison of the efficacy of carbamazepine and chlorpromazine: a double-blind controlled study. Psychopharmacology 1979;66:211–217.
2. Kishimoto A, Okuma T. Antimanic and prophylactic effects of carbamazepine in affective disorders. In Shagass C, Josiassen RC, Bridger W, et al. (eds): Biological Psychiatry 1985. Amsterdam: Elsevier, 1986;883–885.
3. Mitsushio H, Takashima M, Mataga N, et al. Studies on the mechanisms of action of carbamazepine—effects on circadian rhythm and neurotransmitters. Folia Psychiatr Neurol Jpn 1985;39:598–599.
4. Harada T, Otsuki S. Antimanic effect of zotepine. Clin Ther 1986;8:406–414.

5. Kishimoto A, Kunimoto N, Hazama H. An open trial on antidepressive effect of clonazepam in depressed patients. Seishinigaku 1987;29:183–197.
6. Komada A, Kishimoto A, Kamata O, et al. Synergism between lithium and anticonvulsants (carbamazepine, clonazepam) in the prophylaxis of affective disorders. In: Proceedings of the 7th Meeting of the Japanese Society for Lithium Research, Tokyo, 1987.

115. Use of Carbamazepine in Affective Illness

K.D. STOLL, N. GONÇALVES, H.L. KRÖBER, K. DEMISCH, AND W. BELLAIRE

Since 1971 the attention of Japanese investigators[1] has been focused on the tricyclic anticonvulsant carbamazepine (CBZ; Tegretol) as an alternative treatment for acute mania. In addition, a confirming study[2] gave the first evidence of both antidepressant properties and prophylactic effects in manic-depressive illness. The results of these open studies have been validated by a series of controlled trials since 1979 in which CBZ has been shown to be effective in the treatment of acute mania when compared to chlorpromazine[3-5] or placebo[6] and in the treatment of depression when compared to placebo,[6] imipramine,[5] or trimipramine.[7] In controlled trials investigating prophylactic effects, CBZ was superior to placebo[8] or comparable with the efficacy of lithium.[9,10] In the overwhelming number of open studies and case reports in the literature, high CBZ response rates could be observed, but there were also treatment failures. In one study[11] the antimanic effect was better in patients randomly allocated to lithium treatment than in those receiving CBZ (600 mg/day). However, the CBZ group had initially somewhat lower mania scores and significantly higher Brief Psychiatric Rating Scale (BPRS) total scores. Nevertheless, the two patients with the best therapeutic results were treated with CBZ.

Our combined efforts have been directed at clinical trials investigating the effect of CBZ in acute mania as well as for prophylactic treatment. In this chapter we summarize the results of our studies with CBZ in acute mania and give the first report of our multicenter study comparing the prophylactic effect of CBZ and lithium in patients with recurrent affective disorders.

Manic Syndromes

Using *DSM-III*, Research Diagnostic Criteris (RDC), and ICD-9 criteria, inpatients with acute mania (ICD 9: 296.0, 296.2) or schizoaffective episodes (ICD-9: 295.7) were included in our trials and initially treated with 600 mg CBZ (Tegretol 200 t.i.d.) or 800 mg (Tegretol 400 Retard b.i.d.). The daily dosages could be increased stepwise up to 1,200 mg. Neuroleptics could be added if necessary. However, additional drug therapy had to be documented. There were repeated assessments using the Beigel-Murphy scale (also called MS-M).[12] Duration of treatment was 3 weeks.

The first German study,[13] an open one, showed that monotherapy is possible with daily doses up to 1,200 mg CBZ from the third or fourth day on (six patients). Our placebo-controlled study in 12 patients[14] revealed a rapid onset of action, significantly lower MS-M scores ($p < 0.01$, ANCOVA), and significantly less neuroleptic rescue medication ($p < 0.05$, U-test) for the six patients randomly allocated to treatment with CBZ compared to the six placebo cases. A multicenter trial[15] comparing the effect of CBZ and haloperidol (15–30 mg/day) in 58 patients showed both therapies to be equivalent in efficacy (MS-M and global assessment). In the subgroup of schizoaffective patients ($n = 23$), success of treatment was somewhat better with haloperidol (median values of global ratings distributions). Nevertheless, most of the data favor the basic treatment of manic syndromes with CBZ:

1. Significantly ($p < 0.05$, U-test) better therapeutic results in acute mania
2. Better tolerability in terms of global assessment as well as lower frequency, minor severity, shorter duration, and less impairing types of unwanted effects

An open study[16] with a controlled release form of CBZ (Tegretol 400 Retard, on the German market since 1985) in a twice-a-day regimen gives evidence of improved tolerability and therapeutic efficacy comparable to that of conventional CBZ in a three-times-a-day regimen (n = 26 in total, 11 of them assessed using the MS-M).

Prophylaxis of Recurrent Affective Disorders

According to *DMS-III*, RDC, and ICD-9 criteria, and a formal trial plan, 12 centers included a total of 125 patients (Table 115.1) for 1 year of prophylaxis with CBZ given in increasing doses or lithium (salt of free choice) by random allocation. Monthly visits were requested for evaluation, documentation of unwanted effects,

TABLE 115.1. Samples of the prophylaxis study of CBZ versus lithium.

Parameter	CBZ group	Lithium group
Total no. of patients included	65	60
No. of patients <1 year in study (see text)	19	8
No. in prophylaxis 1 year	46	52
No. of men	20 (43%)	18 (35%)
Age (years; mean±SD)	46±15	44±11
Diagnosis		
Bipolar disorder	20	25
Subtype mania		3
Major depression, recurrent	18	15
Schizoaffective disorder	8	9
Duration of illness (years; mean±SD)	8.4±7.4	10.5±8.3
No. of episodes/year (mean±SD)	1.5±1.8	1.1±0.9
No. of episodes last year (mean±SD)	1.76±1.06	1.69±1.02

TABLE 115.2. Results of the prophylaxis study of CBZ versus lithium.

Parameter	CBZ group ($n = 46$)	Lithium group ($n = 52$)
No. of episodes during trial (mean±SD)	0.67±0.54	0.73±0.9
Patients with one episode last year	0.44	0.43
Patients with more episodes last year	0.92	1.07
No. of patients without episodes during trial	22 (48%)	28 (54%
No. with fewer episodes than in previous year	33 (72%)	35 (67%
No. with fewer depressive episodes (35 vs. 34 pts.)	19 (54%)	16 (47%
No. with fewer manic episodes (13 vs. 18 pts.)	11 (85%)	14 (78%
No. with fewer schizoaffective episodes (6 vs. 5 pts.)	4 (67%)	3 (60%
No. with fewer days of illness (34 vs. 33 pts.)	32 (94%)	26 (78%
No. taking antidepressants intermittently during trial	28 (61%)	18 (35%
No. taking neuroleptics intermittently during trial	9 (20%)	15 (29%
Good or very good treatment success (all patients)	41 (89%)	45 (86%)
Bipolar disorder (without subtype mania)	15 (75%)	21 (84%)
Major depression (recurrent)	18 (100%)	12 (80%)
Schizoaffective disorder	8 (100%)	9 (100%
Good or very good tolerability	44 (96%)	45 (86%)
Most frequent side effects	Tiredness (7%)	Tremor (5%)
	Nausea (3%)	Weight gain (3%)
	Others (5%)	Others (11%)
Presence of side effects (predominantly by tendency)	Initially, transient	Lasting

and determination of laboratory values (thrombocytes, leukocytes, transaminases, and drug serum levels).

In each treatment group there were one or two dropouts for the following reasons: unwanted effects, treatment failures, no cooperation, and other non-drug-related causes (e.g., distance to clinic). Two patients in the lithium group and 11 in the CBZ group failed to return for a visit. There is evidence that the package leaflet not mentioning affective illness as an indication for CBZ provoked dropping out.

The main characteristics of the patients and the most important results are displayed in Tables 115.1 and 115.2. Neither global comparisons nor stratifications show marked differences between the two groups, which were comparable with regard to sex, age, history, and severity of illness. The imbalance in the distribution of diagnoses can be adjusted by stratification.

Repeated serum level determinations (carried out in all patients treated with lithium and in the CBZ group, except for five CBZ cases) demonstrated that effective ranges were reached. There was only one patient with lithium levels lower than 0.5 mval/l; all other cases had higher minimum values; the maximum was 1.33 mval/l. In seven patients of the CBZ group, the minimum concentrations were below 4 mg/l. All maximums were over this limit and reached values between 8.0 and 12.5 mg/l in 72% of the cases with determinations; the highest value observed was 12.5 mg/l.

In principal, the prophylactic effects of CBZ and lithium were comparable, but it is obvious that CBZ seemed to be more effective than lithium in patients with a higher frequency of episodes during the year prior to the study (Table 115.2).

Discussion

The results of our studies of acute mania revealed the efficacy of CBZ. The results concerning tolerability are in good concordance with most of the studies mentioned above.

The prophylactic study with 98 patients is, so far as we know, the most extensive comparison between CBZ and lithium. The results are comparable to those of another 1-year study with 29 patients[9] and those of a prophylactic study with 83 patients treated for more than 2 years with a mean duration of about 5 years[10] with either CBZ or lithium.

This picture may be completed by the results of the small-scale study[8] showing the superiority of CBZ to placebo and by data from a series of nine placebo-controlled lithium studies with a total of 659 patients.[17] This reevaluation showed that lithium is superior to placebo to comparable degree.

It may be important that there was a tendency in our study favoring CBZ in patients with a higher frequency of relapses. In general, however, lithium and CBZ may have comparable success rates. Additionally, CBZ seems to have better long-term tolerability.

References

1. Takezaki H, Hanaoka M. The use of carbamazepine in the control of manic-depressive states. Clin Psychiatry (Tokyo) 1971;13:173–183.
2. Okuma T, Kishimoto A, Inoue K, et al. Anti-manic and prophylactic effects of carbamazepine (Tegretol) on manic-depressive psychosis: a preliminary report. Folia Psychiatr Neurol Jpn 1973;27:283–297.
3. Okuma T, Inanaga K, Otsuki S, et al. Comparison of the antimanic efficacy of carbamazepine and chlorpromazine: a double-blind controlled study. Psychopharmacology 1979;66:211–217.
4. Grossi E, Sacchetti E, Vita A, et al. Carbamazepine vs chlorpromazine in mania: a double blind trial. In Emrich HM, Okuma T, Müller AA (eds): Anticonvulsants in Affective Disorders. Amsterdam: Excerpta Medica, 1984;177–187.
5. Sethi BB, Tiwari SC. Carbamazepine in affective disorders. In Emrich HM, Okuma T, Müller AA (eds): Anticonvulsants in Affective Disorders. Amsterdam: Excerpta Medica, 1984;167–176.
6. Ballenger J, Post RM. Therapeutic effects of carbamazepine in affective illness: a preliminary report. Commun Psychopharmacol 1978;2:159–175.
7. Neumann J, Seidel K, Wunderlich HP. Comparative studies of the effect of carbamazepine and trimipramine in depression. In Emrich HM, Okuma T, Müller AA (eds): Anticonvulsants in Affective Disorders. Amsterdam: Excerpta Medica, 1984;160–166.
8. Okuma T, Inanaga K, Otsuki S, et al. A preliminary double-blind study on the efficacy of carbamazepine in prophylaxis of manic-depressive illness. Psychopharmacology 1981;73:95–96.
9. Placidi GF, Lenzi A, Rampello E, et al. Long-term double-blind prospective study on carbamazepine versus lithium in bipolar and schizoaffective disorders: preliminary results. In Emrich HM, Okuma T, Müller AA (eds): Anticonvulsants in Affective Disorders. Amsterdam: Excerpta Medica, 1984;188–197.
10. Kishimoto A. A clinical comparative study of lithium and carbamazepine. Clin Pharmacol Ther 1984;35:251.
11. Moore N, Lerer B, Meyendorff E, et al. Carbamazepine in the acute treatment of mania. In Shagass C, Josiassen RC, Bridger WH, et al (eds): Biological Psychiatry 1985. New York: Elsevier, 1986;726–731.
12. Murphy DL, Beigel A, Weingartner H, et al. The quantitation of manic behavior. Mod Probl Pharmacopsychiatry 1974;7:203–220.

13. Eckmann F. Carbamazepin in Prophylaxe und Therapie affectiver Psychosen. Med Welt 1983;34:984–986.
14. Gonçalves N, Stoll KD. Carbamazepin bei menischen Syndromen. Nervenarzt 1985; 56:43–47,
15. Stoll KD, Bisson HE, Fischer E, et al. Carbamazepine versus haloperidol in manic syndromes: first report of a multicenter study. In Shagass C, Josiassen RC, Bridger WH et al (eds): Biological Psychiatry. New York: Elsevier, 1985;332–334.
16. Kröber HL. Klinische Erfahrung in der Behandlung manischer Syndrome mit einem Carbamazepin-Retardpräparat. Psycho 1987;13:282–290.
17. Greil W, van Calker D. Lithium: Grundlagen und Therapie. In Langer C, Heimann H (eds): Psychopharmaka. New York: Springer, 1983.

116. Action of Carbamazepine Suspension in Acute Manic Syndromes

M. Dose, M. Weber, D. Bremer, C. Raptis, and H.M. Emrich

Although acute antimanic effects of the anticonvulsant iminobenzylderivative carbamazepine have been described in open[1] and controlled[2-4] studies, its use in clinical practice for the treatment of acute manic syndromes still appears to be limited compared to neuroleptics. This limitation is possibly due to the weak sedative properties of carbamazepine and to the fact that it usually is started at low doses and prescribed with small increments. In patients with manic excitement needing an effective and rapid treatment, carbamazepine therefore may appear inadequate, and neuroleptics are regarded as the medication of choice. These compounds, however, have extrapyramidal and motor activity inhibiting side effects, which are especially unpleasant for manic patients; moreover, the possibility of later development of tardive dyskinesia remains a particular problem. Because of this situation, the aim of the present study was to investigate if carbamazepine, formulated as a suspension, can by its pharmacokinetic advantages overcome some of the shortcomings that impede effective acute antimanic treatment with non-suspension carbamazepine in clinical practice.

Methods

Ten patients manifesting a manic syndrome during the course of a bipolar affective or schizoaffective psychosis that had not been treated pharmacologically prior to admission participated in the study after having given informed consent (for details see Table 116.1). Laboratory tests (including carbamazepine serum levels), electrocardiography (ECG), and electroencepholography (EEG) were done before and after the study period of 5 days. Psychopathological examinations were performed daily by a trained psychiatrist using a specific rating scale for manic symptoms (MS-M).[5] Statistical analysis of the MS-M ratings was performed using the Wilcoxon test (two-tailed). Starting with 10–20 ml of carbamazepine suspension (200–400 mg) at the first day of the study, all patients received carbamazepine suspension 30–40 ml/day (600–800 mg) throughout the study. Two patients who had relapsed into a manic episode under lithium prophylaxis continued to take their lithium medication (900 mg lithium carbonate/day). Only lorazepam was additionally allowed as sleep medication.

TABLE 116.1. Data on patients in the study.

Patient N.	Sex	Age (years)	ICD diagnosis	Psychotic features	Additional night medication with lorazepam (mg/day)
1	F	19	295.7	Yes	2.0
2	F	30	295.7	Yes	1.0
3	M	21	295.7	Yes	1.75
4	F	25	295.7	No	—
5	F	48	296.2	No	—
6	M	62	295.7	Yes	0.5
7	M	44	295.7	No	2.0
8	F	24	296.2	No	0.9
9	F	20	296.2	No	0.5
10	M	49	295.7	Yes	—

Results

The trials could be completed in all ten patients included in the study. Although the dosage of carbamazepine was already as high as 600–800 mg/day at the second day of treatment, there were no dropouts due to unwanted side effects or adverse reactions. Transiently blurred vision occurred in one patient for several hours on the second day of treatment with an 800 mg/day dose of carbamazepine and disappeared without any intervention. Blood cell count, liver enzymes, and the other parameters as well as ECG and EEG findings remained normal in all patients before and after the study period. Carbamazepine serum levels of 8.4 ± 0.3 µg/ml (mean ± SEM) were measured 12 h after the first dose of carbamazepine suspension, 12.7 ± 1.0 µg/ml on the third day, and 9.3 ± 0.4 µg/ml on the fifth day. According to the MS-M ratings, the manic symptomatology was decreased by 29% within 3 days and by 35% within 5 days compared with that on the day before entering the study. These changes are statistically significant at the 1% level. Lorazepam medication of the whole study group was 40.75 mg during the study period of 5 days, i.e., 0.8 mg/day/patient. Differentiation between patients with and without psychotic features revealed superior therapeutic effects of carbamazepine suspension in patients without psychotic symptoms (for details see Figure 116.1).

Discussion

The present study demonstrates a statistically significant reduction of manic symptomatology without any severe side effects or adverse reactions in ten patients using carbamazepine suspension. This finding is in line with results of other controlled studies[2,4] regarding the acute antimanic effect of carbamazepine tablets. However, the use of the suspension appears to provide a more rapid onset of antimanic action, which may be useful for clinical practice. In one of the studies,[3] which is comparable to the present investigation, carbamazepine tablets in combination with neuroleptics reduced manic symptomatology by about 25% within 3 days, whereas in the present study a reduction of 29% was induced by the use of carbamazepine suspension and low doses of benzodiazepines (0.8 mg/day) with no neuroleptic co-administration.

This finding may be due to differences of pharmacokinetic properties of tablets and suspension: After administration of tablets, serum peak levels of carbamazepine are usually reached within 4–18 h,[6,7] whereas peak levels after application of the

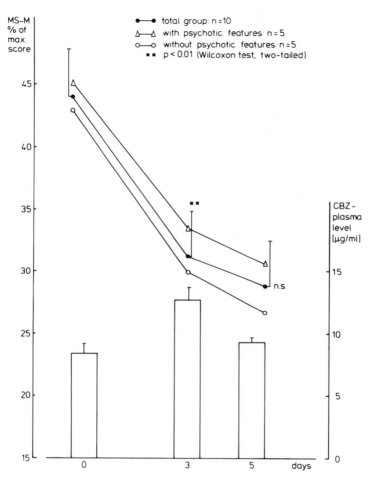

FIGURE 116.1. Mean values (± SEM) of MS-M ratings (% of maximum score) and carbamazepine plasma levels (columns) on days 0, 3, and 5 of the study.

suspension are obtained within 2–3 h.[6] In the present study a serum level of 3 μg/ml was measured 3 h after administration of a single dose of carbamazepine suspension (200 mg). In addition to the earlier and higher peak serum levels induced by the suspension, it has been demonstrated that serum levels also remain higher for 12 h,[6] a finding that could account for its slightly more pronounced antimanic efficacy, obtained here without co-administration of neuroleptics. Interestingly, the therapeutic response was weaker in patients with psychotic features compared with purely manic patients: In patients with psychotic features manic symptomatology was reduced by 28% (day 3) and 32% (day 5), whereas in patients without psychotic features reductions of 31% (day 3) and 38% (day 5) occurred. Because their psychotic symptoms did not respond to carbamazepine and lorazepam alone, additional neuroleptic medication was required for the patients with psychotic features after the study period. Combined treatment with carbamazepine and neuroleptics could, however, help to spare neuroleptics and avoid extrapyramidal side effects in those patients who would otherwise be treated with high dosage neuroleptics alone, as carbamazepine has been shown to be adjunctive in neuroleptic treatment.[8] In conclusion, enhancement of the antimanic and adjunctive efficacy of carbamazepine by administration as a suspension is suggested by the present study.

References

1. Okuma T, Kishimoto A, Inoue K, et al. Anti-manic and prophylactic effects of carbamazepine (Tegretol) on manic depressive psychosis—a preliminary report. Folia Psychiatr Neurol Jpn 1973;27:283—297.
2. Ballenger JC, Post RM. Carbamazepine in manic-depressive illness: a new treatment. Am J Psychiatry 1980;137:782–790.
3. Goncalves N, Stoll KD. Carbamazepin bei manischen Syndromen: eine kontrollierte Doppelblind-Studie. Nervenarzt 1985;56:43–47.
4. Emrich HM, Dose M, Zerssen DV. The use of sodium valproate, carbamazepine and oxcarbazepine in patients with affective disorders. J Affective Disord 1985;8:243–250.
5. Murphy DL, Beigel A, Weingartner H, et al. The quantitation of manic behavior. Mod Probl Pharmacopsychiatry 1974;7:203–220.
6. Wada JA, Troupin AS, Friel P, et al. Pharmacokinetic comparison of tablet and suspension dosage forms of carbamazepine. Epilepsia 1978; 19:251–255.
7. Morselli PL, Monaco F, Gerna M, et al. Bioavailability of two carbamazepine preparations during chronic administration to epileptic patients. Epilepsia 1975;16:759–764.
8. Dose M, Apelt S, Emrich HM. Carbamazepine as an adjunct of antipsychotic therapy. Psychiat Res 1987;22:303–310.

117. Carbamazepine in the Long-Term Treatment of Affective Disorders: Research Strategies

W. Greil, W. Ludwig, D. Huber, and S. Schmidt

The use of lithium in the long-term maintenance treatment of affective disorders is firmly established. However, some patients cannot be treated with lithium because of contraindications, nonresponse, or intolerable side effects. Thus there is a need for alternative treatment strategies.

Increasing evidence indicates that carbamazepine might be an alternative to lithium in the prophylaxis of affective disorders, at least for bipolar and schizoaffective disorders. A few controlled and several open studies (for review see ref. 1) show promising, yet somewhat controversial results concerning the prophylatic efficacy of carbamazepine. Whether carbamazepine will indeed prove to be as effective as lithium or, rather, will be established as a treatment of second choice (e.g., in patients not responding to lithium) is still a matter of debate.

Several questions regarding research strategies that arise with the evaluation of an alternative to a well established maintenance treatment are discussed in this chapter.

1. A simple experimental design, showing the percentage of recurrences under the different treatments, is not sufficient.

2. Research must also try to find additional variables that permit prediction of the patient's response (or nonresponse) to either treatment in order to avoid inefficient treatment attempts.

3. Treatment success should not be measured solely with respect to symptomatology, e.g., number of recurrences and intensity of symptoms. If, for example, lithium and carbamazepine showed equal efficacy in preventing recurrences of affective episodes, the choice between the two drugs should also take into consideration such questions as side effects and risk of intoxication, as well as more subtle effects such as the social functioning of the patients and their subjective feelings of well-being.

Research Strategies: Prediction and Multidimensional Treatment Evaluation

Prediction of Response to Lithium and Carbamazepine

In the past, research has focused on predictors of response or nonresponse to lithium. The results seem to indicate that lithium is most effective in patients with "typical affective disorders," where clear-cut episodes of affective psychoses are followed by complete remission and a symptom-free interval. Patients with continuous cycling, a chronic course of illness, or incomplete remission during intervals often do not respond sufficiently to lithium. Lithium is also less effective in patients with atypical psychotic features such as mood-incongruent delusions.

It has been proposed that lithium-nonresponsive patients might particularly profit from treatment with carbamazepine. For instance, Placidi et al.[2] concluded that carbamazepine might be superior to lithium in patients with "atypical psychoses." This conclusion, however, was based on the finding that patients with schizoaffective or schizophreniform features showed a higher dropout rate when treated with lithium compared to patients treated with carbamazepine. Because the reasons for dropout were not reported, these results should be viewed with caution. Kishimoto[3] and Post and Uhde[4] reported that rapid cyclers, who usually do not respond well to lithium, show good response to carbamazepine. However, these findings too need to be substantiated by further research, as they were derived from uncontrolled studies.

Furthermore, inconsistent results of studies on the efficacy of lithium or carbamazepine in long-term prophylactic treatment might be a consequence of divergent diagnostic criteria between studies. Thus the comparability of studies should be improved by the use of a standardized polydiagnostic approach, allowing diagnoses by different diagnostic systems. The use of a well defined diagnostic evaluation as well as a thorough screening of treatment history are necessary ingredients of future research.

Prophylactic treatment with carbamazepine and with lithium has mainly been studied in patients with high frequencies of previous episodes. Studies in patients exhibiting a milder course of illness are needed, e.g., patients selected according to criteria proposed by Angst (two episodes within 5 years in unipolars, within 4 years in bipolars, and within 3 years in schizoaffectives).[5]

Treatment Evaluation: Beyond Symptomatology

Although assessment of the clinical efficacy of a drug in the prevention of recurrences is the most important aim of a long-term maintenance study, it is not the only variable of interest when comparing two drugs of possibly equal efficacy. Research should also focus on (a) unwanted side effects, (b) minor mood swings between episodes, (c) the influence on the social functioning of the patient, and (d) the patient's feelings of well-being.

1. Unwanted side effects of long-term psychopharmacological treatment should be investigated thoroughly, as long-term side effects may differ in their severity and tolerability between treatments.

2. Aside from clinically relevant illness episodes, minor mood swings that can occur in affective psychoses during symptom-free intervals may be suppressed

by prophylactic treatment. Although this suppression is often welcome to the patient, especially in those with bipolar illness, patients miss those "upward swings," which they experience as episodes of increased creativity. In any case, research should report not only the number and timing of major episodes but should also give an exact and thorough description of the whole course of the illness.

3. Patients usually do not suffer from their illness alone but also from the disturbed social functioning that is in some cases the consequence of the disease (e.g., loss of job or family conflicts). On the other hand, work and family relations may constitute resources from which patients draw social support that helps them during crises. Again, psychopharmacological treatment may affect the patients' social functioning in various ways that should be evaluated carefully.

4. Health means the presence of a positive sense of well-being, as opposed to the more absence of illness. Thus long-term studies should also include measures of the patient's overall satisfaction with the treatment and its effects on his subjective evaluation of his life ("quality of life"). The term "quality of life" means the degree of psychological, social, and vocational well-being as it is felt by the patient. This variable should be of importance for the prognosis as well as for the feasibility of long-term prophylactic treatment.

German Collaborative Study on Maintenance Treatment of Affective Disorders

Some of the issues mentioned will be investigated in a running, randomized, prospective, multicenter study supported by the BMFT (Ministry of Research and Technology of the FRG).* In this study the following treatment regimens will be compared:

1. Bipolar affective disorders: maintenance therapy with lithium or carbamazepine
2. Schizoaffective disorders: maintenance therapy with lithium or carbamazepine (additionally neuroleptics if required)
3. Unipolar depressions: maintenance therapy with lithium or antidepressants as well as an intermittent therapy where antidepressant drugs are applied only in case of the manifestation of significant psychiatric symptoms

Recruitment of patients is based on selection recently developed criteria for prophylactic drug treatment,[5] and thus patients with comparatively few previous episodes will be investigated. Diagnostic and psychometric procedures include a standardized diagnostic interview (German version of SCID extended to include diagnoses according to Research Diagnostic Criteria (RDC) and ICD-10),[6] a standardized interview on social functioning (SIS[7]) and an assessment of family relations according to the concept of "expressed emotions."[8] Additionally, self-rating scales concerning premorbid personality and compliance will be administered.

Treatment outcome will be assessed continuously on several dimensions over a 2.5-year period. In addition to recurrences of the affective disorder, psychic

*Leading center of the study: University of Munich. Project coordinators: W. Greil, W. Ludwig, S. Schmidt. Data preparation and analysis: R. Engel. Treatment centers: Psychiatric university hospitals in Aachen (regional organizer: A. Czernik), Berlin (B. Müller-Oerlinghausen), Düsseldorf (J. Tegeler), Heidelberg (H. Sauer), Lübeck (T. Wetterling), Munich (W. Greil), Münster (G.A.E. Rudolf), Tübingen (H. Giedke) and Würzburg (M. Osterheider).

disturbances of minor degree and unwanted side effects will be documented carefully during this time. Patients' subjective evaluations of the treatment and their social functioning will also be assessed repeatedly.

The main goals of this study are to evaluate the efficacy of the various treatment regimens as well as to provide differential criteria that allow one to select the most appropriate treatment for the individual patient.

References

1. Schmidt S, Greil W. Carbamazepin in der Behandlung affektiver Psychosen. Nervenarzt 1987;58:719–736.
2. Placidi GF, Lenzi A, Lazzerini F, et al. The comparative efficacy and safety of carbamazepine versus lithium: a randomized, double-blind 3-year trial in 83 patients. J Clin Psychiatry 1986;47:490–494.
3. Kishimoto A. A followup prophylactic study of carbamazepine in affective disorders. In Emrich HM, Okuma T, Muller AA (eds): Anticonvulsants in Affective Disorders, Amsterdam: Excerpta Medica, 1984;88–92.
4. Post RM, Uhde TW. Carbamazepine in bipolar illness. Psychopharmacol Bull 1985;21:10–17.
5. Angst J. Ungelöste Probleme bei der Indikationsstellung zur Lithiumprophylaxe affektiver und schizoaffektiver Erkrankungen. Bibl Psychiatr 1981;161:34–44.
6. Wittchen H-U, Zaudig M, Schramm E, et al. Das strukturierte klinische Interview für DSM-III-R (SKID). German Modification of the Structured Clinical Interview for DSM-III-R Patient Version by Spitzer RL, Williams JB, Gibbon M. Weinheim: Beltz, 1987.
7. Hecht H, Faltermaier A, Wittchen H-U. Social Interview Schedule (SIS). Regensburg: S. Roderer Verlag, 1987.
8. Leff J, Vaughn C. Expressed Emotion in Families. New York: Guilford Press, 1985.

118. Plasma Levels of Carbamazepine in Affective Disorder

M. BROEKMAN, W.A. NOLEN, AND G.S. JANSEN

Since the early 1970s many studies have been published about the effectiveness of carbamazepine (CBZ) in affective disorders, first by Japanese investigators[1,2] and later by authors from the United States and Europe.[3–6] At present CBZ has been demonstrated to be effective in mania[7] and depression—not only in the acute phase of these illnesses but also as a prophylactic treatment to prevent new episodes.[4,8–10]

Treatment with CBZ is often accompanied by measurements of plasma levels. Although some authors have not found an additional effect of CBZ in epilepsy beyond plasma levels of 5 mg/l, the generally accepted ranges for therapeutic levels in epilepsy vary between 4 and 12 mg/l.[11–13] Mainly based on these studies, identical therapeutic ranges for plasma levels are advocated in affective disorders. However, no systematic studies have been performed to establish the optimal range of efficacy. Nevertheless, some authors have looked for a relation between plasma levels and effect; some found no correlation,[7,14,15] although one study reported a lower prophylactic effect at plasma levels below 7 mg/l.[9] Despite the lack of supportive evidence, Okuma[16] advised aiming at plasma levels of 6 mg/l, Strömgren and Boller[17] at levels between 4.2 and 7.8 mg/l, and Ballenger and Post[3] at levels between 8 and 12 mg/l. Thus there exists no agreement about an optimal level.

One of the other reasons for measuring plasma levels is the determination of a maximum level above which adverse or toxic effects are likely to occur. Such maximum levels vary in the literature from above 10 mg/l to above 18 mg/l.[18,19] Another problem is that there is no uniform standardization of the measurement of CBZ plasma levels, especially regarding the time of blood sampling. Some take samples 12 h after the last evening intake (so-called trough levels), whereas others take samples 2, 3, or 4 h after (morning) intake (peak levels). The latter procedure is predominantly used by neurologists in Europe when determining optimal levels in epileptic patients.

It seems rational to assume that the therapeutic effect of CBZ is related to its trough level; i.e., it must exceed a certain threshold level, e.g., 5 or 6 mg/l. Therefore trough levels should be measured when determining the dose needed to obtain an optimal therapeutic effect. On the other hand, peak levels should be measured in patients with suspected toxic effects, which are more likely to occur beyond a level of 10–12 mg/l. In some patients it may be necessary to obtain information about both levels, as there are large interindividual variations not only concerning the dose/plasma level ratio but also concerning the course of plasma levels, partly caused by differences in absorption, metabolism, and excretion. Moreover, the daily dosage schedule can influence the course as well.[19]

Aim of the Study

We have studied both trough and peak levels of CBZ in patients with affective disorders in order to determine the course of plasma levels and to obtain information about a possible relation with therapeutic effect and/or adverse effects.

Methods

All patients who were regularly treated with CBZ, i.e., received a stable dose and dosage schedule for at least 3 weeks, were included. Additionally, all patients older than 75 years and/or suffering from a serious somatic illness that might influence the study were excluded. Informed consent was obtained from all patients.

Carbamazepine was given in different dosage schedules, but the last evening dose was given to all patients at 8:00 p.m. At 8:00 a.m. a blood sample was taken to determine the trough level using a high-performance liquid chromatography (HPLC) method.

Immediately after blood sampling all patients received their first dose of CBZ followed by a short neurological examination and an inquiry about subjective experiences, each aimed at detecting possible adverse effects of CBZ. Except for the CBZ intake, the same procedure was repeated at 10:00 a.m. and 12:00 noon.

Results

Altogether 24 patients entered the study. Three of them were excluded when it became evident that they had not taken CBZ according to the time schedule of the protocol. The remaining 21 patients were 13 women and 8 men. Age ranged from 19 to 74 years (mean 49.3 years). They were diagnosed (*DSM-III*) as suffering from a bipolar disorder ($n = 10$), schizoaffective disorder ($n = 3$), major depression ($n = 1$), epilepsy ($n = 1$), bipolar disorder + epilepsy ($n = 3$), and schizoaffective disorder + epilepsy ($n = 1$). None of the patients was in an acute phase of the illness, although some were not completely free from symptoms.

At the time of the study CBZ was used in a stable dose and dosage schedule ranging from 3 weeks to 72 months (mean 16.3 months). The daily doses varied from 300 to 1,200 mg (mean 776 mg) and the dose schedule was two to six times a day. In addition to CBZ, almost all patients ($n = 19$) used other medication, such as neuroleptics ($n = 8$), antidepressants ($n = 5$), lithium ($n = 8$), benzodiazepines ($n = 17$), or other anticonvulsants ($n = 2$).

Trough levels varied from 4.5 to 9.4 mg/l (mean 5.96 ± S.D. 1.20), but no correlation was found with the daily dose of CBZ. Peak levels at 2 and 4 h after the first intake of CBZ varied from 4.7 to 10.6 mg/l (mean 7.40 ± 1.56) and from 4.7 to 10.2 mg/l (mean 7.33 ± 1.49), respectively. A large variation between the patients

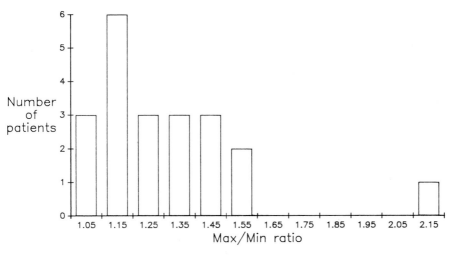

FIGURE 118.1. CBZ concentrations: variation of max/min ratio, i.e., ratio between highest peak level and trough level of CBZ. Samples were taken at 8:00 a.m, 10:00 a.m., and 12:00 noon. First morning dose was taken at 8:00 a.m.

was found in the ratio between highest peak level and trough level, varying from 1.02 to 2.20 mg/l (mean 1.31) (Fig. 118.1).

No correlation was found between trough levels and therapeutic effects, as all patients responded rather well to CBZ. Unwanted effects were observed in many patients, but except for dizziness (ten patients) specific side effects that might have been caused by CBZ were observed in only a few patients: ataxia ($n = 2$), nystagmus ($n = 3$), nausea ($n = 1$), and sedation ($n = 4$). No correlation was found between these effects and the peak levels of CBZ. In addition to CBZ, co-medication might also have been responsible for other adverse effects such as dry mouth ($n = 11$), tremor ($n = 6$), and parkinsonism ($n = 2$).

Discussion

As has already been shown in epilepsy[18,19] we found a large interindividual variation between dose and plasma levels of CBZ. We also found large interindividual differences in the ratio between peak level and trough level. As the therapeutic range for CBZ is rather small and adverse effects might already occur at plasma levels about twice as high as needed for its positive effects, these findings underline the importance of measuring plasma levels of CBZ.

We did not find a correlation between trough levels and therapeutic effect. However, one has to realize that we studied only patients who had already proved to be good or moderate responders to CBZ. Moreover, all patients had trough levels above 4.5 mg/l. We also found no correlation between peak levels and adverse effects, although many patients had unwanted effects. Possible reasons for this finding are that most patients used other medication as well and that peak levels of CBZ did not exceed 10.6 mg/l.

Although no systematic studies concerning optimal plasma levels of CBZ have been performed, some advice can be given. Measuring plasma levels to determine the therapeutic range of CBZ should use trough levels provisionally aimed at 6–8 mg/l. However, more systematic studies are needed. When adverse or toxic effects of CBZ are suspected, one should measure peak levels about 3 h after drug intake, provisionally to be aimed at below 12 (or even 10) mg/l. Because of the high ratio between peak levels and trough levels, as found in some of our patients, the use of slow-release preparations of CBZ should be considered.

References

1. Takezaki H, Hanaoka M. The use of carbamazepine (Tegretol) and the control of manic-depressive psychosis and other manic depressive states. Clin Psychiatry (Tokyo) 1971;13:173–183.
2. Okuma T, Kishimoto A. Anti-manic and prophylactic effects of carbamazepine (Tegretol) on manic depressive psychosis: a preliminary report. Folia Psychiatr Neurol Jpn 1973;27:283–297.
3. Ballenger JC, Post RM. Therapeutic effects of carbamazepine in affective illness: a preliminary report. Commun Psychopharmacol 1978;2:159–175.
4. Ballenger JC, Post RM. Carbamazepine in manic-depressive illness: a new treatment. Am J Psychiatry 1980;137:782–790.
5. Emrich HM, Von Zerssen E, Kissling W, et al. Effect of sodium valproate on mania: the GABA-hypothesis of affective disorders. Arch Psychiatr Nervenkr 1980;229:1–16.
6. Nolen WA. Carbamazepine, a possible adjunct or alternative to lithium in bipolar disorder. Acta Psychiatr Scand 1983;67:218–225.
7. Okuma T, Inaga K, Otsuki S, et al. Comparison of the antimanic efficacy of carbamazepine and chlorpromazine, a double-blind controlled study. Psychopharmacology 1979;66:211–217.
8. Uhde TW, Post RM, Ballenger JC, et al. Carbamazepine in the treatment of neuropsychiatric disorders. In Emrich HM, Okuma T, Müller AA (eds): Anticonvulsants in Affective Disorders. Amsterdam: Elsevier, 1984;132–138.
9. Fawcett J, Kravitz HM. The long-term management of bipolar disorders with lithium, carbamazepine and antidepressants. J Clin Psychiatry 1985;46:58–60.
10. Placidi GF, Lenzi A, Lazzerini F, et al. The comparative efficacy and safety of carbamazepine versus lithium: a randomized, double-blind 3-year trial in 83 patients. J Clin Psychiatry 1986;47:490–494.
11. Schneider H. Carbamazepine; the influence of other anti-epileptic drugs on its serum level. In Schneider H, Janz D, Gardner-Thorpe C, et al (eds): Clinical Pharmacology of Anti-epileptic Drugs. New York: Springer Verlag, 1975;189–195.
12. Eichelbaum M, Bertilsson L, Lund L, et al. Plasma-levels of carbamazepine and carbamazepine-10, 11-epoxide during treatment of epilepsy. Eur J Clin Pharmacokinet 1978;9:417–421.
13. Bertilsson L. Clinical pharmacokinetics of carbamazepine. Clin Pharmacokinet 1978;3:128–143.
14. Okuma T, Inagaka K, Otsuki S, et al. A preliminary double-blind study on the efficacy of carbamazepine in prophylaxis of manic-depressive illness. Psychopharmacology 1981;73:95–96.
15. Kishimoto A, Ogura C, Hazama H, et al. Long-term prophylactic effects of carbamazepine in affective disorder. Br J Psychiatry 1983;143:327–331.
16. Okuma T. Therapeutic and prophylactic efficacy of carbamazepine in manic depressive psychosis. In Emrich HM, Okuma T, Müller AA (eds): Anticonvulsants in Affective Disorders. Amsterdam: Elsevier, 1984;132–138.
17. Strömgren LS, Boller S. Carbamazepine in treatment and prophylaxis of manic-depressive disorder. Psychiatr Dev 1985;4:349–367.
18. Höppener RJ, Kuyer A, Meijer JWA, et al. Correlation between daily fluctuations of carbamazepine serum levels and intermittent side effects. Epilepsia 1980;21:341–350.
19. Tomson T. Interdosage fluctuations in plasma carbamazepine concentration determine intermittent side effects. Arch Neurol 1984;41:830–835.

119. Efficacy and Safety of Lithium–Carbamazepine Combination in Mania

SASHI SHUKLA AND BRIAN L. COOK

Despite the demonstrated efficacy of lithium carbonate during acute episodes of mania and as a prophylactic agent in bipolar disorders, 20–25% of patients fail to respond to this treatment.[1,2] Some clinical predictors of lithium nonresponsiveness have been noted in rapid cycling disorders,[3] mixed manic disorders,[4] and patients with associated neuropsychiatric factors.[4] Often, although there are no controlled studies, such patients are clinically treated with combinations of lithium and neuroleptics. Such patients are subject to the unpleasant side effects and potentially more harmful effects of the tardive dyskinesia[5] associated with neuroleptics. In addition, a significant number of patients clinically fail to respond adequately to even this combined regimen.

The antimanic properties of carbamazepine suggest that the combination of lithium and carbamazepine (CBZ) may be beneficial in some bipolar patients nonresponsive to lithium alone. Open studies by Ballenger and Post[6] and Post et al[7] indicate that this combination may be efficacious in the treatment of acute manic episodes and in the prevention of subsequent relapse. Inuoe et al.[8] found a favorable antimanic response in three and prophylactic benefit in two bipolar patients. Lipinsky and Pope,[9] using the two drugs separately and later in conjunction, demonstrated the superiority of the combination regimen in three acutely manic patients and suggested a synergistic interaction of the two drugs. Nolen[10] found the combination efficacious in four patients. Shukla et al.[11] demonstrated the acute and prophylactic benefit of the combination regimen in seven bipolar patients over 12 months and found the regimen superior to the lithium-neuroleptic trials of the previous year. Maintenance side effects were also significantly lower. Although the efficacy of the combination-drug regimen may represent the additive antimanic effects of the drugs, the exact interactions are not known. Inoue et al.[8] have suggested that CBZ may raise intracellular lithium levels, or alternatively the drugs mutually affect central electrolyte metabolism. Placebo-controlled double-blind trials are required in the future to confirm the preliminary findings that this drug combination may be efficacious in some bipolar patients.

Of concern are reports regarding the safety of these drugs used in combination. Although common side effects of both lithium[12] and CBZ[13,14] are well known in the literature, there have been a few reports implicating this drug combination with neurological phenomena ranging from side effects to toxicity. Ghose[15] noted a 50% dropout rate due to neurological symptoms in ten patients during the active phase of her study involving the addition of CBZ to ten bipolar patients stable on lithium therapy, with lithium plasma levels ranging from 0.8 to 1.2 mEq/l. These symptoms ranged from ataxia, dizziness, frequent blackouts, agitation, restlessness, confusional states, to feelings of unreality. CBZ blood levels were not available. Chaudhry and Walters[16] reported neurotoxicity in a patient who developed a syndrome characterized by unsteady gait, generalized truncal tremors, ataxia, horizontal nystagmus, marked hyperreflexia, muscle fasiculation at lithium and CBZ levels of 1.02 mEq/l and 10.0 μg/ml, respectively. The patient's symptoms abated during separate drug trials and reappeared when the drugs were subsequently prescribed together. Shukla et al.[17] also noted neurotoxic syndromes in five bipolar patients during the addition of CBZ to their lithium regimen. In none of the reports reviewed were permanent neurological sequelae associated on discontinuation of either one drug or both. Some of the predisposing factors appeared to be histories of lithium-related neurotoxicity and the presence of a medical or neurological history in these patients.

Our findings suggested that CBZ enhanced the development of neurotoxicity in patients with underlying central nervous system or metabolic disease. Shopsin et al.[12] have noted that the lithium ion appears capable of modifying brain tissue, which could bring about decreased threshold tolerance or sensitivity to other drugs. Baseline neuropathies predisposed patients to lithium sensitivity at moderately low serum lithium levels. It is of interest to note, however, that two of our patients who developed neurotoxicity[17] on subsequent follow-up did not develop the same syndrome and remained neurologically stable when rechallenged with the addition of CBZ to their lithium regimen at lower CBZ dosages with levels maintained between 6.0 and 8.5 μg/ml. Furthermore, our experience with initial dropout due to neurological side effects during the initiation phase of CBZ therapy only and Ghose's similar data[15] appear to indicate that during the initiation phase of treatment patients already on lithium therapy may be more likely to develop CBZ-related side effects at levels of 9–12 μg/ml. Possibly, CBZ levels recommended by Ballenger and Post[6] of 8–12 μg/ml may represent safe, efficacious levels when CBZ is used alone.

The consensus from the neurological literature also indicates that when used alone CBZ is safe and efficacious at levels ranging from 8 to 12 μg/ml and toxic at levels over 9 μg/ml alone in patients receiving primidone, valproic acid,[18] or phenytoin concurrently.[18,19] Furthermore, our findings of a reduced side effects profile during maintenance with lithium + CBZ compared to lithium neuroleptics in nine patients who completed the study[11] indicate that intolerance to CBZ may be seen only during initiation and may, in some patients, represent what Fogelson[20] has pointed out are common transient side effects seen when CBZ is initiated too abruptly or at levels of more than 9 μg/ml. He explained that patients not previously exposed to CBZ have initial clearance rates 25–50% lower than those on the drug for at least 4 weeks and hence initial serum levels 25–50% higher than those patients on maintenance CBZ. He advised that patients may be unnecessarily denied treatment with CBZ if side effects due to improper dosing are attributed to intolerance to the drug. We recommend that investigators studying the efficacy of lithium and CBZ in combination should attempt gradual dosing of CBZ and maintain levels not higher than 9 μg/ml if clinically possible.

References

1. Stokes PE, Stoll PM, Shamoian CA, et al. Efficacy of lithium as acute treatment of manic depressive illness. Lancet 1971;1:1319–1325.
2. Goodwin FK, Ebert MH. Lithium in mania: clinical trials and controlled studies. In Gershon S, Shopsin B (eds): Lithium: Its Role in Psychiatric Research and Treatment. New York: Plenum Press, 1973;237–252.
3. Dunner DL, Fieve RR. Clinical factors in lithium prophylaxis failure. Arch Gen Psychiatry 1974;30:229–233.
4. Himmelhoch JM, Garfinkel ME. Sources of lithium resistance in mixed mania. Psychopharmacol Bull 1986;22:613–620.
5. Rosenbaum AH, Niven RG, Manson MP, et al. Tardive dyskinesia: relationship with a primary affective disorder. Dis Nerv Syst 1977;38:423–426.
6. Ballenger JC, Post RM. Carbamazepine in manic-depressive illness: a new treatment. Am J Psychiatry 1980;137:782–790.
7. Post RM, Uhde TW, Ballenger JC, et al. Prophylactic efficacy of carbamazepine in manic depressive illness. Am J Psychiatry 1983;140:1602–1604.
8. Inoue K, Arima S, Tanaka K, et al. A lithium and carbamazepine combination in the treatment of bipolar disorder—a preliminary report. Folia Psychiatr Neurol Jpn 1981;35:465–475.
9. Lipinski JF, Pope HG. Possible synergistic action between carbamazepine and lithium carbonate in the treatment of three acutely manic patients. Am J Psychiary 1982;139:948–949.
10. Nolen WA. Carbamazepine, a possible adjunct alternative to lithium in bipolar disorder. Acta Psychiatr Scand 1983;67:218–225.
11. Shukla S, Cook BL, Miller MG. Lithium-carbamazepine versus lithium neuroleptic prophylaxis in bipolar illness. J Affective Disord 1985;9:219–222.
12. Shopsin D, Johnson G, Gershon S. Neurotoxicity with lithium: differential drug responsiveness. Int Pharmacopsychiatry 1970;5:170–182.
13. Reynolds EH. Neurotoxicity of carbamazepine. Adv Neurol 1975;11:345–353.
14. Livingston S, Pauli LL, Berman W. Carbamazepine in epilepsy: nine year follow-up study with special emphasis on untoward reactions. Dis Nerv Syst 1974;35:103–107.
15. Ghose K. Effect of carbamazepine in polyuria associated with lithium therapy. Pharmakopsychiatr Neuropsychopharmakol 1978;11:241–245.
16. Chaudhry RP, Walters BGH. Lithium and carbamazepine interaction: possible neurotoxicity. J Clin Psychiatry 1983;44:30–31.
17. Shukla S, Godwin CD, Long LEB, et al. Lithium-carbamazepine neurotoxicity and risk factors. Am J Psychiatry 1984;141:1604–1606.
18. Kutt K: Clinical pharmacology of carbamazepine in antiepileptic drugs. In Pippenger CE, Penry JK, Kutt M (eds): Quantitative Analysis and Interpretation. New York: Raven Press, 1978.
19. Kutt M, Solomon G, Wasterlain C, et al. Carbamazepine in difficult to control epileptic outpatients. Acta Neurol Scand [Suppl] 1975;60:27–32.
20. Fogelson DL. Using carbamazepine effectively. Am J Psychiatry 1984;141:1130.

V.C. TREATMENT STRATEGIES FOR RESISTANT DEPRESSION

120. Patient Characteristics and Factors Associated with Chronic Depression and Its Treatment

D. Eccleston, J.L. Scott, W.A. Barker, and T.A. Kerr

Depression in most patients remits spontaneously or responds to antidepressant treatment. The few patients in whom it does not form a group who pose a significant therapeutic challenge. Robins and Guze[1] reviewed 20 follow-up studies of affective disorders and concluded that a chronic course supervened in 1–28% of cases (average 12–15%). This wide variation depends on nonuniformity of diagnostic criteria for depression, assessment methods employed, and in particular the intensity of follow-up. In this study the definition used was that of Cassano et al.[2]: "Chronicity refers to symptomatic nonrecovery for a period of 2 or more years and may be a sequel to one or more episodes of depression from which the patient does not recover."

This chapter presents the results of an investigation into the factors associated with chronicity in a sample of 24 patients with primary major depression of 2 years or more in duration admitted consecutively to an inpatient psychiatric unit. They were referred from other hospitals, having received a wide range of antidepressant drugs; many had had electroconvulsive therapy (ECT). The object of the study was twofold: (a) to examine psychosocial factors associated with chronicity; and (b) to use in an open trial a drug regimen that had previously been found in a pilot study to be effective in this type of patient.[3]

Methods

Subjects

All patients met the Research Diagnostic Criteria (RDC)[4] for definite or probable major depression. Severity of depression was assessed using the Hamilton Rating Scale for Depression (HAM-D)[5] and the Beck Depression Inventory (BDI).[6] The control group comprised 20 randomly selected patients suffering from primary major depression at the time of their admission to the inpatient unit.

Through a semistructured interview with the patient and when possible a close relative, and assessment of all previous case records, the following information was obtained and recorded on a specially devised data sheet.

1. Sociodemographic details.
2. Psychiatric history.
3. Family history of psychiatric disorder. These data in first degree relatives were obtained using the RDC—Family History Version,[7] and case notes were examined when possible.
4. Life events. The method described by Akiskal et al.[8] was used. Paykel's questionnaire[9] was used to document life events, and the independence of these events from the depressive illness was established using the method of Brown et al.[10]
5. Personality. The premorbid personality of the patient was assessed using the Eysenck Personality Questionnaire (EPQ).[11]

Statistical Analysis

Results were analyzed using the chi-square test (with Yates's correction applied), Student's t-test, and Fisher's exact probability test.

Treatment Regimen

All patients who successfully completed the washout period of at least 2 weeks were given a combination of drugs: L-Tryptophan 1 g b.d., phenelzine 15 mg t.i.d., and lithium carbonate at a dose sufficient to achieve a plasma level of 0.5–0.8 mmol/l.[12] After 6 weeks on the "serotonin (5-hydroxytryptamine, 5-HT) cocktail" a second drug regimen was added. This second combination, which was continued for another 6 weeks, was designed to lower both total plasma vanadium and the proportion of the pentavalent vanadate ion.[13,14]

Results

Sociodemographic Details

There was no difference between the control group and the chronic depressives in terms of age, sex distribution (female/male approximately 2:1), marital status, and social class.

Family History of Psychiatric Illness

The female chronic depressives had a significantly higher incidence (Fisher's exact test $p < 0.02$) of a family history of affective disorder than the control group.

Severity Ratings

The female chronic patients rated themselves significantly more depressed than the control group on the BDI (39.3 ± 9.5 versus 29.9 ± 5.2; $p < 0.01$ t-test)

Previous Episodes

The female chronic depressives had significantly more ($p < 0.05$, t-test) previous depressive episodes than controls (5.8 ± 4.1 versus 3.2 ± 2.1).

Life Events

The number of individuals reporting independent, undesirable life events during the combined 6 months before and the 2 years after the onset of the depressive episode was significantly higher ($p<0.05$) among the chronic depressives than among the depressives who recovered. Four patients in the chronic group and one in the control group reported independent life events only after the illness had begun. Multiple life events were recorded by 13 patients (9 chronic depressives and 4 recovered depressives).

No differences in personality, as assessed by the EPQ, were found between the chronic and control groups of depressives.

Thyroid Function

Four female chronic depressives had a history of thyroid dysfunction ($p<0.01$, Fisher's exact test).

Treatment Results for the Chronically Depressed Group

During the washout period two patients deteriorated into a severe mixed affective state requiring other therapeutic intervention; they had to be withdrawn from the trial. During the first 6 weeks one patient became severely retarded and required emergency ECT with which he made a good clinical recovery. One patient improved dramatically over the first 3 weeks of treatment and was discharged home. Another patient improved during the first 6 weeks of active treatment and was discharged. Of the remaining 20 patients, seven required a modification of the basic drug regimen. They are analyzed separately as being in the "paratrial." Three of the seven required addition of a major tranquilizer because of the development of paranoid symptoms. The other four "paratrial" patients needed a reduction of the dose of phenelzine because of intolerable side effects.

Trial Patients. Among the trial patients ($n = 13$; 7 female, 6 male), the mean HAM-D on entry was 23.0 ± 7.4 (SD), and at the end of the washout it had not altered significantly. At 6 weeks the mean HAM-D had dropped by a highly significant amount. There was no further change at 12 weeks.

There was a highly significant change in the Beck Depression Inventory (BDI) score by 6 weeks ($t = 3.37, p = 0.006$). As with the HAM-D, there was no further change during the next 6 weeks.

Paratrial Patients. Among the paratrial patients ($n = 8$; 7 female, 1 male), the mean HAM-D on admission was 23.4 ± 5.2 (SD), and it had not changed after the "washout" period. At 6 weeks the mean HAM-D had dropped significantly ($t = 4.9, p = 0.003$) but at 12 weeks it had remained unchanged.

On admission the patients scored themselves on the BDI as moderately severely depressed, and this assessment did not change following withdrawal of drugs. After 6 weeks of active treatment the mean score had fallen significantly ($t = 4.17, p = 0.006$), but there was no further change at 12 weeks.

Discussion

The group examined were characterized by having an illness for at least 2 years that had failed to respond to adequate chemotherapy. Even though 24 patients is a relatively small group, certain factors were significant when compared with 20 depressives who did not become chronic. There was a strong family history of psychiatric disorder of the unipolar type that was significant in the female chronic group. Bipolar disorder showed a trend in the same direction but not significantly so. The number of previous episodes was also significantly higher in the female group, being on average twice that of the controls. Life events were reported almost three times more frequently in the chronic group. There was also a non-significant tendency to report more life events after the onset of the illness, perhaps perpetuating the illness, and to report multiple life events. By contrast, the groups did not differ on the personality characteristics evaluated by the EPQ. Another unexplained variable was the high incidence of thyroid disorder in the history of women in the chronic depression group. Although the cause of chronicity was multifactorial, this group seemed to have a strong genetic background and to have been subject to adverse life events.

Despite the severity of illness, this group proved to be treatable by a particular combination of drugs. Some 60% of all patients entering the study recovered to the extent that the HAM-D value fell to half the initial value. This treatment had to be combined with a major tranquilizer in a group who developed paranoid symptoms, and these symptoms improved significantly. The low vanadium regimen did not contribute to further amelioration in symptoms in these patients. Drug treatment does, however, form the background against which psychotherapy of both the supportive and the cognitive varieties are important, as well as social rehabilitation for those whose role has been lost during many years of absence from the family.

References

1. Robins E, Guze S. Classification of affective disorders—the primary-secondary, the endogenous-reactive and the neurotic-psychotic dichotomies. In Williams TA, Katz MM, Shield JA (eds): Recent Advances in Psychobiology of the Depressive Illnesses. Washington, DC: US Government Printing Office, 1972.
2. Cassano GB, Maggini C, Akiskal H. Short-term, sub-chronic and chronic sequelae of affective disorders. Psychiatr Clin North Am 1983;6:55–68.
3. Loudon JB, Eccleston D. Unpublished observations, 1976.
4. Spitzer RL, Endicott J, Robins E. Research diagnostic criteria: rationale and reliability. Arch Gen Psychiatry 1978;35:773–782.
5. Hamilton M. A rating scale for depression. J Neurol Neurosurg Psychiatry 1960;23:56–62.
6. Beck AT, Ward CH, Mendelson M, et al. An inventory for measuring depression. Arch Gen Psychiatry 1961;4:561–571.
7. Andreasen NC, Endicott J, Spitzer RL, et al. The family history method using diagnostic criteria—reliability and validity. Arch Gen Psychiatry 1977;34:1229–1235.
8. Akiskal HS, King D, Rosenthal T, et al. Chronic depressions. I. Clinical and familial characteristics in 137 probands. J Affective Disord 1981;3:297–315.
9. Paykel ES. Recent life events in the development of depressive disorders. In Depue RA (ed): The Psychobiology of the Depressive Disorders—Implications for the Effects of Stress. New York: Academic Press, 1979.
10. Brown GW, Sklair F, Harris TO, et al. Life events and psychiatric disorders. I. Some methodological issues. Psychol Med 1973:3:74–87.

11. Eysenck HJ, Eysenck SBG. Manual of the Eysenck Personality Questionnaire. London: Hodder & Stoughton, 1975.
12. Barker WA, Eccleston D. The treatment of chronic depression: an illustrative case. Brt J Psychiatry 1984;144:317–319.
13. Naylor GJ, Smith AHW. Defective genetic control of sodium pump density in manic depressive psychosis. Psychol Med 1981;11:257–263.
14. Naylor GJ, Smith AHW. Vanadium: a possible aetiological factor in manic depressive illness. Psychol Med 1981;11:249–256.

121. Resistant Depression: Clinical Characteristics and Response to Treatment

BARUCH SHAPIRA, SETH KINDLER, AND BERNARD LERER

The terms "resistant" or "refractory" depression imply a state of illness that can potentially respond to treatment. The further implication is that conventional therapeutic interventions have been applied at dosages that are adequate and for a sufficient duration to elicit the desired response. In individuals whose depression is labeled "resistant," this situation is not always the case. Furthermore, there is no universally agreed on definition of the term with respect to the number of modalities that should have received an adequate trial. It is also not clear which treatments are regarded as "conventional" and which are not. Whether, for example, electroconvulsive therapy (ECT) falls in the category of conventional therapies is a case in point.

Patients referred, in practice, to a "resistant depression unit" tend to be heterogeneous with regard to the above definitions. They have in common the impression of the referring physician that their illness is sufficiently unresponsive to treatment to warrant specialized care. This impression is frequently influenced by considerations such as the severity of depressive symptoms, the presence of psychotic features or suicidal ideation, and pressure on the part of the patient or family to achieve more rapid therapeutic results.

This chapter briefly reviews the experience of the Jerusalem Mental Health Center–Ezrath Nashim Depression Unit of treating patients referred for resistant depression during the period 1983–1986. The criterion used for including referrals in the data analysis was one of nonresponse to adequate treatment with at least two tricyclic antidepressants (TCAs): a TCA plus a monoamine oxidase inhibitor (MAOI) or a TCA plus ECT. This arbitrary definition is open to criticism by those who regard all three modalities as conventional therapies to which a "refractory" patient should have been exposed. A naturalistic survey of the type reported would lose much of its impact, however, if it excluded subjects whom most referring psychiatrists would regard as refractory and focused only a core group of exceptionally unresponsive patients.

Clinical Characteristics

Fifty-nine patients fulfilling the criterion defined above were referred to the depression unit during the period surveyed. Forty-three were female (age 58.00±11.07 years, mean±SD) and 16 male (age 61.00±7.02 years). This sex and age distribution resembles that reported by other authors.[1] Fifty-one (86.4%) were cases of recurrent depression; in 8 cases (13.6%) it was the first episode of illness. In the recurrent cases the number of previous episodes was 4.4±3.40. The age distribution for the first depressive episode showed peaks at 30–40 years (25.4%) and at 50–60 years (23.7%).

The duration of the current depressive episode was 15.8±18.92 months. All the patients fulfilled *DSM-III* criteria for major depressive disorder; 37 (62.7%) were unipolar, 52 (88.1%) had melancholic features *(DSM-III)*, and 22 (37.3%) fulfilled criteria for psychotic depression (mood congruent delusions and/or hallucinations). It was therefore a group of significantly depressed individuals with prominent endogenous features, a high proportion of concomitant psychosis, and a lengthy period of illness.

Response to Treatment

Forth-four of the 59 patients (74.6%) remitted after treatment in the unit. Remission was defined as an improvement in clinical state sustained for at least 1 month and sufficient to permit discharge from hospital and return to normal, premorbid function. The period to remission in these patients was 3.5±3.17 months. Three patients (5.1%) dropped out prematurely, and 12 did not respond to treatment over a period of 10.6±4.50 months. One of these patients was killed in a motor accident. There were no cases of suicide in the entire sample during the period surveyed.

Tricyclic Antidepressants and Augmenters

Figure 121.1 summarizes the response to treatment trials with TCAs alone and TCAs combined with lithium carbonate and/or neuroleptics. The most frequently used TCA was imipramine (24 trials, 52%) followed by clomipramine (6 trials, 14.3%). A trial considered as adequate lasted a minimum of 4 weeks. TCA serum levels were not monitored, although an attempt was made in all cases to reach the maximum tolerated TCA dosage up to 300 mg/day. Serum level monitoring could well have resulted in some increase in the number of remissions, but it is unlikely to have altered the clear trend toward TCA nonresponse in this group of patients (5 responders in 42 trials, 11.9%).

Lithium supplementation [2,3] was tried in 18 patients on TCA and in 3 patients on TCA + neuroleptic. Thirteen remitted on the TCA + lithium combination (72.2%) and one of three on TCA + neuroleptic + lithium. Remission following lithium supplementation usually required 3–4 weeks of treatment. Four of the responders to TCA + lithium were psychotic, as were the three patients in whom TCA + neuroleptics + lithium was tried (one responder).

Tricyclic antidepressant + neuroleptic treatment was tried in eight patients (all psychotic), two of whom (25%) responded. Other supplements to TCA that were tried were all unsuccessful. The only trial involving substantial numbers was with

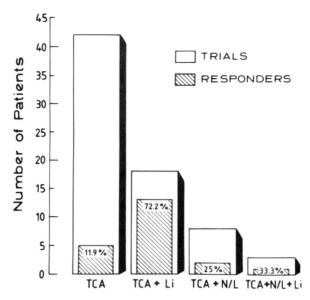

FIGURE 121.1. Treatment outcome: TCA, neuroleptics (N/L), and lithium (Li) augmentation.

estrogen (3.75 mg/day) in 11 cases (one responder). Thyroxine (0.2 mg/day) in six cases, tryptophan (6 g/day) in four cases, and reserpine, phenelzine, and methylphenidate in one or two cases each were all unsuccessful.

Monoamine Oxidase Inhibitors and Augmenters

There were 13 trials of MAOIs (phenelzine in all cases) leading to remission in five cases (38.5%). An attempt was made to reach 90 mg/day in all cases, and treatment was continued at maximum dose for 4 weeks. The percentage inhibition of platelet MAO was not measured and might have improved the response rates.[4] Among five trials of lithium supplementation of phenelzine, only one was successful in achieving remission. A single trial of phenelzine + neuroleptic in a patient with psychotic depression was not successful.

ECT

Electroconvulsive therapy is widely accepted as the treatment of choice in patients nonresponsive to pharmacological treatments of depression.[5] In the present group, ECT was tried in 25 cases and led to remission in 16 (64%). Four responders had undergone unsuccessful ECT trials elsewhere before referral to our unit. ECT was administered bilaterally in all cases using a brief-pulse constant-current apparatus (MECTA model D) with electroencephalography (EEG) and clinical monitoring of seizure duration to ensure a length greater than 25 s. The response rate in our sample (64%) was slightly lower than that reported by Avery and Lubrano[6] in their presentation of the DeCarolis study of ECT efficacy in imipramine nonresponders (72%).

Sixteen of the 25 patients treated with ECT were psychotic; the response rate in this subgroup was 68% (11/16 cases). This figure is also lower than that reported in the DeCarolis study (83%).[6] Differences in the severity of depression and length of illness may partially account for this discrepancy.

It is of interest that patients who do not respond to ECT (or respond partially) may, in our experience, remit following a retrial of antidepressant medication. In the present sample, five of the nine ECT-refractory patients responded to a retrial of TCA alone (clomipramine, four cases; maprotiline, one case) and four to TCAs (clomipramine, three cases; imipramine, one case) potentiated by lithium. In addition, four patients who had not responded to ECT in other centers responded to medication in our unit (phenelzine, one case; imipramine + lithium, two cases; clomipramine + lithium, one case). Medication outcome in ECT-refractory patients is discussed in detail elsewhere,[7] and the possibility that ECT may sensitize refractory patients to antidepressants to which they were previously resistant is considered.

Psychotic Depression

Table 121.1 summarizes the outcome of treatment trials in the 22 patients who were psychotically depressed. Our experience confirms the accepted view that ECT is a highly effective treatment modality for psychotic depression. Response to TCA + neuroleptics was lower than usually reported despite adequate treatment. The effect of lithium augmentation of TCA was striking, remission being achieved in five of six cases, four of them without neuroleptics.

Conclusions

These findings, reflecting the 3-year clinical experience of a unit specializing in the treatment of resistant depression, point to a relatively good prognosis even in patients who have been severely depressed for long periods. The important role of ECT in treating medication-refractory patients was confirmed by our experience. The most important new finding was the striking effect of lithium in potentiating TCA reponse. In this regard three points of interest emerged: (a) efficacy of the combination in patients with psychotic depression even in the absence of concomitant neuroleptics; (b) efficacy in patients refractory to ECT; and (c) the need for a lithium trial longer than that suggested by previous reports.

Acknowledgment. Supported in part by NIMH grant MH-40734.

TABLE 121.1. Treatment outcome in psychotic depression.

Treatment	No. of trials	No. of responders	% Response
ECT	16	11	68.0
TCA + neuroleptic	8	2	25.0
TCA	6	1	16.6
TCA + lithium	4	4	100.0
TCA + neuroleptic + lithium	2	1	50.0

References

1. Roose SP, Glassman AH, Walsh BT, et al. Tricyclic nonresponders: phenomenology and treatment. Am J Psychiatry 1986;143:345–348.
2. Heninger GR, Charney DS, Sternberg DE. Lithium carbonate augmentation of antidepressant treatment. Arch Gen Psychiatry 1983;40:1335–1342.
3. De Montigny C, Cournoyer G, Morissette R, et al. Lithium carbonate addition in tricyclic antidepressant-resistant unipolar depression. Arch Gen Psychiatry 1983;40:1327–1334.
4. Robinson DS, Nies A, Ravaris L, et al. Clinical pharmacology of phenelzine. Arch Gen Psychiatry 1978;35:629–635.
5. Consensus conference, electroconvulsive therapy. JAMA 1985;254:2103–2108.
6. Avery D, Lubrano. A. Depression treated with imipramine and ECT: the DeCarolis study reconsidered. Am J Psychiatry 1979;136:559–562.
7. Shapira B, Kindler S, Lerer B. Medication outcome in ECT-resistant depression. Convulsive Therapy, in Press.

122. Clinical Indicators in Resistant Depressions

H. DUFOUR, P. THERMOZ, AND J.C. SAMUELIAN

Several years after antidepressant drugs came into use general optimism gradually abated. One patient in three does not respond to an initial antidepressant treatment, thus defining the notion of relative resistance. One patient in ten is totally resistant to all proposed therapies, an absolute resistance that invariably leads to chronic depression.

Early in the history of antidepressant drugs, many studies attempted to define the predictive clinical indicators for good response to treatment and hence to guide therapeutic choice. These studies did not always produce the results hoped for.

The retrospective study reported here involved a group of depressed inpatients treated in the Department of Psychiatry, University of Marseille. The aim was to study some predictive indicators of clinical response to one antidepressant treatment during 1985 and 1986.

Methods

The group studied was heterogeneous from a diagnostic point of view. The notion of resistance was defined as total or partial failure of a well managed antidepressant treatment prescribed during hospitalization. This definition is fairly similar to Heimann's notion[1] of relative resistance. Absolute resistance, i.e., failure following several attempts of antidepressant treatment and electroconvulsive therapy (ECT), could not be studied. However, some patients were administered antidepressants and then ECT, after which they were assessed.

The department's computerized files gave us some semeiological characteristics of acute depression, using the ICD-9 diagnostic classification. Initial severity and evoluation under treatment were assessed using a CGI scale. The antidepressants were tricyclic antidepressants (TCAs) prescribed in reported efficacious dosage (without pharmacokinetic control) for 4 weeks or more.

Results

A total of 281 patients were admitted for affective disorder; 52 patients were dropouts, and 33% of the remainder were resistant after a single antidepressant treatment. This percentage is common in the psychiatric literature. Male patients ap-

Table 122.1. Clinical symptoms as resistance indicators.

Symptoms	Resistant	Nonresistant	Total
Restlessness	07 (38.8%)	11	18
Delusion	07 (41.1%)	10	17
Suicidal	20 (33.0%)	40	60
Major anxiety	34 (39.6%)	52	86
Alcohol (chronic)	11 (57.9%)	08	19
Organic disease	12 (28.0%)	32	44
Marital status	51 (38.9%)	80	131

peared more difficult to treat, as in Kuhn's original study with imipramine.[2] The average age of 48 years was the same in the two groups.

Slight and severe depression, with respective percentages of 44% and 38.5%, provided the worst prognosis. Table 122.1 shows the predictive semeiological resistance indicators. Table 122.2 shows the predictive nosographical indicators of resistance. A small group of patients ($n = 10$) did not improve or even worsened on TCAs. Eight improved following an ECT series; among them, five had unipolar melancholia and three bipolar melancholia.

Discussion

Numerous studies have been devoted to clinical data predictive of resistance, but studies substantiating their prediction prior to treatment and giving the actual predictive value of the parameter investigated have been rare. These methodological factors may partially account for the contradictory results often found.[3] However, from the amalgam of uncertain results, some indicators appear interesting.

Phenomenology of Depression

Delusions clearly respond poorly to TCA treatment. Amitriptyline does not worsen delusional symptoms but is no more effective than other TCAs. The repeated failure of TCAs suggests to most authors the immediate use of ECT. According to Davidson et al.,[4] the term "endogenous" is not a useful predictive criterion, as it combines two distinct populations—delusional and nondelusional—who respond differently to TCA drugs. In the opinion of Sweeney et al.,[5] this phenomenon raises the question of the nature of delusional melancholia: Is it a delusional or an affective disorder? This question seems justified, as delusional melancholias always relapse in the same way and are hardly ever standard affective disorders.

Table A 122.2. Nosographical predictive resistance indicators.

Nosography	(O.M.S.)	Resistant	Nonresistant	Total
Total patients		76 (33%)	153	229
Neurotic depression	(300.4)	36 (33%)	73	109
Brief depressive reaction	(309.0)	4 (15.5%)	22	26
Prolonged depressive reaction	(309.1)	6 (30%)	14	20
Unipolar melancholia	(296.1)	18 (39%)	28	46
Bipolar melancholia	(296.3)	5 (35.7%)	9	14
Schizodepressive disorders	(298.0)	5 (41.6%)	7	12
Dysthymia	(301.1)	2 (100%)	0	2

Seriousness is rather difficult to circumscribe or to quantify. Despite these uncertainties, some studies suggest that seriousness and poor response to treatment are not synonymous,[2] and that the best responders have an average score on the Newcastle scale.[6]

Restlessness, anxiety, and the presence of suicidal ideas are much debated response indicators. Age and sex have been reported to be without influence by most authors. Affective disorders in older patients are a problem for the therapist especially because of the semeiological expression they may present. Moreover, the elderly subjects metabolic conditions makes it difficult to manage a treatment with psychotropic drugs. Marital status remain a debated indicator. As a rule, marriage protects from the occurrence of affective disorder. However, Keller et al.'s study[7] shows it as a resistance indicator when depression is already present.

There are few reliable studies concerning associated chronic alcoholism because, as underlined by Leyhman,[8] alcoholics are usually excluded from clinical trials using TCA drugs. This factor has effects on two levels. On the one hand, alcoholic behavior leads to poor compliance and dangerous side effects; on the other hand, it is associated with cerebral consequences that may induce affective disorders.

According to numerous authors,[3] degenerative neurological conditions have frequently been held responsible for resistance. The same applies to hypothyroidism.

Predictive Nosographical Indicators

In 1957, Kuhn, in his initial report on imipramine,[2] stated that endogenous depressions had a better response than nonendogenous ones, an assertion that has been adopted by most authors. The statement is essentially based on imipramine treatment and requires reconsideration when other TCA drugs are used. Today, the well known best response equation with endogenous depression deserves revision. Many authors[9] agree that therapeutic response is statistically equal in different nosographical groups; thus nosography has no predictive value. Moreover, the group with neurotic depression may appear to be without clinical identity. Akistal et al.'s studies[10] on the long-term outcome of neurotic depression indicated the heterogeneity of this group and emphazised the idea of nosographical blur.

Conclusions

Most of our results agree with the data in the literature. However, the nosographical data had surprisingly little value in endogenous depressions. These figures should be moderated, as many of these melancholic patients were already treatment-resistant when they came to us.

Finally, the question of absolute resistance was not investigated in our study. A thorough study of these difficult cases would certainly raise major methodological questions but might shed new light on the concept of resistance.

References

1. Heimann H. Therapy resistant depression: symptoms and syndromes. Pharmacol Psychiatry 1974;7:139–144.
2. Kuhn R. Du traitement des etats depressifs par un dérivé de l'lminodibenzyle (G 22355). J Suisse Med 1957;89-35.36:1135–1140.

3. Zarifian E, Loo H. Les Antidépresseurs. Roche ed., 1982.
4. Davidson J, Mac Leod M. Low Yone B. A comparison of E.C.T. and combined phe-nelzine-amitriptyline in refractory depression. Arch Gen Psychiatry 1978;35:639–642.
5. Sweeney D, Nelson C, Bowers M. Delusional versus non delusional depression: neuro chemical differences. Lancet 1978; 2:200–201.
6. Ramarao, Coppen A. Classification of depression and response to amitriptyline. Psychom Med 1976;6:59–70.
7. Keller MB, Lavori P, Levis. Predictor of relapse in major depressive disorders. JAMA 1983; 250:3299–3304.
8. Leyhman, Therapy resistant depression: a clinical classification. Pharmacopsychiatry 1974;7:156–163.
9. Tissot R. Indicateurs biologiques et prise de décision thérapeutiques. Psychol Med 1984; 16:622–631.
10. Akiskal HS, Bitar AH, Puzantian VR. The nosological statues of neurotic depression: a prospective 3–4 years follow up examination in the light of primary secondary and unipolar-bipolar dichotomies. Arch Gen Psychiatry 1978;35:756–766.

123. Combined MAO Inhibitor and Tri/Tetracyclic Antidepressant Treatment in Therapy-Resistant Depression

M. Schmauss, H.P. Kapfhammer, and P. Hoff

Once rarely prescribed because of the fear of severe complications such as hypertensive crises, hyperthermia, and delirium, the monoamine oxidase (MAO) inhibitors have gained renewed interest for the therapy of depressive disorders. On the one hand, it might be due to the fact that prevention through strong dietary precautions has decreased the incidence of adverse reactions[1,2]; on the other hand, there is evidence that MAO inhibitors may have a unique role in the therapy of many depressed patients who respond poorly to alternative treatments.[1-4] One aspect of using MAO inhibitors—combining them with tricyclic antidepressants in the treatment of therapy-resistant depression—has always been controversially discussed with regard to its unusual toxicity[5-7] and efficacy.[8-12]

Theoretical considerations suggest that such a combined regimen might lead to a more frequent, more rapid, and more pronounced improvement in depressive symptomatology in comparison to a monotherapy. The mechanism, assumed for the possible potentiation of tricyclics by MAO inhibitors, is the combined effect of tricyclic-mediated uptake inhibition and enzyme inhibition following the MAO inhibitor.

The aim of this retrospective study was to obtain detailed information about the safety and efficacy of combined tri/tetracyclic (TCA) and tranylcypromine antidepressant treatment in therapy-resistant depressed inpatients. "Therapy resistant" was defined as at least two unsuccessful single-drug tri/tetracyclic treatments over a period of 3–4 weeks each.

Subjects

A review was made of the charts of all inpatients treated on the combined regimen in the Department of Psychiatry, University of Munich, between January 1977 and June 1981. There were 94 patients; 78 of them were suffering from a depressive episode within a monopolar depression (ICD 296.1), 13 from a depressive episode within a bipolar disorder (ICD 296.3), two from a neurotic depression (ICD 300.4), and one from a depressive syndrome within an organic depression.

Methods

Therapeutic outcome and side effects were measured as described in a previous report.[13]

Results

In all cases tranylcypromine, in a fixed combination with a small amount (1 mg) of the neuroleptic trifluoperazin (Jatrosom), was used as the MAO inhibitor. The procedure used in all cases for administering the combined TCA–MAO inhibitor treatment was the following: After at least 7 weeks of TCA treatment patients received 10 mg of tranylcypromine, gradually increasing this dosage up to a maximum of 30 mg. The daily dosage of tranylcypromine ranged between 10 and 30 mg with a mean dose of 13 mg/day.

Tranylcypromine was combined with amitriptyline in 37 patients, imipramine in 20 patients, dibenzepine in 14 patients, nomifensine in 6 patients, mianserin in 8 patients, doxepine in 4 patients, chlorimipramine in 2 patients, lofepramine in 2 patients, and maprotiline in 1 patient. Mean daily dose and dosage range of these antidepressants did not differ significantly when comparing single with combined antidepressant treatment. Amitriptyline, for example, was administered as a single drug in a mean daily dose of 179.2 mg with a dosage range of 75–250 mg; in combination with tranylcypromine its mean daily dose was 152.8 mg with a dosage range of 75–250 mg. The mean daily dose of imipramine was 193.3 mg when given as a single drug and increased to a mean daily dose of 222 mg in combined therapy, the dosage range in both treatment groups being 50–300 mg.

As to the efficacy of combined antidepressant treatment, within a mean treatment period of 21.9 days 31% of the patients demonstrated a very good and 37% of the patients a good response to combined treatment, the most effective combination being amitriptyline + tranylcypromine, with a very good therapeutic response in 51% and a good therapeutic response in 27% of the patients, followed by the combination of other tricyclics such as imipramine, doxepine, and dibenzepine + tranylcypromine with a very good or good therapeutic response in about 60% of the patients.

In general, the combined treatment produced a slightly but not significantly lower frequency of side effects (1.56 per treatment) than did the single antidepressant treatments (1.84 per treatment). Combining tranylcypromine with chlorimipramine and nomifensine, however, led to an increase of side effects; in the case of nomifensine this increase was especially due to abnormalities in laboratory parameters and vegetative side effects. A reduction of side effects was seen after combining tranylcypromine with dibenzepine, doxepine, and especially amitriptyline. Combining these drugs produced a lower frequency of all classes of side effects—cardiovascular, central nervous system, vegetative, laboratory, and others—than did single amitriptyline treatment.

Throughout all single drug and combined treatments, close monitoring of patients' physical status, including vital signs, uncovered no occurrence of a hyperthermic crisis in any patient.

In four of the 94 patients, however, combined TCA–MAO inhibitor had to be discontinued because of other adverse reactions. A 54-year-old woman treated with 150 mg amitriptyline and 10 mg tranylcypromine complained about severe headache; a 53-year-old woman treated with 150 mg imipramine and 20 mg tranylcypromine indicated a weight gain of 10 kg within 20 days; a 44-year-old woman experienced four orthostatic dysregulations within 24 h after taking 100 mg chlorimipramine and 20 mg tranylcypromine; and a 73-year-old woman treated with 240 mg lofepramine, 20 mg tranylcypromine, and lithium experienced a hypertensive crisis (blood pressure [BP] 200/100). For patients receiving single tri/teracyclic antidepressant treatments there were nonsignificant drops in sitting systolic BP (except a nonsignificant increase in the mianserin group) and nonsignificant changes in sitting diastolic BP compared with baseline. Patients receiving combined treatment demonstrated nonsignificant drops in sitting systolic BP as well as diastolic BP in the amitriptyline, mianserin, doxepin, chlorimipramine, lofepramine, and maprotiline groups and nonsignificant increases in sitting systolic BP as well as diastolic BP in the dibenzepine and nomifensine groups. Only combining imipramine + tranylcypromine produced a significant ($p<0.05$) increase in diastolic BP compared with diastolic BP during single imipramine treatment.

Changes in heart rate reached significance during treatment with both the single tri/tetracyclic and the combined regimens. Weight gain was documented in all single tri/tetracyclic and combined treatments, being significant for the single imipramine ($p < 0.001$) and amitriptyline ($p < 0.01$) treatment and the combined amitriptyline + tranylcypromine ($p < 0.05$) treatment.

Discussion

Our retrospective study supports the general safety of combined TCA–MAO inhibitor treatment and is in agreement with some other studies.[9,14–19] Ananth and Luchins[5] concluded that "from the available evidence it appears that combined treatment if properly administered leads to neither serious complications nor an inordinate number of minor side effects." In these studies a great variety of MAO inhibitors (e.g., isocarboxazid, iproniazid, phenelzine sulfate, and tranylcypromine) and TCAs (e.g., amitriptyline, imipramine, and trimipramine) were used, whereas in our study only one MAO inhibitor, tranylcypromine, was combined with different tri/tetracyclic and "second generation" antidepressants, the most frequently used being amitriptyline, imipramine, and dibenzepine. The incidence of side effects with these drugs was lower on the combined regimen compared to the monotherapy, whereas nomifensine and chlorimipramine demonstrated a higher incidence of side effects in combination therapy. As to chlorimipramine, our results of a small sample size are in agreement with the other clinical findings[20–22] and some pharmacological data,[7,23] indicating that primarily serotonin (5-hydroxytryptamine, 5-HT) reuptake inhibiting tricyclics such as chlorimipramine may have a higher incidence of side effects in combination with MAO inhibitors.

As to the efficacy of combined treatment, our study confirms the results of several open studies[8–11,15,24,25] suggesting that this treatment benefits a great number of patients refractory to alternative treatments. However, these results are not supported by several controlled clinical studies,[26–29] indicating the combined treatment to be only as effective as single TCA therapy alone.

When discussing the results of the controlled studies in comparison to the open studies, however, it must be mentioned that three of the four controlled studies were done in patients not specifically selected as refractory to treatment. This condition might explain the fact that in these studies combined therapy proved as effective as single tricyclic antidepressant treatment. The main indication for combined TCA–MAO inhibitor treatment at present seems to be in refractory depression where several alternative treatments have proved unsatisfactory.[30]

Acknowledgment. This study was supported by the Federal Health Agency (Bundesgesundheitsamt), Berlin, West Germany.

References

1. Tollefson GD. Monoamine oxidase inhibitors: a review. J Clin Psychiatry 1983;44:280–288.
2. Pare CMB. The present status of monoamine oxidase inhibitors. Br J Psychiatry 1985;146:576–584.
3. Outkin F, Rifkin A, Klein DF. Monoamine oxidase inhibitors: a review of antidepressant effectiveness. Arch Gen Psychiatry 1979;36:749–760.
4. White K, Simpson G. Combined MAOI tricyclic antidepressant treatment: a reevalution. J Clin Psychopharmacol 1981;1:264–282.
5. Ananth J, Luchins D. A review of combined tricyclic and MAOI therapy. Compr Psychiatry 1977;18:121–130.
6. Caglieri-Cingolani R, Bencini A. Due case mortali di reazione tossica per assoziazione di farmaci antidepressivi inhibitori delle mono-amino-ossidase e tricyclici. Riv Pat Nerv Ment 1982;103:21–31.
7. Marley E, Wozniak KM. Clinical and experimental aspects of interactions between amine oxidase inhibitors and amine reuptake inhibitors. Psychol Med 1983;13:735–749.
8. Gander DR. The clinical value of monoamine oxidase inhibitors and tricyclic antidepressants in combination, In Garattini S, Dukes MNG (eds): Antidepressant Drugs. Amsterdam: Excerpta Medica, 1967.
9. Goldberg RS, Thornton, WE. Combined tricyclic MAOI therapy for refractory depression: a review, with guidelines for appropriate usage. J Clin Pharmacol 1978;18:143–147.
10. Ray I. Combinations of antidepressant drugs in the treatment of depressive illness. Can Psychiatr Assoc J 1973;18:399–402.
11. Winston F. Combined antidepressant therapy. Br J Psychiatry 1971;118:301–304.
12. Kupfer DJ, Detre TP. Tricyclic and monoamine-oxidase inhibitor antidepressants: clinical use. In Iversen[LL], Iversen[SD], Snyder[SH] (eds): Handbook of Psychopharmacology. Vol. 14. New York: Plenum Press, 1978;199–232.
13. Schmauss M, Kapfhammer, HP, Meyr P, et al. Combined MAO-inhibitor and TCA antidepressant treatment in therapy resistant depression. Pharmacopsychiatry 1986;19:251–252.
14. Ayd FJ Jr. Psychotropic drug combinations: good and bad. In Greenblatt M (ed): Drugs in Combination with Other Therapies. New York: Grune & Stratton, 1975.
15. Kelly D, Cuirgius W, Frommer E, et al. Treatment of phobic states with antidepressants. Br J Psychiatry 1970;116:387–398.
16. Ponto LB, Perry PJ, Liskow BI, et al. Drug therapy reviews: tricyclic antidepressants and monoamine oxidase inhibitor combination therapy. Am J Hosp Pharm 1977;34:955–961.
17. Schuckit M, Robins E, Feighner J. Tricyclic antidepressants and monoamine oxidase inhibitors. Arch Gen Psychiatry 1971;24:509–514.
18. Sethna ER. A study of refractory cases of depressive illness and their response to combined antidepressant treatment. Br J Psychiatry 1974;124:265–272.
19. Snowdon L, Braithewaite R. Combined antidepressant medication. Br J Psychiatry 1974;125:610–611.
20. Beaumont G. Clomipramine in the treatment of pain, enuresis and anorexia nervosa. J Int Med Res 1973;1:435–437.
21. Pare CMB Monoamine oxidase inhibitors in resistant depression. Int Pharmacopsychiatry 1979;14:101–109.
22. von Oefele K, Grohmann R, Rüther E. Adverse drug reactions in combined tricyclic and MAOI therapy. Pharmacopsychiatry 1986;19:243–244.

23. Graham PM, Potter JM, Patterson JW. Combination monoamine oxidase inhibitor tricyclic antidepressant interaction. Lancet 1982;2:440.
24. Spiker DG, Pugh DD. Combining tricyclic and monoamine oxidase inhibitor antidepressants. Arch Gen Psychiatry 1976;33:828–830.
25. Sargant W, Walter CJS, Wright N. New treatment of some chronic tension states. Br Med J 1966;1:322–324.
26. Davidson J, McLeod M, Law-Yone B, et al. A comparison of electroconvulsive therapy and combined phenelzine-amitriptyline in refractory depression. Arch Gen Psychiatry 1978;35:639–642.
27. Young JPR, Lader MH, Hughes WC. Controlled trial of trimipramine, monoamine oxidase inhibitors, and combined treatment in depressed outpatients. Br Med J 1979;2:1315–1317.
28. Razani J, White K, White J, et al. The safety and efficacy of combined amitriptyline and tranylcypromine antidepressant treatment. Arch Gen Psychiatry 1983;40:657–661.
29. White K, Pistole T, Boyd J. Combined monoamine oxidase inhibitor tricyclic antidepressant treatment: a pilot study. Am J Psychiatry 1980;137:1422–1425.
30. White K, Simpson G. Should the use of MAO inhibitors be abandoned. Integr Psychiatry 1985;3:34–45.

124. Management of Resistant Major Depression

P.K. BRIDGES

There is a pervading resistance in psychiatry to the adequate use of medication. Treatment-resistant depressive illnesses are widely accepted as such with little clinical challenge, although a good deal can usually be done to help patients with these distressing conditions. Two possible reasons for this tolerance of apparent untreatability are that (a) psychiatric disorders have a tradition of chronicity and (b) not all clinicians are inspired by the advent of psychopharmacology, which has offered potent treatment for illnesses that were previously hopeless. It is certain that many psychiatrists are mainly interested in psychodynamic approaches, which were likely to have been of prime importance during their training, and they tend to use medication only as adjunctive treatment.

There is confusion as to what are treatment-resistant affective disorders. How can they be defined? The concept obviously has something to do with an illness that responds inadequately to treatment, but it is better expressed as a lack of response to adequate treatment. The next question is, then, what constitutes adequate treatment?

The Geoffrey Knight Unit for Affective Disorders remains one of the few departments still carrying out psychosurgery on a regular basis. The operation used, stereotactic subcaudate tractotomy,[1] is a highly effective treatment of last resort for resistant depression, and this refined technique carries few risks. Its indications have been given by Bartlett et al.[2] Although there is little convincingly scientific evidence of its effectiveness, the clinical results can be remarkable. For example, about a year ago there were admitted almost consecutively, three female patients, two of whom required individual nursing day and night in order to control intense suicidal ideation; the third similarly needed a relative with her during each day. There was a fourth patient, a man, whose weight was down to nearly half the normal for him, and he was dying from chronic, refractory depressive anorexia. One month after the operation, the three female patients could revert to normal nursing and the man was eating well. One year later all had been discharged from hospital, and their depressive illnesses were well controlled. There is understandable reluctance to use surgery for psychiatric illnesses, however, and hence there is a need to ensure that all other reasonable treatments have been tried without success before a patient is referred.

Over a period of about 20 years we have carried out around 1,200 operations, which means that nearly 2,000 patients from all over Britain have been assessed because only two-thirds of those referred are accepted for psychosurgery. It means also that we have unusual experience in terms of what constitutes adequate treatment in the view of a large number of British psychiatrists and which treatments have failed before patients are referred for surgery. There is no doubt that, in the considerable majority of cases the adequacy of therapy is expressed as a function of the number of different antidepressants used, with no emphasis on the highest dose given.[3]

With few exceptions, the highest dose of tricyclic antidepressants tried before referring for psychosurgery is 150 mg daily and about 40% of patients referred have never received more than 100 mg daily. A World Health Organization collaborative study[4] sought to investigate if there were differences in the effects of high and low dose prescribing. The study involved 324 patients at seven centers in five countries. Although no significant differences were found, the study was surely of limited value because the low dose was not more than 75 mg/day and the high dose only up to 150 mg/day.

This underuse and even misunderstanding of medication is psychiatry probably results from the psychodynamic tradition that was firmly established before the advent of modern psychopharmacology during the 1950s and from the considerable influence of the nonmedical and nonnursing professions.[5] Many involved with the treatment of psychiatric disorders have a conviction that help is primarily needed with environmental difficulties, personal conflicts, and social adjustment. Medication is regarded as essentially undesirable and, at best, of only secondary value. Yet there is accumulating evidence that some conditions, especially schizophrenia and the affective disorders, can be brought under control only with medication and that the medication has to be at an adequate dosage. For depressive illnesses not responding to the usual doses of antidepressants, it has been shown that recovery can nonetheless occur with combined medication and with doses of antidepressants well above the usual.[6] Hale et al.[6] reported the value of high dose tricyclic antidepressants, e.g., clomipramine 300–400 mg daily, especially when used with lithium and L-tryptophan.

For the adequate treatment of affective disorders it is important to recognize that psychosurgery is not a bizarre treatment for bizarre psychiatric disorders. It is mainly a treatment for affective disorders and is at the end of the therapeutic continuum beginning with antidepressants (Table 124.1).

If major depression involves a metabolic abnormality, as is often suggested, patients would be best selected for psychosurgery who were positive for a biological marker of the abnormality. There is, however, no reliable marker available at

TABLE 124.1. Treatments for endogenous depression.

Antidepressant medication (introduced during the 1950's): Suppresses symptoms during an episode of depression, but the episode is not terminated; hence relapse occurs if the medication is stopped too soon.

Electroconvulsive therapy (introduced in 1938): Terminates an episode but does not avoid another episode occurring later on.

Psychosurgery (introduced in 1935): Curative. Over a period of weeks or months terminates an episode of depression, and there is usually no recurrence.

present. The dexamethasone suppression test[7] seems to be falling from favor, but a tyramine test is currently showing promise.[8] However, in the absence of such an investigation, we depend to some extent on previous response to antidepressants and/or electroconvulsive therapy. Most patients who do well after psychosurgery have previously responded to these other physical treatments but then fail to respond, whereas most patients with recurrent depression continue to respond variably throughout their lives. We would be unlikely to accept for an operation a patient who had never responded to any physical treatments.

The conclusion is that no severe affective illness can be regarded as treatment-resistant until high dose and combined antidepressants have been tried and until psychosurgery has at least been considered.

References

1. Goktepe EO, Young LB, Bridges PK. A further review of the results of stereotactic subcaudate tractotomy. Br J Psychiatry 1975;126:270–280.
2. Bartlett JR, Bridges PK, Kelly D. Contemporary indications for psychosurgery. Br J Psychiatry 1981;38:507–511.
3. Bridges PK. . . . and a small dose of antidepressant might help. Br J Psychiatry 1983;142:626–628.
4. World Health Organization Collaborative Study. Dose effects of antidepressant medication in different populations. J Affective Disord 1986(suppl 2):51–567.
5. Bridges PK. Psychiatry for all. J R Soc Med 1984;77:911–914.
6. Hale AS, Proctor A, Bridges PK. Clomipramine, tryptophan and lithium in combination for resistant depression: seven case studies. Br J Psychiatry 1987;151:213–217.
7. Carroll BJ. Dexamethasone suppression test—a review of contemporary confusion. J Clin Psychiatry 1985;46:13–24.
8. Hale AS, Walker PL, Bridges PK, Sandler M. Tyramine conjugation deficit as a trait-marker in endogenous depressive illness. J Psychiatr Res 1986;20:251–226.

V.D. ANTIDEPRESSANTS IN CLINICAL PRACTICE: PLACEBO RESPONSE IN DEPRESSION

125. Clinical Characteristics of Placebo Response in Depression

C.J. FAIRCHILD AND A.J. RUSH

Placebo effect went unnoticed for centuries and undoubtedly accounted for the transient popularity of many ineffective medical treatments. Randomized double-blind placebo-controlled drug studies have emphasized the wide range of effectiveness of placebo. It was found to be effective in diseases of every organ system. One-third of major depressives treated with placebo experience decreases in the symptoms of dysphoria, suicidal ideation, insomnia, and weight loss.[1]

Placebo responsiveness is not yet predictable. To characterize which depressives are most likely to respond to placebo, two retrospective descriptive studies were conducted at the University of Texas Health Science Center at Dallas. All subjects met Research Diagnostic Criteria (RDC) for nonpsychotic unipolar major depression, diagnosed by two independent interviewers using the structured diagnostic interview: the Schedule for Affective Disorders and Schizophrenia Lifetime Version[2] (SADS-L). The 17-item Hamilton Rating Scale for Depression[3] (HRSD) was utilized to measure sympton severity.

Study I

The first study compared the characteristics of placebo responders to those of placebo nonresponders. Fifty-five unipolar depressed patients participated in a drug study in which all subjects were treated initially with placebo in a single-blind 1- to 3-week treatment period. Sixteen patients (29%) had a reduction in their HRSD of 50% and were categorized as early placebo responders. The remaining subjects participated in a double-blind treatment in which they were randomly assigned to treatment with an antidepressant or placebo. Five of these placebo-treated patients also had a 50% reduction in HRSD and were categorized as late placebo responders. The remaining subjects, who failed to recover with placebo treatment in either the single- or double-blind placebo treatment, comprised the placebo nonresponder group ($n = 34$). Early and late placebo responders were compared by χ^2 and t-test for all variables. No significance between group differences were found. Early and late responders were combined to form the placebo responder group ($n = 21$).

Placebo responders and nonresponders were compared with regard to demographic, history of illness, diagnostic, and current episode features. Student's t-test and χ^2 were used to compare variables. Discriminant function analysis was used to identify predictors of placebo responsiveness and the relative contribution of these predictors.

Placebo responders and nonresponders did not differ significantly in age, education, marital status, or occupation. Placebo responders reported a significantly shorter history of illness, defined as the time (in months) since the onset of the first episode of major depression (Table 125.1). However, placebo responders and nonresponders reported an equivalent number of episodes of major depression and suicide attempts.

Diagnostic parameters distinguished placebo responders. Ninety-five percent of placebo responders and 50% of the nonresponders were nonendogenous (χ^2 11.7, $p<0.01$). Other psychiatric disorders (either concurrently or in the past) occurred more frequently in placebo responders (85.7%) than nonresponders (44.1%) (χ^2 9.36, $p<0.02$). There was a high frequency of anxiety and abusive disorders among placebo responders.

Features of the current depressive episode also distinguished placebo responders from nonresponders. The speed of onset of the current episode of depression and the length of the current episode did not distinguish placebo responders from nonresponders. Clinician's ratings of symptom severity (HRSD, Covi Global Anxiety Scale,[4] Raskin Depression Scale[5]) also showed no significant differences. However, patients' self-report scales of symptomatology before treatment revealed that responders experienced less severe depression according to the Carroll Rating Scale[6] (CRS) and the Beck Depression Inventory[7] (BDI).

A stepwise discriminant function analysis was performed on the subjects, loading all variables. Items selected included (in weighted order) endogenous/nonendogenous dichotomy, length of illness, and presence of abusive disorders. Placebo responders were more often nonendogenous, with a history of abuse disorders

TABLE 125.1. Study I: Clinical features of placebo responders ($n = 21$) and nonresponders (n 34).

Feature	Responders (mean±SD)	Nonresponders (mean±SD)
History		
Length of illness (months)[a]	40.2±46.1	83.6±99.9
Length of current episode (months)	20.9±16.5	50.1±87.2
Diagnostics		
Nonendogenous[b]	95.2	50.0
Concurrent diagnosis[c]	85.7	44.1
Anxiety disorders[a]	52.4	23.5
Personality disorders	23.8	8.8
Substance abuse[a]	33.3	2.9
Other	9.5	20.5
Severity measures		
HRSD	23.8±4.7	25.5±5.0
BDI[c]	25.6±7.1	32.6±9.1
CRS[a]	29.9±6.2	34.1±6.1

[a]$p<0.05$.
[b]$p<0.001$.
[c]$p<0.01$.

and a shorter length of illness. These three variables correctly classified 85.7% of placebo responders and 76.5% of the nonresponders.

A second stepwise discriminant function analysis was performed on the individual items of the BDI. Two questions (Nos. 15 and 14) discriminated placebo responders from nonresponders: Placebo responders had perceived no change in their personal appearance, whereas placebo nonresponders indicated a deterioration in their personal appearance. Furthermore, nonresponders reported that they frequently had to push themselves very hard to work or to do anything. These two BDI questions correctly classified 75.8% of the placebo responders and 73.8% of placebo nonresponders.

In summary, placebo responders tended to be nonendogenous depressives complicated by other psychiatric diagnoses, lower self-report depression ratings, and a shorter length of illness.

Study II

Placebo responsiveness is reported to be more rapid in onset and less stable in comparison to tricyclic antidepressant responsiveness.[8] Certainly rapid recovery is noted in placebo washout periods in many drugs trials and in study I. Our second study tested the early and unstable placebo remission hypothesis in late placebo responders. The pattern of recovery of unipolar depressed patients treated with amitriptyline versus those treated with placebo were compared by repeated measures analysis of covariance of weekly HRSD and CRS. The study populations consisted of two groups of unipolar depressives who participated in a 6-week randomized double-blind drug study. Subjects who did not recover during the study period were eliminated from the final analysis.

The final study population consisted of 14 subjects treated with amitriptyline and nine subjects treated with placebo. The groups were similar with regard to age and sex. Diagnostically, the placebo responders of this study population were similar to the first study population. Endogenous depression occurred in 92.8% of the amitriptyline remitters and 44% of the placebo remitters. A previous or concurrent psychiatric diagnosis was identified in 77.7% of the placebo-treated subjects and 35.7% of the amitriptyline-treated patients.

Weekly HRSDs were analyzed by repeated measures analysis of covariance with the pretreatment HRSD covariant. No group differences were detected across time, nor was there a significant interaction of group and time (Table 125.2).

TABLE 125.2. Study II: Mean weekly severity measures in amitriptyline ($n = 14$) and placebo ($n = 9$) remitters.

	HRSD		CRS	
Week	Amitriptyline	Placebo	Amitriptyline	Placebo
0	25.7	22.7	27.4	25.8
1	15.9	12.8	20.4	16.2
2	9.6	8.9	16.8	13.0
3	9.8	8.8	14.1	11.6
4	7.1	6.1	11.0	9.4
5	6.7	8.1	9.4	9.9
6	4.1	4.5	8.1	7.6

Similarly, the weekly CRSs were analyzed by repeated measures analysis of convariance with pretreatment CRS covariant. No significant group differences were detected across time, nor was there a significant interaction of group and time.

Conclusions

Depressed patients who respond to placebo are likely to be of any age, sex, marital status, or occupation. Demographic features do not distinguish the placebo responder. To the clinician, placebo responders appear as ill as placebo nonresponders; clinician severity scales do not distinguish placebo responders from nonresponders. Additionally, late placebo responders recover from depression in a manner similar to that of patients treated with a tricyclic antidepressant. Placebo responders distinguished themselves from placebo nonresponders in several ways. Placebo responders endorsed less severe depressive symptomatology on self-report symptom scales, the BDI and CRS. A history of other psychiatric diagnoses also distinguished placebo responders and nonresponders, especially those with anxiety and substance abuse disorders.

The endogenously depressed patients did not respond to placebo as frequently as the nonendogenous patients, a finding that has been frequently reported in the literature. The lack of endogenous features does not ensure placebo response, however, as 50% of the placebo nonresponders were nonendogenous.

Finally, the length of illness discriminated placebo responders from nonresponders. Those with a shorter length of illness were more likely to be placebo responders. Perhaps the longer persistence of symptoms (if first episode) or the recurrence of symptoms results in more frequent treatment exposure, which over time reduces the incidence of placebo responders. Placebo is less effective in more chronic than acute depressions.

The value of extended placebo research lies in the evaluation of new pharmacological treatments of depression, where the question in whether a response is primarily biochemical or psychological. If placebo responsiveness is viewed as the opposite side of the treatment coin, presumably placebo research can help the physician decide who is not a candidate for drug treatment. The conclusion of this study is that the endogenously depressed patient uncomplicated by another diagnosis is the most likely candidate for antidepressant treatment.

References

1. Ansom C, DeBacker-Dierch G, Vereechen JLTM. Sleep disorders in patients with severe mental depressions: double-blind placebo-controlled evaluation of the value of pipamperone (Dipiperon). Acta Psychiatr Scand 1977;55:116–122.
2. Endicott J, Spitzer RL. A diagnostic interview: the Schedule for Affective Disorders and Schizophrenia—Lifetime Version. Arch Gen Psychiatry 1978;35:837–844.
3. Hamilton M. A rating scale for depression. J Neurol Neurosurg Psychiatry 1960;23:56–62.
4. Covi L, Lipman R, McNair DM, et al. Symptomatic volunteers in multicenter drug trials. Prog Neuropsychopharmacol 1979;3:521–533.
5. Raskin A, Shulterbrandt JG, Reating N, et al. Differential response to chlorpromazine; imipramine and placebo: a study of subgroups of hospitalized depressed patients. Arch Gen Psychiatry 1970;23:164–173.

6. Carroll BJ, Feinberg M, Smouse PE, et al. The Carroll Rating Scale for depression. I. Development, reliability and validity. Br J Psychiatry 1981;138:194–209.
7. Beck AT, Ward CH, Mendelson M, et al. An inventory for measuring depression. Arch Gen Psychiatry 1961;4:561–571.
8. Quitkin FM, Rabkin JG, Ross D, et al. Identification of true drug response to antidepressants: use of pattern analysis. Arch Gen Psychiatry 1984;41:782–786.

126. Pretreatment Pituitary-Adrenocortical Status: Prediction of Placebo Response in Depression

WALTER A. BROWN

The high placebo response rate in depressed patients creates a dilemma for the clinician and can obscure the evaluation of new treatment modalities. Individual symptoms or symptom profiles clearly predictive of response to placebo treatment have not been identified among patients who meet *DSM-III* criteria for major depression of moderate or greater severity.

A substantial subgroup (30–60%) of patients with major depression have a dysregulation in pituitary-adrenocortical function in the direction of hyperactivity or disinhibition. The pathophysiology and site of this dysregulation, assessed most often in recent years with the dexamethasone suppression test (DST), is unknown, and its specificity for depressive illness is unclear; but it is indisputable that a subgroup of depressed patients have a state-dependent pituitary-adrenocortical abnormality similar in quality and in some instances in degree to that seen in Cushing's disease.

Implicit to the early notion, since called into question, that this endocrine dysfunction is selectively associated with endogenous "biological" depression was the seemingly ingenuous idea that depressed patients with this endocrine "biological" disturbance require a "biological" treatment. Antidepressant treatment studies in the aggregate do show a somewhat better response rate in DST nonsuppressors (76–82%) than in suppressors (64–74%), but this difference is neither statistically nor clinically significant.[1]

To directly assess the relative necessity for pharmacological treatment in depressed patients with and without pituitary-adrenocortical dysfunction, Brown et al.[2] examined pretreatment DSTs in relation to placebo response and found that, among outpatients with major depression treated with placebo for 2–6 weeks, 10 of 22 (45%) normal suppressors recovered as opposed to none of the nine nonsuppressors. Of the four independent studies subsequently examining this issue,[3–6] three have confirmed this difference between suppressors and nonsuppressors in placebo response.[3–5] This chapter presents data on the author's entire sample of placebo-treated patients to date and reviews the findings of related studies.

Subjects and Methods

Subjects were 39 outpatients, 22 men and 17 women, ranging in age from 20 to 45 with a mean age of 30.8; they all met the *DSM-III* criteria for major depression and scored at least 18 on the 21-item Hamilton Rating Scale for Depression (HRSD). They participated in studies of new antidepressants, were assigned on a double-blind basis to placebo treatment for up to 6 weeks, and completed a minimum of 4 weeks. A placebo response was defined as a greater than 50% decrease in HRSD score and a final score of 10 or less.

The DST was carried out while patients were drug-free during the week before they were assigned on a double-blind basis to placebo. Patients took dexamethasone (1 or 2 mg) at 11:00 p.m., and a blood sample was obtained between 4:00 and 5:30 p.m. the next day for measurement of cortisol by radioimmunoassay. A serum cortisol concentration greater than 4 μg/dl was the criterion for nonsuppression.

Results

Of the 12 subjects who underwent a 2-mg DST, (17%) were nonsuppressors; and of the 27 who underwent a 1-mg DST, 10 (37%) were nonsuppressors. The combined nonsuppression rate was 31%. Of the patients who underwent a 2-mg DST, 8 of the 10 (80%) suppressors responded to placebo in contrast to neither of the two nonsuppressors (χ^2 4.80, p <0.05). For those who underwent a 1-mg DST, 8 of the 17 (47%) suppressors in contrast to 1 of the 10 (10%) nonsuppressors responded to placebo (χ^2 3.89, p <0.05). Combining the data from these groups, 16 of 27 (59%) suppressors responded to placebo in contrast to 1 of 12 (8%) nonsuppressors (χ^2 8.76, p <0.01). The combined placebo response rate was 44%. Suppressors and nonsuppressors did not differ significantly in age (31.4 versus 29.2 years), sex distribution, or initial HRSD scores (25.4 versus 29.1).

Discussion

These observations substantiate the findings of our initial report,[2] which were based on a subsample of these subjects. Since the initial report, four independent additional studies examining pretreatment DST results in relation to placebo response have appeared.

Georgotas et al.[6] in a study of elderly depressed outpatients, found an unusually low placebo response rate and no difference between suppressors and nonsuppressors; one of seven (14.3%) nonsuppressors and one of ten (10%) suppressors responded to 5–7 weeks of placebo treatment. Consistent with our findings, however, Peselow et al.[3] found that, among depressed outpatients treated with placebo for 3–6 weeks, 7 of 12 (58%) suppressors in contrast to none of seven nonsuppressors responded; and in a separate study of depressed inpatients treated with placebo for 3–6 weeks 7 of 12 (58%) suppressors in contrast to none of five nonsuppressors responded.[4] Preskorn et al.[5] found that among 30 inpatient depressed prepubertal children suppressors did not differ in response to imipramine and placebo, whereas nonsuppressors improved with imipramine but not with placebo.

Because placebo response is usually defined as clinical improvement or recovery within the standard 4- to 6-week clinical trial, the time in which a drug response is expected, the author limited his patient sample to those treated with placebo for a minimum of 4 weeks. Not surprisingly, the proportion of placebo responders increases with the length of time on placebo treatment. Twelve patients entered into the study completed 3 weeks or less of placebo treatment; one was a nonsuppressor and the rest suppressors. Most dropped out for "side effects" or lack of efficacy. None met criteria for placebo response.

Likewise, there is a low rate of placebo response during the 1 week of single-blind placebo treatment often preceding double-blind assignment in antidepressant clinical trials. Typically, placebo "response" during this week is defined as a greater than 20% improvement. Using this criterion, the author found that 5 of 65 (7.7%) suppressors and 1 of 25 (4%) nonsuppressors were placebo responders during the "baseline" week; and Peselow et al.[4] that 5 of 37 (14%) suppressors and 1 of 24 (4%) nonsuppressors were placebo responders. Coryell and Turner[7] reported that 8 of 29 (28%) suppressors but only 1 of 9 (11%) nonsuppressors showed a 1-week placebo response (30% or more improvement). None of these differences between suppressors and nonsuppressors in early placebo response is statistically significant; and this early placebo "response" is not necessarily predictive of the response to a full course of placebo. Nonetheless, the consistently higher 1-week placebo response rate in suppressors is congruent with and adds validity to the observed difference between suppressors and nonsuppressors in the 4- to 6-week placebo response.

The author is aware of two preliminary studies examining pretreatment pituitary-adrenocortical status in relation to psychosocial treatment. Rush[8] examined the response to cognitive therapy alone in outpatients with major depression. Eight of nine (89%) suppressors, all of whom who were nonendogenous by Research Diagnostic Criteria (RDC), but none of the five nonsuppressors, all of whom were endogenous, recovered with cognitive therapy alone. D. Robbins (personal communication, 1986) examined the response of inpatient depressed adolescents to several months of psychosocial treatment. Eighteen of 31 (58%) suppressors but none of the seven nonsuppressors responded to inpatients psychosocial interventions alone. Six of the seven nonsuppressors subsequently responded to treatment with antidepressants. Because patients in these studies were neither randomly assigned to treatment nor blindly assessed, these observations require cautious interpretation. Nevertheless they are intriguingly consistent with the double-blind placebo treatment studies in suggesting that without psychopharmacological treatment nonsuppressors are likely to remain depressed for more than a month.

The replicated observation of relatively poor placebo response in nonsuppressors, the preliminary data suggesting that nonsuppressors do not recover with psychosocial treatment alone, and the consistent finding that nonsuppressors respond to antidepressants as well as, if not better than, suppressors strongly suggest that nonsuppressors require antidepressant treatment whereas suppressors are far more variable in their treatment requirements, about (50%) improving with placebo. Furthermore, the "true" drug response rate for nonsuppressors may lie between 75 and 80%, whereas that for suppressors hovers around 15%.

In the context of depression, pituitary-adrenocortical hyperfunction appears to be associated with a relatively tenacious illness that is unlikely to improve with placebo and is likely to require and respond to antidepressant medication.

References

1. Arana GW, Baldessarini RJ, Ornsteen M. Commentary: the dexamethasone suppression test for diagnosis and prognosis in psychiatry. Arch Gen Psychiatry 1985;42:1193–1204.
2. Brown WA, Arato M, Shrivastava RK. DST nonsuppression predicts poor placebo response in depression. In: Proceedings of the 16th International Congress of the International Society of Psychoneuroendocrinology, Japan, 1985.
3. Peselow ED, Stanley M, Fieve RR. Plasma cortisol and clinical response to antidepressants and placebo in depressed outpatients. In: Proceedings of the Annual Meeting of the American College of Neuropsychopharmacology, Maui, Hawaii, 1985.
4. Peselow ED, Lautin A, Wolkin A, et al. The dexamethasone suppression test (DST) and response to placebo. J Clin Psychopharmacol 1986;6:286–291.
5. Preskorn SH, Weller EB, Huges CW, et al. Depression in prepubertal children: DST nonsuppression predicts differential response to imipramine versus placebo. Psychopharmacol Bull 1987;23:128–133.
6. Georgotas A, Stokes P, McCue RE, et al. The usefulness of DST in predicting response to antidepressants: a placebo-controlled study. J Affective Disord 1986;11:21–28.
7. Coryell W, Turner R. Outcome with desipramine therapy in subtypes of nonpsychotic major depression. J Affective Disord 1985;9:149–154.
8. Rush AJ. A phase II study of cognitive therapy of depression. In Williams JBW, and Spitzer RL (eds): Psychotherapy Research. New York: Guilford Press, 1984;216–234.

127. Clinical Features, DST, and Response to Placebo in Depressed Outpatients

ERIC D. PESELOW, MICHAEL STANLEY,
ADAM WOLKIN, CLIVE ROBINS, FAOUZIA
BAROUCHE, AND RONALD R. FIEVE

The efficacy of tricyclic antidepressants in treating acute depression has been well established. Morris and Beck[1] suggested that antidepressants alleviate depressive symptoms in approximately 70% of depressed patients. However, they also noted that 40% of depressed individuals respond to placebo over a 3- to 4-week period.

The purpose of this study was to evaluate this drug–placebo difference. We examined life events, dysfunctional attitudes, personality traits, clinical symptoms of depression, and plasma cortisol levels before and after dexamethasone suppression test (DST) administration in order to determine if any of these factors plays a role in predicting placebo response. We also assessed the above factors in predicting drug response.

Methods

Since June 1984 our group has conducted three outpatient drug studies involving 6-week trials of: (a) flouxetine HCl (dose 20–60 mg/day) versus placebo; (b) flouxetine HCl (dose 5–40 mg/day) versus placebo; or (c) clovoxamine HCl (dose 200–350 mg/day) versus imipramine HCl (dose 140–245 mg/day) versus placebo. Overall, 157 patients who met *DSM-III* criteria for major depressive disorder gave voluntary informed consent to participate in one of these three studies. All patients in these trials had a minimum score of 16 on the Hamilton Depression Scale.

At the onset of entry into any of the three studies, patients were rated with the Hamilton Depression Scale, Beck Self-Rating Scale, Clinical Global Scale, Raskin Depression Scale, and an Endogenous Symptom Scale abstracted from the SADS-C. If the patient fulfilled the above criteria for entry into one of studies, they were then placed on single-blind placebo over 5–10 days.

During the single-blind period the patients returned for various other assessments, including the number of life events, their meanings to patients, and the degree of social service supports the patient received during the year prior to treatment (rated on a 1–7 point scale). Also assessed were the degree of congnitive dysfunction as measured by the Dysfunctional Attitude Scale of Weissman,[2] a 40-item scale measuring cognitive dysfunction on a 1–7 point scale, and the degree of deviant personality traits as measured by the Structured Interview for *DSM-*

III Personality Disorders (SIDP) adapted by Pfohl et al.[3] The latter is a structured interview of the 11 *DSM-III* personality disorders, allowing one to rate individual personality traits on a 0–2 point scale and achieve a personality score for each disorder and a total score.

During the 1-week single-blind placebo period, we evaluated hypothalamic-pituitary-adrenal activity in these patients by means of the DST. Individuals had initial morning (8–9 a.m.) and afternoon (4 p.m.) plasma cortisol samples drawn. They were then given 1 mg of dexamethasone to take at 11 p.m. that night. They returned the next day to have post-DST morning and afternoon blood samples drawn in order to measure plasma cortisol. All patients who participated in the studies were free of medical illness, endocrinopathy, or current substance abuse.

Following the 1-week single-blind placebo period, patients were reassessed with the above scales. If the patient's Hamilton score did not drop more than 20% below its value prior to single-blind placebo and if it remained above 16, the patient was entered into one of the three double-blind trials. The patients were rated weekly and at the end of the 6-week course (or final endpoint analysis). The response to treatment, defined as a final Hamilton + Beck reduction of 50% or greater from baseline, was determined.

In order to analyze the above factors with respect to drug response, we combined the flouxetine, clovoxamine, and imipramine groups into a single "antidepressant drug group" based on evidence in the literature that suggested antidepressant efficacy for flouxetine[4] and clovoxamine.[5] The placebo group consisted of the three placebo groups from the individual studies.

Response to treatment in our evaluation was based on individuals receiving an adequate trial, which we defined as being treated during the double-blind period with either active agent or placebo for a minimum of 3 weeks. Of the 157 patients who entered one of the three drug trials, 137 were treated under double-blind conditions for at least 3 weeks. We obtained complete data 112 of the 137 patients (81.8%) prior to double-blind entry. From this group we studied clinical symptoms, dysfunctional attitudes, personality traits, life events (and their meanings), and the DST for predicting response to placebo and antidepressants.

Results

When the code was broken it was noted that 77 of the patients had been randomized to drug (flouxetine, clovoxamine, or imipramine) and 35 patients to placebo. Of the 77 patients (53.2%) randomized to drug, 41 were classified as responders by our criteria, whereas only 11 of 35 patients (31.4%) randomized to placebo were classified as responders. This difference was statistically significant [chi-square (χ^2) 3.86,1 df, $p < 0.5$)].

Table 127.1 evaluates differences in initial clinical traits, life events, dysfunctional attitudes, and personality traits between both placebo and drug responders versus nonresponders. There was no difference between initial clinical symptoms, life events and their meanings, and personality traits for placebo responders versus nonresponders. Placebo responders had a nonsignificant trend toward lower DAS scores than placebo nonresponders. Drug responders showed no difference in clinical symptoms versus drug nonresponders, but drug responders had lower DAS scores and lower total personality traits than drug nonresponders. Drug responders

TABLE 127.1. Clinical factors affecting drug and placebo response.

Factor	Patients randomized to drug (N = 77) (fluoxetine, clovoxamine, imipramine)		Patients randomized to placebo (N = 35)	
	Responders (n = 41)	Nonresponders (n = 36)	Responders (n = 11)	Nonresponders (n = 24)
Clinical symptoms				
Hamilton scale	23.73	23.86	25.09	24.33
Deck inventory	24.39[a]	29.61[a]	25.36	26.75
Raskin scale	9.68	10.19	9.90	10.67
CGI	4.17	4.25	4.36	4.50
Endogenous symptoms	33.07	33.61	33.81	35.25
Life events				
No. of events	2.02	3.03	1.55	1.96
Severity of events	3.83[a]	4.86[a]	3.35	3.74
Requested social support	3.10[a]	4.35[a]	3.00	3.29
Received social support	3.05[a]	2.06[a]	2.55	2.30
Received − requested	−0.05[b]	−2.29[b]	−0.45	−0.99
Beliefs that life events				
Precipitated illness	3.34	4.00	3.72	3.25
Predisposed to illness	2.90[a]	3.89[a]	2.54	2.92
Dysfunctional attitudes				
DAS pretreatment	140.29[b]	171.47[b]	134.09	148.25
DAS posttreatment	111.80[b]	172.19[b]	119.27[a]	145.70
PreTX − postTX	+28.49[b]	−0.72[b]	+14.82[b]	+2.45
Personality traits				
Paranoid	0.90[b]	2.89[b]	1.82	3.25
Schizoid	0.32[a]	0.81[a]	0.45	1.29
Schizotypal	0.95[b]	2.25[b]	1.00	2.67
Compulsive	1.39	1.78	1.27	2.04
Histrionic	2.22	3.78	2.45	1.63
Dependent	1.54[a]	2.53[a]	1.27	2.25
Antisocial	1.56	2.53	1.82	2.25
Narcissistic	1.54	2.61	2.73	1.46
Avoidant	3.05	3.80	3.09	0.92
Borderline	2.95	4.39	2.64	3.38
Passive-aggressive	1.59[b]	4.11[b]	3.27	2.04
Total score	18.05[b]	31.42[b]	21.82	2.54
				23.46

[a]Statistically significant: $p < 0.05$ responders vs. nonresponders.

were less disturbed by life events and received greater social service supports for the life events than drug nonresponders.

Table 127.2 evaluates the DST results. Placebo responders had significantly higher post-DST plasma cortisol levels than placebo nonresponders. Only one of the 13 placebo-treated patients with an initial positive DST responded to placebo versus 10 of 22 with an initial negative DST (χ^2 3.88, 1 df, $p < 0.5$). There was no correlation between initial DST and drug response and no correlation between initial pre-DST plasma cortisol and both drug and placebo response.

Discussion

Though much has been written about placebo effectiveness in depression,[6] there have been only a few reports in the literature suggesting variables predictive of placebo response in depression. Ansoms et al.[7] noted significant decreases in dysphoria, suicidal ideation, initial, middle, and terminal insomnia, and weight loss in acute unipolar and bipolar depressives treated with placebo. Fairchild et al.,[8] studying 55 depressed patients 21 of whom responded to placebo over 1 week, noted shorter length of illness, presence of concomitant anxiety, panic disorder, substance abuse, and lower initial pretreatment Beck Depression Inventory score as predictive of placebo response.

In addition to demographic and clincal variables, the DST has been studied in terms of predicting treatment outcome. Though there have been conflicting reports concerning a positive or negative role for DST in predicting response to drug,[9] two studies have evaluated the DST's role in predicting response to placebo. Shrivistava et al.[10] and Peselow et al.,[11] examining the DST within the context of a placebo-controlled trial, noted that nonsuppressors (patients with a positive DST) had a significantly poorer response to placebo than suppressors (patients with a negative DST). However, a study by Georgatas et al.[12] noted that a positive or negative DST did not predict response to placebo or drug.

It is interesting to note that there have been few data evaluating clinical symptoms, life events, cognitive dysfunction, and personality traits in predicting drug responsiveness, which is surprising as many believe that these factors play a role in the decision to prescribe antidepressants. Many studies aimed at identifying clinical and demographic variables that predict drug responsiveness show con-

TABLE 127.2. Plasma cortisol before and after DST versus drug and placebo response.

Subject	8 a.m. Pre-DST	4 a.m. Pre-DST	8 a.m. Post-DST	4 p.m. Post-DST	Positive DST (No.)
Drug-treated patients (flouxetine, clovoxamine, imipramine) ($n = 77$)					
Responders ($n = 41$)	19.66	8.84	5.13	4.89	16/41
Nonresponders ($n = 36$)	16.73	8.17	3.82	4.09	12/36
Placebo-treated patients ($n = 35$)					
Responders ($n = 11$)	17.62	10.45	1.55[a]	3.14[a]	1/13[a]
Nonresponders ($n = 24$)	15.88	9.26	6.78[a]	7.53[a]	10/22[a]

[a]Statistically significant: $p < 0.04$ (placebo responders versus nonresponders for both a.m. and p.m. plasma cortisol and for frequency of abnormal DSTs).

flicting results.[13] The best controlled study attempting to evaluate this problem was done by Stewart et al.,[14] who examined 103 depressed outpatients treated with desipramine or placebo in double-blind fashion. Nonreactivity (autonomy) of depressed mood, pervasive anhedonia, and a diagnosis of major depressive disorder predicted a greater drug–placebo difference (i.e., the patients were more likely to respond to drug and not likely to respond to placebo). Individuals with less severe depressive illness, particularly situational depression, were more likely to respond to placebo.

The literature contains numerous references to life events and the onset of depressive illness but few on if the presence of a specific event affects antidepressant treatment.[15] Cognitive dysfunction has long been thought to play a role in the etiology of depressive illness, and numerous investigators have found cognitive therapy equal to pharmocotherapy in the outpatient treatment of depression.[16] However, there have been few studies that have quantified the degree of cognitive dysfunction and correlated it with prospective response to drug or placebo.[17]

Though much has been surmised concerning the existence of personality traits in patients with major depression and their effect on treatment response, little has been done in the way of controlled trials. Tyrer et al.[18] and Pfohl et al.[19] noted a poor response to antidepressants among individuals with depression plus a coexistent personality disorder, in agreement with our findings. It is interesting to note that individual and total personality scores did not correlate with placebo response in our evaluation.

The most powerful factor in predicting placebo response was the initial post-DST plasma cortisol level. Although one might interpret this finding to mean that the presence of a positive DST suggests the need for active treatment, we believe that it might not mean much clinically. The above 112 patients presented with major depressive symptoms, which remained constant after a week of single-blind placebo. It seems that such patients should be treated with somatic therapy on a clinical basis regardless of the results of this test.

Summary

Depression is an illness with many etiologies. It is clear that before initiating treatment one must evaluate clinical symptoms, life events, dysfunctional attitudes, personality traits, and possibly the DST before proceeding. Further studies are needed to clarify the role of these factors in predicting response to placebo or drug.

References

1. Morris JB Beck AT. The efficacy of antidepressant drugs—a review of research (1958–1972). Arch Gen Psychiatry 1974;30:667–674.
2. Weissman AN. The Dysfunctional Attitude Scale: A Validation Study Thesis. Philadelphia: University of Pennsylvania Graduate School of Arts & Sciences, 1979.
3. Pfohl B, Stangl D, Zimmerman M. The Structured Interview for DSM-III Personality Disorders (SIDP). Iowa City: Department of Psychiatry, University of Iowa, 1982.
4. Stark P, Hardison CD. A review of multicenter controlled studies of fluoxetine vs. imipramine and placebo in outpatients with major depressive disorder. J Clin Psychiatry 1985;46(3):53–58.
5. Gelenberg AJ, Wojcik JD, Newell C, et al. A double blind comparison of clovoxamine vs. amitriptyline in the treatment of depressed outpatients. J Clin Psychopharmacol 1985;5:30–34.

6. Downing RW, Rickels K. The prediction of placebo response in depressed & anxious outpatients. In Wittenborn JR, Goldberg SC, May PRA (eds): Psychopharmacology & the Individual Patients. New York: Raven Press, 1970;160–168.
7. Ansoms C, DeBacker-Dierich G, Vereecken JLTM. Sleep disorders in patients with severe mental depressions. Acta Psychiatr Scand 1977;55:116–120.
8. Fairchild CJ, Rush AJ, Vasavada N, et al. Which depressions respond to placebo. Psychiatry Res 1986;18:217–226.
9. Arana GW, Baldessarini R, Ornsteen M. The dexamethasone suppression test for diagnosis & prognosis in psychiatry. Arch Gen Psychiatry 1985;42:1193–1204.
10. Shrivastava RK, Schwimmer R, Brown RA, et al. The DST predicts poor placebo response in depression. Scientific Proceedings of the American Psychiatric Association, Dallas, 1985. New research abstract No. 94.
11. Peselow ED, Lautin A, Wolkin A, et al. The dexamethasone suppression test and response to placebo. J Clin Psychopharmacol 1986;6:286–291.
12. Georgatas A, Stokes P, McCue RE, et al. The usefulness of DST in predicting response to antidepressants: a controlled study. J Affective Disord 1986;11:21–28.
13. Bielski RJ, Friedel RO. Prediction of tricyclic antidepressant response. Arch Gen Psychiatry 1976:33:1479–1489.
14. Stewart JW, Quitkin FM, Liebowitz MR, et al. Efficacy of desipramine in depressed outpatients. Arch Gen Psychiatry 1983;40:202–207.
15. Garvey MJ, Schaeffer CB, Tuason V. Comparison of pharmacological treatment response between situational and non-situational depressions. Br J Psychiatry 1984;145:363–365.
16. Beck AT, Hollon SD, Young JE. Treatment of depression with cognitive therapy and amitriptyline. Arch Gen Psychiatry 1985;42:142–148.
17. Silverman JS, Silverman JA, Eardley DA. Do maladaptive attitudes cause depression? Arch Gen Psychiatry 1984;41:28–30.
18. Tyrer P, Casey P, Gall J. Relationship between neurosis and personality disorder. Br J Psychiatry 1983;142:404–408.
19. Pfohl B, Stangl D, Zimmerman M. The implication of DSM-III personality disorder for patients with major depression. J Affective Disord 1984;7:309–318.

V.D. ANTIDEPRESSANTS IN CLINICAL PRACTICE: PLASMA LEVELS OF ANTIDEPRESSANTS

128. Antidepressant Drug Measurement: Review of Methods for Clinical Application

TREVOR R. NORMAN AND GRAHAM D. BURROWS

Although antidepressants are widely used for the treatment of depressive illness, they are not effective in every patient. In clinical trials as many as 20–30% of patients may fail to respond to adequate doses of drugs administered for an adequate length of time. As an attempt to improve treatment for these nonresponders, Brodie[1] suggested that the measurement of plasma concentrations may be of benefit. Given the assumptions it entails, the search for plasma antidepressant–clinical response relations has been vigorously pursued with varying degrees of success. Even the advocates of a "no simple relation" position have defended the value of plasma level monitoring in certain situations.[2] A crucial element in the study of these relations is the method of drug analysis. The methods for antidepressants are reviewed.

Collection, Storage, and Stability of Samples

For clinical studies the most widely used biological fluid has been plasma, although serum, whole blood, erythrocytes, or cerebrospinal fluid may be equally suited. Problems have arisen with the use of Vacutainers for the collection of plasma samples. Several studies have shown lowered plasma concentrations in samples collected in these tubes compared to glass or polystyrene containers.[3] The reduction in concentration is caused by displacement of the drug from plasma proteins, principally α_1-acid glycoprotein by a plasticizer in the Vacutainer stopper. The increased free drug is redistributed between plasma and erythrocytes. Similarly, problems may be observed using indwelling needles flushed with heparin to collect multiple blood samples during pharmacokinetic studies.[4] Serum concentrations show a 1:1 correspondence with plasma,[5] and their use may obviate the problem.

Assay Methodologies

Analyses of antidepressent drugs based on spectrophotometric or fluorimetric methods are not described in this review. Although such methods have sometimes demonstrated adequate assay characteristics, they are not frequently used on a routine basis nor are they the method of choice in research studies.

Isotope Derivative Dilution Analysis

Historically, the first practical assays for desipramine (DMI) and nortriptyline (NT) were described by Hammer and Brodie using the isotope derivative approach.[6] The principle of the method is based on the formation of a derivative of the drug to be measured with a radioactive reagent of known specific activity. The radioactive derivative is separated and purified, the radioactivity measured, and the amount of drug calculated from the stoichiometry. In practice, for a single isotope assay it is necessary to construct a standard curve to account for procedural losses. Both secondary and tertiary amines can be determined by this method. Secondary amines are readily derivatized with ^{3}H-acetic anhydride, whereas for tertiary amines quarternary ammonium salts can be formed with labeled methyliodide. The first approach was utilized for DMI and NT, and the latter was used for imipramine (IMI) determination. Early studies of the plasma level–response relation for NT utilized this method extensively and demonstrated the wide interindividual variability in steady-state concentrations in patients receiving the same oral dose. The major weakness of the method is its lack of selectivity, as any of the primary or secondary amine metabolites of the tricyclics could undergo derivatization. Inclusion of a chromatographic step improves selectivity but increases assay time. The use of reagents such as salicylaldehyde to block derivative formation with primary amines by formation of Schiff bases also improves selectivity but contributes to procedural losses.

The incorporation of a second isotope, the so-called double isotope derivative dilution assay, can correct for losses due to the method. The approach is particularly suited to secondary amines, although tertiary amines can be determined after appropriate chemical modification.[6] Selectivity of the assay can be improved using a thin-layer chromatography step after derivative formation. Furthermore, calibration curves are unnecessary, as the known specific activity of the derivatizing agent can be used to calculate mass.[6] This methodology has been applied to the determination of NT, maprotiline (MAP), and chlomipramine (CMI) for plasma level and pharmacokinetic studies.

Chromatographic Analysis

Antidepressant analysis by chromatographic techniques has been widely applied to clinical situations, with the most recent emphasis on high performance liquid chromatographic (HPLC) methods.[4] Gas-liquid chromatography (GLC), combined gas chromatography–mass spectrometry (GC-MS), and thin-layer chromatography (TLC) have many features that suit them to clinical applications. Almost invariably chromatographic analyses require extensive preparation of plasma samples. Usually an extraction of the drug (and metabolites) from basic solution (pH > 10) into an organic solvent followed by back-extraction into a mineral acid and then extraction into the organic solvent after neutralization of the acid is required. Occasionally, chromatographic separations, at least for GLC or GC-MS, may be improved by derivatization of secondary amines. Another approach has been the use of C_{18}-bonded phase columns for sample clean-up. Equivalent results have been demonstrated for column and three-step extractions, with the columns providing a more rapid extraction process. Further development of the columns will no doubt prove useful in the future.

Gas-Liquid Chromatography. Gas-liquid chromatography is a selective analytical technique and, depending on the type of detector used, has sufficient sensitivity for most measurements. The flame ionization detector (FID) is the least sensitive of detectors and requires large plasma volumes to be extracted in order to ensure adequate assay characteristics. Column packing is another consideration in the analysis. A common choice has been 3% OV-17, which provides satisfactory resolution of tertiary and secondary amines in a reasonable run time. Derivatization significantly improves the tailing of secondary amine peaks. The limit of detection of FID methods is around 10–20 μg/l. Selectivity, accuracy, precision, and sensitivity are acceptable for steady-state monitoring and forensic applications but not for single-dose kinetic studies.

A lower detection limit and increased sensitivity is afforded by the electron capture detector (ECD). A limitation of its use is the need to convert drugs to a species that readily captures electrons, usually a halogenated compound. The technique has been utilized for the determination of most antidepressants. Despite its somewhat more difficult technical demands, ECD is well suited to most clinical applications.

The nitrogen-phosphorus (N-P) detector is a modification of a conventional flame ionization detector with a high selectivity for compounds containing nitrogen or phosphorus and a much lower detection limit than FID. Until recently N-P detectors represented the most widely applied technique of measurement for antidepressants. All of the most recently published methods have satisfactory characteristics for routine monitoring and pharmacokinetic studies. A number of stationary phases have been used including 3% OV-17, 3% OV-101, and 3% SP-2250, which give equivalent results. Capillary column technology has not been widely used as yet, but coupled with the N-P detector, represents a significant advance for the analysis of antidepressants with better chromatographic resolution of peaks and lower limits of detection.

Mass Fragmentography. The coupling of a mass spectrometer as a detector for the effluent of a gas chromatograph provides the most sensitive and specific assays for antidepressants. Simultaneous and continuous monitoring of mass spectral ions representing mass fragments of the drug to be quantitated gives both total ion and single ion chromatograms. Most GC-MS combinations can monitor six or more ions simultaneously, which is usually sufficient to quantitate parent drug and metabolites. Mass fragmentography has been widely applied to antidepressant measurement with assay characteristics suitable for single-dose and steady-state studies. The amount of plasma required is small (about 1 ml), but a three-step extraction procedure for sample clean-up is necessary. GC-MS allows the use of stable-isotope-labeled drugs as internal standards with obvious advantages. Both electron impact (EI) and chemical ionization (CI) procedures have been used to produce mass fragments. Because CI maintains greater structural integrity of the molecule it may be the technique of choice. The coupling of HPLC to a mass spectrometer is a new development and has not yet been applied to drug analysis extensively. Capillary column GC is also available coupled to the MS, and developments with these instruments are awaited with interest.

High Performance Liquid Chromatography. The technique of HPLC has been increasingly applied to antidepressant measurement to the extent that it now rivals GC-NP as that most commonly used. Prior extraction of the drug from plasma before application to the column is required. The type of chromatography performed has varied, but reversed-phase methods have received wide attention. Normal-phase (adsorption) chromatography is equally applicable. HPLC methods that simultaneously measure parent drug and all active metabolites, including the hydroxymetabolites, have been described for all the commonly prescribed antidepressants. Quantitation is most often achieved using an ultraviolet detector, but fluorimetric or electrochemical detectors can be used. Generally, lower limits of detection can be achieved with the latter detectors.

Thin-Layer Chromatography. Detection of substances on thin-layer plates can be achieved by an elution process or in situ measurement of compounds on the plates. Only direct evaluation (densitometry) of the plates has sufficient sensitivity, precision, and accuracy necessary for quantitative analysis. The proper choice of solvents and plate-coating materials determines the success of separations.

Application to antidepressant measurement was first demonstrated for IMI and DMI. After a one-step extraction from 5 ml of plasma, IMI and metabolites were separated on the TLC plate and quantified by densitometry of the intense yellow spots formed on reaction with nitrous gases. Similar methods for the quantitation of amitriptyline (AT) and NT and the separation of AT, IMI, and their metabolites have been described. High-performance thin-layer chromatography (HPTLC) has also been applied to antidepressant determination. The plates used in this technique provide better resolution and sensitivity than conventional TLC plates. As little as 2 μg/l from 1 ml of plasma can be detected. Adequate selectivity, precision, and sensitivity has been demonstrated, and the methods are widely applied to routine monitoring and pharmacokinetic studies.

Biological Methods

Radioimmunoassay (RIA) and radioreceptor assay (RRA) are two potentially important biological methods of drug assay that have not been utilized as fully as perhaps they might for antidepressant analysis. The reasons are both intrinsic to the assay methods themselves and perhaps due to the chronology of development: Workable, specific GC methods were already available when suitable RIAs or RRAs were being developed.

Radioimmunoassay. Radioimmunoassays have been developed for several antidepressants. The principle of RIAs involves competition between radiolabeled and unlabeled drug for the antiserum, with increasing amounts of the unlabeled drug lowering the amount of labeled drug bound. The free and bound ligand are physically separated prior to counting either fraction. Concentration of drug in a patient specimen is determined from a calibration curve. Antisera have been prepared by injection of the drugs coupled to bovine serum albumin into rabbits or sheep. The antigenic determinants for the tricyclic antidepressants are the nucleus and the aliphatic side chain. Slight structural modifications can produce major changes to the cross-reactivity of the antiserum to the drug and its metabolites. Most antisera show little or no cross-reactivity to the 2- or 10-hydroxymetabolites, but the cross-reactivity to secondary or tertiary amine tricyclics is significant. This lack of specificity of the antisera so far produced has been a major factor limiting their use. Sensitivity and precision of most RIAs are adequate for clinical applications. Furthermore, the assays require only small amounts of plasma and can be often be used as direct assays.

Radioreceptor Assays. Radioreceptor assays measure the amount of drug in plasma that binds to specific receptors prepared from brain tissue membranes. The particular substance competes with a radiolabeled drug of high specific activity for the receptor site. Antidepressants bind to muscarinic-cholinergic and α-adrenergic receptors in brain defined by ^{3}H-quinuclidinylbenzilate (^{3}H-QNB) and WB-4101, respectively. An assay for nortriptyline based on displacement of these ligands from rat cortical membranes has been described.[7] Plasma samples were extracted and aliquots of the reconstituted sample used. Calculations were performed from log-probit plots of the percent inhibition of QNB or WB-4101 versus concentration. Results from split samples were compared with a GC method. The RRA consistently overestimated steady-state drug levels, indicating a lack of specificity.

The RRAs offer limited usefulness as routine or research methods. Interference with binding by co-prescribed drugs and the inability to simultaneously quantitate parent drug and metabolites will see other methods remain at the forefront.

Enzyme Immunoassay. Enzyme immunoassay techniques (EMIT) utilize the principle of competitive protein binding. A drug bound to an enzyme competes with drug in patient samples for binding to an antibody raised against the drug. After an incubation period, the activity of the enzyme–drug–antibody or enzyme–drug complex is measured. Drug concentrations are correlated with enzymic activity. A double-antibody immunoassay procedure has been described for NT.[8] It is a time-consuming procedure; it requires a 20-h incubation but has sufficient precision and sensitivity for most clinical applications. Its specificity is poor, however, showing cross-reactivity with other tricyclics as well as some NT metabolites. A single-antibody EMIT procedure (marketed by Syva Inc.) requires only 20 min for incubations but is currently only a qualitative assay. At present enzyme immunoassays are not suitable for routine applications.

Conclusions

Antidepressant drug monitoring remains an important part of clinical practice, and doubtless as new technologies evolve they will be applied to this purpose. For the present, GLC with nitrogen phosphorous detection or HPLC are the techniques within the reach of most laboratories and, as noted, are well suited to analysis of this important group of drugs. GC-MS is also well suited, but the cost of the apparatus precludes its use in many laboratories. HPTLC may offer advantages in terms of the speed of sample processing; it is adequate for routine analysis, and the cost is low by comparison to other apparatus. The ultimate decision of which piece of equipment to buy will no doubt be determined by its utility for measuring other drugs and the anticipated demand for antidepressant analysis.

References

1. Brodie BB. Physico-chemical and biochemical aspects of pharmacology. JAMA 1967; 202:600–609.
2. Norman TR, Burrows GD. Plasma concentrations of antidepressant drugs and clinical response. In Burrows GD, Norman TR, Davies B (eds): Drugs in Psychiatry, Vol. 1: Antidepressants. Amsterdam: Elsevier, 1983;111–120.
3. Brunswick D, Mendels J. Reduced levels of tricyclic antidepressants in plasma from Vacutainers. Commun Psychopharmacol 1977;1:131–134.

4. Norman TR, Maguire KP. Analysis of tricyclic antidepressant drugs in plasma and serum by chromatographic techniques. J Chromatogr 1985;340:173–197.
5. Saady JJ, Bloom VL, Narasimhachari N, et al. A comparison of plasma and serum levels of two tricyclic antidepressants: imipramine and desipramine. Psychopharmacology 1981;75:173–174.
6. Scoggins BA, Maguire KP, Norman TR, et al. Measurement of tricyclic antidepressants. 1. A review of methodology. Clin Chem 1980;26:5–17.
7. Smith RC, Vroulis G, Misra CH, et al. Receptor techniques in the study of plasma levels of neuroleptics and antidepressant drugs. Commun Psychopharmacol 1980;4:451–465.
8. Al-Bassam MN, O'Sullivan MJ, Gnemmi E, et al. Double-antibody enzyme immunoassay for nortriptyline. Clin Chem 1978;24:1590–1594.

129. Relation Between Plasma Antidepressant Concentrations and Clinical Effects

Graham D. Burrows, Iain M. McIntyre, Kay P. Maguire, Bruce A. Scoggins, and Trevor R. Norman

Studies of the plasma levels of antidepressant drugs may improve the treatment of depression and related disorders. It is approximately 20 years since plasma levels of the tricyclic antidepressant drugs first began to be measured. There are close to 100 plasma tricyclic level clinical response studies in the literature today. About one-third find a relation and two-thirds do not. The reasons for this controversy are reviewed and some directions for future research presented.

Methodological Issues

The relation between plasma concentration and clinical effect can be influenced by a number of variables, including the following.

1. Nature and severity of the illness studied, i.e., patient variables
2. Laboratory assay methods
3. Method of data analysis
4. Age of the patient
5. Sex of the patient
6. Concurrent medications used and consequent drug interactions
7. Adequate methods for the assessment of severity and change in severity
8. Pharmacokinetic variability of the drugs used and the relation of plasma sampling times to account for this variability
9. Definition of treatment endpoints
10. Size of the sample studied

Relation Between Plasma Concentration and Clinical Response

The plasma concentration–clinical response issue for antidepressant drugs has been widely debated and reviewed.[1-7] A detailed critique of all of the studies is not presented here; rather, some individual examples are discussed.

Nortriptyline was the first drug studied in plasma concentration–response relations and immediately produced two studies with conflicting results. A curvilinear relation suggested a "therapeutic window," or range of nortriptyline concentrations of 50–140 µg/l. Kragh-Sorensen et al.[8,9] confirmed the curvilinear nature of the relation but modified the upper limit to 150 µg/l. On the other hand, Burrows et al.[10–12] were unable to demonstrate a simple correlation between plasma concentration and clinical response for the total group. For 12 patients in whom plasma levels were alternately raised and lowered, a correlation for individuals was demonstrated.[12] A number of subsequent studies have supported one or the other of these opposed views. More studies have corroborated a curvilinear than no simple relation.

Demonstration of a curvilinear relation for nortriptyline suggests that routine monitoring of plasma concentrations should be undertaken in patients receiving this drug. However, the meaning of a therapeutic range needs some consideration. It is well recognized that the therapeutic range of plasma lithium concentrations is 0.5–1.2 mmol/l. Above 1.5 mmol/l toxic symptoms are often experienced. It is also clearly recognized that for some patients lithium concentrations outside the "therapeutic window" are necessary to achieve satisfactory clinical response. Some individuals do not respond to lithium irrespective of plasma concentrations. The therapeutic range is then an initial goal, with any further adjustments of plasma concentration being dictated by the clinical response of the patient. The same may be said of nortriptyline plasma concentrations. The upper therapeutic limit of nortriptyline is now regarded as 200 µg/l. This figure is based on the findings of Burrows et al.[13] that cardiotoxicity is associated with nortriptyline concentrations above 200 µg/l. Not all patients have conduction defects above this concentration, and some patients with plasma concentrations below this figure experience cardiac changes; i.e., 200 µg/l should not be regarded as an absolute upper limit. In most patients plasma monitoring is unnecessary, as adjustment of dosages is made on the basis of clinical response.

For other antidepressant drugs the relation between plasma concentrations and clinical response is as confused as that for nortriptyline. Studies have suggested that a minimum of 45 µg/l for imipramine and 75 µg/l for desipramine is necessary for recovery[14]; no upper limit has been reported. Other studies of imipramine have found either no correlation[15] or negative correlations, i.e., suggesting a curvilinear relation.[16] For amitriptyline all of the above types of relation have been found. Limited studies of maprotiline, protriptyline, butriptyline, doxepin, mianserin, clomipramine, nomifensine, dibenzepin, lofepramine, dothiepin, and viloxazine have produced conflicting findings.

In summary, our studies of the plasma level–response relations of several tricyclic drugs show for groups that there is no simple relation between plasma level of a tricyclic drug and the clinical response. For given individuals, however, there may be a range that is important. This situation is not surprising because it is the same with most other drugs in medicine. There are only approximate guidelines for therapeutic levels of most drugs, e.g., the anticonvulsants.

These studies have brought about a change of prescribing habits. Most of the antidepressants now are given in a single dose at night or perhaps as one-third in the morning and two-thirds at night. During the 1970s, three or four times a day was more the rule, and 75 mg of an antidepressant was common. Now many of the drugs are prescribed up to 300–500 mg/day. Studies of plasma level–effect relations have largely been responsible for an improvement in patient care.

Plasma Drug Concentrations and Cardiac Effects

Cardiovascular side effects attributed to antidepressants include hypotension, postural hypotension, hypertension, tachycardia, aggravation or precipitation of congestive cardiac failure and angina pectoris, cardiac arrhythmia, myocardial infarction, atrioventricular block, and increased incidence of sudden death among cardiac patients. Most concerns regarding cardiotoxicity focused on the tricyclic antidepressants, whereas the monoamine oxidase inhibitors, with the exception of hypo- and hypertension, have generally been regarded as less cardiotoxic. The "new" antidepressants introduced in recent years are claimed to be less cardiotoxic than the older tricyclic drugs.

Some studies have attempted to relate changes in cardiological parameters to concentration of drug in plasma. Freyschuss et al.[17] studied 40 depressed patients treated with nortriptyline. Heart rate and blood pressure increased in all patients during treatment, but the increase was not correlated with plasma drug concentrations.

Plasma nortriptyline concentrations and the electrocardiogram (ECG) were recorded in 20 patients who received the drug for a minimum of 2 weeks.[18] The PR interval and heart rate increased in all subjects after drug administration, but this change was not correlated with plasma drug concentration.

There is some evidence that plasma nortriptyline concentrations in excess of 200 μg/l are associated with cardiac effects. Burrows et al.[13] have shown, using ECG and H_{is} Bundle Electrography (HBE) studies, that significantly more patients receiving nortriptyline had increased H-V intervals and broadened QRS width than patients receiving doxepin. Vohra et al.[18] demonstrated that four of five patients receiving nortriptyline who experienced ECG and HBE changes had plasma drug levels in excess of 200 μg/l. In general, this finding has been confirmed. Zeigler et al.[19,20] have demonstrated an association of plasma nortriptyline or plasma amitriptyline concentration and increased heart rate. Veith et al.[21] have shown an association between plasma desipramine concentration and the heart rate and QRS and QT_c intervals. There were no correlations between plasma concentrations and change in the variables. Plasma drug concentrations varied over a wide range, 13–882 μg/l. These authors did not comment on the association of high plasma levels with ECG changes.

It can be concluded from these studies that dosages of the antidepressants within the usual range lead to ECG and HBE changes in some patients. These changes are most likely to be associated with high plasma concentrations of the drug. On the other hand, plasma concentration monitoring is not necessarily a guide to ECG and HBE changes.

Cardiovascular Effects of Antidepressants: Overdose

The effects of tricyclic poisoning are unpredictable: Serious complications have been observed in some patients who ingest only small amounts of the drug, whereas no or mild symptoms may occur in those who ingest 2 g or more. Generally, acute ingestion of 1 g is clinically serious, and doses of 2 g or more are frequently fatal. Often antidepressants are combined with other drugs on overdosage, and adverse effects may be due to the antidepressant per se or to drug interactions.

Common ECG abnormalities on overdosage include sinus or supraventricular tachycardia, prolongation of the Q-T interval, intraventricular conduction defects, and ST and T wave changes. Tachycardia has been attributed to the anticholinergic effects of the drugs. Intracardiac conduction studies of patients with tricyclic antidepressant overdose have shown prolongation of the H-V interval (conduction through the main His bundle to the Purkinje fibers) but a normal A-H interval (conduction through the atria and the atrioventricular node) and prolonged QRS duration. Similar changes are produced by quinidine. Studies have shown a strong correlation between maximum QRS duration and total tricyclic levels and have demonstrated that intraventricular conduction delays are more common with plasma levels in excess of 1,000 μg/l.[22] Prolongation of the QRS width by 100 ms or more is a reliable and readily available clinical index of tricyclic overdosage.

Conclusions

Plasma level monitoring has its main role in research: pharmacokinetics, pharmacodynamics, investigation of side effects, and evaluation of drug interactions. In the clinical situation plasma level monitoring does have some specific roles. With therapeutic failures, monitoring may indicate poor compliance or rapid metabolism and the need to increase the dose. Certainly they are helpful for investigation of troublesome side effects and cardiotoxicity, when drugs are being prescribed chronically or for prophylaxis, when many drugs are precribed concomitantly, and in patients with gastrointestinal, cardiovascular, or renal disease. There has been an expansion of commercial laboratories around the world that routinely measure plasma tricyclic levels. Whether such knowledge has altered clinical improvement for many patients is debatable. Plasma levels do have a role to play, as discussed, but for a given individual therapeutic levels are difficult if not impossible to define a priori. Obviously, too little drug produces no response, and too much produces side effects. The definition of therapeutic ranges requires more well designed studies.

References

1. Burrows GD. Plasma levels of tricyclics, clinical response and drug interactions. In Burrows GD (ed): Handbook of Studies on Depression. Amsterdam: Excerpta Medica, 1977;173–194.
2. Burrows GD, Davies B, Norman TR, et al. Should plasma level monitoring of tricyclic antidepressants be introduced in clinical practice? Commun Psychopharmacol 1978;2:393–408.
3. Risch SC, Huey LY, Janowsky DS. Plasma levels of tricyclic antidepressants and clinical efficacy: review of the literature. Part I. J Clin Psychiatry 1979;40:4–16.
4. Risch SC, Huey LY, Janowsky DS. Plasma levels of tricyclic antidepressants and clinical efficacy: review of the literature. Part II. J Clin Psychiatry 1976;40:58–69.
5. Norman TR, Burrows GD. Plasma levels of psychotropic drugs and clinical response. In Burrows GD, Werry J (eds): Advances in Human Psychopharmacology. Vol. 1. Greenwich. JAI Press, 1980;103–140.
6. Scoggins BA, Maguire KP, Norman TR, et al. Measurement of tricyclic antidepressants. Part 2. Applications. Clin Chem 1980;26:805–815.
7. Burrows GD, Norman TR. Tricyclic antidepressants: plasma levels and clinical response. In Burrows GD, Norman TR (eds): Psychotropic Drugs, Plasma Concentration and Clinical Response. New York: Marcel Dekker, 1981;169–204.
8. Kragh-Sorensen P, Eggert-Hansen C, Larsen N, et al. Longterm treatment of endogenous depression with nortriptyline with control of plasma levels. Psychol Med 1974;4:174–180.

9. Kragh-Sorensen P, Hansen CE, Baastrup PC, et al. Self inhibiting action of nortriptyline antidepressive effect at high plasma levels. Psychopharmacology 1976;45:305–312.
10. Burrows GD, Davies BM, Scoggins BA. Plasma concentration of nortriptyline and clinical response in depressive illness. Lancet 1972;2:619–623.
11. Burrows GD, Scoggins BA, Turecek LR, et al. Plasma nortriptyline and clinical response. Clin Pharmacol Ther 1974;16:639–644.
12. Burrows GD, Maguire KP, Scoggins BA, et al. Plasma nortriptyline and clinical response—a study using changing plasma levels. Psychol Med 1977;7:87–91.
13. Burrows GD, Vohra J, Dumovic P, et al. Tricyclic antidepressant drugs and cardiac conduction. Prog Neuropsychopharmacol 1977;1:329–334.
14. Gram LF, Reisby N, Ibsen I, et al. Plasma levels and antidepressive effect of imipramine. Clin Pharmacol Ther 1976;19:318–324.
15. Ballinger BR, Presley A, Reid AH, et al. The effects of hypnotics on imipramine treatment. Psychopharmacology 1974;39:267–274.
16. Bhanji S, Lader MH. The electroencephalographic and psychological effects of imipramine in depressed inpatients. Eur J Clin Pharmacol 1977;12:349–354.
17. Freyschuss U, Sjoqvist F, Tuck D, et al. Circulatory effects in man of nortriptyline, a tricyclic antidepressant drug. Pharmacol Clin 1978;2:68–71.
18. Vohra JK, Burrows GD, Sloman G. Assessment of cardiovascular side effects of therapeutic doses of tricyclic antidepressant drugs. Aust NZ Med J 1975;5:7–11.
19. Ziegler VE, Co BT, Biggs JT Plasma nortriptyline and ECG findings. Am J Psychiatry 1977;134:441–443.
20. Ziegler VE, Co BT, Biggs JT. Electrocardiographic findings in patients undergoing amitriptyline treatment. Dis Nerv Syst 1977;38:697–699.
21. Veith RC, Friedel RO, Bloom V, et al. Electrocardiogram changes and plasma desipramine levels during treatment of depression. Clin Pharmacol Ther 1980;27:796–802.
22. Sloman JG, Norman TR, Burrows GD. Clinical studies of antidepressant cardiotoxicity. In Burrows GD, Norman TR, Davies B (eds): Drugs in Psychiatry, Vol. 1: Antidepressants. Amsterdam: Elsevier, 1983;173–186.

130. Clinical Implications of the Tricyclic Antidepressant Hydroxy-Metabolites

J. Craig Nelson

Metabolism of the tricyclic antidepressants results in the production of hydroxylated compounds (OH-TCAs) that are then conjugated and excreted. Although concentrations of hydroxyimipramine and hydroxyamitriptyline are low in human subjects relative to their parent compounds, levels of 2-hydroxydesipramine (OH-DMI) are commonly half that of DMI and levels of 10-hydroxynortriptyline (OH-NOR) are comparable to that of the parent compound. In some individuals plasma concentrations of OH-NOR and OH-DMI exceed those of the parent drug. OH-TCAs appear to be less protein-bound in plasma than their parent compounds, and the OH-DMI/DMI and OH-NOR/NOR ratios are higher in cerebrospinal fluid (CSF) than in plasma. Thus OH-DMI and OH-NOR are present in appreciable levels in plasma and CSF and, if active, could contribute to the clinical effects of the TCAs. During the late 1970s it was demonstrated that the OH-TCAs block reuptake of norepinephrine and serotonin and that they have behavioral effects in animals similar to those of the TCAs, but it was not clear that they have antidepressant effects.

Antidepressant Effects of OH-NOR

Antidepressant activity of the OH-TCAs was first reported by Breyer-Pfaff and associates in 1982.[1] They treated 27 inpatients with amitriptyline (AT) 150 mg/day for 4 weeks. Responders were more likely to have AT levels of 50–125 ng/ml and nortriptyline (NOR) levels below 95 ng/ml, or AT levels within this interval and NOR + OH-NOR levels less than 150 ng/ml. Although OH-NOR levels appeared to be related to response, a complicated post hoc analysis was necessary to uncover this relationship.

Robinson et al.,[2] who subsequently examined outpatients treated with AT 150 mg/day for 6 weeks, did not find evidence of a lower threshold for response and concluded that response was unrelated to drug levels. However, in the 27 patients for whom all levels were available, response was less likely if total levels of AT, NOR, OH-AT, and OH-NOR exceeded 200 ng/ml, suggesting that hydroxy levels might affect response.

It is surprising that OH-NOR has not been studied more during administration of NOR, as it presents a simpler analysis than when AT is given. OH-NOR/NOR ratios are highest among the TCAs, and clinical effects of this hydroxy-metabolite would be most obvious. These data might explain why effective levels of NOR are lower than those of other TCAs. Recent findings for OH-NOR during NOR administration are presented elsewhere in this book (see Ch. 131).

Antidepressant Activity of OH-DMI

We examined OH-DMI in 28 melancholic inpatients who underwent a 3-week fixed-dose (2.5 mg/kg/day) DMI trial.[3] DMI levels were significantly higher in responders than nonresponsders (200 versus 73 mg/ml; $t = 4.04$, $p < 0.001$), but mean OH-DMI levels were identical in the two groups (46 ng/ml). Total DMI + OH-DMI levels were less closely related to response than were DMI levels alone. The findings did not indicate that OH-DMI was inactive but that OH-DMI levels contributed little to response during a fixed-dose trial.

Amsterdam et al.[4] studied outpatients who met Research Diagnostic Criteria for endogenous depression and were treated with mean DMI doses of 185 mg/day for 4 weeks. Response was not associated with plasma levels of DMI, OH-DMI, or total drug in 54 completers whose drug levels were available. Because no drug levels were related to response, it is unclear if the findings reflect the activity of OH-DMI or if in that sample response was less dependent on drug treatment.

Kutcher et al.[5] described a naturalistic, variable-dose DMI study in 19 elderly depressed outpatients. Response was more frequent above a threshold DMI level but was not associated with OH-DMI.

Distinguishing the effects of OH-DMI and DMI during a fixed-dose study is difficult, as OH-DMI levels are usually one-half that of DMI; and patients who have high OH-DMI/DMI ratios and for whom OH-DMI might be expected to play a important role are the ones who rapidly metabolize the drug and thus have low DMI and low total DMI + OH-DMI drug levels. In two samples[4,6] OH-DMI/DMI ratios inversely correlated with DMI levels (r −0.75 and −0.63, respectively). This inverse relationship mitigates against finding a significant relationship for OH-DMI and response in a *fixed-dose study*.

We examined the relationship of OH-DMI and response during a *fixed plasma level* study. Nonpsychotic, unipolar inpatients with major depression underwent a 4-week DMI trial. Dose was rapidly adjusted to achieve a DMI plasma concentration within a therapeutic range using 24-h blood levels to calculate the dose.[7] Twenty-nine patients completed the trial. With this method, DMI plasma concentrations were substantially less variable (94–314 ng/ml) than in the fixed-dose study (20–934 ng/ml), but the variability in OH-DMI blood levels (6–110 ng/ml) was similar to that of the fixed-dose study. On every measure of response—the Hamilton Depression Rating Scale (HDRS), the Clinical Global Improvement Scale (CGI), and an eight-item Tricyclic Response in Melancholia Scale (TRIM) we developed to specifically assess drug response—total drug levels (DMI + OH-DMI) were more strongly correlated with outcome than were DMI levels alone. On the HDRS and TRIM scales, endpoint scores were significantly associated with total DMI + OH-DMI levels but not with DMI levels alone. In this study, in which the variability of DMI levels was restricted, OH-DMI concentrations appeared to contribute to response.

We had expected that OH-DMI might play an important role in patients with elevated OH-DMI/DMI ratios who might develop very high OH-DMI levels with dosage increase. In the fixed-dose study[6] 7 of 47 patients had OH-DMI/DMI ratios greater than 0.7. However, in the fixed plasma level study, only 1 of 40 patients had a ratio above 0.7. It appeared that nonlinear changes in DMI levels after dosage increase decreased the frequency of elevated OH-DMI/DMI ratios. Nonlinear changes in DMI concentrations are most apt to occur after dose change in patients whose DMI levels on a standard dose are low.[8] These patients rapidly hydroxylate DMI and have high OH-DMI/DMI ratios. However, if dosage is increased to reach a therapeutic DMI concentration, nonlinear changes in DMI levels result in lower OH-DMI/DMI ratios. To some extent, it limits the clinical importance of OH-DMI.

Adverse Effects

We examined OH-DMI concentrations in patients who had major adverse reactions that interrupted DMI treatment.[9] Among 84 patients treated with DMI, 13 developed major adverse reactions and 11 had plasma samples available for determination of OH-DMI. Neither DMI nor OH-DMI levels were elevated in the patients experiencing major adverse reactions. Orthostatic hypotension, the only common major side effect, often occurred at low levels.

The OH-DMI levels were also examined in relation to 23 subjective complaints and a 14-item subjective complaint total in 37 inpatients treated with DMI 2.5 mg/kg/day.[3] OH-DMI concentrations were not associated with the 14-item total or any of the individual symptoms, including dry mouth, the most common complaint. Amsterdam et al.[4] noted similar findings. It is not surprising that the OH-TCAs do not contribute to anticholinergic side effects as they have only 3–6% of the affinity for muscarinic receptors displayed by their parent compounds.[10] In addition, the only side effects that occur commonly during DMI treatment, dry mouth and orthostatic hypotension, do not appear to have a dose-dependent relation to DMI at therapeutic levels.[9,11]

Electrocardiogram (ECG) changes have been reported to be associated with OH-DMI[12] and OH-NOR[13] levels but not with levels of the parent TCAs. A case of heart failure associated with high OH-NOR levels was also described.[14] These cardiac findings are particularly important for the treatment of the elderly, in whom OH-NOR/NOR ratios are elevated.[15] Elevated OH-DMI/DMI ratios have also been reported in elderly patients,[16] but in that study the four elderly patients received lower DMI doses and achieved lower DMI plasma levels than the younger patients. At comparable doses and levels, nonlinear changes may result in lower OH-DMI/DMI ratios. In our fixed plasma level sample, the 12 patients over 60 years of age who received doses and achieved levels similar to the 33 younger patients had comparable OH-DMI/DMI ratios.

Conclusion

Research to date, exploring clinical relations of the OH-TCAs, have examined correlations of hydroxy levels with clinical variables in the presence of the parent drug. These findings are of value for understanding the clinical implications of OH-TCAs during treatment with the parent drug; however, the pharmacology of the OH-TCAs could be more directly studied by administration of the OH-TCAs themselves. This approach is currently being employed by Bertilsson, Nordin, and their associates and promises interesting results.[17]

References

1. Breyer-Pfaff U, Gaertner HJ, Kreuter F, et al. Antidepressive effect and pharmacokinetics of amitriptyline with consideration of unbound drug and 10-hydroxynortriptyline plasma levels. Psychopharmacology 1982;76:240–244.
2. Robinson DS, Cooper TB, Howard D, et al. Amitriptyline and hydroxylated metabolite plasma levels in depressed outpatients. J Clin Psychopharmacol 1985;5:83–88.
3. Nelson JC, Bock J, Jatlow P. The clinical implications of 2-hydroxydesipramine in plasma. Clin Pharmacol Ther 1983;33:183–189.
4. Amsterdam JD, Brunswick DJ, Potter L, et al. Desipramine and 2-hydroxydesipramine plasma levels in endogenous depressed patients: lack of correlation with therapeutic response. Arch Gen Psychiatry 1985;42:361–364.
5. Kutcher SP, Shulman KI, Reed K. Desipramine plasma concentration and therapeutic response in elderly depressives: a naturalistic pilot study. Can J Psychiatry 1986;31:752–754.
6. Bock JL, Nelson JC, Gray S, et al. Desipramine hydroxylation: variability and effect of antipsychotic drugs. Clin Pharmacol Ther 1983;33:190–197.
7. Nelson JC, Jatlow PI, Mazure C. Rapid desipramine dose adjustment using 24-hour levels. J Clin Psychopharmacol 1987;7:72–77.
8. Nelson JC, Jatlow PI. Nonlinear desipramine kinetics: prevalence and importance. Clin Pharmacol Ther 1987;41:666–670.
9. Nelson JC, Jatlow PI, Bock J, et al. Major adverse reactions during desipramine treatment: relationship to drug plasma concentrations, concomitant antipsychotic treatment and patient characteristics. Arch Gen Psychiatry 1982;39:1055–1061.
10. Wagner A, Ekqvist B, Bertilsson, et al. Weak binding of 10-hydroxy-metabolites of nortriptyline to rat brain muscarinic acetylcholine receptors. Life Sci 1984;35:1379–1383.
11. Nelson JC, Jatlow P, Quinlan DM. Subjective side effects during desipramine treatment. Arch Gen Psychiatry 1984;41:55–59.
12. Kutcher SP, Reid K, Dubbin JD, et al. Electrocardiogram changes and therapeutic desipramine and 2-hydroxy-desipramine concentrations in elderly depressives. Br J Psychiatry 1986;148:676–679.
13. Young RC, Alexopoulos GS, Shamoian CA, et al. Plasma 10-hydroxy-nortriptyline and ECG changes in elderly depressed patients. Am J Psychiatry 1985;142:866–868.
14. Young RC, Alexopoulos GS, Shamoian CA, et al. Heart failure associated with high plasma 10-hydroxynortriptyline levels. Am J Psychiatry 1984;141:432–433.
15. Young RC, Alexopoulos GS, Shamoain CA, et al. Plasma 10-hydroxy-nortriptyline in elderly depressed patients. Clin Pharmacol Ther 1984;35:540–544.
16. Kitanaka I, Ross RJ, Cutler NR, et al. Altered hydroxydesipramine concentrations in elderly depressed patients. Clin Pharmacol Ther 1982;31:51–55.
17. Bertilsson L, Nordin C, Otani K, et al. Disposition of single oral doses of E-10-hydroxynortriptyline in healthy subjects, with some observations on pharmacodynamic effects. Clin Pharmacol Ther 1986;40:261–267.

131. Disposition and Effects of E-10-Hydroxynortriptyline— An Active Metabolite of Nortriptyline

CONNY NORDIN AND LEIF BERTILSSON

Of the various tricyclic antidepressants available, the secondary amine nortriptyline (NT) is one of the most thoroughly studied from the clinical pharmacological point of view.[1] The major metabolite of NT, 10-hydroxynortriptyline (10-OH-NT), has two isomers (E- and Z-10-OH-NT) of which E-10-OH-NT is the quantitatively dominant one.[2,3] Compared with NT, the 10-hydroxymetabolites have about half the potency to inhibit the uptake of norepinephrine (NE) in vitro.[4] Thus the clinical and biological effects attributed to NT in earlier studies might at least partly be accounted for by 10-OH-NT.

Role of 10-OH-NT During Treatment of Depression with NT

In a group of 30 primarily depressed inpatients treated with NT, the clinical and biochemical effects were related to the concentrations of NT and 10-OH-NT in plasma and cerebrospinal fluid (CSF).[5] In most of the patients a debrisoquine (D) hydroxylation test was performed.[6] We found a correlation between the debrisoquine metabolic ratio (D/4-hydroxy-D) and the steady-state plasma concentration of NT (but not 10-OH-NT). The lack of correlation to 10-OH-NT indicates that its plasma concentrations are not only determined by the rate of NT hydroxylation but also by further elimination (metabolism and excretion).[6]

After 3 weeks of NT treatment the mean plasma and CSF concentrations of 10-OH-NT (599 and 67 nM, respectively) were higher than the corresponding levels of the parent drug NT (433 and 39 nM, respectively). There was a correlation ($p < 0.001$) between the CSF and plasma concentrations of both NT (r 0.92) and 10-OH-NT (r 0.77).[7] A correlation was found between the amelioration of depression and the plasma and CSF concentrations of NT (but not 10-OH-NT). However, the nine patients who recovered completely had plasma concentrations of NT and 10-OH-NT ranging from 358 to 728 nM and from 428 to 688 nM, respectively. A hypothetical "therapeutic area" within these two plasma concentration ranges has been suggested, indicating a contribution of 10-OH-NT.[5] Treatment with NT for 3 weeks decreased the NE metabolite 4-hydroxy-3-methoxyphenylglycol (HMPG) by a mean of 31%. It was not possible to evaluate to what extent this decrease was caused by NT and 10-OH-NT. However, the ratio between NT and 10-OH-NT in CSF correlated to the reduction of HMPG ($p < 0.05$) and the amelioration ($p < 0.001$), which might indicate that NT and 10-OH-NT interact with the NE system in a nonadditive way. A 15% mean decrease in the CSF concentration of the serotonin metabolite 5-hydroxyindoleacetic acid (5-HIAA) was mediated by NT itself.[5] The mean decrease of the dopamine metabolite homovanillic acid (HVA) was influenced by 10-OH-NT.

Disposition and Effects of E-10-OH-NT in Healthy Subjects

The major isomer of 10-OH-NT, E-10-OH-NT, has been administered in single doses to healthy subjects in three studies. We found that oral E-10-OH-NT was completely absorbed as shown by an urinary recovery of 86%.[8] About 50% of the given dose was recovered as conjugated E-10-OH-NT and about 25% as unchanged compound in urine. The mean plasma half-life of E-10-OH-NT was 8.8 h.

In a later double-blind crossover study aimed to assess the reduction of saliva flow, placebo and equimolar doses of E-10-OH-NT and NT were given to eight healthy men.[9] NT significantly depressed saliva flow compared with both placebo ($p<0.01$) and E-10-OH-NT ($p<0.05$). By contrast, there was no significant difference between E-10-OH-NT and placebo (Fig. 131.1).[9] Preliminary data indicate that E-10-OH-NT increases heart rate compared with NT and placebo.

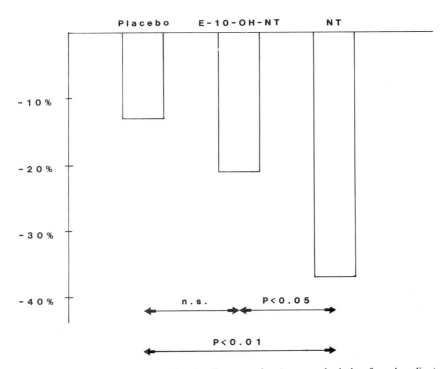

FIGURE 131.1. Changes in unstimulated saliva secretion (percent deviation from baseline).

TABLE 131.1. Properties of NT and E-10-OH-NT.

Property	NT	E-10-OH-NT
Disposition	Mainly hydroxylation	50% Glucuronidation 25% Renal excretion
Individual variation in disposition	Pronounced	Little
Inhibition of NE	+ + +	+ +
Inhibition of serotonin uptake	+	−
Anticholinergic effects	Yes	No
Antidepressant effect	Yes	To be evaluated

Conclusion

Certain properties of NT and E-10-OH-NT are compared in Table 131.1. A major problem with the use of NT as an antidepressant is its pronounced interindividual variation in metabolism.[1] The rate of metabolism (10-hydroxylation of NT) is genetically regulated.[3] E-10-OH-NT is mainly glucuronidized, and there seems to be little variation between individuals. The weak anticholinergic effects of E-10-OH-NT and its selective effects on NE uptake imply that the drug is a more specific tool than NT for evaluating the role of NE in the mechanism of antidepressant drug action. The potential clinical utility of E-10-OH-NT should be further evaluated in depressed patients and healthy subjects.

Acknowledgment. The studies were supported by grants from the Swedish Medical Research Council (3902), the Karolinska Institute, and the Söderström-König Foundation.

References

1. Sjöqvist F, Bertilsson L, Asberg M. Monitoring tricyclic antidepressants. Ther Drug Monit 1980;2:85–93.
2. Bertilsson L, Alexanderson B. Stereospecific hydroxylation of nortriptyline in man in relation to interindividual differences in its steady-state plasma level. Eur J Clin Pharmacol 1972;4:201–205.
3. Mellström B, Bertilsson L, Säwe J, et al. E- and Z-hydroxylation of nortriptyline: relationship to polymorphic debrisoquine hydroxylation. Clin Pharmacol Ther 1981;30:189–193.
4. Bertilsson L, Mellström B, Sjöqvist F. Pronounced inhibition of noradrenaline uptake by 10-hydroxymetabolites of nortriptyline. Life Sci 1979;25:1285–1292.
5. Nordin C, Bertilsson L, Siwers B. Clinical and biochemical effects during treatment of depression with nortriptyline—the role of 10-hydroxynortriptyline. Clin Pharmacol Ther 1987;42:10–19.
6. Nordin C, Siwers B, Benitez J, et al. Plasma concentrations of nortriptyline and its 10-hydroxy-metabolite in depressed patients—relationship to the debrisoquine hydroxylation metabolic ratio. Br J Clin Pharmacol 1985;19:832–835.
7. Nordin C, Bertilsson L, Siwers B. CSF and plasma levels of nortriptyline and its 10-hydroxy metabolite. Br J Clin Pharmacol 1985;20:411–413.
8. Bertilsson L, Nordin C, Otani K, et al. Disposition of single oral doses of E-10-hydroxynortriptyline in healthy subjects with some observations on pharmacodynamic effects. Clin Pharmacol Ther 1986;40:261–267.
9. Nordin C, Bertilsson L, Otani K, et al. Little anticholinergic effect of E-10-hydroxynortriptyline compared with nortriptyline in healthy subjects. Clin Pharmacol Ther 1987;41:97–102.

132. Genetic Polymorphism in Drug Oxidation: Implications for the Clinical Use of Tricyclic Antidepressants

L.F. GRAM AND KIM BRØSEN

Tricyclic antidepressants have been well characterized in terms of their pharmacokinetics. They are typical "high-clearance" drugs with elimination largely (> 97%) by hepatic biotransformation, high systemic clearance (0.2–1.2 l/min), and accordingly substantial elimination by first-pass metabolism.[1] The metabolism takes place primarily by demethylation, hydroxylation, and glucuronide conjugation.[2] Tricyclic antidepressants were among the first classes of drugs for which pronouned interindividual variations in pharmacokinetics, in particular clearance and steady-state levels on fixed doses, were shown.[2,3] The clinical consequences of this variability for therapeutic and unintended effects have been reviewed elsewhere.[4]

In a clinical fixed-dose study with imipramine we found an interindividual variation with a factor of 25–30 in steady-state levels of imipramine and the formed metabolite desipramine.[5] Interestingly, there was no intersubject correlation between imipramine and desipramine levels, indicating that demethylation (imipramine→desipramine) and 2-hydroxylation of both compounds vary among subjects in an independent way. The considerable advances in experimental and clinical research on drug oxidation permits a much better understanding of the mechanisms underlying this type of variability.

Drug Oxidation and Cytochrome P-450 Isozymes

Oxidation is often the rate-limiting step in the elimination of many drugs. The microsomal cytochrome P-450 monooxygenase, which is the major enzyme system for drug oxidation, consists of a series of isozymes with the same catalytic moiety (cytochrome P-450) but with different protein structures.[6-8] Isozymes differ by exhibiting a varying degree of stereoselective substrate specificity and regioselective drug oxidation; i.e., a given drug may be oxidized at different sites of the molecule by different isozymes. In addition, the function of cytochrome P-450 depends on the availability of oxygen, cofactors, and associated enzyme systems (cytochrome P-450 reductase, etc). Induction, by which certain chemicals or drugs cause an increase in the amount of enzyme by transcriptional activation of the corresponding P-450 genes, is a characteristic of some but not all cytochrome

P-450 isozymes.[9] The number of drug-oxidizing isozymes in human liver is unknown but probably amounts to more than 30.[9]

Genetic Polymorphism

The cytochrome P-450 isozymes appear to be controlled by separate genes.[9] The presence of different alleles (normal and variant) at one of these gene loci carries the possibility of a monogenetically determined polymorphic drug oxidation, provided the variant gene product (isozyme) has properties discernible from that of the normal gene.[7]

Clinical pharmacokinetic studies have revealed four or five independent polymorphic drug oxidations in man. This feat has been accomplished primarily by population studies demonstrating bimodal distribution in the formation of oxidized drug metabolites. The first and far best studied of these metabolic actions is the debrisoquine/sparteine oxidation polymorphism demonstrated independently for the two probe drugs and subsequently shown to represent one entity.[10] Among caucasians 6–10% of the population have a severely impaired ability to oxidize sparteine and debrisoquine. Family studies have shown that this abilit is an autosomal recessively inherited variant,[11,12] and the recipient is designated a "poor metabolizer" (PM); the remainder, representing home- and heterozygotes of the dominant gene, are designated "extensive metabolizers" (EMs). The frequency with which PMs appear seems to indicate distinct interethnic differences, with much lower frequencies in noncaucasian populations in Africa and Far East Asia.[8]

Other genetically independent polymorphisms include the oxidation of mephenytoin, tolbutamide, nifedipine, S-carboxymethyl-cysteine, and possibly others.[8] No widespread clinical significance has been demonstrated so far for the latter polymorphisms.

Phenotyping is usually carried out by having the subject ingest a nonpharmacological dose of the probe drug followed by measurement of the parent compound and oxidized metabolites in urine collected for 8–24 h. Results are expressed as the metabolic ratio (MR), i.e., the ratio between parent compound and oxidized metabolite(s). This measure exhibits bimodal distribution in population studies. PMs are characterized by very high MR values, and the distribution antimode is used as a cutoff point between PMs and EMs.[13]

Clinical Significance of the Debrisoquine/Sparteine Oxidation Polymorphism

The debrisoquine/sparteine MR has been shown to correlate strongly with the oxidation of several types of drugs, including several β-blockers, probably all tricyclic antidepressants, and some other drugs.[8,10] The relation to other types of drugs such as neuroleptics (see below) remains to be established. To become quantitatively important, the oxidation mediated by the debrisoquine/sparteine oxygenase must be a major pathway of elimination of the drug. It is the case for tricyclic antidepressants, where hydroxylation is the rate-limiting step before final elimination via glucuronide conjugation and urinary excretion. This is exemplified by our panel study with imipramine/desipramine single-dose kinetics[14] (Table 132.1). The primary metabolic pathways of imipramine are demethylation to desipramine, 2-hydroxylation of imipramine and desipramine, and subsequent glucuronide con-

TABLE 132.1. Imipramine and desipramine kinetics after single oral dose (100 mg): Mean values in groups of six healthy volunteers.

| Metabolizing Status | Sparteine MR | Imipramine | | | Desipramine | |
| | | $t_{1/2}$(h) | Clearance (l/min) | | $t_{1/2}$(h) | Clearance, (l/min) total[a] |
			Demethylation	Other pathways[a]		
Rapid EM	0.2–0.3	16	1.42	1.13	17	1.64
Slow EM	0.7–1.0	16	1.60	0.69[b]	21[b]	1.03[b]
M	60–180	23	1.09	0.26[b,c]	97[b,c]	0.19[b,c]

(EM) extensive metabolizers. (PM) poor metabolizers.
[a] Largely hydroxylation.
[b] Different from rapid EM ($p < 0.05$).
[c] Different from slow EM ($p < 0.05$).
Data are from ref. 14.

jugation of these two hydroxy-metabolites. The administration of imipramine and desipramine on separate occasions permits estimation of imipramine clearance as demethylation clearance and clearance via other pathways (largely hydroxylation).

Demethylation is the major pathway of elimination of imipramine, and it is not influenced by sparteine oxidase (Table 132.1). In contrast, 2-hydroxylation appears to be largely determined by the sparteine oxygenase with considerably lower clearance values in PMs and a significant difference between the two EM subgroups. Sparteine oxygenase thus exhibits regioselective oxidation (2-hydroxylation), and the demethylation is probably mediated by a different cytochrome P-450 isozyme.

For desipramine the major elimination pathway is 2-hydroxylation, and here the total clearance as well as elimination half-life (t_i) is heavily influenced by the sparteine oxidation phenotype. Treatment of a PM subject with standard doses of imipramine results in an almost immediate pronounced rise in the desipramine level; and many of these patients probably stop medication at an early stage due to severe side effects.[15] The logical solution would be to administer a very low dose (25–50 mg imipramine per day), in contrast to the very high doses required by some of the most rapid EMs (350–450 mg/day).[16]

Dose-Dependent Kinetics

The interindividual variability in EMs seems to be augmented as a consequence of dose-dependent kinetics, as shown for imipramine/desimipramine in clinical studies.[17,18] A dose increase thus results in a disproportionate rise in steady-state levels of, in particular, desipramine. This rise seems to be related to partial saturation at the 2-hydroxylation step,[18] which probably occurs mainly during first-pass metabolism (Brøsen and Gram[19]), when the drug concentration is particularly high in the liver.

Interaction Between Neuroleptics and Antidepressants

The pronounced inhibiting effect of neuroleptics on the metabolism of tricyclic antidepressants was reported many years ago[1,4,20] and was later confirmed by several groups. Studies with human liver microsomal preparations have shown that tricyclic antidepressants are potent inhibitors of sparteine oxidation (Ki 15–50 μM), and several neuroleptics (haloperidol, chlorpromazine) appear to be even stronger inhibitors (Ki 1–7 μM).[21] Metabolite studies further substantiate that the debrisoquine/sparteine oxygenase, in fact, is the site of this interaction, which affects the hydroxylation of imipramine/desipramine.[1,18] It remains to be shown if neuroleptics also are substrates of this isozyme and thus may exhibit the same type of oxidation polymorphism as was shown for the tricyclic antidepressants.

Conclusion

The debrisoquine/sparteine cytochrome P-450 isozyme mediates the rate-limiting step (hydroxylation) in the metabolism and elimination of all major tricyclic antidepressants and thus influences their pharmacokinetics and clinical use in several ways.

1. *Genetic polymorphism* accounts for the extreme variation in elimination rate, PM subjects being at risk of developing nearly toxic levels if they are given standard doses of tricyclic antidepressants.
2. *Dose-dependent kinetics* yield a disproportionate rise in steady-state levels with increasing doses, and thus pharmacokinetic variability is augmented.
3. *Drug–drug interactions* occur at this isozyme, notably the strong inhibitory effect of neuroleptics on the metabolism of tricyclic antidepressants.

This pattern of pronounced intersubject pharmacokinetic variability underlines the importance of careful drug level monitoring and the phenotyping of patients to be treated with tricyclic antidepressants. Depressed patients who are PMs should be offered phenotyping for family members, who are at substantial risk of developing depressions and at the same time of being PMs.

Acknowledgments. Recent studies discussed in this review were supported by grants from the Lundbeck Foundation.

References

1. Gram LF. Factors influencing the metabolism of tricyclic antidepressants: studies on interactions and first pass elimination (thesis). Dan Med Bull 1977;24:81–89.
2. Gram LF. Metabolism of tricyclic antidepressants: a review. Dan Med Bull 1974;21:218–231.
3. Hammer W, Sjöqvist F. Plasma levels of monomethylated tricyclic antidepressants during treatment with imipramine-like compounds. Life Sci 1967;6:1895–1903.
4. Gram LF. Plasma level monitoring of tricyclic antidepressants. Clin Pharmacokinet 1977;2:237–251.
5. Gram LF, Søndergaard I, Christiansen J, et al. Steady state kinetics of imipramine in patients. Psychopharmacology 1977;54:255–261.
6. Nebert DW, Negiski M. Multiple forms of cytochrome P-450 and the importance of molecular biology and evolution. Biochem Pharmacol 1982;14:2311–2317.
7. Al-Dabbagh SG, Smith RL. Species differences in oxidative drug metabolism: some basic considerations. Arch Toxicol [Suppl 7] 1984;219–231.
8. Kalow W. Genetic variation in the human hepatic cytochrome P-450 system. Eur J Clin Pharmacol 1987;31:633–641.
9. Nebert DW, Gonzalez J. Cytochrome P-450 gene expression and regulation. TIPS 1985;160–164.

10. Eichelbaum M. defective oxidation of drugs: pharmacokinetic and therapeutic implications. Clin Pharmacokinet 1982;7:1–22.
11. Price Evans DA Mahgouba, Sloan IP et al. A family and population study of the genetic polymorphism of debrisoquine oxidation in a white British population. J Med Genet 1980;17:102–105.
12. Brøsen K, Otton SV, Gram LF. Sparteine oxidation polymorphism: a family study. Br J Clin Pharmacol. 1986;21:661–667.
13. Brøsen K, Otton SV, Gram LF. Sparteine oxidation polymorphism in Denmark. Acta Pharmacol Toxicol 1985;57:357–360.
14. Brøsen K, Otton SV, Gram LF. Imipramine demethylation and hydroxylation: impact of the sparteine oxidation phenotype. Clin Pharmacol Ther 1986;40:543–549.
15. Gram LF, Bjerre M, Kragh-Sørensen P, et al. Imipramine metabolites in blood of patients during therapy and after overdose. Clin Pharmacol Ther 1983;33:335–342.
16. Brøsen K, Klysner R, Gram LF, et al. Steady state concentrations of imipramine and its metabolites in relation to the sparteine/debrisoquine polymorphism. Eur J Clin Pharmacol 1986;30:679–684.
17. Bjerre M, Gram LF, Kragh-Sørensen P, et al. Dose dependent kinetics of imipramine in elderly patients. Psychopharmacology 1981;75:354–357.
18. Brøsen K, Gram LF, Klysner R, et al. Steady-state levels of imipramine and its metabolites: significance of dose-dependent kinetics. Eur J Clin Pharmacol 1986;30:43–49.
19. Brøsen K, Gram LF. First-pass metabolism of imipramine and desipramine: impact of the sparteine oxidation phenotype. Clin Pharmacol Ther 1988;43:400–406.
20. Gram LF, Fredricson Overø K. Drug interaction: inhibitory effect of neuroleptics on metabolism of tricyclic antidepressants in man. Br Med J 1972;1:463–465.
21. Inaba T, Jurima M, Mahon WA, et al. In vitro inhibition studies of two isozymes of human liver cytochrome P-450. Drug Metab Dispos 1985;13:443–448.

V.D. ANTIDEPRESSANTS IN CLINICAL PRACTICE: ADVERSE EFFECTS OF ANTIDEPRESSANTS

133. Overdosage of Antidepressants

P. KRAGH-SØRENSEN

Most clinicians encounter patients seriously poisoned by antidepressants. These potentially life-threatening poisonings occur in three ways: accidentally, e.g., in children, a phenomenon that seems to be increasing[1]; intentionally, as with suicide attempts; and unintentionally, e.g., overdosage by the prescribing physician. The latter example is due to wide interindividual variability in the metabolism of these drugs, a problem with which many physicians are still not familiar.[2]

Risk of Lethality

From a formal clinical point of view, it is perhaps not surprising that antidepressants are frequently taken in overdose, as the indication for their use is depressive illness, a condition associated with a high incidence of self-poisoning and successful suicide. The problem is illustrated by data from the Office of Population and Censuses Survey (OPCS),[3] where facts on fatal poisonings in England and Wales from 1977 to 1984 are given. These data indicate that a high percentage (15%) of deaths involving antidepressants are registered. What is surprising and equally disturbing is that the total and percent of deaths involving antidepressants remained remarkably constant during the same period. The data also shows that the relative incidence per million patients for the individual drug largely reflects market share and prescribing figures. The data do not indicate the greater safety of a particular tricyclic antidepressant (TCA) compared with the remainder; however, mianserin (a tetracyclic antidepressant) seems to be less dangerous in overdosage, although mianserin alone or in combinations with other drugs can be lethal.

Prevention of Overdosage

The OPCS data[3] indicate that despite the considerable volume of literature available and the annual mortality statistics warning of the dangers of the older TCAs especially, they continue to be widely prescribed; data from sales statistics in many countries show that sales figures have even increased.[4] The widespread use of the older TCAs probably reflects the fact that the efficacy of these agents in depressive illness has long been recognized and appreciated by clinicians, whereas antidepressants of a more novel structure are not universally viewed as having convincingly demonstrated an efficacy in line with that of TCAs.

It is evident from sales figures[4] that the preparations most often prescribed are those with a pronounced sedative effect, e.g., amitriptyline and doxepin. Sales figures may then be an indication of how antidepressants are used. As only 5–10% of the use of antidepressants pertains to the treatment of manic-depressive disorders,[4] which is their proved indication, the high prescription figures for antidepressants with sedative effect could indicate that they probably are used as sedatives for other mental afflictions displaying certain depressive symptoms. This point is a serious one, as most of the deaths occur outside the hospital.

Data from many studies have indicated that a major reduction in mortality depends on prevention rather than on any improvements in management.[1] When a suicide risk is obvious it has been recommended that only a limited number of tablets should be left in the possession of the patient. The conventional guideline with the potentially suicidal patient is that no more than 1,000–1,200 mg, or about a 1 week's supply, should be given at one time. With many patients, however, it is misleading to think in terms of a "safe supply" limit, as the toxic dose for many does not greatly exceed the daily dose because of the tremendous interindividual variability in plasma levels and in the toxic response to a given dose. As at present there is no way of predicting which patients will or will not have a severely toxic response to overdosage, the patient's supply should be limited to less than 500 mg. Alternative treatment should be considered carefully in patients not suffering from manic-depressive disorders, as it is well known that affective reactions often are seen in these cases and a more or less unintended suicide attempt with drugs can follow on these reactions.[5]

Management of Overdosage

Self-poisoning with antidepressants is an economic problem, not only for the patient and his or her family but also for the society. It is estimated that each year 10,000 people in the United Kingdom poison themselves with antidepressants. In many countries all such patients are hospitalized routinely, and many require intensive care because of coma, perhaps ventilatory support, or treatment for seizures and/or cardiac complications.

The frequencies of major complications, taken from six published sources,[5–10] are shown in Table 133.1. The disparity in the frequencies reported in the various studies is probably not as interesting as the conclusions regarding future policy on cardiac monitoring following antidepressant overdose. There is still disagreement on the number of days in hospital necessary to ensure sufficient cardiac monitoring following overdose of antidepressants. Such disagreement exists because poisoning with these medications can cause specific toxic cardiovascular symptoms, e.g., broadening of the QRS complex, without simultaneously affecting consciousness. It has been claimed that in the case of patients suspected of overdose ingestion monitoring for 3–5 days after electrocardiogram (ECG) normalization is necessary. Although late deaths after recovery from TCAs have been reported, data from well controlled studies have shown that most deaths occurred within the first 24 h after admission, and late death was due to consequences of cerebral anoxia or to pulmonary complications, not to cardiac arrhythmias.[1]

TABLE 133.1. Frequency of major complications of TCA overdose.

Complication	Frequency (%)					
	Serafimovski et al.[6] ($n = 68$)	Thorstrand[7] ($n = 153$)	Petit et al.[8] ($n = 40$)	Marshall & Forker[9] ($n = 28$)	Pedersen et al.[5] ($n = 29$)	Goldberg et al.[10] ($n = 75$)
Coma	38	57	48	46	35	32
Supportive ventilation	34	23	40	7	45	57
QRS duration > 100 ms	—	73	50	44	30	23
Cardiac arrhythmias	—	3	18	11	8	4
Bundle branch block	—	—	15	17	0	0
Convulsions	19	11	20	11	15	12
Hypotension	29	26	15	11	11	7
Cardiac arrest	12	3	8	0	0	4
Death	7	3	5	0	0	3

These results have been further elucidated in plasma level monitoring studies.[5,8,10] Patients with total TCA levels above 1,000 µg/l have a higher incidence of coma, seizures, cardiac arrest, arrhythmias, and artificial ventilations. All patients having plasma levels above 1,000 µg/l experience impaired intracardiac conduction with a QRS duration above 100 ms, but these changes in the QRS can also be seen at plasma levels well below 1,000 µg/l. Plasma drug estimations have also been shown to be useful in patients with severe, unusual, and prolonged symptoms. In our 1982 study[5] we found that in some patients with severe and prolonged amitriptyline intoxication a high plasma level was sustained several days probably because of saturation kinetics. Conversely, plasma drug estimations were also useful for identifying patients in whom the diagnosis was uncertain.

These data indicate that when an overdose with antidepressants occurs continuous ECG monitoring is required for those patients who are comatose, are hypotensive, have arrhythmias, have prolongation of the QRS interval of more than 100 ms, or have plasma levels of more than 400–500 µg/l. Intensive cardiac monitoring may be discontinued if a normal level of consciousness and normal ECG have been observed for a period of 12–24 h or when the plasma concentration falls below 400 µg/l. Finally, there is little evidence to suggest that TCAs differ in their toxicity, and it seems that some novel nontricyclic agents are safer than TCAs in overdose situations.

Conclusion

Tricyclic antidepressants undeniably are highly toxic, and unfortunately overdosage frequently occurs. Therefore a substantial decrease in their usage could have been expected, but no such decrease has occurred. The persistence of clinicians in using these drugs surely reflects the fact that TCAs are regarded as effective drugs and as more effective than many of the new, though possibly safer, antidepressants.

Therefore we must face the benefit-risk aspect. We know that the risk of suicide attempt is great for patients suffering from severe depression, that TCAs are therapeutically effective for two-thirds of those suffering from so-called endogenous depression, that a substantial number of these and other psychiatric patients use these drugs in attempts at self-poisoning, and that many of these patients are hospitalized with severe intoxication. We also know that the cost of treating these patients is high and that, even so, TCAs will remain the drug of choice for treatment of many depressed patients for many years to come. We recognize that the risk of lethality is small once the patient has been hospitalized, but we also recognize that many patients die before they can be hospitalized. At the moment, the only way out of this dilemma is to focus on prevention.

References

1. Crome P. Antidepressant overdosage: Drugs 1982;23:431–461.
2. Kragh-Sørensen P. Monitoring Plasma Concentration of Nortriptyline: Methodological, Pharmacokinetic and Clinical Aspects. Copenhagen: Laegeforeningens Forlag, 1984;1–31 (thesis).
3. Office of Population and Censuses Survey. Death from Solid and Liquid Poisoning. London: HMSO, 1984; DH 4 No. 8.
4. Nordic Council on Medicines. Nordic Statistic on Medicines 1981–1983. Uppsala: NCM publications, 1986;4;187–198.
5. Pedersen OL, Gram LF, Kristensen CB, et al. Overdosage of antidepressants: clinical and pharmacokinetic aspects. Eur J Clin Pharmacol 1982;23:513–521.
6. Serafimovski N, Thorball N, Asmussen I, et al. Tricyclic antidepressive poisoning with special reference to cardiac complications. Acta Anaesthesiol Scand [Suppl] 1975;57:55–63.
7. Thorstrand C. Clinical features in poisonings by tricyclic antidepressants with special reference to the ECG. Acta Med Scand 1976;199:337–344.
8. Petit JM, Spiker DG, Ruwitch JF, et al. Tricyclic antidepressants plasma levels and adverse effects after overdose. Clin Pharmacol Ther 1977;21:47–51.
9. Marshall JB, Forker AD. Cardiovascular effects of tricyclic antidepressant drugs: therapeutic usage, overdose, and management of complications. Am Heart J 1982;103(3):401–414.
10. Goldberg RJ, Capone RJ, Hunt JD. Cardiac complications following tricyclic antidepressant overdose. JAMA 1985;13:1772–1775.

134. Risk-Benefit Assessment of Deaths from Adverse Drug Reactions and Overdosage with Antidepressants

STUART A. MONTGOMERY AND M.T. LAMBERT

When a drug is newly released onto the market there is relatively careful reporting of possible adverse drug reactions (ADRs). As the drug becomes established, the incidence of drug reactions reported is seen to fall. This fall does not necessarily imply a reduction in the true incidence of ADRs but, rather, reflects the less careful observation of patients that comes with familiarity. This gradual decrease of ADR reporting is a well known phenomenon. It makes it difficult to compare directly the ADRs reported for a new drug with those reported for an old drug without taking into account the selective underreporting produced by this effect.

When calculating the relative risk of a new class of drugs compared with an old one, it is therefore desirable not to rely only on a comparison of ADRs with the problems attendant on such an analysis. It is helpful, if possible, to take a measure of morbidity that is not related to voluntary reporting. A useful approach when analyzing relative risks of the new compared with the old antidepressants is to take a classic problem associated with each of the groups of drugs, e.g., deaths from blood dyscrasias and deaths from overdose.

It is difficult to determine the true incidence of ADRs because of underreporting. However, attention drawn to the occurrence of blood dyscrasias with mianserin by the medical press and the Committee on Safety of Medicines (CSM)[1] makes it likely that an accurate picture of dyscrasias with mianserin is now available. There has been less stimulus to report accurately the dyscrasias with other antidepressants so it is still not possible to make valid comparisons.

The most accurate reporting of ADRs is likely to be seen when there is an associated death, and we have taken this endpoint as a measure. Dyscrasias are more commonly seen in some countries than others.[2] It is unlikely that there are major differences in reporting between countries, and the variation in rates probably reflects a true national susceptibility. It may be that prescribing habits in some countries lead to selective use of mianserin for the physically ill and elderly, and in this case a higher incidence of dyscrasias would be expected.

In the United Kingdom hematological adverse reactions for mianserin, including aplastic/hypoplastic anemia, agranulocytosis, granulocytopenia, and thrombocytopenia, amounted to 18 per million prescriptions by the end of 1985.[1] There has been a sharp rise in the incidence of dyscrasias in the over-65 age group, rising from 11 per million to 30 per million prescriptions. The 12 fatal reactions were predominantly due to leukopenia or agranulocytosis, to which the elderly are particularly susceptible, the mean age for bone marrow suppression being 70 years and in fatal cases 75 years.

With antidepressants a convenient measure of ADRs that is independent of voluntary reporting is the data taken from death certificates following overdose (Table 134.1). The drugs that are named in the death certificate give a fairly accurate measure of the toxicity of those drugs in overdose. A crude measure of the toxicity of the drug may be obtained from the number of times a drug is cited in deaths from overdose with multiple drugs. A more accurate measure is provided where the drug is cited on its own as the single drug associated with death in overdose.

Assuming that overdoses are randomly distributed, a measure of the toxicity of a drug in overdosage can be obtained from the relation between the cumulative deaths from 1977–1984 [Office of Population and Censuses Survey (OPCS) data] and the market share of a particular drug. There are several ways of approaching this problem, and in this analysis the total sales in kilograms divided by the average dose and duration of treatment has been calculated. For the tricyclic antidepressants (TCAs) the average daily dose of 112.5 mg and for mianserin 45 mg is used. The average duration of treatment is taken as 60 days for all drugs.

It is helpful to sum the data over a number of years to allow for minor fluctuations on a yearly basis. The analysis is limited, as only those drugs that have been available for the whole period may be compared. It is clear from this analysis that in general the TCAs are associated with a substantial mortality rate as an ADR to overdose. Using this calculation the most dangerous TCAs are amitriptyline and dothiepin, with 166 and 143 deaths per million patients, respectively. The mean toxicity for the TCAs in this calculation is 106 fatalities per million patients, a figure that is disturbingly high. Maprotiline, which is a bridged tricyclic, is clearly associated with the same risk seen with the other tricyclics. Clomipramine appears

TABLE 134.1. Fatalities following self-poisoning with antidepressants, intentional or accidental: England and Wales, 1977–1984.

Drug	No. of fatalities[a]		Single-drug fatalities/ million patients[b]	Fatal ADR[c]/ million prescriptions
	Single drug	Multiple drugs		
Amitriptyline	808	447	166	< 1
Dothiepin	453	159	143	< 1
Imipramine	201	102	106	1–2
Doxepin	67	42	106	< 1
Maprotiline	60	24	103	< 1
Trimipramine	109	85	87	< 1
Clomipramine	34	35	32	5
Mianserin	27	53	13	2–3

[a]Cumulative figures from the Office of Population Censuses and Surveys (1977–1984).
[b]The number of patients was calculated on the basis of total sales in kilograms (IMS market statistics) divided by the average dose and duration of treatment. For the tricyclic antidepressants an average daily dose of 112.5 mg and for mianserin 45 mg was used, with an average duration of treatment of 60 days for all. (Data from Montgomery and Pinder.[3])
[c]Data from Committee of Safety of Medicines.[1]

to be an exception in the tricyclic group, with only 32 single death fatalities per million patients. This analysis does not yield an explanation for the difference, but one can speculate that clomipramine tends to be used in England and Wales for a somewhat different category of depression. Clomipramine has become established as the drug of choice in obsessive complusive disorder. This group of patients has been reported to be less at risk from overdose.[4] The newer antidepressant mianserin appears to be associated with considerably less toxicity in overdose, with only 13 fatalities per million patients.

In the risk-benefit analysis it is clear that the deaths from the toxicity of the drugs in overdosage exceed the deaths from ADRs from all other causes. It appears that TCAs are associated with more deaths than are the newer antidepressants, and clinicians should include these data in their assessment of relative risk and benefit.

References

1. Committee on Safety of Medicines. CSM update. Br Med J 1985;291:1638.
2. The International Agranulocytosis and Aplastic Anaemia Study. Risks of agranulocytosis and aplastic anaemia. JAMA 1986;256:174–1757.
3. Montgomery SA, Pinder RM. Do some antidepressants promote suicide? Psychopharmacology 1987;92:265–266.
4. Kringlen E. Obsessional neurotics—a long term follow up. Br J Psychiatry 1965;111:709–722.

135. Assessing the Safety of Antidepressant Drugs After Marketing: A U.S. View

CHARLES ANELLO

Before a new drug may be approved for marketing in the United States, evidence must be submitted to the Food and Drug Administration (FDA) in the form of a New Drug Application[1] (NDA) to show that the drug is effective and safe for use under the conditions of use claimed in its labeling. If the FDA concludes that the NDA meets the appropriate standards, the product is approved for marketing.

The limited scope of premarketing testing and evaluation, however, necessarily restricts the degree of assurance that can be given about any drug's freedom from rare and/or delayed-onset untoward events. Consequently, an active program of postmarketing surveillance is deemed a central and critical part of domestic drug regulations in the United States. In conjunction with the 1985 revision of the New Drug Regulations,[2] the Epidemiology and Biostatistics Office has developed and implemented an innovative set of procedures to screen and evaluate reports of adverse drug reactions.

This chapter focuses on (a) the FDA's monitoring system, using examples of selected antidepressant drugs; and (b) the "time-less risk" phenomenon, a phrase coined by Dr. Paul Leber to characterize the failure of published reports to indicate unit of time associated with cited adverse drug reaction rates.

The FDA method of monitoring adverse drug reactions (ADRs) is used to illustrate the importance of ADRs being submitted to a central point. Three drugs and their ADRs are discussed: amoxapine (Asendin; Lederle) and tardive dyskinesia; maprotiline (Ludiomil; Ciba) and seizures; and trazodone (Desyrel; Meade-Johnson) and priapism.

Monitoring in the United States

As soon as a new antidepressant agent is approved for marketing in the United States the FDA immediately begins tracking its clinical use and collects and evaluates reports of ADRs.[3] Through a contractual arrangement with IMS America, a pharmaceutical marketing research firm, the FDA has access to national estimates

---

The opinions expressed are those of the author and not necessarily those of the Food and Drug Administration.

of the antidepressant drug's use. The details of the IMS data base are discussed elsewhere.[4]

From these sources, much can be learned about the patterns of drug use. An examination of the trends in the use of antidepressant drugs shows that antidepressant drugs in 1976 comprised 18% of all prescriptions for psychotherapeutic drugs, whereas in 1984 the percentage was 26% (Fig. 135.1) The number of prescriptions for all psychotherapeutic drugs fell from 161.2 million to 130.6 million during this time period, however, even though the ratio of antidepressant drug use to psychotherapeutic drugs increased.

Other IMS data provide information on patterns of use: (a) indication; (2) demographic characteristics of the users of each drug; and (c) characteristics of the prescriber. The estimates of drug use obtained from IMS America also provide crude denominators for estimating reporting rates.

Adverse Drug Reaction Reports

The numerators used to estimate ADR reporting rates come from the FDA's spontaneous reporting system.[5] The FDA begins to receive ADR reports spontaneously from the medical community and routinely from the manufacturer immediately after a drug is marketed. Most of the ADRs being reported are a result of the drug firm's compliance with regulation 21 CFR 314.80. The FDA revised its regulations governing the reporting of ADRs by manufacturers in 1985. These regulations have had a profound impact on the U.S. manufacturers' reporting patterns. The average number of ADR reports entered into the FDA's computer file has grown from 10,000 per year to about 50,000 per year. The objective of the FDA's postmarketing reporting requirement is to signal potential serious safety problems with marketed drugs, especially those that are newly marketed. The following explains how regulation 314.80 works.[6]

An *adverse drug experience* is an adverse reaction (ADR) that occurs in the course of use of a drug in professional practice. (It could include overdose, abuse, withdrawal, and failure of expected pharmacological action.)

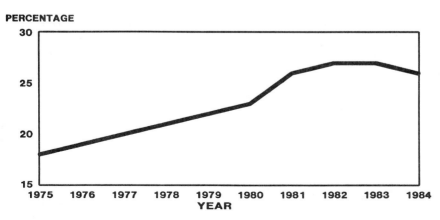

FIGURE 135.1. Percentage of antidepressant drugs compared to all psychotherapeutic drugs. (From IMS America national prescription audit.)

A *serious ADR* is an adverse drug reaction that results in death, disability, hospitalization, or prolonged inpatient hospitalization; requires prescription drug therapy; or involves death, congenital anomaly, cancer, or overdose.

An *unexpected ADR* means that it is not mentioned on the approved drug label (unlabeled).

A *15-day report* is a requirement to submit within 15 days an individual report (using form 1639) on any adverse drug reaction meeting both definitions of serious and unlabeled.

A *15-day report* is a requirement to submit within 15 days an individual report (using form 1639) on any adverse drug reaction meeting both definitions of serious and unlabeled.

A *15-day increased frequency report* is a requirement to submit a narrative to the FDA within 15 days of detection of an increase in the relative number of reports of serious labeled ADRs when suitable adjustments for marketing shall have been made.

A *periodic ADR report* is a requirement of the NDA holder to summarize the ADRs at regular intervals from the date of marketing of a drug. The reporting interval is quarterly for the first 3 years and annually thereafter.

The *1639 form* is a reporting form made available to drug manufacturers in the United States and other interested persons on which information related to suspected ADRs can be submitted to the FDA in a standardized manner.

The primary vehicle for reporting ADRs to the FDA is the FDA-1639 form. The form has five components: (a) reaction information (including outcome); (b) suspect drug(s) information; (c) concomitant drugs and (medical) history; (d) manufacturer-related information; and (e) initial reporter identity (which is confidential). The 1639 form clearly states that "submission of a report does not necessarily constitute an admission that the drug caused the adverse reaction." The 1639 form is intended to be filled out for each patient and is not used for submission of aggregated reports.

During the first 3 years of marketing, the manufacturer must submit a report quarterly. After 3 years of marketing the reporting period is extended to annual reporting.

To illustrate the use of the ADR reporting process, consider the drugs amoxapine, maprotiline, and trazodone. The reports received through the spontaneous reporting system (SRS) for each drug by year from the date of marketing to 1986 are presented in Table 135.1. (This information is contained in our on-line computer file, which maintains the current 5 years of data for direct access.) Amoxapine and maprotiline show the usual patterns of an initial increase in reporting for a new drug followed by a decline. The trazodone pattern is somewhat unusual because of the usual decline followed by an increase in reports to the FDA.

TABLE 135.1. Reports to the FDA spontaneous reporting system: All sources by drug and seriousness.

ADR	Amoxapine	Maprotiline	Trazodone
Total No.	1,029	1,332	1,814
Serious ADR	195 (19%)	183 (14%)	190 (10%)
Death	92	67	67
Hospitalization	120	125	132
Disability	3	2	6

By FDA's criteria for seriousness (i.e., death, hospitalization, and disability) from all sources, including foreign and study, the percentage of serious reports were 19% for amoxapine compared to 14% for maprotiline and 10% for trazodone.

It is often informative to restrict attention to domestic reports and to incorporate the IMS data in order to obtain crude estimates of reporting rates per 10^6 prescriptions (Rx) per year. To illustrate this idea, attention is restricted to those ADRs that are noted as unique on the drug's label. For amoxapine, consider tardive dyskinesia. The reporting rate in 1982 was $8/10^6$ Rx/year and declined to $6/10^6$ Rx/year in 1985: Maprotiline seizures; the reporting rate was $70/10^6$ Rx/year in 1982 and declined to $13/10^6$ Rx/year in 1985. On the other hand, trazodone-induced priapism is of interest. These data show that reporting rates for priapism increased from $3/10^6$ Rx/year in 1982 to $15/10^6$ Rx/year in 1985.

These examples illustrate that the FDA's spontaneous reporting system, when coupled with drug use data, does provide a method to monitor the ADRs of marketed drugs. Because manufacturers differ in their reporting patterns, however, one does not want to make too much out of comparisons across drugs in the same class from spontaneous reports. The FDA uses the spontaneous reporting system to generate hypotheses but relies on epidemiological studies to test hypotheses. The methods discussed so far relate to a spontaneous reporting system where only numerator data have been collected and only crude denominator data are available to the FDA. The rates calculated are reporting rates *(not incidence rates)* and cannot provide direct evidence of causal relations.

Leber's Time-Less Risk Phenomenon

Dr. Paul Leber, Director of the Division of Neuropharmacologic Drug Products at the FDA, introduced the phrase "time-less risk"[7] to call attention to a "common failing" in reporting risks of adverse reactions. As Leber stated, "One might hope that after more than two decades of extensive clinical experience with antidepressant drug therapy, the literature might contain sufficient information to answer . . ." practical comparative questions. Unfortunately, the cited estimates of drug risk vary by as much as 50-fold. (In regard to seizures, Peck et al.[8] reported 0.06% for amitriptyline; and Burley, cited by Trimble,[9] reported 3% for clomipramine.) Many authors offer sensible explanations for the variation, pointing to obvious differences in clinical pharmacological conditions under which the data in various reports were collected.[7]

Uncritical acceptance of a time-less risk, "that is a *risk without stated units of time,*" can itself pose a risk to the reader's ability to interpret the results. For example, a risk depicted as 0.005 per month is identical to one depicted as 0.06 per year. However, if stated in the literature without time units, e.g., 6% versus 0.5%, the former figure is likely to terrify the reader whereas the latter figure seems reassuring, when in fact these two risks are identical.

Conclusions

The manner by which the FDA collects and evaluates information reported to us on the adverse effects of antidepressant drugs, especially the incorportion of drug use information in relation to ADR reporting rates has been outlined. It is also noted that there are various methods to calculate the risk of an adverse event.

Special emphasis was placed on the importance of clearly specifying the time units in any published risk estimates if Leber's "time-less risk" is to be avoided and the scientific literature is to be more helpful as a source of comparative information of antidepressant drugs.

References

1. 21 CFR 312.0, New Drugs for Investigative Use. April 1986./
2. 21 CFR 314.80, Federal Register, New Drugs and Antibiotic Regulations, final rule. February 22, 1985.
3. Faich GA. Adverse Drug Reactions, FDA Office of Epidemiology and Biostatistics, 1984.
4. Baum C, Kennedy DL, Knapp DE, et al. Drug Utilization in the U.S.—1985. NTIS No. PB87-149902/AS. FDA Office of Epidemiology and Biostatistics, 1986.
5. Draft Guideline for Postmarketing Reporting of Adverse Drug Reactions. FDA Docket No. 850-0249, August 23, 1985.
6. Nelson RC, Baum C. Maprotiline and Seizures; An Analysis of FDA's Adverse Reaction System. Presented at the American Public Health Association Annual Meeting, Washington, DC, 1985.
7. Leber P. Time-less risks (a hazard of risk assessment; examples of seizure and antidepressants). Psychopharmacol Bull 1985;21(2)334–338.
8. Peck AW, Stern WC, Watkinson C. Incidence of seizures during treatment with tricycle antidepressant drugs and bupropin. J Clin Psychiatry 1983;44:197–201.
9. Burley, cited in Trimble MR. Non-monoamine inhibitors antidepressants and epilepsy, a review. Epilepsia 1978;19:241–250.

136. Tricyclic Antidepressants, Electroconvulsive Therapy, and Memory in Depressed Patients

A. CALEV, E. BEN-TZVI, BARUCH SHAPIRA, AND BERNARD LERER

It is well known that tricyclic antidepressants have relatively potent anticholinergic effects.[1] Anticholinergic activity is known to adversely affect memory performance,[2,3] and it is therefore reasonable to expect that tricyclic antidepressants produce memory deficits.

Conversely, depression itself is a cause of a transient but severe memory impairment.[4,5] As tricyclic antidepressants improve depressive symptoms,[5,6] they are also likely to improve memory function in depressives, thus acting against their own anticholinergically induced adverse effect on memory. Table 136.1 presents, in summary, a review of the literature, which addresses both the effect of lifting of depression on memory and the direct effect of tricyclic antidepressants on memory and other cognitive functions.

Table 136.1 shows that long-term memory (sometimes termed "secondary memory") is impaired during the course of tricyclic treatment. It should be noted that given the memory impairment caused by depression and the expected improvement in memory with the alleviation of depressive symptoms, an unchanged memory performance may be regarded as indicating impairment. If so, one can reasonably conclude that tricyclic antidepressants adversely affect long-term memory. It is well known, however, that long-term memory is not a pure memory function. It depends on processes that control the effectiveness of encoding, long-term retention, and proper retrieval. Examples of these processes are the ability to integrate to-be-remembered elements into a superordinate meaningful structure or context[7] and the ability to integrate the to-be-remembered material in an affective way.[8] Memory tasks that do not involve these processes, such as short-term memory tasks (sometimes referred to as "primary memory")[9] are not always impaired in subjects receiving tricyclic antidepressants (Table 136.1). Unlike long-term memory, this memory function depends on rehearsal, or on keeping a simple sensory trace of an event. Short-term memory is least affected by tricyclic antidepressants, in the same way that it is least affected by amnesic conditions such as senile dementias and Korsakoff's syndrome.

The present study was designed (a) to evaluate the impairment in long-term memory relative to short-term memory and remote memory (e.g., memory for events from the distant pretreatment past) following 3 weeks of treatment with

TABLE 136.1. Effect of tricyclic antidepressants on cognitive function.

Study	Anterograde memory				Attention		Other cognitive tasks	
	Long-term memory		Short-term memory					
	Directly observed deficit	Deficit inferred[a]	Directly observed deficit	Deficit inferred[a]	Directly observed deficit	Deficit inferred[a]	Directly observed deficit	Deficit inferred[a]
Belmont et al. (1963)[b]		−						−
Zung et al. (1968)[b]	−							
Henry et al. (1973)[b]	−							
Wittenborn et al. (1976)					−			
Legg & Stiff (1976)[b]	−							
Sternberg & Jarvik (1976)[b]	−			+				
Bye et al. (1981)					−		−	
Glass et al. (1981)			+					
Staton et al. (1981)			+					
Branconnier et al. (1982)[b]	−				−			
McNair et al. (1984)[b]	−				−	−		
Moskowitz & Burns (1986)					−			
Jones et al. (1986)					−	−	−	

(+) Improvement. (−) Deficit.

[a]Inferred from the fact that with improvement in depressive symptoms there was no improvement in cognition and memory.

[b]Studies involving long-term-memory tasks.

TABLE 136.2. Effects of imipramine and ECT on various memory tasks.

Treatment	Anterograde memory tasks			Retrograde memory tasks	
	Short-term memory (digits span)	Long-term memory		Public events recall	Autobiographical events recall
		Verbal (paired associates recall)	Visual (complex figure reproduction)		
Imipramine (200 mg)	Not impaired	Impaired	Not impaired	Not impaired	Not impaired[a]
ECT (seven treatments)	Not impaired	Impaired	Not impaired	Impaired	Impaired[a]

[a]For imipramine patients it was impaired relative to a normal control group, probably due to depression rather than treatment. ECT patients also showed better recall of the distant than the more recent past. The most recent past (events related to the last hospitalization) was least well remembered.

200 mg imipramine per day, and (b) to compare these impairments with those caused by a series of seven electroconvulsive therapy (ECT) treatments (using a minimum dose, bilateral procedure). The fact that the tricyclic group did not respond to treatment provided a unique opportunity to evaluate the effects of imipramine in a situation independent of alterations in memory function related to alleviation of depressive symptoms.

There were 16 patients in the ECT group and 10 in the imipramine group.

Age (mean ± SD): 60.4 ± 9.03 and 54.4 ± 14.06, respectively
General intellectual functioning assessed by the Quick test, form I, IQ (mean ± SD): 86.0 ± 24.05 and 91.0 ± 11.7, respectively

Baseline testing was conducted while the subjects were drug-free for at least 10 days and then about 14 h after the seventh ECT treatment or during the fourth week of imipramine treatment. Hamilton Depression Scale scores (mean ± SD) indicated an improvement for ECT patients (from 29.92 ± 5.5 to 14.76 ± 8.7; t = 5.430, $p < 0.0002$) and no improvement for imipramine patients (from 24.11 ± 7.7 to 22.00 ± 9.3; NS).

The results of the study are presented in Table 136.2, which shows that imipramine did not impair a short-term-memory task (digit span) that depended on an echoic trace and rehearsal. Nor did it impair retrograde remote memory, the encoding of which was done before treatment. It had, however, a clearly adverse effect on anterograde long-term memory for verbal material encoded during treatment. In this respect only was there a resemblance to the adverse effects of ECT on memory. Both ECT and imipramine patients showed faster forgetting of newly learned information after treatment than before treatment. The visual long-term-memory task did not appear to be impaired in either imipramine- or ECT-treated patients. This situation was probably due to the extreme difficulty of this task, which produced a floor effect for many of these severely ill, resistant depressive patients. However, ECT produced a clear impairment in memory for both distant public events and distant autobiographical events, whereas imipramine did not adversely affect this type of material, which had been encoded in the distant past. The ECT-induced deficit was characterized by better recall of distant autobiographical events than of more recent events, i.e., there was an amnesic gradient.

These results are in line with the literature review on the effects of tricyclics on memory.[5,6,10–20] They are based on the study of treatment-resistant patients whose depression was not alleviated by imipramine. The results show an impairment in long-term memory (paired-associates recall and forgetting speed) and, in line with the literature, no immediate (short-term) memory deficit (digits span). Although anterograde tasks were similarly affected by the two treatments, the effect of imipramine on retrograde memory was qualitatively different from that of ECT. ECT-treated, but not imipramine-treated, patients showed evidence of retrograde amnesia, i.e., impairment in remembering events that were encoded before treatment commenced.

Acknowledgment. Supported in part by NIMH grant MH40734.

References

1. Snyder SH, Yamamura HI. Antidepressants and the muscarinic acetylcholine receptor. Arch Gen Psychiatry 1977;34:236–239.

2. Crow TJ, Grove-White IG. An analysis of the learning deficit following lyoscine administration to man. Br J Pharmacol 1973;49:322–327.
3. Tune LE, Strauss ME, Lew MF, et al. Serum levels of anticholinergic drugs and impaired recent memory in chronic schizophrenic patients. Am J Psychiatry 1982;139:1460–1462.
4. Cohen RM, Weingartner H, Smallberg SA, et al. Effort and cognition in depression. Arch Gen Psychiatry 1982;39:593–597.
5. Sternberg DE, Jarvik ME. Memory functions in depression. Arch Gen Psychiatry 1976;33:219–224.
6. Zung WWK, Rogers J, Krugman A. Effects of electroconvulsive therapy on memory in depressive disorders. Recent Adv Biol Psychiatry 1968;10:160–179.
7. Mandler G. Organization of memory. In Spence KW, Spence JT (eds): The Psychology of Learning and Motivation. New York: Academic Press, 1967;327–372.
8. Koh SD, Grinker RR, Marusarz TZ, et al. Affective memory and schizophrenic adbedonia. Schizophr Bull 1981;7:292–307.
9. Baddeley AD. The Psychology of Memory. New York: Basic Books, 1976.
10. Belmont I, Pollack M, Willner A, et al. The effect of imipramine and chlorpromazine on perceptual analytic ability, perceptual responsivity and memory as revealed in Rorschach responses. J Nerv Ment Dis 1963;137:42–50.
11. Henry GM, Weingartner H, Murphy DL. Influence of affective state and psychoactive drugs on verbal learning and memory. Am J Psychiatry 1973;130:966–971.
12. Witterborn JR, Flaberty CF, Mc-Gough WE, et al. A comparison of the effects of imipramine, nomitensine and placebo on psychomotor performance of normals. Psychopharmacology 1976;51:85–90.
13. Legg JF, Stiff MP. Drug related test patterns of depressed patients. Psychopharmacology 1976;50:205–210.
14. Bye C, Clubley M, Peck AW. Drowsiness impaired performance and tricyclic antidepressants. Br J Clin Pharmacol 1978;6:55–161.
15. Glass RM, Uhlenhuth EH, Hartel FW, et al. Cognitive dysfunction and imipramine in outpatient depressives. Arch Gen Psychiatry 1981;38:1048–1051.
16. Branconnier RJ, Cole JO, Ghazvinian S, et al. Treating the depressed elderly patient: the comparative behavioral pharmacology of mianserin and amitriptyline. In Costa R (ed): Typical and Atypical Antidepressants: Clinical Practice. New York: Raven Press, 1982;195–212.
17. Staton RD, Wilson H, Brumback KA. Cognitive impairment associated with tricyclic antidepressant treatment of childhood major depressive illness. Percept Motor Skills 1981;53:219–234.
18. McNair DM, Kohn RJ, Frankenthalaer LM, et al. Amoxapine and amitriptyline. II. Specificity of cognitive effects during brief treatment of depression. Psychopharmacology 1984;83:134–139.
19. Moskowitz H, Burns MM. Cognitive performance in geriatric subjects after acute treatment with antidepressants. Neuropsychobiology 1986;15(1):38–43.
20. Jones DM, Allen EM, Griffiths AN, et al. Human cognitive function following binadaline (50 mg and 100 mg) and idmipramine (75 mg): results with a new battery of tests. Psychopharmacology 1986;89:198–202.

V.E. GABA-Mimetics as Antidepressants

137. GABA Theory of Depression and Antidepressant Drug Action

G. BARTHOLINI, K.G. LLOYD, B. SCATTON, AND B. ZIVKOVIC

Double-blind trials have shown that γ-aminobutyric acid (GABA)-mimetic agents such as progabide* and fengabine,† compared to tricyclic antidepressants (TCAs), exhibit an antidepressant action of shorter onset and have a lower incidence of side effects (see Chs. 138–140). GABA-mimetics affect norepinephrine (NE) and serotonin (5-hydroxytryptamine, 5-HT) neurons and their postsynaptic cells (for the pharmacological spectrum of GABA-mimetics, see ref. 1). Thus the question is whether GABA-mimetics—similar to TCAs and monoamine oxidase (MAO) inhibitors—act via monoamines or directly trigger the antidepressant effect. Three types of evidence are discussed: (a) the alterations of monoamine-related parameters induced by GABA-mimetics; (b) how these changes differ from those induced by TCAs; and (c) the involvement of the GABA system in the antidepressant action.

Effects of GABA-Mimetics on the NE System

On acute administration, GABA-mimetics (progabide, fengabine, muscimol, THIP) enhance, by a picrotoxin-sensitive mechanism, the liberation of NE in rat brain areas.[2,3] This effect probably results from the activation of NE neurons, as it is prevented by interruption of the impulse flow (injection of tetrodotoxin in the ascending bundle).[3,4] On sustained treatment, GABA-mimetics do not down-regulate β_1-receptors,[5] at variance with TCAs. However, fengabine (and progabide associated with desipramine) desensitizes β_1-receptor-linked adenylate cyclase; uncoupling the enzyme from the β_1 site may result from a direct postsynaptic effect of the drug.[6,7]

Serotonergic System

In the rat, the turnover of cerebral 5-HT is decreased by GABA-mimetics on both acute and repeated administration. This bicuculline-sensitive effect probably results

---

*4-[(4-Chlorophenyl)(5-fluoro-2-hydroxy-phenyl)-methylene] amino butanamide.
†2-[(Butylamino)(2-chlorophenyl)methyl]-4-chlorophenyl.

from a primary reduction in firing rate of 5-HT neurons.[4] Progabide also enhances the density of 5-HT$_2$ receptors.[8] At variance with progabide and muscimol, fengabine does not affect the 5-HT system, possibly because of its kinetic features.[6]

Mode of Antidepressant Action of GABA-Mimetics as Related to Monoamines

Whereas TCAs and MAO inhibitors enhance NE and 5-HT concentrations by inhibition of reuptake and metabolism, respectively, GABA-mimetics (a) primarily affect the firing rate of monoamine neurons, (b) cause opposite changes on NE and 5-HT systems, and (c) elicit postsynaptic alterations different from those observed with conventional antidepressants (Table 137.1). These heterogeneous patterns suggest that monoamine changes are not a common mechanism of the two classes of compounds and that an additional or alternative mechanism—possibly GABAergic in nature—is involved.

Involvement of GABA

In models specifically predictive of antidepressant drug action—olfactory bulbectomy and learned helplessness—GABA-mimetics and conventional antidepressants reverse the behavioral deficit.[6,9] The reversal by GABA-mimetics (a) occurs after acute administration whereas TCAs have to be administered repeatedly and (b) is blocked by bicuculline. Also, bicuculline antagonizes the reversal by TCAs (e.g., imipramine),[6,10] indicating that their mode of action involves a GABA$_A$-receptor-mediated mechanism.

Moreover, up-regulation of GABA$_B$ receptors is induced in rat frontal cortex on repeated administration of GABA-mimetics and all clinically effective antidepressants, independently of their chemical structure and mechanism of action: (a) inhibitors of dopamine, NE, or 5-HT uptake; (b) MAO inhibitors iprindole, and mianserine; and (c) electroshock.[11,12,13]

Psychotropic classes other than antidepressants do not affect GABA$_B$ receptors. The mechanism of this change and the possible relation between GABA$_B$ and GABA$_A$ receptors are still unknown. However, it appears that the GABA system plays a main role in the mode of antidepressant action of not only GABA-mimetics but also of other types of antidepressant.

TABLE 137.1. Effect of monoamine uptake inhibitors and GABA agonists on NE- and 5-HT-related parameters.

Antidepressant	Postsynaptic changes			Transmission	
	β_1	AC	5-HT$_2$	NE	5-HT
Monoamine uptake inhibitors					
NE + 5-HT	−	−	−	+	+
Specific NE	−	−	=	+	=
Specific 5-HT	=	=	−	=	+
GABA agonists					
Progabide	=	−	+	+	−
Fengabine	=	−	=	+	=

(+) increase. (−) decrease. (=) no change. (AC) adenylate cyclase.

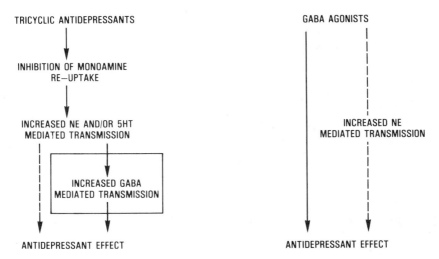

FIGURE 137.1. Modes of action of conventional antidepressants (e.g., monoamine uptake inhibitors) and GABA agonists.

Other data further suggest a role of GABA. Thus in hippocampal slices of rats in a learned helplessness situation, depolarization-induced GABA liberation is reduced compared to controls; imipramine corrects the behavioral deficit[10] (see above) along with the biochemical alteration.[14] Also, injection of GABA into the frontal cortex prevents,[10] whereas hippocampal injection of bicuculline induces,[14] learned helplessness. Moreover, desipramine enhances thalamic GABA liberation (push-pull cannula),[13] an effect that may be linked to GABA reuptake inhibition by TCAs.[15] Finally, GABA concentrations are reduced in the plasma[16] and cerebrospinal fluid[17–20] of depressed patients.

Conclusion

The following conclusions can be drawn: (a) A deficit in GABA function is involved in models in which the behavioral alteration is specifically reversed by antidepressants. (b) A GABAergic mechanism is involved in the mode of action of conventional antidepressants (Fig. 137.1); this mechanism may be triggered by the activation of monoamine (possibly NE)- mediated transmission, which could explain the longer onset of action of TCAs versus that of GABA-mimetics in both animal models and depressed patients. (c) GABA agonists, compared to conventional antidepressants, may lead more directly to the relief of depressive symptoms; additionally, provided that activation of NE neurons enhances GABA-mediated transmission, the GABA-mimetic-induced NE changes may reinforce the effect of the direct stimulation of GABA receptors. (d) These hypotheses are supported by the antidepressant action of GABA-mimetics in clinical trials.

References

1. Bartholini G, Scatton B, Zivkovic B, et al. GABA receptor agonists as a new therapeutic class. In Bartholini G, Bossi L, Lloyd KG, et al, (eds): Epilepsy and GABA Receptor

Agonists: Basic and Therapeutic Research (L.E.R.S. Monograph Series, Vol. 3). New York: Raven Press, 1985;1–30.

2. Scatton B, Zivkovic B, Debek J, et al. γ-Aminobutyric acid (GABA) receptor stimulation. III. Effect of progabide (SL 76 002) on norepinephrine, dopamine and 5-hydroxytryptamine turnover in rat brain areas. J Pharmacol Exp Ther 1982;220:678–688.

3. Dennis T, Curet O, Nishikawa T, et al. Further evidence for, and nature of the facilitatory GABAergic influence on central noradrenergic transmission. Naunyn Schmiedebergs Arch Pharmacol 1985;331:225–234.

4. Scatton B, Nishikawa T, Dennis T, et al. GABAergic modulation of central noradrenergic and serotonergic neuronal activity. In Bartholini G, Lloyd KG, Morselli PL (eds): GABA and Mood Disorders: Experimental and Clinical Research (L.E.R.S. Monograph Series, Vol. 4). New York: Raven Press, 1986;67–75.

5. Zivkovic B, Scatton B, Dedek J, et al. GABA influence on noradrenergic and serotonergic transmissions: implications in mood regulation. In Langer SZ, Takahashi R, Segawa T, et al (eds): New Vistas in Depression. Oxford: Pergamon Press, 1982;195–201.

6. Zivkovic B, Lloyd, KG Scatton B, et al. The pharmacological and neurochemical spectrum of fengabine, SL 79 229, a new antidepressant agent. In Bartholini G, Lloyd KG, Morselli PL (eds): GABA and Mood Disorders: Experimental and Clinical Research (L.E.R.S. Monograph Series, Vol. 4). New York: Raven Press, 1986;85–95.

7. Scatton B, Lloyd KG, Zivkovic B, et al. Fengabine, a novel antidepressant GABAergic agent. II. Effect on cerebral noradrenergic, serotonergic and GABAergic transmission. J Pharmacol Exp Ther 1987;241:251–257.

8. Langer SZ, Arbilla S, Scatton B, et al. Progabide and SL 75 102: interaction with GABA receptors and effects on neurotransmitter and receptor systems. In Bartholini G, Bossi L, Lloyd KG, et al (eds): Epilepsy and GABA Receptor Agonists: Basic and Therapeutic Research (L.E.R.S. Monograph Series, Vol. 3). New York: Raven Press, 1985;81–90.

9. Lloyd KG, Morselli PL, Depoortere H, et al. The potential use of GABA agonists in psychiatric disorders: evidence from studies with progabide in animal models and clinical trials. Pharmacol Biochem Behav 1983;18:957–966.

10. Sherman AD, Petty F. Neurochemical basis of the action of antidepressants on learned helplessness. Behav Neurol Biol 1980;30:119–134.

11. Pilc A, Lloyd KG. Chronic antidepressants and GABA receptors: a GABA hypothesis of antidepressant drug action. Life Sci 1984;35:2149–2154.

12. Lloyd KG, Thuret F, Pilc A. Up-regulation of γ-aminobutyric acid (GABA) B binding sites in rat frontal cortex: a common action of repeated administration of different classes of antidepressants and electroshock. J Pharmacol Exp Ther 1985;235:191–199.

13. Korf J, Venema K. Desmethylimipramine enhances the release of endogenous GABA and other neurotransmitter amino acids from the rat thalamus. J Neurochem 1983;40:946–950.

14. Petty F, Sherman AD. GABAergic modulation of learned helplessness. Pharmacol Biochem Behav 1981;15:567–570.

15. Harris M, Hopkins M, Neal MJ. Effect of centrally acting drugs on the uptake of γ-aminobutyric acid (GABA) by slices of rat cerebral cortex. Br J Pharmacol 1973;47:229–239.

16. Petty F, Schlesser MA. Plasma GABA in affective disorders. J Affective Disord 1981;3:339–343.

17. Gold BI, Bowers MB, Roth RH, et al. GABA levels in CSF of patients with psychiatric disorders. Am J Psychiatry 1980;137:362–364.

18. Gerner RH, Hare TA. CSF GABA in normal subjects and patients with depression, schizophrenia, mania and anorexia nervosa. Am J Psychiatry 1981;138:1098–1101.

19. Kasa K, Otsuki S, Yamamoto M, et al. Cerebrospinal fluid γ-aminobutyric acid and homovanillic acid in depressive disorders. Biol Psychiatry 1982;17:877–883.

20. Gerner RH, Fairbanks L, Andersen GM, et al. CSF neurochemistry in depressed, manic and schizophrenia patients compared with that of normal controls. Am J Psychiatry 1984;141:1533–1540.

138. GABA-Mimetic Agent Fengabine in the Treatment of Depression: An Overview

B. MUSCH AND M. GARREAU

The development of antidepressant drugs has traditionally been based on the potentiation of central monoaminergic synaptic activity. In order to dissociate the classic undesirable effects of antidepressants related to monoamine potentiation from the antidepressant effect, attempts have been made to discover new antidepressant drugs with other mechanisms of action. One of these new approaches suggests the involvement of γ-aminobutyric acid (GABA) in the pathogenesis of depression.[1]

The potential antidepressant efficacy of a new GABA-mimetic drug fengabine has been investigated in depressed patients to better elucidate the role of GABA agonists in the treatment of depression. This chapter presents the results of ten open pilot studies and three double-blind comparative trials versus reference drugs performed in Europe with fengabine.

Open Pilot Studies in Depressed Patients

The antidepressant effect of fengabine was evaluated initially in ten open pilot studies conducted according to the same study design under open conditions.[2,3] Fengabine was administered orally three times a day at flexible daily doses of 400–2,400 mg for a period of 3–4 weeks.

A total of 108 patients were included in the ten studies, 34 men and 74 women aged 18–68 years, with a mean age of the entire population of 48.4 years. The characteristics of the population were as follows: A group of 75 patients were suffering from major depression (13 patients with a single episode, 62 with recurrent episodes), 16 patients had bipolar disorder, and 17 patients had dysthymic disorder. Duration of disease was more than 6 years in 60% of patients, 1–5 years in 27%, and less than 1 year in the remaining 13%.

Eighty-five patients (78.7%) completed the trial according to the protocol; five patients dropped out because of inefficacy, six patients because of side effects, three for both inefficacy and side effects, and nine for reasons not related to fengabine treatment.

Clinical efficacy was assessed using rating scales for depression: Montgomery Asberg Depression Rating Scale (MADRS)[4] and Hamilton Rating Scale for

Depression (HRSD).[5] The overall clinical response was assessed by the investigators according to a clinical global impression scale (CGI).[6]

Ninety-seven patients were taken into consideration for the evaluation of efficacy. The therapeutic response was judged good or excellent by the investigator in 60 patients (61.9%) and as a partial response in 13 patients (13.4%); 24 patients (24.7%) remained unchanged. In all centers the decrease of the total scores on the MADRS or HRSD at the end of study was significant ($p < 0.05$ or $p < 0.01$, depending on the center). The initial scores on the rating scales were reduced in responders by 40.1–84.5%. Of the 80 patients suffering from a major affective disorder according to *DSM-III* classification, 49 (61.2%) had a good or excellent response; a similar response was observed in 11 of the 16 patients (68.8%) suffering from dysthymic disorders. The response rate (excellent or good), according to the maximum daily dose received, was higher in the group of patients treated with a maximum daily dose of 1,200–1,400 mg fengabine. In eight of the ten studies, the mean total scores of rating scales were significantly reduced ($p < 0.05$) at day 7 of the treatment period, suggesting a short onset of action. In the remaining two centers the mean total scores decreased significantly at day 14.

In regard to clinical safety, headache was the most frequent side effect (12%); nausea and vomiting (11.1%), somnolence (8.3%), abdominal pain (7.4%), and diarrhea (6.5%) were also reported. No abnormalities were detected in the electrocardiogram or vital signs. An increase in γ-GT, consistent with the liver-enzyme-inducing properties of the molecule (in 30 patients) and a slight increase of transaminases (SGOT and SGPT) (in 2 patients) were the only abnormal findings in laboratory tests. None of these abnormalities was associated with clinical signs or symptoms.

Comparative Studies: Fengabine Versus Reference Drugs

Fengabine was compared to reference drugs in three double-blind parallel group studies in depressed patients. A total of 238 patients were included, 115 of whom received fengabine. The results are discussed study by study.

Fengabine Versus Imipramine

In this study[7] fengabine was compared to imipramine over 4 weeks. Drugs were administered at flexible, increasing doses with a comparative dose ratio of 200 mg fengabine versus 10 mg imipramine. The study was performed in 81 outpatients suffering from neurotic depression (*DSM-III* 300.40) with a prestudy HRSD total score of more than 25. A group of 38 patients received fengabine and 43 imipramine; the mean doses were 1,460 mg fengabine and 75 mg imipramine. Reasons for dropouts were inefficacy (one fengabine, two imipramine), side effects (three fengabine, ten imipramine), others (two fengabine, eight imipramine).

Both fengabine and imipramine reduced the Hamilton Depression Rating Scale total score; but no statistical difference was shown between treatments. The CGI scale at the end of the study showed that 89% of the patients had a good or excellent response in the fengabine group in contrast to 73.7% in the imipramine group; this better response rate of fengabine versus imipramine did not reach statistical significance.

Fengabine appeared to be better tolerated than imipramine; the therapeutic index of the CGI was slightly in favor of fengabine, and side effects were less frequent after fengabine. Major complaints in the fengabine group were dry mouth (16%) and nausea (10.5%); in the imipramine group 46.5% of patients reported dry mouth, 23.3% constipation, and 18.6% tremor and anxiety.

Multicenter Trials: Fengabine Versus Clomipramine

In two multicenter studies[8,9] fengabine was compared to clomipramine for 4 weeks. Both studies were conducted according to the same protocol: The dose regimen was flexible, with a comparative dose ratio of 300 mg fengabine versus 25 mg clomipramine. The depression scale used was the Montgomery Asberg Depression Rating Scale (MADRS). The patients included in the two studies are reported in Table 138.1.

In the first study, fengabine was administered at the mean daily dose of 1,400 mg and clomipramine at 115 mg/day. Thirty-seven patients in the fengabine group and 39 in the clomipramine group completed the trial period. Dropouts for inefficacy were, respectively, five and two; for side effects two and six; three and two patients, respectively, dropped out for reasons not drug-related, and five in the fengabine group and seven in the clomipramine group were discontinued due to recovery from the depressive state.

The curves representing the mean MADRS total scores during the course of the study (Fig. 138.1) were superimposable. Both treatments significantly reduced the mean total scores, and no significant difference was observed between treatments.

Comparison on the CGI did not demonstrate any significant difference between the two groups: 67.6% responded (good or excellent response) in the fengabine group and 74.4% in the clomipramine group.

In the second study doses ranged from 1,200 to 1,800 mg (mean 1,400 mg) for fengabine and from 50 to 150 mg (mean 110 mg) for clomipramine. Eighty-one patients were included: 40 received fengabine and 41 clomipramine. Seven patients dropped out of the study in the fengabine group: one for adverse events and six for reasons not treatment-related. In the clomipramine group six patients discontinued treatment: one for inefficacy, two for adverse events, and three for reasons not treatment-related.

Results from this study confirmed those obtained in the previous one. The antidepressant activity of fengabine was comparable to that of clomipramine: reduction of the MADRS total score in both groups was superimposable at all study intervals. According to the CGI, 78.4% of patients responded to fengabine (good or excellent response) and 82.1% responded to clomipramine.

TABLE 138.1. Characteristics of the population.

Characteristic	Fengabine	Clomipramine	Total
Patients (No.)	77	80	157
Age (mean; years)	43.1	46.6	
Sex	51 F/26 M	50 F/30 M	101 F/56 M
Diagnosis *DSM-III*[a]			
296.2	13	15	28
296.3	41	49	90
296.5	23	16	39

[a]296.2: major depression, single episode. 296.3: major depression, recurrent episode. 296.5: bipolar disorder, depressed.

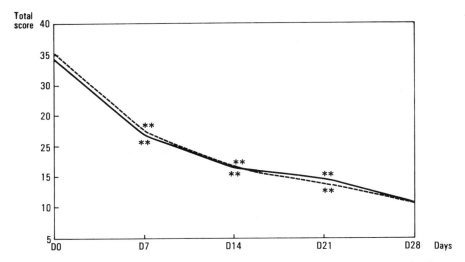

Figure 138.1. MADRS total score in fengabine versus clomipramine study. Solid full line: fengabine. Dotted line: clomipramine.

In both studies fengabine appeared to be better tolerated than clomipramine: 63.6% of patients treated with fengabine presented adverse events, as did 83.7% in the clomipramine group. The more frequent adverse events, dry mouth and postural hypotension, were present in 47.5% of patients in the clomipramine group and in 21.0% of patients in the fengabine group. There were no significant variations in the vital signs of either group.

Conclusions

Pharmacological treatment of depression is still based mainly on use of tricyclic antidepressant drugs. Some new drugs have been introduced during the last two decades. Some of them have been withdrawn from the market because of toxic reactions (nomifensine, indalpine), some of them have not shown a clear-cut effect in major depression so far (mianserine, trazodone), and some have been on the market for too short a time to represent an alternative to tricyclics.

Although tricyclic antidepressants are considered to be active, their use is not devoid of serious problems, i.e., delay in the onset of action and disturbing side effects. New drugs with a faster onset of action and a better safety profile are consequently needed.

GABA agonists represent a new approach to the treatment of depression. Their suggested mechanism of action has opened new vistas on the pathogenesis of depression, and their effect in depressed patients has provided important evidence of the fact that the proposed mechanism may have a real impact in the therapy of depression. The available clinical data demonstrate the antidepressant activity of fengabine and support the hypothesis of a new approach to the drug treatment of depression by means of GABA-mimetic agents.

References

1. Lloyd KG, Morselli PL, Depoortere H, et al. The potential use of GABA agonists in psychiatric disorders: evidence from studies with progabide in animal models and clinical trials. Pharmacol Biochem Behav 1983;18:957.
2. Musch B, Garreau M. An overview of the antidepressant activity of fengabine in open clinical studies. In Proceedings of the IVth World Congress of Biological Psychiatry, Philadelphia, 1985.
3. Musch B. Antidepressant activity of fengabine: a critical overview of the present results in open clinical studies. In Bartholini G, Lloyd KG, Morselli PL (eds): GABA and Mood Disorders: Experimental and Clinical Research (L.E.R.S. Monograph Series, Vol. 4). New York: Raven Press, 1986;171–177.
4. Montgomery SA, Asberg M. A new depression scale designed to be sensitive to change. Br J Psychiatry 1979;134:382–385.
5. Hamilton M. Development of a rating scale for primary depressive illness. Br J Psychiatry 1967;6:278–296.
6. Guy W. ECDEU Assessment Manual for Psychopharmacology. Rockville, MD: National Institute of Mental Health, 1976.
7. Brion S, Gailledreau J, Garreau M., et al. Double blind study of fengabine versus imipramine in depression. In preparation.
8. Bourgeois M, Escande M, Lepine JP, et al. Multicenter double blind study of fengabine versus clomipramine in major affective disorders. In preparation.
9. Samuelian JC, Ballereau J, Bordarier V, et al. Fengabine, a new GABA-mimetic agent, and clomipramine in the treatment of major depression—a double blind study. Submitted for publication.

139. Antidepressant Activity of Progabide and Fengabine

P.L. MORSELLI, P. PRIORE, C. LOEB, C. ALBANO, N.P. NIELSEN, C. SERRATI, AND B. MUSCH

Evidence suggests the involvement of the GABAergic (γ-aminobutyric acid) system in affective disorders and the therapeutic action of GABA-mimetic agents, e.g., progabide (PGB) and fengabine (FGB), in depressive states.[1-3] The hypothesis of a novel pathogenetic mechanism of depression is interesting on both the heuristic and pragmatic levels, and it may lead to a better understanding of some of the biochemical alterations underlying depressive disorders. Moreover, it may open new therapeutic possibilities in an area where the available medication is still far from optimal. We report here an overview of the clinical data available for PGB as well as data on FGB.

Controlled Clinical Studies with Progabide

Open clinical studies in several neuropsychiatric syndromes suggested the possibility of a mood-elevating effect of progabide.[2] As a consequence, a series of controlled clinical trials was carried out.[4-6] We report here a meta-analysis of these studies, which were all conducted according to a similar, randomized, parallel group design, with blinding obtained by the "double dummy" technique. Patients corresponded to the diagnostic criteria defined in the *DSM-III* for major depressive illness; the total score on the Hamilton Rating Scale for Depression (HRSD) was above 23, with a duration of at least 3 months for the depressive episode.

Following a washout period of 4–8 days, all patients were treated for 4 weeks. The reference drugs tested were imipramine (IMI) in two studies and nortriptyline (NT) in the third one. Initial doses were 2.5 mg/kg/day for IMI, 1.75 mg/kg/day for NT, and 20 mg/kg/day for PGB. Observations were carried out on 118 patients: 59 received PGB, 50 IMI, and 9 NT.

Efficacy was assessed by mean of the Hamilton Rating Scale for Depression (HRSD), Zung self-rating scale, Comprehensive Psychopathological Rating Scale (CPRS), and Global Clinical Rating (GCR). Safety was assessed by means of the patient's spontaneous reports, a side effects checklist, biological controls, and electrocardiography (ECG) carried out at regular intervals. Statistical analysis was performed on the basis of the scores obtained in the pretreatment and treatment phases of the drug trial.

Therapeutic results were considered *excellent* when disappearance of the mood disturbance and of the depressive symptomatology was observed. Results were rated as *good* in those patients who experienced a marked improvement in mood and a decrease in symptoms (HRSD < 15) and who were able to resume their daily activities. The efficacy was considered *insufficient* when the effect on mood was moderate or nil, with persistence of most symptoms of the depressive syndrome.

Diagnostic groups included 46 MDSE (*DSM-III* 296.2X), 25 MDRE (*DSM-III* 296.3X), 17 BD (*DSM III* 296.5X), 29 DD (*DSM-III* 300.40), and 3 AD (*DSM-III* 296.86) equally distributed among the three treatments.

Progabide and the tricyclic antidepressants (TCAs) were equally effective in various diagnostic groups. The global results are summarized in Table 139.1. It can be observed that 77% of the patients improved (excellent or good ratings by GCR) on PGB and 71% on TCAs and that the number of dropouts was significantly higher in the TCA group. Similarly, the incidence of less severe side effects was higher in the TCA than in the PGB group. It may also be of interest to underline that three manic switches were observed with TCA and none with PGB. No clinically significant alterations were observed at the biological level.

Controlled Clinical Studies with Fengabine

Fengabine is a novel benzylidene derivative active in behavioral models of depression. At the biochemical level[7] it is devoid of effects on the serotonin (5-hydroxytryptamine (5-HT) system, accelerates norepinephrine (NE) turnover, and causes desensitization of isoprenaline-stimulated adenylate cyclase but fails to cause down-regulation of β-adrenoceptor binding sites. After repeated treatment (6 days), it causes, as do all clinically effective antidepressant agents, up-regulation of rat cortical $GABA_B$ receptors.

Open pilot studies have suggested that the drug exerts an antidepressant effect with a more rapid onset of action than TCAs, a significant clinical improvement being noticeable in some cases as early as after 3–4 days of treatment.[8]

On this basis, a series of controlled double-blind trials were initiated with the aim of comparing the activity of FGB to that of major TCAs. So far four studies have been completed. We report here on the results of two of these studies, which were conducted according to a similar protocol: a 4-week treatment period, where FGB was compared to either clomipramine (CLOMI)[9] or amitriptyline (AMI).[10]

Inclusion and assessment criteria were similar to those described above for PGB except for the first evaluation of efficacy on the third day of treatment and

TABLE 139.1. Therapeutic efficacy of progabide in depression: Analysis of three controlled clinical trials versus TCAs.

Treatment group	No. of patients	Analyzed for efficacy	Improved	Dropouts due to inefficacy	Dropouts due to ADRs	Incidence of ADRs (dropouts excluded) (%)	Total No. side effects
TCA	59	57	42 (71%)	11	10[a]	64	97
PGB	59	57	46 (77%)	9	2	45	57
Total population	118	114	88	20	12	54	154

[a] $p < 0.05$ versus PGB.

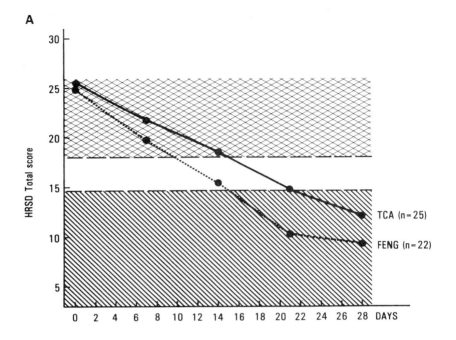

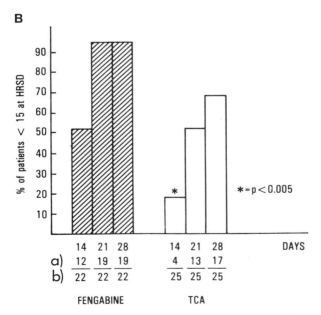

FIGURE 139.1. Comparison of the efficacy of TCAs and fengabine in depressive syndromes. A: HRSD total scoring at various times of treatment in the two therapeutic groups (FENG vs. TCA, $p < 0.05$). B: Percent of patients having an HRSD total score of less than 15 at days 14, 21, and 28. a) Number of patients improved. b) Total number of patients.

the evaluation of clustered items at HRSD for "anxiety/somatization," "cognitive disturbance," "retardation," and "sleep disturbance."

A total of 60 depressed patients (HRSD > 23) entered the studies: 20 were suffering from MDE (10 FGB and 10 TCA), 6 from BD (2 FGB and 4 TCA), 3 from AD (1 FGB and 2 TCA), and 31 from DD (17 FGB and 14 TCA). Initial doses were 12–16 mg/kg/day for FGB, 1.0 mg/kg/day for CLOMI, and 0.7–1.0 mg/kg/day for AMI. The doses were then adapted to the patient's need: with maximal final doses of 1,500 mg/day for FGB, 150 mg/day for CLOMI, and 100 mg/day for AMI.

Twenty-five patients completed the 28 days' treatment in the TCA group and 23 in the FGB group. Reasons for dropouts were intercurrent diseases (one FGB), bad compliance (two FGB), inefficacy (one FGB and two TCA), ADRs (one FGB and two TCA), and administrative reasons (three FGB and one TCA).

In both studies FGB appeared to exert an antidepressant action comparable or superior ($p < 0.05$ versus CLOMI) to that of the reference drug. Moreover, when analyzing the recovery rate and the number of patients with an HRSD score of more than 15 on days 14 and 21, a significant ($p < 0.05$) difference in favor of FGB becomes evident (Fig. 139.1). For instance, whereas at day 14 about 55% of the patients were ameliorated with FGB, only 16% were improved on TCA. Furthermore, considering the analysis of various clustered items of HRSD, FGB appears to act more specifically on such factors as "cognitive disturbance" and "retardation," with a more rapid normalization of these items.

On the GCR 82% of the patients in the FGB groups were rated as improved as were 72% in the TCA groups. Side effects were experienced by 14 patients in the FGB group and by 24 in the TCA group, with a number of adverse events reported (30 and 84, respectively).

Conclusion

The two sets of clinical data reported here on PGB and FGB confirm that GABA-mimetic drugs have a significant therapeutic action in various depressive syndromes. This antidepressant action is accompanied by an incidence of ADRs lower than that observed with TCAs. Furthermore, up to now no manic switches have been observed in more than 280 patients treated with either PGB or FGB in open and controlled trials.

The most interesting point, however, appears to be the rapid onset of action of FGB, with normalization of the psychic picture observed already at day 14 in about 50% of the cases. This fact and the specific effect on "cognitive disturbance" and "retardation" point toward a primary involvement of the GABAergic system in the etiopathogenesis of depression. The reported data, confirming the validity of the GABA hypothesis of depression, stress the necessity of further experimental work at a biochemical level for a better understanding of the alterations underlying the depressive disorders.

References

1. Bartholini G, Lloyd KG, Scatton B, et al. The GABA hypothesis of depression and antidepressant drug action. Psychopharmacol Bull 1985;21:385–387.
2. Morselli PL, Bossi L, Henry JF, et al. On the therapeutic action of SL 76002 a new GABAmimetic agent: preliminary observations in neuropsychiatric disorders. Brain Res Bull 1980;5:411–414.

3. Lloyd KG, Morselli PL, Depoortere H, et al. The potential use of GABA agonists in psychiatric disorders. Pharmacol Biochem Behav 1983;18:957–966.
4. Morselli PL, Fournier V, Macher JP, et al. Therapeutic action of progabide in affective disorders: a controlled clinical trial. In Bartholini G, Lloyd KG, Morselli PL (eds): GABA and Mood Disorders: Experimental and Clinical Research (L.E.R.S. Monograph Series, Vol. 4). New York: Raven Press, 1988;118–125.
5. Perris C, Tjalldem G, Bossi L, et al. Progabide versus Nortriptiline in depression: a controlled trial. In Bartholini G, Lloyd KG, Morselli PL (eds): GABA and Mood Disorders: Experimental and Clinical Research (L.E.R.S. Monograph Series, Vol. 4). New York: Raven Press, 1988;135–138.
6. Weiss E, Brunner H, Clerc G, et al. Multicentre double blind study of progabide in depressed patients. In Bartholini G, Lloyd KG, Morselli PL (eds): GABA and Mood Disorders: Experimental and Clinical Research (L.E.R.S. Monograph Series, Vol. 4). New York: Raven Press, 1988;127–133.
7. Scatton B, Lloyd KG, Zivkovic B, et al. Fengabine a novel antidepressant GABAergic agent: effect on central noradrenergic, serotoninergic and GABAergic transmission in the rat. J Pharmacol Exp Ther 1987;241:251–257.
8. Musch B. The antidepressant activity of fengabine (S1 79229): a critical overview of the present results in open clinical studies. In Bartholini G, Lloyd KG, Morselli PL (eds): GABA and Mood Disorders: Experimental and Clinical Research (L.E.R.S. Monograph Series, Vol. 4). New York: Raven Press, 1988;118–126.
9. Nielsen NP, Priore P, Morselli PL. Double blind study of fengabine versus chlorimipramine in depressed patients. 1989; submitted for publication.
10. Albano C, Loeb C, Priore P, et al. Fengabine versus amitriptyline in depressed patients: a double blind study. 1989; submitted for publication.

140. Activity of Fengabine, a GABAergic Drug, in Depression

Julien Mendlewicz, M. Ansseau, M. Toscano,
J. Wilmotte, J.-L. Evrard, J.E. De Wilde,
C.J.H.M. Mertens, R. Coupez-Lopinot,
and P.H. Hermanns

Fengabine is a new γ-aminobutyric acid (GABA)-mimetic drug with atypical antidepressant activity in various models of depression (reduces the behavioral effects of 5-hydroxytryptophan and the behavioral deficits secondary to olfactory bulbectomy and learned helplessness). Like the conventional antidepressants, fengabine delays the appearance of paradoxical sleep and reduces its total duration in rats.[1,2] On the basis of these results, the potential antidepressant action of fengabine and its effects on sleep parameters versus the effects of amitriptyline were assessed in a controlled clinical trial.

Patients and Methods

The trial was a multicenter double-blind parallel-groups study. Six centers were included. Following a washout period of 2 weeks, patients were randomly assigned to fengabine or amitriptyline. The duration of treatment was 4 weeks. Fengabine doses ranged from 1,200 to 2,400 mg/day and amitriptyline doses from 100 to 200 mg/day.

Inclusion criteria were the following: Patients were of either sex, were 16–65 years of age, and had endogenous bipolar or unipolar depression (as defined in the *DSM-III*). The total score for the Hamilton Rating Scale for Depression (HRSD) 26 items had to be superior to 25, and the depressive episode had to be of at least 2 weeks and less than 6 months duration.

The exclusion criteria were concomitant severe somatic or neurological disorders, psychotropic drugs during the preceding 7 days, electroshock therapy during the previous 3 months, treatment with lithium during the last month, history of drug or alcohol abuse, or pregnancy.

Clinical assessment was carried out on days 0, 3, 7, 14, 21, and 28. The main criteria of assessment were the HRSD and the Global Clinical Impression.

Sleep recordings were performed in 20 patients (ten in each treatment group) on nights −3, −2 (baseline) and nights 1, 2, 25, and 26. The selected sleep parameters were sleep latency, total sleep duration, sleep efficiency, delta sleep duration, rapid-eye-movement (REM) duration, and REM latency.

A total of 88 patients entered the trial after giving their informed consent. The characteristics of the patients are given in Table 140.1. The two treatment groups were comparable for age, sex, weight, type of depression, and mean total score of the HRSD at entry.

Statistical Analysis

The comparability of the two treatment groups on day 0 was analyzed by means of Student's t-test or by the chi-square test. The global efficacy of treatment was assessed using an analysis of variance (ANOVA) with two factors (treatment, period). If a significant overall effect was observed, Tukey's multiple comparison method was applied to compare the different levels two by two. Mean values are given with standard deviation (SD).

Results

A total of 83 patients completed the treatment period; five patients (three in the fengabine group and two in the amitriptyline group) prematurely discontinued treatment. Lack of efficacy was the cause of dropout in one patient in the fengabine group. Adverse events caused discontinuation of treatment in two patients in the fengabine group and in two patients in the amitriptyline group.

Antidepressant Action

Figure 140.1 illustrates the comparative evolution of total scores of the HRSD in the two treatment groups. The rate of improvement is parallel in the two groups, with a significant difference versus the baseline values as early as day 3 ($p < 0.01$); and it persisted for at least 28 days ($p < 0.01$). No difference could be demonstrated between the two treatments. The final total HRSD score was 15 ± 11.5 versus 36 ± 5.4 at entry in the fengabine group and 13.2 ± 9.4 versus 35.6 ± 6.4 at entry in the amitriptyline group.

Effects on Sleep Parameters

There was a significant decrease ($p < 0.001$) of sleep latency in the two treatment groups. Sleep duration and sleep efficiency increased significantly ($p < 0.001$) in

TABLE 140.1. Characteristics of patients in the study.

Characteristic	Fengabine ($n = 44$)	Amitriptyline ($n = 44$)	p
Sex			
Male	15	18	N.S.
Female	29	26	
Age (years)	42.2 ± 2.2	43.6 ± 2.2	N.S.
Weight (kg)	71.2 ± 1.4	69.4 ± 2.2	N.S.
Diagnosis			
Bipolar disorder, depressed	2	0	N.S.
Major depression, single episode	3	4	N.S.
Major depression, recurrent	5	6	N.S.
Hamilton score on day 0	33.1 ± 1.1	34.4 ± 1.6	N.S.

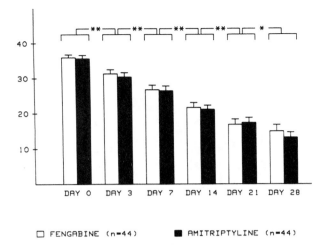

FIGURE 140.1. Time course of scores (mean ± SD) of the HRSD in the two treatment groups. *$p < 0.05$; **$p < 0.01$.

both groups. The effects of amitriptyline and fengabine on these parameters were identical. No significant difference between the two drugs could be demonstrated. The delta sleep (stages 3 and 4) increased significantly during both treatments ($p < 0.001$), but no significant difference between the two treatments could be observed. A significant decrease in REM duration occurred ($p < 0.001$) in both groups, but there was no significant difference between amitriptyline and fengabine, both drugs being equally efficacious. Fengabine and amitriptyline also induced a significant increase of REM latency ($p < 0.001$), with no difference between the two drugs.

Sleep Parameters According to Treatment Response

A good response to treatment was defined as a total HRSD score at the end of the study at least 75% lower than the score at baseline. The percent change between nights 25–26 and baseline (nights −3, −2) in REM latency and delta sleep duration were significantly higher in the group of good responders than in the nonresponders (86.7 ± 15.4% versus 35.7 ± 6.0%, $p < 0.01$, for REM latency; and 49.7 ± 16.8 versus 7.2 ± 5.8%, $p < 0.05$, for delta sleep duration). No significant difference in the percent change in REM duration was observed between the good responders and the nonresponders.

Safety

Considering the safety aspect, there was a trend for fengabine to be associated with fewer adverse events than amitriptyline (Table 140.2).

Comments

The results of this study showed that fengabine was as effective as amitriptyline in the treatment of depression (major depression, recurrent and single episode,

TABLE 140.2. Adverse events reported by patients in the two treatment groups.

Events	Fengabine group (No.)	Amitriptyline group (No.)
Total events	18	39
Dry mouth	4	18
Sleep disturbances	1	9
Gastrointestinal disturbances	7	6
Vertigo	5	5
Confusion	1	1

or bipolar disorder of the *DSM-III* classification). Each drug induced a significant reduction in the HRSD total score ($p < 0.001$), without significant difference between the two treatments at any time during the study.

It is now well established that sleep abnormalities occur in depressed patients and that most clinically used antidepressants reduce the time spent in paradoxical sleep (PS) and lengthen the PS latency in animals as well as in man. In this study, fengabine and amitriptyline presented the same profile of action on sleep parameters, particularly a reduction of PS duration and an increase of PS latency and delta sleep duration ($p < 0.001$). No significant difference was observed between the two treatment groups.

A good correlation was found between treatment response and the percent change in REM latency and delta sleep duration. In contrast to the findings of Kupfer et al.,[3,4] we could not find any early predictive value of REM latency, REM duration, or delta sleep duration after acute antidepressant treatment (1–2 days of treatment) for therapeutic response (at day 28).

Conclusion

These observations indicate that fengabine may act on sleep physiology through a GABAergic mechanism, which may have some relevance to the pathophysiology of depressive illness.

References

1. Zivkovic B, Lloyd K, Scatton B, et al. Pharmacological and neurochemical spectra of fengabine (SL 79229), a new antidepressant agent. In Bartholini G, Lloyd KG, Morselli PL (eds): GABA and Mood Disorders: Experimental and Clinical Research (L.E.R.S. Monograph Series, Vol.4). New York: Raven Press, 1986;85–95.
2. Depoortere H, Riou-Merle F. Pharmaco-EEG profiles of progabide and fengabine compared with classical antidepressants. In Bartholini G, Lloyd KG, Morselli PL (eds): GABA and Mood Disorders: Experimental and Clinical Research (L.E.R.S. Monograph Series, Vol. 4). New York: Raven Press, 1986;97–99.
3. Kupfer D, Spiker D, Coble P, et al. Depression, EEG sleep and clinical response. Compr Psychiatry 1980;21:212–220.
4. Kupfer D, Spiker D, Coble P, et al. Sleep and treatment prediction in endogenous depression. Am J Psychiatry 1980;138:429–434.

141. Depression in Children and Adolescents: A Controlled Study of Progabide Versus Imipramine

M. Dugas

Parents, and such as have the tuition and oversight of children, offend many times in that they are too stern, always threatening, chiding, brawling, whipping or striking; by means of which, their poor children are so disheartened and cowed, that they never after have any courage, a merry hour in their lives, or take pleasure in anything.

These observations made by Robert Burton[1] (1577–1640) suggest that the existence of mood disorders in children has been recognized for a long time. In 1867 Maudsley[2] described monomania, choreic delirium, cataleptoid insanity, epileptic insanity, mania, melancholia, and moral insanity in children. He took a developmental perspective, pointing out that as the child's mind developed its more elaborate organization permitted more elaborated phenomena such as hallucinations and delusions to occur.

Yet a hundred years later, psychiatric writing bearing on childhood depression remained surprisingly scarce.[3] Although depression in children was vaguely thought to exist, for decades it was for the most part ignored. Until the 1970s the concept of depression in children was completely denied. Psychoanalysts, exemplified by Rie[4] and Mahler,[5] believed that the immature personality structure (specifically, an incompletely formed superego) of the child does not permit development of a depressive neurosis. They argued that children are less affected by object loss than adults, which would diminish the possibility of developing a depressive neurosis.

Another point of view, denying the existence of childhood depression, was that of Lefkowitz and Burton,[6] who viewed symptoms of childhood depression as developmental phenomena. They claimed that depressive symptoms in children dissipated as a function of time and cited longitudinal and epidemiological data to support their position. According to them, the prevalence of depressive symptoms in "normal" children is too high to be considered statistically deviant.

In recent years there have been three other schools of thought concerning depression in children. The first school of thought is that childhood and adult depressive disorders have a number of similarities, but childhood depression has additional unique features such as temper tantrums, enuresis, encopresis, and somatic complaints. The second school of thought is that childhood and adult depressive disorders differ in that adult disorders are manifest but childhood disorders are masked. The numerous symptoms that "mask" childhood depression include acting out, truancy, decreased school performance, school phobia, somatic complaints, temper tantrums, moodiness, accident proneness, phobias, running away, and fire-setting. The final and major school of thought concerning childhood depression is that it is similar to adult depression and can be diagnosed using adult-type criteria.

The possibility of adolescents having a clinical depression was never as much in doubt as it was with prepubertal children. Nevertheless, many clinician-theorists opined that the more or less classic indicants of depressive illness were absent or exceptional in this age group. Current approaches have veered away from impressionistic and theoretical views to more rigorous investigation that builds on the wide range of advances in our understanding of adult affective illness.

An increasing number of studies have been published on childhood and adolescent depression leading to the development of diagnostic criteria. In fact, when one compares the diagnostic criteria proposed, one finds that the various suggested lists share numerous common points. Nevertheless, it does not mean that those patients who are selected from one or the other of these lists make up identical groups. Despite the absence of a sufficient number of studies on the reliability and validity of *DSM-III* criteria[7] for the diagnosis of childhood and adolescent depression, the most recent studies make reference to these criteria, which, at least in adults, have a good interrater reliability.

With regard to the diagnosis of depression, the poor agreement that exists between clinicians who examine children in their usual way has led to the development of semistructured interviews. These interviews make it possible to do a detailed assessment of the depressive syndrome and reach diagnoses that fit *DSM-III* criteria, as is the case for affective disorders.[8-11] For purposes of research and more specifically for pharmacological studies, there was a need to create homogeneous groups of patients and to assess the course of their symptoms. This structuring has encouraged the development of instruments geared to: (a) identify children with a clinically significant depression, (b) provide a psychiatric diagnosis, (c) measure or obtain data on the degree of response to therapeutic agents. Among the 17 scales cited in the *Psychopharmacology Bulletin*,[12] seven are self-evaluation scales; one is a sociometric scale (peer-nomination, index of depression; PNID); nine are scales that are filled out by outside observers; and one is a parent interview scale.

Until now, few controlled studies have been conducted on the treatment of childhood depression with antidepressant drugs. In Puig-Antich et al.'s study,[13] response to placebo was higher than to imipramine (IMI); however, all subjects whose IMI blood level was higher than 150 ng/ml were responders. In Kashani et al.'s study,[14] which involved nine subjects, there was a trend for amitriptyline (AMI) to be superior to placebo ($.05 < p < .08$). Preskorn et al.'s study[15] is interesting because it is the first study that found, in children, a superiority of IMI versus placebo. When the plasma drug concentration was monitored between 125 and 250 ng/ml, the drug response rate approached 80%. In contrast, the placebo response rate in that study is less than 30%.

When we conduct drug studies, we establish diagnoses on the basis of *DSM-III* criteria. For inclusion in the study, we currently use an observer scale: the Children's Depression Rating Scale Revised (CDRS-R), by Poznanski et al.[16] and adapted from Hamilton's scale. This scale has the least questionable validity and reliability of all existing scales and can be used in children between the ages of

6 and 12 years. To assess the course of the illness, we use the CDRS-R, which is sensitive to change; a self-report scale, the Children Depression Inventory (CDI) by Kovacs,[17] which is also sensitive to change; and the Children's Global Assessment Scale (CGAS) by Shaffer et al.[18]

For children 13 years of age and over we use as inclusion criteria a score of 25 and above on the MADRS. To assess the course of the illness, we currently use the MADRS scale,[19] a self-report scale (the Beck Depression Inventory),[20] and the Clinical Global Impression Scale (CGI). As one can see, assessment of childhood depression has greatly improved, and psychiatrists who treat children and adolescents can now use as many assessment tools as their colleagues who deal with adults.

The results presented below deal with a preliminary study of a GABAergic drug, progabide, versus imipramine in the treatment of childhood and adolescent depression. For this study, the inclusion criteria were as follows: (a) boys and girls 6–19 years of age; (b) hospitalized for a minimum of 10 days since the beginning of the study; (c) fulfilling the *DSM-III* criteria for major depressive episode; (d) a CDRS-R score of 35 or above for children 6–13 years, a MADRS score of 25 or above for adolescents who are 13 years or older; (e) must have discontinued antidepressant therapy for at least 15 days; (f) informed consent given by the patient (if older than 16 years) or by the parents.

To assess the course of the illness we used (a) the CDRS-R score for children under 13 years and MADRS score for adolescents who are 13 years or older; (b) a Depression Self-Rating Scale, the Birleson Depression Self-Rating Scale[21] (DRSR) for children under 13 years or a Visual Analog Scale if patients were 13 years old or older; (c) the score from the CGI, a four-point scale; (d) a clinical global assessment of efficacy by responding yes/no; and for side effects a Somatic Scale, the AMDP-5.[22]

The design of the study was a doubleblind randomized distribution to progabide or imipramine. The characteristics of our study were as follows.

The mean (±SD) age was 15.3 ± 2.6 (range 9–19) years for the progabide group and 14.3 ± 1.7 (range 11–19) years for the imipramine group. The sex distribution was 13 girls and 9 boys. Nine subjects were treated by progabide and ten by imipramine. Of these subjects, two dropped out in the progabide group, none for a treatment-related reason. We had 17 completed cases: seven in the progabide group and ten in the imipramine group. Daily dosage was 1,256 ± 343.2 mg (range 900–1800 mg) for the progabide group and 116 ± 24.9 mg (range 80–160 mg) for the imipramine group. All the patients were treated by monotherapy. The initial

TABLE 141.1. Progabide versus imipramine: Therapeutic effect.

Effect	Progabide	Imipramine
No. of patients	7	10
CGI therapeutic effect		
Very good	0	2 (20%)
Good	1 (14.3%)	4 (40%)
Weak	6 (85.7%)	3 (30%)
Null	0	1 (10%)
% Responders	14.3%	60%
Efficacy as assessed by investigator (Is drug effective?)		
Yes	3/7 (42.9%)	8/10 (80%)
No	5/7 (57.1%)	2/10 (20%)

Table 141.2. MADRS: Evolution of scores (mean ± SD).

Drug	Day 0	Day 7	Day 14	Day 21	Decrease (%)
Progabide (n = 6)	33 ± 7.0	29.7 ± 6.8	28.6 ± 8.8	23.7 ± 6.4	28.2
Imipramine (n = 7)	35.5 ± 8.9	23 ± 7.5	15.4 ± 6.2	15.1 ± 10.3	57.5

dosage for progabide was 150 mg and for in order to achieve imipramine 20 mg 7.5 mg/kg/24 h. In case of inefficacy at day 10, dosage was increased by 30%.

The results are shown in Table 141.1. The global therapeutic effect, assessed by CGI scores, was estimated as good (responders) in 14.3% for progabide versus 60% for imipramine. For treatment efficacy, the investigator judged the drug to be effective three times out of seven (42.9%) for progabide and eight times out of ten (80%) for imipramine. These results for imipramine are in agreement with the data available in the literature.

A more precise assessment of the evolution was made using observer rating scales. Because of the small number of subjects under 13 years of age (four) we consider the data for the MADRS only (Table 141.2). For the progabide group, at day 21 the decrease of the mean MADRS score was 28.2%, and for the imipramine group it was 57.5%. Side effects were twice as frequent in the imipramine group as in the probagide group. In the latter group we observed one case of orthostatic hypotension, one case of dry mouth, one case of fatigue, and one case of elevated transaminase levels.

When presenting the results obtained from this initial study on the action of a GABAergic drug in the treatment of child and adolescent depression, we are fully aware of its inherent weaknessess. We nevertheless present it for the following reasons: (a) Existing controlled studies on the treatment of child depression are, as yet, scarce. (b) We wanted the public to be aware that child psychiatrists now have access to diagnostic criteria and evaluation scales that make it possible to carry out investigations according to a methodology that has already been well tested in adults. Finally, (c) we wanted the psychiatric and medical community to know and accept the fact that depressive illness exists in children and adolescents, that it is a painful and lasting affliction that involves risks of relapse, and that it must be treated with all available means known to be efficient, chemotherapy being one of them.

References

1. Burton R. The Anatomy of Melancholy: New Impression. London: Chatto & Winders, 1927.
2. Maudsley H. Insanity of early life. In: Physiology and Pathology of the Mind. London: Macmillan, 1981;259–268.
3. Dugas M, Mouren MC. Les Troubles de l'Humeur Chez l'Enfant de Moins de 13 Ans. Paris: Presses Universitaires de France, 1980.
4. Rie HE. Depression in childhood: a survey of some pertinent contributor. J Am Acad Child Psychiatry 1966;5:653–685.
5. Mahler MS. Notes on the development of basic moods. In Newman L, Schur M, Solnit A (eds). New York: International Universities Press, 1966;152–168.
6. Lefkowitz MM, Burton N. Childhood depression: a critique of the concept. Psychol Bull 1978;85:716–726.
7. American Psychiatric Association. Diagnostic and Statistical Manual of Mental Disorders, DSM-III. 3rd Ed. Washington, DC: APA, 1980.

8. Herjanic B, Reich W. Development of a structured psychiatric interview for children: agreement between child and parent on individual symptoms. J Abnorm Child Psychol 1982;10:307–324.
9. Kovacs M. The Interview Schedule for Children (ISC): interrater and parents–child agreement. Unpublished manuscript, 1983.
10. Puig-Antich J, Chambers WJ. Schedule for affective disorders and schizophrenia for school-age children (6–16 years)—Kiddie-SADS. Unpublished manuscript. New York: New York State Psychiatric Institute, 1978.
11. Hodges K, Kline J, Stern L, et al. The development of a Child Assessment Interview for research and clinical use. J Abnorm Child Psychol 1982;10:173–189.
12. Raskin A (ed). Rating scales and assessment instruments for use in pediatric psychopharmacology research. Psychopharmacol Bull 1985;21:713–1125.
13. Puig-Antich J, Perel JM, Lupatkin W, et al. Imipramine in prepubertal major depressive disorders. Arch Gen Psychiatry 1987;44:81–89.
14. Kashani J, Shekin WO, Reid JC. Amitriptyline in children with major depressive disorder: a double blind cross-over pilot study. J Am Acad Child Psychiatry 1984;23:348–351.
15. Preskorn SH, Weller E, Hughes C, et al. Plasma monitoring of antitricyclic anti-depressants: defining the therapeutic range for imipramine in depressed children. Clin Neuropharmacol (special issue) 1986;265–267.
16. Poznanski EO, Grossman JA, Buchsbaum Y, et al. Preliminary studies of the reliability and validity of the Children's Depression Rating Scale. J Am Acad Child Psychiatry 1984;23:191–197.
17. Kovacs M. The Children's Depression Inventory (CDI). Psychopharmacol Bull 1985;21:995–998.
18. Shaffer D, Gould MS, Brasic J, et al. A children's global assessment scale. Arch Gen Psychiatry 1983;40:1228–1231.
19. Montgomery SA, Asberg M. A new depression scale designed to be sensitive to change. Br J Psychiatry 1979;134:382–389.
20. Beck AT, Ward CH, Mendelson M, et al. An inventory for measuring depression. Arch Gen Psychiatry 1961;4:561–571.
21. Birleson P. The validity of depressive disorder in childhood and the development of self-rating scale: a research report. J Psychol Psychiatry 1981;22:73–88.
22. Le Manuel AMDP. Association de méthologie et de documentation en psychiatrie, section francophone. In: Bobon DP (ed): Book Title. Liége: Presses Universitaires de Liége, 1981.

V.F. Therapeutic Variations in ECT Administration

142. Electrode Placement and Stimulus Waveform: Conceptual and Practical Issues

R.D. WEINER AND C.E. COFFEY

The establishment of the safest, most effective means to administer electroconvulsive therapy (ECT) has been a goal of many clinical researchers. Dating back to the early days of ECT, a variety of modifications in ECT technique have been investigated in this regard. Two areas of particular contemporary relevance are stimulus electrode placement and stimulus waveform. In this chapter we present data from recent and ongoing clinical studies that have focused on the relative safety and efficacy of these modifications in ECT technique. It is concluded that consideration of electrode placement and waveform effects can lead to a significant diminution of adverse cerebral effects, while, at least for most patients, allowing a high level of therapeutic efficacy.

The positioning of stimulus electrodes has long been known to affect the nature and degree of memory dysfunction occurring with ECT.[1] Specifically, placement of stimulus electrodes over the nondominant cerebral hemisphere (ULND) is associated with significantly less verbal memory impairment than when stimuli are applied bifrontotemporally. Unfortunately, there has been less consistency with respect to the relative efficacy of ULND versus bilateral ECT. Though most studies have observed no apparent differences, a significant minority have reported at least a trend favoring bilateral ECT.[2,3]

Much less research effort has focused on stimulus waveform. Because early studies were confounded by concomitant differences in electrode placement, it was not until recent years that data appeared suggesting that less confusion and memory loss occur with the use of intermittent stimuli, such as the brief pulse, as opposed to the continuous sinewave stimulus.[4] Though, again, only a few relevant studies are available, the various stimulus waveforms appear to be equivalent in efficacy, except for extremely brief pulses.

Our work in this area has addressed the following issues.

1. When carried out with state-of-the-art technique, is ULND ECT as effective as bilateral ECT, and is brief pulse ECT as effective as sinewave treatments?
2. What are modality-dependent differences in memory function and pathophysiological electroencephalographic (EEG) changes in terms of acute and long-term effects?

3. Is there an interaction between electrode placement and stimulus waveform with respect to either beneficial or adverse effects?
4. To what extent are any of the above differences associated with alterations in induced seizure activity?

In an initial study, 53 hospitalized patients referred to ECT treatment of major depression were randomly assigned to either ULND or bilateral electrode placement and, simultaneously, to either brief pulse or sinewave stimuli. Subjects were tested prior to ECT and 2–3 days and 6 months after completion of the ECT course with a battery of therapeutic, memory, and EEG outcome measures. A clinically matched group of 21 depressed inpatients not referred for ECT were tested at analogous time intervals.

In terms of efficacy, no modality-dependent differences were observed in Hamilton Depression Scale ratings, global clinical ratings, or self-ratings on the Zung depression scale. In this case, equivalent therapeutic potency for ULND ECT compared with bilateral ECT may have been a product of the relatively optimum ULND placement chosen.[5]

Acute amnestic effects were found to be greater for both bilateral and sinewave ECT.[6] This phenomenon was present for both retention of newly learned material and items learned prior to the ECT course. By 6 months post-ECT, nearly all evidence of electrode placement and stimulus waveform effects on memory function had disappeared, except for some increased residual forgetting of autobiographical memory for subjects given bilateral ECT. Interestingly, no modality-dependent effects were observed for self-rated memory function. Instead, most ECT subjects reported memory function to have improved post-ECT, with the degree of improvement highly correlated with the extent of clinical response but not with objective memory measures. These data indicate that self-ratings of memory function after ECT may not offer an adequate reflection of actual memory changes.

Bilateral and sinewave ECT were also found to be associated with larger acute increases in EEG slowing.[7] This observation, which was highly correlated with the extent of impairment in memory function, suggests that, at least acutely, a global encephalopathic disturbance coexists with the more specific amnestic changes. After 6 months, all intergroup differences in EEG slowing had disappeared, though several bilateral/sinewave subjects still showed evidence of mild residual increases in this measure.

For both memory function and EEG slowing, the interaction between electrode placement and stimulus waveform was observed to be additive in nature, with unilateral pulse treatments showing little or no impairment. Bilateral/sinewave ECT, on the other hand, was associated with the greatest amount of acute dysfunction.

The etiology of the above electrode placement and stimulus waveform differences is unclear. Visual analysis of single-channel ictal EEG monitoring revealed that bilateral/sinewave treatments were particularly likely to be followed by postictal EEG suppression. This finding suggests that bilateral/sinewave ECT is associated with the most intense seizure activity. On the other hand, sinewave, but not brief pulse, ECT showed a significant positive correlation between stimulus intensity levels and degree of memory impairment. The latter relation points to the stimulus itself as a potential factor in the occurrence of memory dysfunction with ECT.

In order to replicate our findings and to more effectively investigate underlying mechanisms, we began a new study. The experimental design for this ongoing protocol is similar to that described above, except that more sensitive multichannel EEG measurement is carried out both before and after the ECT course, as well as during some of the induced seizures. In addition, the neuroendocrine response to individual seizures is monitored.

Preliminary analysis of EEG data thus far collected has tended to corroborate earlier electrode placement and stimulus waveform results and has, in addition, provided evidence for the existence of regional cerebral differences. Acutely following the ECT course, ULND ECT is associated with greater right-sided than left-sided slowing, whereas bilateral treatments produce either symmetrical or left-sided changes. By 1 month post-ECT, the right-sided slowing in ULND subjects appears to have largely disappeared, whereas a small amount of residual left-sided slowing persists in at least some bilateral and sinewave subjects. These findings clarify the nature of EEG changes following ECT and suggest a more rapid disappearance of pathophysiological alterations with ULND and brief pulse treatments. The significance of the persistence of left-sided slowing is unclear but may reflect a higher sensitivity of the left cerebral hemisphere to induced cerebral dysfunction.

Nineteen-channel ictal EEG recording carried out in some subjects has suggested the presence of more intense seizure activity with sinewave than with brief pulse stimuli. In addition, ULND ECT seizures are higher in amplitude on the right, at least in anterior regions, and so far show relative sparing of left mid and posterior temporal regions. The latter result is consistent with our observed pre-ECT/post-ECT differences in both memory function and EEG slowing and suggests that the extent of seizure generalization plays a role in the development of adverse cerebral effects with ECT.

Further support for this hypothesis comes from an analysis of postictal serum prolactin secretion data thus far collected. In this case a trend toward higher prolactin levels 15–30 min poststimulus was observed with bilateral electrode placement and with sinewave stimuli. Particularly because prolactin is generally believed to be a good marker of seizure generalization, this relation between prolactin and ECT type is certainly compatible with the existence of modality-dependent differences in ictal intensity and/or distribution.

The results of our data combined with the work of others indicate that there is a clear advantage for ULND electrode placement and brief pulse stimulus waveform in terms of a reduced level of induced cerebral impairment with ECT. In addition, intrinsic differences in therapeutic efficacy can be minimized through use of optimum electrode placement and stimulus dosing techniques.

References

1. Lancaster NP, Steinert RR, Frost I. Unilateral electroconvulsive therapy. J Ment Sci 1958;104:221–227.
2. d'Elia G, Raotma H. Is unilateral ECT less effective than bilateral ECT? Br J Psychiatry 1975;126:83–89.
3. Abrams R. Is unilateral electroconvulsive therapy really the treatment of choice in endogenous depression? Ann NY Acad Sci 1986;462:50–55.
4. Weiner RD. The role of stimulus waveform in therapeutic and adverse effects of ECT. Psychopharmacol Bull 1982:18:71–72.

5. Weiner RD, Coffey CE. Minimizing therapeutic differences between bilateral and unilateral nondominant ECT. Convulsive Ther 1986;2:261–265.
6. Weiner RD, Rogers HJ, Davidson JRT, et al. Effects of stimulus parameters on cognitive side effects. Ann NY Acad Sci 1986;462:315–325.
7. Weiner RD, Rogers HJ, Davidson JRT, et al. Effects of electroconvulsive therapy upon brain electrical activity. Ann NY Acad Sci 1986;462:270–281.

143. Unilateral and Bilateral Electroconvulsive Therapy in Depressive Illness

D. GILL

There has rightly been concern in recent years about demonstrating scientifically the effectiveness of electroconvulsive therapy (ECT). Such concern has arisen for two reasons. First, ECT was introduced to psychiatry before controlled trials of treatment were widely used; hence its efficacy was never properly tested. Second, scientific evaluation has become necessary because of a frequent outcry by the public against what seems to be a primitive and even barbaric form of treatment—a view too often shared by fellow professionals of nonmedical disciplines.

In the United Kingdom there have been several important studies published since 1978.[1-5] In our 1978 study[1] we looked at two groups of patients with depressive illness. One group was given brief pulse stimulus ECT (unilateral) applied to the nondominant hemisphere, and a second matched group was given simulated ECT. The brief pulse unilateral method was chosen to produce a fit and yet cause no memory upset, so that the blind rating procedure could be more strictly maintained. Both groups did well, and only a nonsignificant trend in favor of ECT could be demonstrated.

In the 1980 Northwick Park study[3] of similiar design, the more traditional, high energy, sinusoidal waveform current was applied bilaterally. In this case ECT produced a superior effect in depressive illness, but again a remarkably high placebo effect was noted in the simulated group. At the end of the trial period ECT had demonstrated only a small advantage.

Because these studies challenged so seriously the status of ECT and particularly the paramount importance of the convulsion produced, we embarked on a second study[5] to replicate and intensify the work undertaken in these two trials. At the same time there seemed an opportunity to compare bilateral, unilateral, and simulated techniques.

Of the 564 patients admitted to the Nottingham Psychiatric Hospital between August 1981 and February 1983 with an International Classification of Disease diagnosis of depressive illness (ICD 9), 40% were referred for ECT. Those who gave their consent and were suitable were admitted to a well designed study and assigned randomly to three treatment groups to receive bilateral, unilateral, or simulated ECT, respectively, according to usual hospital procedures and after administration of a standardized anesthetic. The electrical current was delivered by an Ectron Duo Pulse Mark 2 machine producing 70 joules of energy at each application. Of the patients available to the study, 69 were entered and 49 were rejected because consent was refused or they suffered from physical illness. This selection at least gave us the opportunity to compare those entered with those who were not entered so as to assess their comparability. They were found to be similar in general biographical characteristics and depression scores using the Montgomery and Asberg depressive rating scale (MADRS); the results of the Hamilton Depressive Rating Scale (HDRS) and the Psychological Impairments Rating Scale (PIRS) were also comparable. We found a comparable spread of delusions and agitation, two items that in our earlier study[1] had seemed to be the best predictors of responsiveness to ECT.

The 69 patients who were allocated to the three treatment groups were also well matched for age, sex, previous episodes, family history, length of present episode, prescription of antidepressants, and presence of delusions and agitation. The degree of depression before and during treatment in the three groups is recorded in Figure 143.1.

The score changes on the MADRS were used to compare the three groups and were analyzed using analysis of variance by Scheffe (AOVS). Marked significance of change was demonstrated after six treatments between the simulated and the

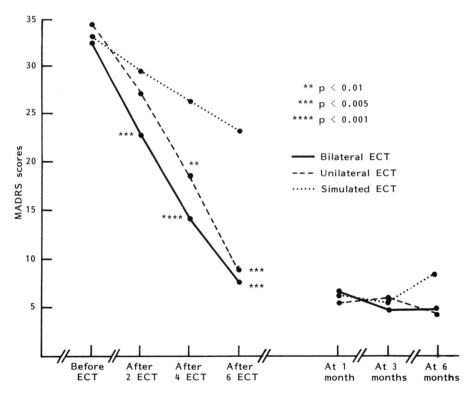

FIGURE 143.1. Depression scores before and after treatment in three comparable groups of patients assessed using the Montgomery and Asberg Depression Rating Scale (MADRS). [Reprinted from ref. 5, with permission.]

unilateral group and the simulated and the bilateral group, whereas there was no significant difference in change between the unilateral and bilateral groups. When we studied the MADRS scores after two, four, and six treatments and analyzed them using Students *t*-test (two-tailed), however, it is seen that after two treatments there is a difference between the simulated and unilateral groups although it is nonsignificant; the difference between the simulated and bilateral groups, on the other hand, is highly significant. After four treatments the amount of change in the unilateral group has become significant, and in the bilateral group it has become highly significant. After six treatments, as already mentioned, the change in both unilateral and bilateral groups has attained high and comparable significance. One other important observation may also be made. After six treatments there has been a change in the MADRS score in the simulated group, and it is also statistically significant. Although not demonstrated in Figure 143.1, the changes in the HDRS follow a similar pattern.

Discussion

In this and the other studies carried out in the United Kingdom in recent years, it has been possible to demonstrate unequivicably that ECT is an effective treatment for severe depressive illness. A criticism of ECT studies often made in the past has been that patients studied are not truly representative and there is hence bias in the sample, or there has not been a proper comparison with a control group. In our studies we have used samples where no significant difference could be demonstrated between the patients in the study and those who could not be included in the study for various reasons, and we have used a simulated controlled group matched in every respect to the two groups who received "active" treatment.

Bilateral and unilateral ECT were both highly significantly better than simulated ECT, which has also been demonstrated in other studies. We could demonstrate no difference in overall outcome between bilateral ECT and unilateral ECT, although bilateral ECT gave a speedier response. This difference probably explains why the unilateral group received, on average, 8 treatments (7.91) and the bilateral group received 6.5 (6.59) treatments. Hence there is a difference between these two methods.

We must note, in addition, that the placebo response is also important, a finding that has been demonstrated throughout our studies and in those conducted at Northwick Park by Johnstone and her colleagues.[3] In our last study,[5] simulated ECT produced changes in depressive scores that were statistically significant.

It now seems possible to understand why we obtained such a different result in our first study in 1978,[1] where we compared unilateral and simulated ECT groups and found no significance. Clearly, the placebo response was an important factor, but with unilateral ECT the patient takes longer to respond as well; in the 2-week study period we did not allow enough time for this response to develop. It seems now that the most important factor was that we gave a low energy stimulus of only 10 joules compared with 70 joules in our later study; hence, despite obtaining a fit of reasonable length, we were not obtaining the same therapeutic efficacy. This interesting finding was also described by Robin and DeTissera[6]; their comment is pertinent: "Whilst the emergence of a convulsion is necessary to see a therapeutic effect with ECT it is not certain that the convulsion produces that response. . . . An alternative possibility is that when measures are taken to produce the response, a convulsion is unavoidable."

Summary

It has been possible in recent years to demonstrate the value of ECT in modern practice, and some differences and similarities between unilateral and bilateral ECT have been noted. We still need to understand more of the nature of placebo, which also plays a significant role in the change ECT brings about, and to learn why the passage of electricity is more important than the convulsion it produces. Perhaps even now we should begin to talk of electrocerebral or even electrolimbic therapy, rather than electroconvulsive therapy.

References

1. Lambourn J, Gill D. A controlled comparison of simulated and real ECT. Br J Psychiatry 1978;133:514–519.
2. Freeman CPL, Basson JV, Creighton A. Double-blind controlled trial of electroconvulsive therapy (ECT) and simulated ECT in depressive illness. Lancet 1978;1:738–740.
3. Johnstone EC, Deakin JFW, Lawler P, et al. The Northwick Park electroconvulsive therapy trial. Lancet 1980;2:1317–1320.
4. Brandon S, Cowley P, McDonald C, et al. Electroconvulsive therapy: results in depressive illness from the Leicestershire trial. Br Med J 1984;288:22–25.
5. Gregory S, Shawcross CR, Gill D. A double-blind comparison of bilateral, unilateral and simulated ECT in depressive illness. Br J Psychiatry 1985;146:520–524.
6. Robin A, DeTissera S. A double-blind controlled comparison of the therapeutic effects of low and high energy electroconvulsive therapies. Br J Psychiatry 1982;141:357–366.

144. ECT: Rising Trends and Current Policy

ASHLEY ROBIN, J. DROGO MONTAGU,
ANTHONY G. JOLLEY, AND BRYAN CORRIDAN

Only 4 years after electroconvulsive therapy (ECT) was introduced, Friedman and Wilcox[1] described a method of modifying current form and electrode position that should have ended the concept of ECT as a unitary treatment and necessitated the individual assessment of an infinitely variable group of treatments in the same way that analogues are treated in pharmacology. The first British apparatus to produce pulses was described by Strauss and McPhail,[2] but because of the rugged construction and extended half-life of earlier ECT apparatus, shown by Pippard and Ellman[3] to run into decades, it enjoyed little currency. It was only during the 1970s that a pulse apparatus became generally available, the Ectron Duopulse. This apparatus, because of the clinically observed therapeutic variability of its four waveforms, and the reputation that the pulse form derived from its use in the only published controlled trial which did not show an advantage for ECT over placebo,[4] caused a renewal of interest in the use of electrical currents in Britain.

An initial inquiry[5] simply examined the duration of courses of treatment ordered by "blind" prescribers. In a series of 128 patients, 70% treated with narrow (0.34 ms) pulses and a charge of 50 millicoulombs (mC) had six or fewer treatments in contrast to 90% of patients treated with a 60% sine wave current and a charge of 700 mC. A prospective inquiry[6] compared McPhail's wide (5-ms) pulses, which delivered 250 mC (despite a rapid drop in voltage as the capacitor discharged), with the narrow pulses and "chopped" sinewave already described. Ratings of depression showed the narrow pulse, low energy treatment to be less therapeutic than either of the others. No differences were noted among the groups in terms of duration of observed fits in this trial, and a hypothesis was proposed that demanded closer examination of the ictal response. This phase was undertaken in a within-patient comparison of the same three treatments,[7] which were administered in random order to each patient. Although therapeutic outcome could not be studied in this design, a variety of significant differences were observed in the immediate electrophysiological and hormonal responses, although again no differences were seen in the duration of observed fits. Eight-channel electroencephalograms (EEGs) contained a longer duration of epileptiform activity than the visible convulsion in two-thirds of treatments, and the duration of the EEG discharge was longest in narrow-pulse treatments. On the other hand, this waveform produced significantly lower amplitudes in the epileptic discharge in the centroparietal channel as well as less isoelectric EEG and burst suppression after the fit. The mean prolactin ratio (20 min posttreatment level/baselevel) was lowest with narrow pulses. Holmberg's[8] observation that second and subsequent treatments showed restricted responses in comparison to the first treatment was confirmed, and it was also observed that age was positively correlated with postictal EEG disturbance and negatively correlated with duration of fit.

Clearly a trial was needed that included both clinical-psychiatric ratings and electrochemical indices of the first treatment of the series to see if predictive relations might be described. By now, however, a Department of Health working group on electrical safety prompted many centers to renew their apparatus, and the only British manufacturer, Ectron, had produced a new constant-current apparatus delivering trains of 1.25-ms pulses of 850 mamp (thus generating about 1 mC per pulse). Piloting work soon showed that the charge, virtually always capable of inducing a convulsion with very narrow pulses, rarely induced one now; at least 80 mC were required. Even then we later found that one-third of patients failed to convulse at the first, second, or third treatment and had to be switched to either a higher dose or an alternative treatment form.

For pragmatic reasons our ongoing comparative trial randomly allocates patients to low dose (80 mC) pulses (LEP) or high dose (250 mC) (HEP) pulses using the same waveform, thus meeting the valid criticism made by Malitz et al,[9] that we had confused waveform and energy level in our earlier trial. The third treatment used was again variable-current fixed-voltage "chopped" sine wave (CSW) as it had been used in virtually every British ECT versus placebo trial subsequent to 1978. The design included pre-, within, and posttreatment EEGs; prolactin, cortisol, growth hormone assays; estimates of C-reactive protein; clinical ratings; and cognitive tests. All treatments were administered bilaterally as in the earlier trial; but acceding to the policy of the hospital, treatment was administered thrice weekly and not as before, twice weekly. To date, 42 patients have entered the trial, and as always a high level of ambition correlates strongly with the amount of missing data, particularly in the EEG field. The results are therefore tentative.

The three treatment groups were found retrospectively to match for age and sex. The five patients who failed to convulse with the first low energy treatment were older than the rest of the low energy group and have been excluded from consideration. The groups were comparable for the number of precipitating life events, the proportion to have had previous ECT, for the duration of the current episode, and for the reasons for the choice of ECT (which, regrettably, even at this stage was commonly the failure of pharmacological treatment rather than a primary indication). The groups matched on both the diagnostic and ECT indices of Carney et al.[10] and Hobson's[11] prognostic scale.

Hamilton's[12] rating for depression showed the three groups to match before treatment (Table 144.1), and the initial ratings closely resembled scores in the earlier trial, although the possibility exists that the scores were composed in different ways. Patients did not improve to the same degree as in the previous trial, even with the "chopped" sinewave, which was used in both trials. (In fact, some surprise has been expressed at the extent of the improvement previously reported.) Different raters were involved in this trial (and of course the treatment intervals were different). It may be noted that the scores over the same time (2 weeks) resemble each other more closely than those after the same number of ECTs.

TABLE 144.1. Group mean Hamilton scores with different currents.

Condition	1.25 ms LEP 80 mC	(0.34 ms) (LEP) (50 mC)	1.25 ms HEP 250 mC	(5 ms) (HEP) (250 mC)	CSW	(CSW)
Pretreatment	25	(25)	28	(23)	29	(24)
After ECT × 2	18	(19)	20	(15)	21	(14)
After ECT × 4 (i.e. after 2 weeks 1982)	18	(15)	16	(11)	15	(8)
After ECT × 6 (i.e. after 2 weeks 1987)	17	(12)	11	(4)	11	(5)

The data from the study of Robin and De Tissera are in parentheses.

On inspection, HEP was as effective as "standard" CSW treatment (which is confirmed statistically), and comparison of the effects of the two similar waveform pulse treatments shows the effect of energy in therapeutic efficacy. No differences were noted until after six treatments, when (using the median test) HEP was significantly more effective than LEP at the 5% level of probability; 27 ictal EEGs were reported blind. Mean duration of both clinical fit (31–33 s) and EEG epileptiform discharge (45–49 s) was similar for the three groups and considerably shorter than in the earlier trial (47–54 s for the observed fit and 57–77 s on the EEG). Excluding one maverick result, the range of amplitudes on the centroparietal channel at 15 s after treatment was 70–420 μV; the mean amplitude of epileptiform discharges was 140 μV with LEP, 190 μV with HEP, and 245 μV with CSW. The difference in amplitude between the LEP and the HEP group was significant at the 5% level using the Mann Whitney U-test. Five of the eight LEP postictal records showed no isoelectric phase in contrast to two of the 11 HEP records and one of the CSW records. Nonsignificant trends were noted for the duration of burst suppression, and the total duration of the EEG disturbance was less with LEP than the other treatments. The mean group score for the prolactin ratio and cortisone ratio (40 min post-ECT level/base level) rose according to the energy supplied (Table 144.2).

Whereas prolactin and cortisone inevitably peaked after treatment, growth hormone behaved inconsistently: It rose, fell, or remained unchanged. All the trends observed, apart from fit duration, were similar to those previously reported and may now be related to energy. Because all the results were subject to large individual variability, it is unlikely that any single measure predicts effective treatment, a fact that applies to fit duration as well as to the others. Certainly, a lower charge is required for therapeutic efficiency with a pulse waveform compared to a sinewave, but there seems little doubt that in all cases supramarginal currents are required rather than the induction of "generalised seizure activity with a minimum electric energy."[13] Available energy may explain the reduced effect that Malitz et al.[9] described with low dosage unilateral ECT, where interelectrode energy loss may be critical at low energy levels. Bayles et al.'s[14] rider that the "least amount of any therapeutic agent (should be) *consistent with maximum benefit to*

TABLE 144.2. Prolactin and cortisone ratios with different currents.

Ratio	LEP (80 mC)	HEP (250 mC)	CSW	CSW (1982)
Prolactin	6.6	10.5	13.3	(13.8)
Cortisone	1.5	1.9	2.1	

the patient'' may predict a move away from low dosage schedules in everyday treatment practice toward supramarginal currents.

Acknowledgment. The authors thank Ms. Amanda Green for technical assistance in recording the EEGs.

References

1. Friedman E, Wilcox PH. Electrostimulated convulsive doses in intact humans by means of undirectional currents. J Nerv Ment Dis 1942;96:56–63.
2. Strauss EB, McPhail A. Steep wave electroplexy. Lancet 1946;2:896–899.
3. Pippard J, Ellam L. Electroconvulsive Treatment in Great Britain. Ashford, Kent: Headley Brothers, 1980.
4. Lambourn J, Gill D. A controlled comparison of stimulated and real E.C.T. Br J Psychiatry 1978;133:514–519.
5. Robin AA. E.C.T.: current status. In Palmer RL (ed): Electroconvulsive Therapy: An Appraisal. Oxford: OUP, 1981;65–78.
6. Robin AA, de Tissera S. A double blind controlled comparison of the therapeutic effects of low and high energy E.C.T.'s. Br J Psychiatry 1982;141:357–366.
7. Robin AA, Binnie CD, Copas JB. Electrophysiological and hormonal responses to three types of E.C.T. Br J Psychiatry 1985;147:707–712.
8. Holmberg G. Effect on electrically induced convulsions of the number of previous treatments in a series. AMA Arch Neurol Psychiatry 1954;71:619–623.
9. Malitz S, Sackeim HA, Decina P, et al. The efficacy of E.C.T.: dose-response interactions with modality. Ann NY Acad Sci 1986;462:56–64.
10. Carney MWP, Roth M, Garside RF. The diagnosis of depressive syndromes and the prediction of E.C.T. response. Br J Psychiatry 1965;111:659–674.
11. Hobson RF. Prognostic factors in electro-convulsive therapy. J Neurol Neurosurg Psychiatry 1953;16:275–281.
12. Hamilton M. A rating scale for depression. J Neurol Neurosurg Psychiatry 1960;23:56–62.
13. D'Elia G, Ottoson JO, Stromgren LS. Present practice of electroconvulsive therapy in Scandinavia. Arch Gen Psychiatry 1983;40:577–581.
14. Bayles S, Busse EW, Ebaugh FG. Square waves (BST) versus sine waves in E.C.T. Am J Psychiatry 1950;107:34–41.

145. Pharmacological Manipulation of Seizure Duration: A New Direction in ECT Technology

SETH KINDLER, BERNARD LERER,
BARUCH SHAPIRA, AND HEINZ DREXLER

The use of caffeine sodium benzoate to prolong electroconvulsive therapy (ECT)-induced seizures was first prompted by preclinical studies in our department on the effect of electroconvulsive shock (ECS) on adenosine receptors of the A_1 subtype. Newman et al.[1] found an increase in maximal binding (Bmax) of [^{3}H]cyclohexyladenosine to these receptors in rat cerebral cortex after repeated ECS. Because A_1 adenosine receptors have been linked to anticonvulsant effects,[2] enhancement of their sensitivity or number could play a role in the increase in seizure threshold and reduction in seizure duration, which are frequent concomitants of an ECT course. Methylxanthines inhibit A_1 adenosine receptors and increase seizure duration[3]; administration of caffeine prior to ECT therefore seemed a plausible method for enhancing the efficacy of the treatment. The intervention would be of greatest potential importance in patients whose seizure threshold rises during ECT to an extent that results in short, clinically ineffective seizures.

In a preliminary report on a single patient with treatment-refractory depression, Shapira et al.[4] found that administration of caffeine sodium benzoate (250–1,000 mg i.v.) prior to ECT increased seizure length and improved therapeutic outcome. In a subsequent study, Shapira et al.[5] examined the effect of caffeine pretreatment on ECT-induced seizure length under more controlled conditions. Eight patients receiving bilateral ECT for major depressive disorder participated in a research protocol in which seizure threshold was determined by a method of limits procedure[6] and seizure length was monitored centrally and peripherally. At least once during ECT treatment phases 2–4, 6–8, and 10–12, caffeine sodium benzoate (500–2,000 mg) was administered intravenously 10 min before ECT administration. As shown in Figure 145.1, seizure length was found to increase significantly compared to that seen with the immediately preceding treatment, which was unmodified by caffeine ($p<0.05$ during treatment 5–8, $p<0.01$ during treatment 9–12). Another three patients were administered caffeine when seizure threshold increased during their ECT course to an extent that precluded seizure elicitation at maximal stimulation. In each case, caffeine administration facilitated seizure induction. During subsequent treatments, seizure length again dropped but could be increased above 20 s by raising caffeine dosage. Caffeine administration was not associated with

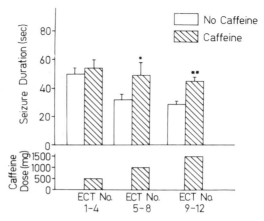

FIGURE 145.1. Effect of pretreatment administration of caffeine on seizure duration (mean ± SEM) during ECT. *$p < 0.05$; **$p < 0.01$. [Reprinted from Lerer B, et al. Pharmacological manipulation of ECT-induced seizure duration. Clinical Neuropharmacology 1986; 9 (supplement 4), by permission of Rowen Press.]

significant anxiogenic effects or with exacerbation of the cognitive adverse effects of ECT.

The seizure-prolonging effects of caffeine observed by us have since been confirmed by Hinkle et al.,[7] who also reported no clinically significant adverse effects. It remains to be established, however, whether caffeine administration or increased current intensity is the preferred method for dealing with seizure threshold increases and short seizure duration during ECT. Relative severity of cognitive adverse effects is likely to be the most important criterion in this regard. Caffeine dosage is an additional issue that is as yet unclear. We have observed considerable individual variability in this regard. Furthermore, dosage requirement appears to rise during the ECT course, probably as a consequence of threshold increase.[5]

When further analyzing hemodynamic data from our controlled study,[5] we have observed interesting correlations with seizure duration that may provide a lead in predicting dosage requirements. For six patients who participated in the study, full details were available on blood pressure and pulse rate before and 10 min after caffeine administration and immediately after the seizure. On the first occasion that caffeine was administered to these subjects, systolic blood pressure (BP) increased from 150±31.6 mm Hg at baseline to 155±28.1 mm Hg 10 min later (paired $t = 1.167$, $p > 0.10$), diastolic blood pressure from 80±11.1 mm Hg to 91±9.8 mm Hg ($t = 2.071$, $p = 0.10$) and pulse rate from 84±15.5 beats/min to 87±25.5 beats/min ($t = 0.71$, $p > 0.10$). The corresponding values immediately following the seizure compared to baseline were as follows: systolic blood pressure 177±49.9 mm Hg (paired t versus baseline $= 1.46$, $p > 0.10$), diastolic blood pressure 101±21.3 mm Hg ($t = 2.18$, $p = 0.09$), and pulse rate 92±11.6 per minute ($t = 1.79$, $p = 0.09$). Table 145.1 shows the degree of correlation between seizure duration and these hemodynamic parameters. Seizure duration was significantly correlated with the increase in systolic blood pressure 10 min after caffeine, with systolic blood pressure after the seizure, and with the increase in systolic blood pressure after the seizure compared to the systolic blood pressure before caffeine

TABLE 145.1. Relation of seizure length following caffeine administration to hemodynamic parameters.[a]

Measurement	Correlation	p (two-tailed)
Ten minutes after caffeine		
Systolic BP	0.295	NS
Systolic BP increase[b]	0.849	0.01
Pulse rate	−0.323	NS
Pulse rate increase[b]	−0.497	NS
Immediately after seizure		
Systolic BP	0.860	0.03
Systolic BP increase[c]	0.922	0.01
Pulse rate	0.217	NS
Pulse rate increase[c]	−0.134	NS

[a]Partial correlations, excluding influence of caffeine dose, performed on values from the first caffeine administration in six subjects (NS = $p > 0.10$).
[b]Systolic BP and pulse rate 10 min. after caffeine minus values before caffeine.
[c]Systolic BP and pulse rate after seizure minus values before caffeine.

administration. Caffeine dose was not significantly correlated with seizure duration or with any of the hemodynamic parameters.

Although these findings are preliminary, they suggest a relation between the small increases in systolic blood pressure induced by caffeine and the effect of the drug on seizure duration. If this relation is substantiated, caffeine could be administered independently of ECT and the dosage requirement for administration in conjunction with ECT calculated on the basis of the blood pressure increase observed. These suggestions require further investigation. It is, however, clear from the studies reported by our group[4,5] and by Hinkle et al.[7] that pharmacological manipulation of seizure duration represents a potentially valuable tool for enhancing the efficacy of ECT, particularly when successful treatment is impeded by extreme increases in seizure threshold and consequent reduction in seizure duration below therapeutically effective levels.

Acknowledgment. Supported in part by NIMH Grant No. 40734.

References

1. Newman M, Zohar J, Kalian M, et al. The effects of chronic lithium and ECT on A_1 and A_2 adenosine receptor systems in rat brain. Brain Res 1984;291:188–192.
2. Dunwiddie TV, Worth T. Sedative and anticonvulsant effects of adenosine analogs in mouse and rat. J Pharmacol Exp Ther 1982;220:70–76.
3. Albertson TE, Joy RM, Stark LG. Caffeine modification of kindled amygdaloid seizures. Pharmacol Biochem Behav 1983;19:339–343.
4. Shapira B, Zohar J, Newman M, et al. Potentiation of seizure length and clinical response to ECT by caffeine pretreatment. Convulsive Ther 1985;1:58–60.
5. Shapira B, Lerer B, Gilboa D, et al. Facilitation of ECT by caffeine pretreatment. Am J Psychiatry 1987;144:199–1202.
6. Sackeim H, Decina P, Prohovnik I, et al. Seizure threshold in electroconvulsive therapy. Arch Gen Psychiatry 1987;44:355–360.
7. Hinkle PE, Coffey CE, Weiner RD, et al. Use of caffeine to lengthen seizures in ECT. Am J Psychiatry 1987;144:1143–1148.

146. "Isoflurane Narcotherapy" in Depression: Methodological Issues

GRETA KOINIG, GERHARD LANGER,
AND REGINA DITTRICH

Preliminary observations of our study on the therapeutic effects of deep anesthesia with insoflurane in psychiatric patients have been reported elsewhere.[1] After awakening from the first anesthesia, antidepressant effects were observed in 9 of the 11 patients, who had been classified as depressives (by Research Diagnostic Criteria, RDC) refractory to conventional antidepressant drug therapy. The therapeutic effect diminished gradually over several days unless another session of "isoflurane narcotherapy" (ISONAR) was given. That study was uncontrolled; currently, a double-blind controlled study comparing the efficacy of electroconvulsive treatment (ECT) with ISONAR is in preparation. A synopsis of methodological and theoretical considerations is presented here as a consequence of many observations and discussions in this explorative state of affairs. If a potentially new mode of treatment such as ISONAR is to be given an optimal chance for proof of efficacy, it is important that the appropriate clinical indication and administration procedure be established (the two most important factors in pharmacological therapy).

ISONAR: Methodological Considerations

The theoretical background of our decision to explore the possible therapeutic usefulness of ISONAR in psychiatric patients has been presented elsewhere.[2] For the purpose of this overview the notion may suffice that we were primarily motivated by the idea of a substitute treatment for ECT; that is, we looked for a method that would possibly yield rapid therapeutic effects comparable to those of ECT yet without the unwanted implications of electric current and grand mal seizures and without signs and symptoms of an acute organic brain syndrome. In a further analogy with ECT, we postulated that the anesthesia should be performed with isoflurane (Forane), which , aside of being an established and well tolerated inhalation anesthetic, also has the ability to suppress ("flat line") the cortical electroencephalogram (EEG) in concentrations[3] that appear nontoxic for any body including the brain.[4]

Optimal Indication

At this point of the investigation the optimal clinical indication for ISONAR has not yet been established. Our original selection of patients, i.e., treatment-refractory depressives of a more chronic course, was guided by the analogy of clinical practice of ECT; i.e., in Central Europe severely depressed patients who show no benefit from several drug therapies are ultimately given a trial with ECT. It is conceivable, however, that chronically ill, drug-treatment-resistant patients may not represent the optimal indication of ISONAR, as (a) the overall profiles of effects of ECT and ISONAR do not overlap sufficiently (see below) to establish a complete analogy of indication and (b) the rapid elimination of isoflurane from the body (see below) leaves little to continuously counteract a chronic pathological process.

It is thus conceivable that patients presenting with acute and reversible psychotic episodes of prominent affective and/or other psychopathological features might benefit most from ISONAR. Uncontrolled observations by us favor this hypothesis. In these patients the conventional psychiatric therapy would be the administration of neuroleptics and/or antidepressants at a moderate to high dosage for at least several weeks. ISONAR could possibly reduce the period to clinical remission and permit a lower dose regimen of psychopharmacological drugs; furthermore, more favorable conditions could be provided for a psychotherapeutic doctor-patient relationship when the psychosis fades away (see below).

Pharmacological Profile

Upon awakening from the first anesthesia a high proportion of depressed patients showed marked improvement of the entire psychopathological syndrome; this rapid therapeutic effect was reproducible by repeated ISONARs.[1] Nevertheless, the typical profile of therapeutic effects of ISONAR is not yet established; it appears to extend to psychotic and nonpsychotic states other than the depressive syndrome, but our preliminary observation requires controlled evaluation.

Unlike ECT, ISONAR does not appear to produce major psychoorganic signs and symptoms; in particular, no amnesia was recognized either by complaints from the patient (as in ECT) or objectively by the doctor. Quite to the contrary, some of the patients experienced a certain quality of "clear mind" without euphoric or uncritical features, and they felt strong enough to constructively discuss with the doctor their long neglected problems. This finding is in line, for example, with observations by Klaesi and others regarding "barbiturate narcotherapy" some 70 years ago—that patients were particularly amenable to psychotherapeutic doctor-patient interaction shortly after anesthesia.

The unwanted effects of ISONAR appear to be essentially limited to the well known effects during anesthesia, e.g., lowered blood pressure.[1] The possible lack of major long-lasting side effects of ISONAR could be due in part to the fact that isoflurane is completely eliminated from the body shortly after awakening, without being metabolized or tightly bound to tissue. Isoflurane can induce a "flat line" in the EEG, an effect that does not appear to be accompanied by side effects noticeable either shortly after anesthesia or even several months later. This important question, however, requires substantial documentation by controlled investigations of important psychometric and psychobiological parameters.

Optimal Administration

The procedure and the dosage of isoflurane administration that should be optimal for therapeutic efficacy have not yet been established. Based on our data in 15 patients with a total of 40 anesthesias, the following tentative conclusions can be drawn from the exploratory statistical analysis: (a) It appears beneficial if the patient quickly(!) reaches the EEG state of "burst suppression." Taking this state as a goal, the time from initiation of isoflurane administration (Fig. 146.1) seems to be of greater therapeutic benefit than the time from thiopental (the barbiturate thiopental is used to initiate anesthesia shortly before isoflurane is given). (b) The dosage of isoflurane that effects a "burst suppression" pattern in the EEG may be of greater therapeutic benefit than the slightly higher dose that effects the anesthesia state of continuous "flat line" in the EEG. (c) The speed of awakening following the discontinuation of isoflurane does not appear to play a major role for the therapeutic benefit. (d) If the conditions described in (a) and (b) were fulfilled, the entire anesthesia appeared to be more beneficial if it lasted for a rather short time (median time 36 min). These tentative findings need confirmation or rejection by a controlled study.

Concluding Remarks

There is a long history describing the use of "narcotherapy" with hypnotics (e.g., barbiturates and other anesthetics) in the treatment of psychiatric patients. The

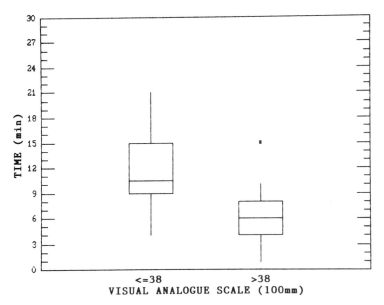

FIGURE 146.1. "Isoflurane narcotherapy" and isoflurane administration. Relation between acute therapeutic response (quantified by a visual analogue scale) and time of isoflurane administration necessary to reach the EEG state of "burst suppression." The frequency distribution of therapeutic responders (> 38 mm) and poor responders (≤ 38 mm) is expressed in "box plots" (median and quartiles).

advent of modern psychopharmacology has rendered most of such "sleep cures" obsolete. Thanks to the exceptional pharmacological properties of isoflurane, the old idea of "narcotherapy" may be reevaluated for certain indications.

Our idea emerged in the conceptional context of ECT and was aimed at a probable substitute for ECT; however, it is possible that ISONAR and ECT are therapeutically different to the degree that one cannot substitute for the other or, if so, only in a special subpopulation of patients. Thus the question of optimal indication for ISONAR remains open.

As to the optimal dosage of isoflurane, exploratory evaluation of our uncontrolled data points to the possibility that the original regimen may be modified as follows: The slightly lower dose of isoflurane necessary for maintaining the EEG state of "burst suppression" might be therapeutically superior to the EEG state of continuous "flat line" for several minutes.

As to the issue of unwanted side effects, anesthesias with isoflurane, even with concentrations that induce a "flat line" in the EEG for several minutes, appear to be tolerated well as judged by both patients and physicians. This lack of apparent side effects is in contrast to the experience with ECT. Nevertheless, the possible risks and benefits of ISONAR remain to be established and need to be compared with those of alternative treatment modalities.

Unlike most psychopharmacological agents, isoflurane is completely eliminated from the body within minutes after awakening from anesthesia. This pharmacokinetic fact may be theoretically advantageous or problematical depending on the patients selected for treatment. Certainly it may explain the early relapse of several patients unless another ISONAR is being given. To counterpart the relapse, additional psychopharmacological drugs are to be given in the interval between the anesthesias to maintain symptomatic remission. The therapeutic advantage of ISONAR—if the method passes the test of efficacy for a defined indication and dose regimen—may lie in a considerable improvement of psychobiological therapy of a certain population of psychiatric patients, i.e., quick symptomatic remission of reversible disorders with earlier access of psychotherapeutic intervention and earlier initiation of a lower dosage psychopharmacological maintenance regimen.

Acknowledgment. Supported in parts by "Fonds zur Foerderung der wissenschaftlichen Forschung," grant 5785 (Dr. Langer et al.).

References

1. Langer G, Neumark J, Koinig G, et al. Rapid psychotherapeutic effects of anesthesia with isoflurane (ES narcotherapy) in treatment-refractory depressed patients. Neuropsychobiology 1985;14:118–120.
2. Langer G, Koinig G, Neumark J. "Narcotherapy" with isoflurane anesthesias: psychotherapeutic profile, "flat-line" in EEG and other observations. Clin Neuropharmacol 1986;9(suppl 4):450–452.
3. Eger EI, Stevenson WC, Cromwell TH. The electroencephalogram in men anesthetized with Forane. Anesthesiology 1971;35:504–508.
4. Eger EI. Isoflurane: a review. Anesthesiology 1981;55:559–576.

V.G. Psychotherapy of Depression

147. Response to Combined Pharmacotherapy and Psychotherapy Among Recurrent Depressives

ELLEN FRANK AND DAVID J. KUPFER

The treatment of recurrent depression can be thought of as occurring in three phases. In the first phase, acute treatment, the goal is symptom remission and the time frame is one of weeks. The second phase, continuation treatment, has as its goal the prevention of relapse and has a time frame of months. The final phase, maintenance treatment, is aimed at preventing a recurrence of illness in those who have remained well for several months. The time frame of maintenance treatment may be years or a lifetime. Klerman and colleagues have demonstrated the efficacy of interpersonal psychotherapy[1] as both an acute and a continuation treatment. We are currently involved in a study that attempts to demonstrate its usefulness as a maintenance treatment for patients with recurrent illness.

Interpersonal Psychotherapy as Acute and Continuation Treatment

This chapter addresses the usefulness of interpersonal psychotherapy (IPT) as both an acute and a maintenance treatment for major depressive disorder. As its originators have described. IPT is a brief (16–20 weeks) manual-based psychotherapy that adheres to a medical model while emphasizing interpersonal functioning in the present as the key to recovery from major depressive disorder.

Weissman and Klerman have conducted two studies of IPT, the first with 150 female patients[2] and the second with 81 male and female patients.[3] The first study involved a 3×2 design following 1 month of amitriptyline treatment. Patients were assigned to one of three drug conditions (amitriptyline, placebo, or no pill) and one of two psychotherapy conditions (IPT or low contact). The second study of IPT was a four-cell, 16-week, acute treatment study in which IPT alone was compared with amitriptyline alone, IPT plus amitriptyline, and a nonscheduled treatment format, a limited-attention control. In both studies, IPT and amitriptyline were found not to differ with respect to treatment efficacy; however, in the second study the combined treatment was superior to either treatment alone.

A third test of IPT occurred in the Treatment of Depression Collaborative Research Project.[4] In this three-center study, IPT was one of four 16-week interventions. It was compared with cognitive behavior therapy, imipramine offered in a specified medical management modality, and placebo offered in the same medical management modality. Whether assessed using self-report, therapist, or independent evaluator ratings, IPT was found to be as effective as medication in this 16-week trial.

IPT in a Maintenance Trial

Acute Phase

Our study[5] involves the treatment of recurrent outpatients with a diagnosis of either unipolar or biopolar II depression. Patients are treated acutely with a combination of IPT and imipramine (150–300 mg) weekly for 12 weeks, then every other week for 8 weeks, and finally monthly until they achieve the 20-week stabilization that is required for entry into the maintenance phase. The maintenance treatments being studied are maintenance interpersonal psychotherapy (MIPT) alone; MIPT + active imipramine; MIPT + placebo; medication clinic + active imipramine; or medication clinic + placebo. Maintenance treatment is continued for 3 years or until the patient experiences a recurrence of illness. Patients are evaluated once every 3 months. Baseline evaluations involve the collection of psychiatric, psychosocial, and biological data from the patient as well as information from a family member or significant other. All subsequent evaluations replicate the initial evaluation with the exception that personality is assessed at subsequent evaluation points.

The 230 patients entered into this study were primarily female ($n = 180$), although, a substantial number of men ($n = 50$) have also been studied. The population is relatively young (39.5 ± 10.6). They entered the study with a mean Hamilton Rating Scale for Depression score of 22.1 ± 4.6 and had been ill for an average of 23.2 ± 17.2 weeks at the time of initial assessment. Although only two previous episodes were required, the mean number of previous episodes was 7.4 ± 12.1, and the median was 4.3.

Early in the study we noted that the study participants appeared to divide into three groups in terms of their manner of responding to the combined acute treatment regimen. Approximately one-third of the population could be characterized as "normal" responders, individuals who were well by 8 weeks and remained well through 16 weeks of treatment. Another one-third of the population could be characterized as "slow" responders. These individuals demonstrated a slow or erratic treatment course, but nonetheless were considered well (i.e., Hamilton ≤ 7, Raskin ≤ 5) by 16 weeks of treatment. A third group, whom we have called "partial" responders, did not respond fully to the combination of imipramine and IPT within the first 16 weeks of the study. As we have noted elsewhere,[6] normal responders tended to be distinguished by their rather more disturbed baseline biology and relatively healthy personality adjustment. More specifically, the normal responders tended to be characterized by poor sleep maintenance, high rapid-eye-movement (REM) density, high emotional stability, high objectivity, low neuroticism, and low ratings on avoidant and dependent features.

Continuation Phase

Interestingly, there were no differences between normal responders and slow responders in terms of their "response" during continuation treatment. Members of both groups were equally likely to complete the continuation phase and be assigned to the maintenance phase. Thus the combined treatment appears to be equally effective in keeping both groups of patients well during a continuation treatment phase.

Maintenance Phase

Maintenance IPT differs slightly from IPT in terms of some of its basic principles, but not in others. With MIPT the emphasis continues to be interpersonal relationships in the here and now, and treatment strategies parallel those employed in IPT. However, the goals of MIPT differ from those of IPT; the therapist seeks to maintain the patient in the remitted state, emphasizing both preexisting and newly acquired interpersonal skills. Both the therapist and the patient watch for early warning signs of an impending recurrence of illness. Although multiple treatment foci are possible in the brief format of IPT, generally speaking, therapists restrict interventions to one or, at most, two of the treatment foci. However, with MIPT multiple treatment foci are almost an inevitabilty, as patients continue in MIPT for 3 years in the present treatment protocol. As noted above, MIPT sessions are scheduled on a once-a-month rather than a once-a-week basis.

At the time the present protocol was designed a number of questions were raised about MIPT by the investigators themselves and by the reviewers of the protocol. These questions included the following: (a) Is monthly psychotherapy possible? (b) Does MIPT serve as an active treatment or an adjunct to pharmacotherapy? (c) Does MIPT help prevent recurrences of illness? (d) Does MIPT improve the quality of the patients' lives between episodes? (e) Does MIPT improve study participation rates? At present, because the study is still several years from completion, we can address only some of these questions and then only partially.

As can be seen in Table 147.1, we have at least partial answers to the first question: Is monthly psychotherapy possible? The table shows mean scores on a therapy rating scale designed to tap four dimensions of therapeutic intervention: interpersonal, somatic, cognitive behavioral, and psychodynamic. After training, blind raters listened to 7-min segments of audiotaped treatment sessions. Individuals assigned to MIPT and MIPT + pill conditions receive a treatment that is significantly different ($p < 0.01$) from that of patients assigned to a medication clinic condition in terms of the interpersonal content of the sessions, suggesting that when the treatment assignment is MIPT both patient and therapist are able to continue in a psychotherapeutic mode despite the relative infrequency of sessions.

It would be premature to say that MIPT serves as an active treatment, prevents recurrence, or improves the quality of patients' lives between episodes, as only ten patients have completed the full 3 years of the study. However, it appears already that MIPT has an effect in that it improves study participation rates. Of

TABLE 147.1. Scores on therapy rating scale (mean ± standard deviation).

Treatment condition	Total rating scale dimension scores			
	Interpersonal	Somatic	Cognitive behavioral	Psychodynamic
Medication clinic + pill	1.43 ± 0.59	2.08 ± 0.86	1.17 ± 0.23	1.01 ± 0.10
MIPT alone	1.82 ± 0.76	1.45 ± 0.65	1.18 ± 0.24	1.03 ± 0.18
MIPT + pill	2.00 ± 0.78	1.51 ± 0.60	1.35 ± 0.32	1.09 ± 0.37

the 51 patients entered into an MIPT + pill condition, only three have dropped out compared with eight of the patients entered into a medication clinic + pill condition. Put another way, the mean number of weeks in maintenance for medication clinic patients thus far is 47.3 versus 62.2 for the MIPT + pill patients (p <0.05).

It will be several years before we can make definitive statements about the relative efficacy of medication, psychotherapy, and their combination in the prevention of recurrence in a population of recurrent unipolar depressives; however, early results suggest that MIPT is possible and that it has a beneficial effect in terms of the prevention of attrition from treatment. If MIPT proves to have no other effect than this one, it may well be considered a valuable adjunct to treatment. If it can be demonstrated that MIPT reverses or ameliorates the social adjustment difficulties typically seen in recovered recurrent depressives, it will be an even stronger argument for its use in maintenance treatment.

References

1. Klerman GL, Weissman MM, Rounsaville BJ, et al. Interpersonal Psycotherapy of Depression. New York: Basic Books, 1984.
2. Klerman GL, Dimascio A, Weissman M, et al. Treatment of depression by drugs and psychotherapy. Am J Psychiatry 1974:131:186–191.
3. Weissman MM, Prusoff BA, Dimascio A, et al. The efficacy of drugs and psychotherapy in the treatment of acute depressive episodes. Am J Psychiatry 1979;136:555–558.
4. Elkin I, Parloff MB, Hadley SW, et al. NIMH Treatment of Depression Collaborative Research Program: Background and research plan. Arch Gen Psychiatry 1985;42:305–316.
5. Frank E, Jarrett DB, Kupfer DJ, et al. Biological and clinical predictors of response in recurrent depression: a preliminary report. Psychiatry Res 1984;13:315–324.
6. Frank E, Kupfer DJ, Jacobs M, et al. Personality features and response to acute treatment in recurrent depression. J Pers Dis 1987;1:14–26.

148. Cognitive Therapy for Major Depressive Disorder: Current Status

JOHN D. TEASDALE

The view that psychological treatments have little to offer to the management of major depressive disorder is still not uncommon. A decade ago the evidence from clinical trials was broadly consistent with that view: The few trials that had been conducted generally indicated the relative ineffectiveness of traditional psychotherapies in producing symptomatic improvement in major depression. However, more recently encouraging evidence has been reported for the effectiveness of a new generation of highly structured psychological treatments, often incorporating a behavioral or cognitive-behavorial approach. Such evidence now convincingly demonstrates that in outpatients with major depressive disorder some of these treatments can achieve symptomatic reduction on average as great as that shown with tricyclic antidepressants. There is also some evidence to suggest that, compared to antidepressants, these psychological treatments can have a prophylactic effect in preventing relapse or recurrence following termination of treatment.

Cognitive therapy has been the most extensively studied of this new range of structured psychological treatments but by no means the only one for which there is evidence of effectiveness. Cognitive therapy is based on Beck's cognitive model of depression,[1] which suggests that the negative thinking shown by depressed patients contributes substantially to the maintenance of their depression, by both maintaining depressive symptomatology and undermining problem-solving efforts directed at symptomatic relief or the resolution of life problems. Cognitive therapy is a complex, highly structured problem-oriented treatment involving both behavioral and cognitive components. It aims to help patients, by identifying and modifying negative thinking, to learn methods for achieving symptomatic relief, solving life problems, and preventing recurrence and relapse. A detailed manual describing the treatment procedures is available,[1] and scales have been developed to assess the quality of cognitive therapy from video- and audiotapes of therapy sessions.

Outcome Studies

At least five randomized controlled trials have compared the effectiveness of cognitive therapy with tricyclic antidepressant medication. In all cases, the patients studied have been outpatients meeting Research Diagnostic Criteria (RDC), or the equivalent, for nonbipolar major depressive disorder, as well as further criteria of severity of depression. Outcome of treatment has been assessed using both the Hamilton Rating Scale (completed by a psychiatric assessor) and the Beck Depression Inventory (completed by the patient).

A consistent picture has emerged from all these trials: The reduction in depression in patients receiving cognitive therapy has always been significant—and not statistically significantly different from that shown by patients receiving tricyclic antidepressant medication. On the whole, cognitive therapy and pharmacotherapy achieve comparable reductions; the superiority of cognitive therapy reported in the first comparative trial to be published[2] was generally not repeated in subsequent studies of psychiatric outpatient populations. Three criticisms were directed at this initial study: (a) antidepressant medication was discontinued prior to posttreatment assessment; (b) in the absence of monitoring of plasma levels, it was possible that pharmacotherapy patients may not have complied with their treatment regimen; and (c) the patients were an unrepresentative sample, being, on average, well educated and fee-paying, and attending the center in Philadelphia where cognitive therapy had been developed. All subsequent studies have maintained pharmacotherapy up to posttreatment assessment. Monitoring of plasma levels has shown that cognitive therapy is as effective as antidepressants taken in therapeutic dosage.[3,4] These last two studies were conducted on patients drawn from predominantly working class areas, suggesting that cognitive therapy is a generally applicable psychological treatment, a conclusion strengthened by the positive results of Blackburn and her colleagues working in Scotland.[5] Thus when the criticisms of the initial study are met, the results of methodologically adequate studies still show that cognitive therapy is at least as effective, on average, as tricyclic antidepressants. The preliminary findings of the recent large U.S. National Institute of Mental Health (NIMH) Treatment of Depression Collaborative Research Study[6] also showed that cognitive therapy and tricyclic medication achieve significant reductions in depression that are not statistically different between the two conditions. However, the variability in response to cognitive therapy across treatment sites suggests that definitive conclusions from this study should await further analysis.

In addition to the demonstrated effectiveness of cognitive therapy in reducing symptoms of the presenting episode, follow-up of patients in three of the above studies[4,7,8] has shown that cognitive therapy is significantly superior to pharmacotherapy in preventing relapse or recurrence following termination of treatment.

The evidence for the effectiveness of cognitive therapy appears compelling. However, it has by no means been universally accepted. It is thus worth briefly examining some of the criticisms of these studies that might be raised.

Possible Criticisms

Patient Selection

It might be objected that the patients included in trials of cognitive therapy are in some way unrepresentative of typical outpatients with major depressive disorder. If true, this would cast doubt on both the generalizability of the research findings and the validity of using tricyclic antidepressants as a comparison condition.

There seems no basis for this criticism. As well as meeting diagnostic criteria for major depressive disorder, patients in trials of cognitive therapy seem comparable to those normally included in trials of antidepressants in both severity and diagnostic composition: On the 17-item Hamilton Rating Scale the mean score of the 493 patients in the five trials reviewed was 20, and in the two trials reporting the proportion of patients meeting criteria for definite endogenous depression these figures were 38% and 42%, respectively. These figures are comparable to those typically reported in outpatient trials of pharmacotherapy.

Specificity of Effects

In trials comparing cognitive therapy and pharmacotherapy, patients undergoing cognitive therapy receive considerably more therapist time than those receiving drugs. Could the benefits of cognitive therapy merely reflect the nonspecific effects of extra attention of any form? This seems unlikely because, for the type of patients studied, merely spending time with them in an activity labeled therapeutic does not necessarily produce symptomatic improvements: (a) As already noted, earlier trials of traditional psychotherapy failed to show benefit for such patients. (b) Furthermore, there is evidence for the differential effectiveness of psychological treatments even when equated for therapist contact; for example, McLean and Hakstian[9] showed that a structured behavioral treatment was superior to traditional short-term psychotherapy provided by experienced psychotherapists in reducing major depression. Thus the nature of the psychological contact seems important. However, cognitive therapy is not unique in its effectiveness on depression: Other structured, problem-focused treatments such as McLean and Hakstian's behavioral approach and interpersonal psychotherapy[6] have also shown promising evidence of efficacy. The specific components of effective psychological treatments have yet to be identified.

Cost-Effectiveness

In its present form, cognitive therapy is clearly not as cost-effective as tricyclic antidepressants in the short-term. However, given the promising evidence of a prophylactic effect of cognitive therapy in preventing relapse, it may prove to be more effective than antidepressants in the long term. Further research aimed at identifying the specific therapeutic components within cognitive therapy may lead to the development of briefer, more efficient forms of this treatment. This, coupled with research leading to more appropriate patient selection, may yield further gains in cost-effectiveness.

References

1. Beck AT, Rush AJ, Shaw BF, et al. Cognitive Therapy of Depression. New York: Guilford Press, 1979.
2. Rush AJ, Beck AT, Kovacs M, et al. Comparative efficacy of cognitive therapy and pharmacotherapy in the treatment of depressed out-patients. Cognitive Ther Res 1977;1:17–38.
3. Murphy GE, Simons AD, Wetzel RD, et al. Cognitive therapy and pharmacotherapy, singly and together in the treatment of depression. Arch Gen Psychiatry 1984;41:33–41.
4. Hollon SD, Evans MD, De Rubeis RJ. Final report of the cognitive-pharmacotherapy trial. Presented at World Congress on Behavior Therapy, Washington, DC, 1983.
5. Blackburn IM, Bishop S, Whalley LJ, et al. The efficacy of cognitive therapy in depression: a treatment trial using cognitive therapy and pharmacotherapy each alone and in combination. Br J Psychiatry 1981;139:181–189.

6. Elkin I, Shea T, Watkins J, et al. NIMH Treatment of Depression Collaborative Research Program: comparative treatment outcome findings. Presented at the American Psychiatric Association Annual Meeting, 1986.
7. Simons A. Murphy GE, Levine JL, et al. Cognitive therapy and pharmacotherapy of depression: sustained improvement over one year. Arch Gen Psychiatry 1986;43:43–50.
8. Blackburn IM, Eunson KM, Bishop S. A two-year naturalistic follow-up of depressed patients treated with cognitive therapy, pharmacotherapy and a combination of both. J Affective Disord 1986;10:67–75.
9. McLean PD, Hakstian AR. Clinical depression: comparative efficacy of out-patient treatments. J Consult Clin Psychol 1979;47:818–836.

149. Use of Reminiscing in the Psychotherapy of Depression

EYTAN BACHAR, HAIM DASBERG,
AND BARUCH SHAPIRA

As early as 1917 Freud[1] pointed out the contrast between normal reaction and adaptation to loss and the pathological responses of depressed patients. Focusing on mechanisms that can ward off sorrow in normals is one of the major contributions of Arieti's work.[2] In line with this quest for normal self-healing processes, we suggest harnessing reminiscing—the mental activity of dwelling on the past— in the psychotherapy of depression, specifically in aging patients.

Butler[3] pointed out the universality of reminiscing in aging people and viewed the behavior as an exploration of unresolved conflict that can facilitate the assimilation of forgotten aspects of past life. Similarly, Pollock[4] saw a resemblance between the repeated recounting of the past by the aging person and the working-through process in psychoanalytical treatment. He also pointed to a resemblance between reminiscing and mourning work, in which the expression of memories plays a significant role in the self-healing process. The many losses experienced by aging people necessitate such devices. Thus Lieberman[5] viewed reminiscing as an adaptive mechanism for maintaining a sense of identity in a changing and alienating environment that includes declining health, social status, and income.

The adaptive role of reminiscing for combating depressed mood during later adulthood has been demonstrated experimentally by Fallot's work with normal subjects.[6] Fallot randomly assigned participants, aged 45 years and older, into two groups. In individual interviews participants in the first group were asked to speak about their past and in the second group about their present and future. After the interview, participants in the second group rated themselves on a mood scale as having significantly more depressed mood than the participants in the first group.

We have investigated the use of reminiscing in the psychotherapy of depression. The study was conducted in a group psychotherapy framework in the Ezrath Nashim Resistant Depression Unit. For research purposes the group was run in two phases of 3 months each, with a 2-month break between the phases. The group was guided by two male therapists (a psychologist and a psychiatrist) and consisted of four to ten participants. The group was open, i.e., the patients could join or leave in accordance with their stay in the ward. There were no patients who participated in fewer than five sessions. Many patients participated in both phases of the group.

In the first phase the group was guided using a conventional, unstructured group psychotherapy approach. The second phase was the reminiscing phase. Patients were told that the purpose of the group sessions was to reminisce, i.e., to share memories of more than 5 years ago. Whenever new patients joined the group, they were told about the purpose of the group by the therapists or the participants. Patients enthusiastically stuck to the instructions to reminisce and willingly related stories, mostly about the era of the establishment of the State of Israel or their immigration to it. The atmosphere was one of active, pleasurable participation, which was in contrast with the heavy, depressed mood of the first phase. This impression was demonstrated empirically.

At the beginning of each session patients were asked to rate the extent of their depression on a nine-point scale. At the end of every session they were asked to repeat that procedure and to rate, on an additional nine-point scale, the extent to which they felt that the group was of benefit to them. The difference in the patients' ratings of their depression before and after sessions in the two phases varied signficantly (paired $t = 2.33$, $p < 0.04$). Patients in the reminiscing phase rated themselves after sessions as less depressed and in the regular, unstructured phase as more depressed. Patients rated the group psychotherapy in its reminiscing phase as significantly more beneficial than the regular, unstructured phase (Table 149.1).

Therapists' evaluations were consistent with those of the patients. The therapists rated patients in the reminiscing phase as having significantly benefited and as having been more involved than during the first phase. They also rated patients as signficantly less depressed after the reminiscing phase, in comparison to the effect of regular, unstructured psychotherapy (Table 149.1).

Indirect support for the idea of using reminiscing in the psychotherapy of depression can be derived from viewing the effect that changes in depression have on reminiscing. It was found[7] that prior to treatment depressed patients reminisced significantly less than normals ($t = 5.76$, $p < 0.0000$). When effective treatment was given (electroconvulsive therapy in the aforementioned study) and depression was removed to a great extent, reminiscing returned to normal levels (Table 149.2). The patients treated with antidepressant medication were not improved after 21 days of treatment. These patients had significantly decreased their amount of re-

TABLE 149.1. Patients' and therapists' evaluations of regular and reminiscing group psychotherapy.

Parameter	Regular group psychotherapy (11 sessions)	Reminiscing group psychotherapy (11 sessions)	paired t value	p
Patients' evaluation of benefit	2.45 ± 0.77	4.07 ± 0.59	5.33	< 0.0004
Therapists' evaluation of benefit	2.08 ± 0.51	4.72 ± 0.65	10.8	< 0.0000
Therapists' evaluation of depression after sessions	5.10 ± 0.75	4.23 ± 0.41	3.11	< 0.01
Therapists' evaluation of participation	2.20 ± 0.65	4.69 ± 0.87	12.2	< 0.0000

Scores are derived from nine-point scales. Higher scores represent greater benefit, more severe depression, or increased participation.

TABLE 149.2. Reminiscing scores (mean ± SD) of normals, ECT patients, and drug therapy patients in first and second interviews.

Subjects	First interview	Second interview	Paired t value	p
Normals (n = 12)	53.6 ± 10.1	40.4 ± 14.3	3.4	< 0.0005
ECT patients (n = 10)	13.9 ± 15.8	42.3 ± 23.5	3.7	< 0.005
Drug therapy patients (n = 8)	29.9 ± 24.6	7.3 ± 7.5	2.3	< 0.05

Eighteen patients in two treatment groups (ECT and tricyclic antidepressants), mean age 62.17 ± 8.9 (SD), and 12 normals matched by age, sex, socioeconomic status, and education were administered an open interview to assess the extent of reminiscing during natural conversation. Reminiscing data are presented in percentages, expressing the proportion of sentences related to the past (more than 5 years ago).

miniscing at the second interview. Remaining hospitalized without significant change in their condition could well have increased concern for and precoccupation with their present and future situation and further reduced their tendency to reminisce.

The normal decrement in reminiscing at the second interview (which was far less than that of the drug therapy patients) can be attributed to the communicative value of reminiscing in old age. "Presenting a calling card" is one of the functions fulfilled by reminiscing.[8-11] It is likely that after presenting that "card" at the first meeting, the need to introduce it again had decreased.

These observations, along with the group psychotherapy data, suggest that reminiscing may usefully contribute to the psychotherapy of depression. Moreover, the patient's family can, by encouraging him or her to reminisce, play a natural therapeutic role. As a natural, adaptive mechanism, reminiscing may also help to prevent recurrent depressive episodes.

References

1. Freud S. Mourning and Melancholia. Standard Edition. London: Hogarth Press, 1957[orig. 1917];14:243–258.
2. Arieti S. Individual psychotherapy. In Paykel ES (ed): Handbook of Affective Disorders. New York: Guilford Press, 1982;297–306.
3. Butler RN. The life review: an interpretation of reminiscence in the aged. Psychiatry 1963;26:65–76.
4. Pollock G. Reminiscences and insight. Psychoanal Study Child 1981; 36:279–287.
5. Lieberman M. Adaptive processes in late life. In Datan N, Ginsberg L (eds): Life-Span Developmental Psychology—Normative Life Crisis. New York: Academic Press, 1975;135–159.
6. Fallot R. The impact on mood of verbal reminiscing in later adulthood. Int J Aging Hum Dev 1979–1980;10:385–400.
7. Bachar E, Dasberg H, Shapira B, et al. Reminiscing in depressed, aging patients: effect of ECT and antidepressants. Submitted for publication.
8. Lewis C. Reminiscing and self-concept in old age. J Gerontol 1971;26:240–243.
9. Lewis C. The adaptive value of reminiscing in old age. J Geriatr Psychiatry 1973;6:117–121.
10. Revere V, Tobin S. Myth and reality: the older person's relationship to his past. Int J Aging Hum Dev 1980–1981;12:15–26.
11. Beaton SR. Reminiscence in old age. Nurs Forum 1980;19:271–283.

Index